Ian K Ritchie
5th May 1988

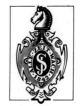

Joseph Schatzker Marvin Tile

The Rationale of Operative Fracture Care

With a Foreword by M.E. Müller

With 396 Figures in 1132 Separate Illustrations,
Some in Color

Springer-Verlag
Berlin Heidelberg NewYork
London Paris Tokyo

JOSEPH SCHATZKER, M.D., B.Sc. (Med), F.R.C.S. (C)
Orthopedic-Surgeon-in-Chief, Sunnybrook Medical Centre
Professor of Surgery, University of Toronto

MARVIN TILE, M.D., B.Sc. (Med), F.R.C.S. (C)
Surgeon-in-Chief, Sunnybrook Medical Centre
Professor of Surgery, University of Toronto

Sunnybrook Medical Centre
2075 Bayview Avenue
Toronto, Ontario M4N 3M5, Canada

ISBN 3-540-10675-8 Springer-Verlag Berlin Heidelberg New York Tokyo
ISBN 0-387-10675-8 Springer Verlag New York Berlin Heidelberg Tokyo
ISBN 4-431-10675-8 Springer Verlag Tokyo Berlin Heidelberg New York

Library of Congress Cataloging-in-Publication Data. Schatzker, Joseph. The rationale of operative
fracture care. Includes bibliographies and index. 1. Fractures – Surgery. I. Tile, Marvin. II. Title.
[DNLM: 1. Fractures – surgery. WE 175 S312r] RD101.S28 1987 617′.15 87-12693
ISBN 0-387-10675-8 (U.S.)

Reproduction of the figures: Gustav Dreher GmbH, D-7000 Stuttgart
Typesetting, printing and bookbinding: Universitätsdruckerei H. Stürtz AG, D-8700 Würzburg
2124/3130-543210

This book is dedicated to our families
for their patience, devotion, and understanding.

To the Schatzker clan:
Valerie, Erik, Adam, and Mark

To the Tile clan:
Esther, Gary, Rosemary, Stephen, Christine,
Steve, Deborah, and Andrew

Foreword

After the publication of the AO book *Technique of Internal Fixation of Fractures* (Müller, Allgöwer and Willenegger, Springer-Verlag, 1965), the authors decided after considerable discussion amongst themselves and other members of the Swiss AO that the next edition would appear in three volumes. In 1969, the first volume was published (the English edition, *Manual of Internal Fixation*, appeared in 1970). This was a manual of surgical technique which discussed implants and instruments and in which the problems of internal fixation were presented schematically without radiological illustrations. The second volume was to be a treatise on the biomechanical basis of internal fixation as elucidated by the work done in the laboratory for experimental surgery in Davos. The third volume was planned as the culminating effort based upon the first two volumes, treating the problems of specific fractures and richly illustrated with clinical and radiological examples. It was also to discuss results of treatment, comparing the results obtained with the AO method with other methods. The second and third volumes were never published.

The second edition of the AO *Manual* appeared in 1977. It dealt in greater detail with the problems discussed in the first edition, although it still lacked clinical examples and any discussion of indications for surgery. Like the first edition, it was translated into many languages and was well received.

Finally, after 22 years, the much discussed and much needed third volume has appeared. Two Canadian surgeons have successfully undertaken the challenging task of filling this gap in the AO literature.

Joseph Schatzker and Marvin Tile first came into contact with AO methods of internal fixation in 1965. Impressed by the results of the method, they set themselves to learn it in minute detail and before long became masters of the technique and strong exponents of its effectiveness. They appeared often as lecturers and instructors in AO courses in Switzerland, and North America. Their numerous publications and lectures have greatly contributed to the wide acceptance of the operative method of fracture care.

Joseph Schatzker translated the first and second editions of the *Manual* from German into English, and has, in addition to these excellent translations, achieved distinction as a teacher of the AO method. Both he and Marvin Tile participate annually as instructors in the instructional courses at the American Academy of Orthopedic Surgeons.

With their long association with AO techniques and tremendous clinical experience, these two distinguished surgeons were eminently qualified to undertake the monumental task of defining the specific indications for operative fracture care. In this book they present not only their own views but also a synthesis of the thoughts and writings of other AO members. The book is outstanding and far exceeds the goals originally envisaged for the projected third volume.

The authors have been careful in choosing examples and the appropriate radiological illustrations to delineate the mechanism of injury, the biomechanical problems, the indications for treatment, and the actual execution of surgical procedures. They always guide the reader to the essence of the problem, clearly emphasizing the principles of fracture treatment, a deductive approach through analysis to the clinical decision.

Schatzker and Tile speak of fractures having a "personality." This "personality" is a key concept requiring careful definition: it includes not only a careful analysis of the fracture and all of its soft tissue components, but also a thoughtful assessment of the patient, his or her age, occupation, health, and expectations of treatment, as well as a critical appraisal of the skill of the surgeon and the supporting surgical team and environment. This analysis, combined with the knowledge of what constitutes a reasonable result, allows the authors to formulate a guide to treatment. They also provide useful advice about avoiding technical difficulties and pitfalls, about planning correct postoperative care, and about the treatment of complications which may arise.

The book is superbly illustrated with many drawings skillfully employed to clarify and emphasize essential techniques. The style is easy to understand, clear and unambiguous, giving a lucid presentation of complex and difficult concepts. It will certainly become a standard reference work for everyone involved in the treatment of fractures.

Berne, July 1987   MAURICE E. MÜLLER

Preface

The purpose of this book is to describe our philosophy of fracture care, which reconciles both the closed and open methods of fracture treatment. We do not regard these two methods as representing opposing points of view, but as complementary to each other. Some surgeons, who tend to treat fractures by closed methods, often imply that the open method is dangerous. By "conservative treatment" they imply a nonoperative method and suggest that it is well thought out, tried, and safe, and will yield results equal to if not superior to those achieved by surgery. "Conservative" as defined by the Oxford dictionary means "characterized by a tendency to persevere or keep intact and unchanged." The surgeons who continue to view the open method of fracture treatment as the last resort, and who will do anything, no matter how extreme, to avoid opening a fracture, are indeed characterized by a tendency to keep unchanged an attitude whose prevalence was justified when the methods of internal fixation were inadequate and the results of surgical treatment often worse than those of nonoperative care.

However, the founding of the Swiss AO, an association for the study of problems in internal fixation, by Müller, Allgöwer, Willenegger and Schneider in 1958 ushered in a new era in fracture treatment. These pioneer surgeons developed new principles of stable internal fixation along with new implants. Their methods of open reduction and internal fixation, performed by atraumatic techniques, produced sufficient stability to allow early functional rehabilitation without an increase in the rate of malunion or nonunion. The results of treatment changed so dramatically that new standards of care and assessment had to be adopted. Nowadays, an excellent result means the full recovery of function, a painless extremity, a normal mechanical axis, and full joint stability with a normal range of motion. Anything less can no longer be considered excellent, as it has been in reports in the past. Operative fracture care has become safe, scientific, and predictable. It is now based on a firm foundation of biomechanical and clinical data.

Although it has become clear from clinical reviews that open fracture care in certain fractures gives far better results than closed treatment of that same fracture, we emphasize again and again that the indication for surgery for a particular patient must be based on a clear definition of the "personality of the fracture." The personality of a fracture depends upon many factors, including the age, medical condition, and expectations of the patient, the nature of the injury, and the skill of the health care team and surgical environment in which the fracture is to be treated.

Once the decision has been made that open reduction and stable fixation will afford the patient the best end result, we progress to the execution of the surgical procedure. We describe fully the methods of treatment that are best for each particular fracture based on the principles of stable internal fixation. The details of preoperative investigation and planning so essential to successful surgery are stressed. Technical details are also described, including the surgical approach, the selection of the best implant, the methods of inserting the implant, and the common pitfalls the surgeon may encounter.

Since the operative treatment of fractures demands so-called functional aftertreatment, the details of postoperative care have become as important as the steps of the operative procedure. We therefore describe not only the details of postoperative treatment, but also the danger signals of common complications and their treatment.

We hope that this book will become a guide for all surgeons treating fractures in this era of advanced technology, and that inadequate internal fixation, once so commonly encountered, will become history. Internal fixation should no longer be viewed as a last resort or as a more dangerous form of treatment, but as safe, scientific and predictable, and as the best form of treatment for those cases in which it is indicated.

Toronto, June 1987   JOSEPH SCHATZKER
                                                                              MARVIN TILE

Acknowledgements

This book, a labor of love, could not have been completed without the unselfish support and hard work of many individuals. We are especially grateful to:

Our families for their patient understanding during this period

Valerie Schatzker for her help in the English editing

Our orthopedic teachers at the University of Toronto, who roused our interest in orthopedic trauma and have encouraged us to complete the task

Our orthopedic colleagues at Sunnybrook Medical Centre, Stanley Gertzbein, Jim Kellam, and Bob McMurtry, for contributing cases and helpful suggestions, and especially to Gordon Hunter, who read most of the manuscript, for his helpful criticism

The founding members of the AO-ASIF for recognition and support of our efforts

Maurice Müller for reading the manuscript and for his kind remarks in the Foreword

Instructional Media Services at the Wellesley Hospital and Sunnybrook Medical Centre in Toronto for their contribution, especially to Patsy Cunningham who did some of the artwork, and to Jim Atkinson and his staff in Medical Photography

The staff of Springer-Verlag, Heidelberg, for their efficiency and expertise in producing and publishing this volume

Mr. Pupp of Springer-Verlag, Heidelberg, to whom we are indebted for many of the new drawings in this book

Our secretaries, Shirley McGovern and Joan Kennedy, for their constant support

Jan King and Ronda Klapp for typing the manuscript

Carol Young for typing the manuscript and helping with the index

Shirley Fitzgerald for her devotion to detail in both the editing and the completion of the index

Contents

Part II. Fractures of the Upper Extremity

Part III. Fractures of the Pelvis and Acetabulum

Part IV. Fractures of the Lower Extremity

18   Fractures of the Distal Tibial Metaphysis Involving the Ankle Joint: The Pilon Fracture. M. TILE

**Part I
General Aspects of Stable Fixation**

1 Principles of Stable Internal Fixation

J. SCHATZKER

1.1 Introduction

1.1.1 Mechanical Properties of Bone

The principal mechanical function of bone is to act as a supporting structure and transmit load. The loads which bone has to withstand are those of pure compression, those of bending, which result in one cortex being loaded in tension and the other in compression, and those of torque, or twisting. Bone is strongest in compression and weakest in tension. Fractures as a result of pure compression are therefore rare and occur only in areas of cancellous bone with a thin cortical shell. Thus, we find pure compression fractures in such areas as the metaphyses, vertebral bodies, and the os calcis. Transverse, oblique, and spiral are the common fracture patterns seen in tubular bone.

Transverse fractures are the result of a direct bending force (Fig. 1.1). They may be associated with a small triangular fragment, which rarely extends the full width of the diameter of the bone and is always found on the compression side. Because it is extruded from bone under load, it retains little of its soft tissue attachment and has therefore, at best, a precarious blood supply. This must be kept in mind when one is planning an internal fixation. Attempts to secure fixation of such extruded fragments may result in their being rendered totally avascular. If very small they may be ignored. If larger, it is best to leave them alone and fill the defects created with cancellous bone.

Spiral and oblique fractures are the result of an indirect twisting force (Fig. 1.1). They often occur in combination with butterfly fragments of corresponding configuration. These fragments are larger and retain their soft tissue attachment. It is frequently possible to secure them with lag screws without disrupting their blood supply. Many fractures are the result of a combination of forces: thus, their pattern may be mixed.

1.1.2 Types of Load and Fracture Patterns

Bone is a viscoelastic material. Fractures are therefore related not only to the force but also to the rate of force application. Much less force is required to break the bone if the force is applied slowly and over a long period of time than if it is applied rapidly: bone is better able to withstand the rapid application of a much greater force. This force is stored, however, and when failure finally occurs and the bone breaks, it is dissipated in an explosive fashion, causing considerable damage to the soft tissue envelope. A good example of this is the skier who walks away from a spectacular tumble, only to break his leg in a slow, twisting fall. We therefore distinguish between low- and high-velocity injuries.

Low-velocity injuries have a better prognosis. In high-velocity injuries the fractures are not only more comminuted but also associated with a much greater damage to the enveloping soft tissues, because of the higher energy dissipation and because of the direct application of force. Low-velocity injuries are more commonly spiral, without excessive comminution.

1.1.3 Effects of Fracture

When a bone is fractured it loses its structural continuity. The loss of the structural continuity renders it mechanically useless because it is unable to bear any load.

1.1.4 Soft Tissue Component

We have alluded to the poorer prognosis of high-velocity injuries because of the greater damage to the soft tissue envelope. Long-term disability following a fracture is almost never the result of damage to the bone itself; it is the result of damage to the soft tissues and of stiffness of neighboring joints.

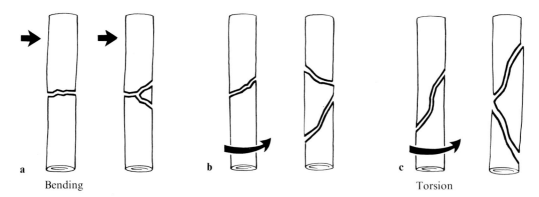

Bending   Torsion

Fig. 1.1 a–c. Types of fracture patterns. A lateral bending force results in a *transverse fracture,* which may have a small triangular fragment as well as longitudinal fissures on the concave or compression side. *Oblique* and *spiral fractures* may have butterfly fragments of corresponding shape. They are the result of a twisting force

Brüggemann 1976; Tscherne and Östern 1982; Tscherne and Gotzen 1984).

1.2 Aims of Treatment

The loss of function of the soft tissue envelope due to scarring and secondary joint stiffness can be prevented only by early mobilization. Thus, modern fracture treatment does not focus on bone union at the expense of function but addresses itself principally to the restoration of function of the soft tissues and adjacent joints. A deformity or a pseudarthrosis is relatively easy to correct in the presence of good soft tissue function, while scarring, obliteration of the soft tissue gliding planes, and joint stiffness are often permanent. The modern fracture surgeon will therefore direct his treatment to the early return of function and motion, with bone union relegated to secondary importance.

Modern functional fracture treatment does not denote only operative fracture care. It makes use of specialized splinting of the bone in special braces which allow an early return of function and motion. There are, however, limitations to the nonoperative system, which we will address as we discuss the different fractures. It can be applied to fractures where angulation, rotation, and shortening can be controlled. Thus, it is limited only to certain long bone fractures. Its application to intra-articular and periarticular fractures is very limited.

Early return of full function following fracture can be achieved only by absolute anatomic reduction of fractures and early resumption of motion with partial loading. This, in turn, can be achieved only by absolutely stable, strong, and lasting internal fixation. With non-functional methods full return of function is rarely achieved and then only after a prolonged period of rehabilitation.

In a closed fracture the injury to the surrounding tissue evokes an acute inflammatory response, which is associated with an outpouring of fibrinous and proteinaceous fluid. If, after the injury, the tendons and muscles are not encouraged to glide upon one another, the inflammatory response leads to the obliteration of tissue planes and to the matting of the soft tissue envelope into a functionless mass.

In an open fracture, in addition to the possible scarring from immobilization, there is direct injury to the muscles and the effects of infection if this develops. Indeed, infection is the most serious complication of trauma because, in addition to the scarring related to the initial trauma, infection compounds the fibrosis as a result of the prolonged immobilization frequently necessary until the infection is cured.

Stiffness in adjacent joints in nonarticular fractures is also the result of immobilization. Prolonged immobilization leads to atrophy of the articular cartilage, to capsular and ligamentous contractures, and to intra-articular adhesions. The joint space normally filled with synovial fluid becomes filled with adhesions which bind the articular surfaces together. Added to the local effects is, of course, the tethering effect of the scarred soft tissues.

Although the significance of the open fracture with regard to the soft tissue component of the injury has been recognized for a long time, only in the past decade has the soft tissue component of closed injuries been classified (Tscherne and

1.3 Previous Experience with Internal Fixation

Internal fixation is not a new science. The past 50 years have permitted ample documentation of the results of unstable internal fixation. Surgery has frequently proved to be the worst form of treatment. It destroyed the soft tissue hinges, interfered with biological factors such as the blood supply and the periosteum, and was never sufficiently strong or stable to permit active mobilization of the limbs with partial loading. Supplemental external plaster fixation was often necessary. The emphasis was on bone healing and not on soft tissue rehabilitation. Healing became evident when callus appeared. Unfortunately, unstable internal fixation was unpredictable and uncertain, and it frequently resulted in delayed union, nonunion, or deformity. When union did occur, instead of signifying the end of treatment it merely signaled the beginning of a prolonged phase of rehabilitation designed to regain motion in the soft tissue envelope and in the stiff joints. The ravages of this prolonged nonfunctional form of treatment were such that open reduction and internal fixation were looked upon as the last resort in the treatment of a fracture.

1.4 Rigidity and Stability

The introduction of compression introduced stability. Stability was achieved not by rigidity of the implant, but by impaction of the fragments. The intimate contact of the fragments brought about by compression restored structural continuity and stability and permitted the direct transfer of forces from fragment to fragment rather than via the implant. Stable fixation restores load-bearing capacity to bone. This greatly diminishes the stresses borne by the implant and protects the implant from mechanical overload or fatigue failure.

Key (1932) and Charnley (1953) were the first to make use of compression in order to achieve stable fixation. Both applied it to broad cancellous surfaces by means of an external compression clamp. Similar attempts to achieve union of the cortex failed. The resorption around the pins of the external fixator employed to stabilize the cortical fragments was thought to be due to pressure necrosis of the cortex. Cancellous surfaces under compression united rapidly, and it was thought initially that compression provided an osteogenic stimulus to bone. The failure of the cortex to unite

led to general acceptance of the thesis that cancellous and cortical bone behaved differently, and that they probably united by different mechanisms.

Since then it has been demonstrated that, under conditions of absolute stability, both cancellous and cortical fragments heal by primary direct or vascular bone union (primary bone healing). The simple external fixator of Charnley, applied close to broad, flat cancellous surfaces of an arthrodesis, was able to achieve absolute stability. The same system applied to diaphyseal bone, where tubular fragments rather than broad, flat surfaces were in contact, resulted in a system of relative instability with micromotion between the fragments. The resorption around the pins and at the fracture was due to motion and not due to pressure necrosis.

Danis in 1949 (Müller et al. 1970) was the first to demonstrate that cortical fragments stabilized by a special plate, which was able to exert axial compression and bring about absolute stability at the fracture, united without any radiologically visible callus. Danis referred to this type of union as "primary bone healing." Studies on experimental models by Schenk and Willenegger (1963) revealed a different type of union than that commonly associated with the healing of fractures. Rather than by callus and endochondral ossification, union occurred by direct formation of bone. Different events were seen where bone was in contact and where gaps were present.

In areas of contact the healing was seen to be the result of proliferation of new osteons which arose from remaining open haversian systems. The osteons grew parallel to the long axis of the bone, through the necrotic bone ends, and then across the fracture. These osteons can be viewed as a myriad of tiny bone dowels which reestablished the continuity of bone. The capillary buds which sprang from the capillaries became cutting cones. These consisted of osteoclasts, followed by the capillary bud, surrounded by a cuff of osteoblasts which were laying down bone. In this way, there was simultaneous bone resorption and deposition. This bridging of a fracture line by osteons, which gives rise to an osteonal union, can occur only where bone is in direct contact and where there is absolute stability of the fragments without any movement at the interface. In this type of union there is no net resorption at the fracture interface. For every bit of bone removed, new bone is laid down. Under these circumstances, internal fixation does not lead to a relative distraction of the fragments, because no absolute resorption occurs.

Areas of bone separated by gaps demonstrated first of all an invasion of the gaps by blood vessels with surrounding osteoblasts. The osteoblasts laid down osteoid which served to bridge the gaps and to permit stage two to begin. Stage two is identical to contact healing, described above. Examination of human material (R. Schenk, personal communication) from autopsies of patients who had had fractures operated upon revealed that the experimentally noted phenomena of contact and gap healing also occurred clinically. Material from patients whose fractures had zones of comminution revealed that although healing seemed undisturbed, free fragments whose blood supply had been interfered with lagged very much behind in their degree of revascularization and remodeling. Thus, the rate of revascularization and union was seen to be influenced by the severity of comminution, the degree of initial displacement — for this has a bearing on the severity of devitalization of the fragments — and by the presence of the soft tissue lesion and its degree. This last observation is of particular importance when one considers implant removal, for not every fracture, nor all areas of the same fracture, will have advanced to the same degree of remodeling at a given time from injury. With primary bone healing we see a different biological phenomenon to healing under conditions of relative instability which is associated with the formation of callus. Primary bone healing is not necessarily better, and certainly in the early stages of healing it is weaker than bone bridged by a peripheral concentric callus.

1.5 Methods of Stable Fixation

1.5.1 Lag Screw

Compression exerts its beneficial effect on bone union by creating an environment of absolute stability where no relative micromotion exists between the bone fragments. Interfragmental compression results in impaction of the fragments and in a marked increase in frictional resistance to motion. It is therefore the most important and efficient method of restoring functional and structural continuity to bone. It also greatly diminishes the forces borne by an internal fixation because the load transfer occurs directly from fragment to fragment. Stability is thus achieved, not by rigidity of the implant, but by compression and bone contact.

The simplest way of compressing two fragments of bone together is to lag them together with a *lag screw*. The lag screw is the simplest and most efficient implant in use to secure interfragmental compression (Fig. 1.2).

The insertion of a screw into bone results in local damage which incites immediate repair. This is seen histologically as the formation of new bone which closely follows the profile of the screw threads. Thus, after the insertion of a screw, as healing occurs the holding power of the screw increases, reaching its peak between the 6th and 8th weeks. The holding power then gradually declines to a level well above what it was at the time of insertion (Schatzker et al. 1975b). This occurs because, as the bone matures and becomes organized, much of the newly laid-down woven bone around the screw is resorbed.

Screws may be either self-tapping or non-self-tapping. It was formerly thought that self-tapping screws provided a poorer hold in bone because they created more damage at the time of insertion and became embedded in fibrous tissue rather than in bone (Müller et al. 1979). This has been shown to be incorrect. The fibrous tissue forms as a result of instability and motion between the implant and bone. Instability is seen histologically as bone resorption and the formation of fibrous tissue, with occasional islands of cartilage and synovial-like cells (Schatzker et al. 1975a). Size for size, the different thread profiles of self-tapping and non-self-tapping screws have almost the same holding power. The advantage of the non-self-tapping screws is that they can be inserted into bone with far greater ease and precision, particularly when the screw comes to lie obliquely through thick cortex.

In order to exert the most efficient degree of interfragmental compression, lag screws must be inserted into the center of fragments and at right angles to the fracture plane (Fig. 1.3). A single lag screw is never strong enough to achieve stable fixation of diaphyseal fragments. A minimum of two, and preferably three screws are required. This means that only long oblique and long spiral fractures can be stabilized with lag screws alone. This can be done only in short tubular bones such as phalanges, metacarpals, metatarsals, or malleoli. If lag screws alone are used for the fixation of long bones such as the femur or the humerus, they almost always end in early failure because of mechanical overload. Therefore the most common use of lag screws in the fixation of shaft fractures is in combination with neutralization, buttress, or

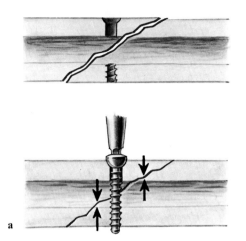

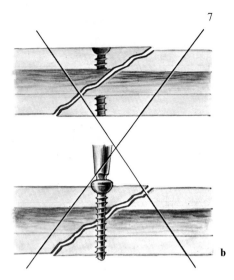

Fig. 1.2a, b. The lag screw. **a** The hole next to the screw head is larger than the diameter of the thread. This is the *gliding hole*. The hole in the opposite cortex is the *thread hole*. As the screw is tightened the two fragments are pressed together.

b Both holes are *thread holes*. The fragments cannot be compressed. (From Müller et al. 1979)

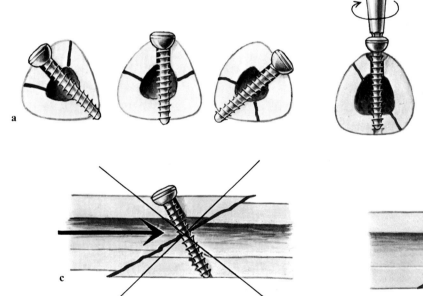

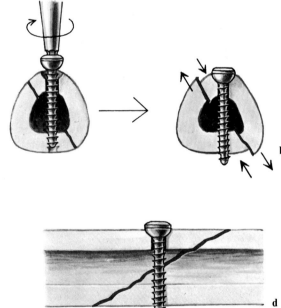

Fig. 1.3a, b. In order to exert the most efficient degree of compression, lag screws must be inserted into the center of the fragments and at right angles to the fracture plane. If they are off-center or angled, the fragments may displace on tightening of the screw, and reduction will be lost. **c** A lag screw inserted at a right angle to the fracture plane results in the best compression but does not provide the best stability under axial load, because the fragments may glide upon one another as the screw tips in the thread hole. **d** A lag screw at right angles to the long axis of the bone may cause tendency for the fragments to displace as the screw is tightened, but it provides the best resistance to displacement under axial load. Displacement can occur only if the thread rips out of the thread hole or the screw head sinks into the gliding hole. (From Müller et al. 1979)

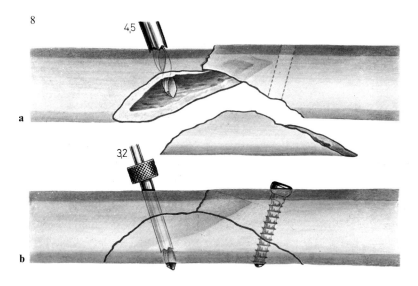

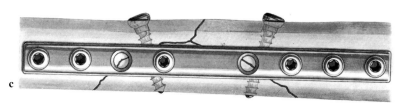

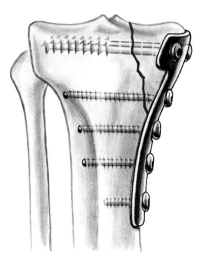

Fig. 1.4a–c. The neutralization plate. The two lag screws provide interfragmental compression (**a, b**). The neutralization plate in **c** bridges the fracture zone and protects the lag screw fixation from bending and torsional forces. (From Müller et al. 1979)

tension-band plates which protect the screw fixation from mechanical overload.

1.5.2 Lag Screw, Neutralization, and Buttressing

Neutralization plates or *protection plates* are used to protect the primary lag screw fixation. They conduct part or all of the forces from one fragment to the other. In this way they protect the fracture fixation from the forces of bending shear and rotation (Fig. 1.4).

In metaphyseal areas the cortex is very thin, and if subjected to load it can fail. Such failures result in deformity and axial overload of the joint. Therefore, internal fixation in metaphyseal areas requires protection with plates which support the underlying cortex. These are referred to as *buttress plates* (see Fig. 1.5).

1.5.3 Tension Band Plate

Short oblique or transverse fractures do not lend themselves to lag screw fixation. In mid-diaphyseal regions of the tibia and femur, as will be seen in the section on splinting, we prefer intramedullary nailing for fixation. There are many transverse or short oblique fractures of diaphyses, such as

of the radius and ulna, of the humerus, or of long bones close to or involving the metaphyses, which do not lend themselves to intramedullary nailing. Yet these fractures require stable fixation. Such fracture patterns can be stabilized by compression, but the compression has to be in the long axis of the bone. Such compression can be generated only by a plate. If a fracture is reduced and a plate is applied to the bone in such a way that axial compression is generated, either by means

Fig. 1.5. The buttress plate. The T plate buttresses the cortex and prevents axial displacement. (From Müller et al. 1979)

of the tension device or by the self-compressing principle of the dynamic compression (DC) plates, the plate is referred to as a *compression plate* (Fig. 1.6a, b).

Certain bones such as the femur are eccentrically loaded. This results in one cortex being under compression and the other under tension (Müller et al. 1979; Schatzker et al. 1980). If a plate is applied to the tension side of a bone and placed under tension which causes the cortex under the plate to be compressed, such a plate not only achieves stability because of the axial compression it generates, but also, because of its location on the tension side of the bone, as bending forces are generated under load, it is capable of increasing the amount of axial compression. Such a plate is referred to as a *tension band plate* (Fig. 1.7).

1.5.4 Splinting

1.5.4.1 External Skeletal Fixation

As we have seen from the classical experiments of Key and Charnley, axial compression can be applied by means of pins which traverse bone and are then squeezed together. This type of fixation is stable over only a short length of the bone and only when broad, flat, cancellous surfaces are being compressed. When applied to tubular bone, such fixation is relatively unstable. Although not absolutely stable, the external fixator, either as a full frame or as a half frame, is extremely useful under certain clinical circumstances, such as in the treatment of open fractures not suitable for internal fixation, or in the treatment of infected fractures or infected nonunions. Under these circumstances the external fixator provides sufficient stability to permit functional use of the extremity while maintaining the bones in their reduced position. The stability is sufficient in fresh fractures to render the extremity painless and encourage soft tissue rehabilitation. Because external skeletal fixation does not result in absolute stability, it behaves similarly to unstable internal fixation in retarding or discouraging bone union. Therefore, when it is used as the definitive mode of fixation it should almost always be combined with bone grafting.

1.5.4.2 Intramedullary Nailing

The manner in which an intramedullary nail splints and bestows stability is best likened to a

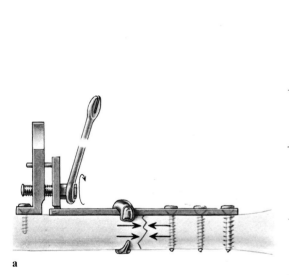

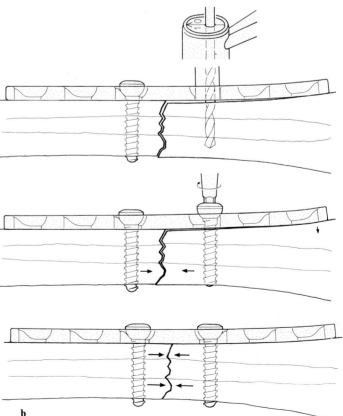

Fig. 1.6. a As the tension device is tightened, the plate is brought under tension and the bone under compression. (From Müller et al. 1979). b The dynamic compression plate. As the load screw is tightened it moves from its eccentric position to the center of the screw hole. This movement of screw and bone toward the fracture results in axial compression. (From Allgöwer et al. 1973)

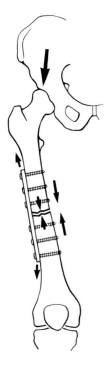

Fig. 1.7. Tension band plate. In an eccentrically loaded bone, not only does a compression plate secure a degree of compression at rest, but also, when the bone is loaded, the bending force so generated is converted by the action of the plate into further compressive stresses. Such a plate is called a "tension band plate" and the force generated, "dynamic compression". The essence of dynamic compression is that although the compressive force fluctuates in magnitude it never reverses direction.

tube within a tube. The nail is therefore dependent upon the length of contact for its resistance to bending, and upon friction and the interdigitation of fracture fragments for rotational stability. Intramedullary reaming is frequently employed to enlarge the area of contact. This enlarges the medullary canal sufficiently to permit the insertion of a nail which is not only large enough to provide stability but also strong enough to take over the function of the bone. Small nails adapted to the size of the medullary canal were frequently limited in size to the diameter of the isthmus, which in young patients is frequently narrow. As a result, they were rarely strong enough and usually too flexible. Their use led to complications such as nail migration, nail bending, nail fracture, delayed union, and nonunion.

The biological expression of unstable fixation is the formation of external callus. The instability associated with intramedullary nailing is reflected in the amount of callus produced. A large intramedullary nail may, when tightly wedged, provide sufficient stability to result in primary bone healing without discernible callus. Most often, however, a variable amount of periosteal callus is seen.

As a mode of fixation of weight-bearing extremities, intramedullary nailing has distinct advantages. Because it is a load-sharing device and much stronger than a plate, the nail enables a much earlier return to weight bearing than is possible to achieve with other means of fixation.

An intramedullary nail, because of the mode of its application and the manner in which it renders stability, is best suited for fractures which occur in the middle one-third of the femur and of the tibia. The proximal and distal ends of tubular bones widen into broad segments of cancellous bone. In these areas the nail can provide neither angular nor rotational stability. Axial stability of a nailed fracture depends on cortical stability and on the ability of the cortex to withstand axial loads. Thus, certain fracture patterns are not ideally suited for intramedullary nailing. These are: long oblique and long spiral fractures, and comminuted fractures, fractures where the cortex in contact is less than 50% of the diameter of the bone at that level.

An intramedullary nail has distinct mechanical and biological advantages. Because of its design and mode of application it is much stronger than a plate. Consequently, it will withstand loading for a much longer period of time than a plate will before failure. Reaming combined with closed insertion of the nail without disturbing the soft tissues surrounding the fracture has been associated with a much more rapid and more abundant appearance of callus. Thus, it is an ideal device for tubular bones. The limitations imposed on the conventional nail by the location of the fracture and its pattern or comminution have given rise recently to the development of a interlocking medullary nail. After closed insertion, the nail is locked proximally, distally, or both by the insertion of bolts which traverse bone and the nail. This technique, although still in the stages of clinical definition, seems to have greatly enlarged the scope of intramedullary nailing (Kempf et al. 1985).

1.6 Implant Failure and Bone Grafting

Metal plates or other devices, no matter how rigid or how thick and strong, will undergo fatigue failure and break if subjected to cyclical loading. Metal is best able to withstand tension. Bone is best able to withstand compression. Thus, in an ideal internal fixation, the biomechanical arrangement should be such that the bone is loaded in compression and the metal in tension. If a defect is present in the cortex opposite the plate, and the bone is under bending load, the fulcrum will move closer and closer to the plate until it eventually falls within the plate (Fig. 1.8). Consequently, with repetitive loading, even if due only to muscular contrac-

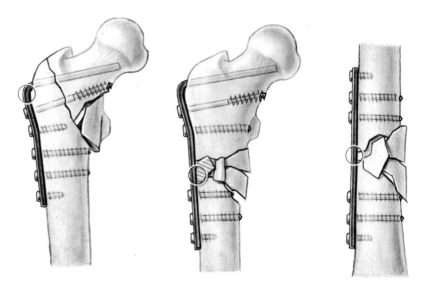

Fig. 1.8. Examples of deficiencies of the cortex opposite the plate which will result in cyclic bending of the plate and in its ultimate failure. (From Müller et al. 1979)

tion, the implant is repeatedly cycled and may fall. Internal fixation can therefore be viewed as a race between bone healing and implant failure.

In order to prevent the possibility of implant failure, whenever there is comminution, whenever there is a defect in the cortex opposite the plate, whenever there is devitalization of fragments (as is frequently the case in high-velocity injuries), and whenever enormous forces have to be overcome, as in plating of femoral shaft fractures, the fracture should be bone grafted. Such a graft, once it becomes incorporated into an osteoid bridge opposite the plate, rapidly hypertrophies and matures because it is subjected to compressive stresses. As soon as it reestablishes the continuity of bone opposite the plate it acts as a second plate and prevents the cycling and inevitable fatigue failure of the implant (Fig. 1.9).

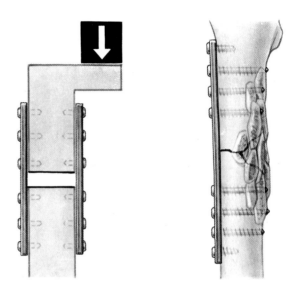

Fig. 1.9. Once it becomes incorporated into an osteoid bridge, a bone graft, if it is under compression, rapidly matures and hypertrophies. It reestablishes the continuity of the bone opposite the plate and prevents further cycling of the plate and its failure. (From Müller et al. 1979)

1.7 Implant Removal

Early on after fracture, bone which has united by primary bone healing is weaker than that united by callus. A callus, because of its spatial disposition, is further away from the central axis of bone than a plate, and therefore in a mechanically more advantageous position to withstand force. The osteons of primary healing are closer to the central axis and the union is therefore mechanically weaker.

Early on, primary bone healing is also weaker than that by callus because it undergoes a tremen-

dous remodeling, which is manifested by a proliferation of haversian canals. Thus, such bone, although unchanged in its cross-sectional diameter, contains less bone per cross-sectional area because of the haversian proliferation. This continues until the accelerated remodeling ceases and the architecture gradually returns to normal. Based on their studies, Matter et al. (1974) suggested that the intense remodeling subsides some 12 months or so after fracture. Factors which prolong the remodeling phase are the patient's age, the degree of comminution, the degree of devitalization, the size of the gaps, the accuracy of the reduction, the stability of the fixation, and whether the fracture was bone grafted or not. Furthermore, it is important to note whether there were any signs of instability during the time of healing, or whether the fracture progressed uneventfully to union.

All these factors must be borne in mind when implant removal is being contemplated. If the implant is removed prematurely the bone will fail and a refracture will occur. We feel that most implants should be left in place for 2 years before their removal is contemplated. This timing may be modified by factors indicated in the preceding paragraph.

Following removal of an implant the bone must be protected from overload. The screw holes act as stress raisers, and if the bone is suddenly loaded before the screw holes have filled in — a process which takes 6–8 weeks in experimental animals — the bone may fail. Similarly, the ridges which frequently develop on each side of the plate should not be osteotomized, as this further weakens the bone and may contribute to its failure.

Implant removal is advised in younger patients, particularly in the lower extremity, even if the implant is completely nonirritating. Such implants clearly change the physical property of the bone and expose the individual to the dangers of fracture at the point where the plate ends and normal bone begins.

References

Allgöwer M, Matter P, Perren SM, Rüedi T (1973) The dynamic compression plate. Springer, Berlin Heidelberg New York

Charnley J (1953) Compression arthrodesis. Livingstone, Edinburgh

Kempf I, Grosse A, Beck G (1985) Closed locked intramedullary nailing. J Bone Joint Surg 67A:709–720

Key JA (1932) Positive pressure in arthrodesis for tuberculosis of the knee joint. South Med J 25:909–915

Matter P, Brennwald J, Perren SM (1974) Biologische Reaktion des Knochens auf Osteosyntheseplatten. Helv Chir Acta [Suppl] 12

Müller ME, Allgöwer M, Willenegger H (eds) (1970) Manual of internal fixation, 1st edn. Springer, Berlin Heidelberg New York, p 10

Müller ME, Allgöwer M, Schneider R, Willenegger H (eds) (1979) Manual of internal fixation, 2nd edn. Springer, Berlin Heidelberg New York

Schatzker J, Horne JG, Sumner-Smith G (1975a) The effects of movement on the holding power of screws in bone. Clin Orthop 111:257–263

Schatzker J, Sanderson R, Murnaghan P (1975b) The holding power of orthopaedic screws in vivo. Clin Orthop 108:115

Schatzker J, Manley PA, Sumner-Smith G (1980) In vivo strain gauge study of bone response to loading with and without internal fixation. In: Uhthoff H (ed) Current concepts of internal fixation of fractures. Springer, Berlin Heidelberg New York, pp 306–314

Schenk R, Willenegger H (1963) Zum histologischen Bild der sogenannten Primärheilung der Knochenkompakta nach experimentellen Osteotomen am Hund. Experientia 19:593

Tscherne H, Brüggemann H (1976) Die Weichteilbehandlung bei Osteosynthesen, insbesondere bei offenen Frakturen. Unfallheilkunde 79:467

Tscherne H, Gotzen L (1984) Fractures with soft tissue injuries. Springer, Berlin Heidelberg New York Tokyo, pp 1–9

Tscherne H, Östern HJ (1982) Die Klassifizierung des Weichteilschadens bei offenen und geschlossenen Frakturen. Unfallheilkunde 85:111

2 Intra-articular Fractures

J. Schatzker

Intra-articular fractures may result in stiffness, deformity, pain, and post-traumatic arthritis. In order to avoid deformity and stiffness it is necessary to secure an anatomical reduction and begin early motion. Sir John Charnley stated that "perfect anatomical restoration and perfect freedom of joint movement can be obtained simultaneously only by internal fixation" (Charnley 1961). At the time that Charnley wrote *The Closed Treatment of Common Fractures,* sufficiently stable and sufficiently strong internal fixation which would allow early motion was not available. Indeed, the results of internal fixation were so discouraging because of stiffness, deformity, delayed union, and nonunion that Charnley argued in favor of nonoperative treatment. His sentiments were soon echoed by Stewart et al. (1966) and Neer et al. (1967), who published the results of treatment of a major intra-articular fracture, the supracondylar fracture of the femur in the adult. Even with limited criteria of excellence which today would be thought unacceptable, such as the acceptance of 70° knee flexion as satisfactory (Neer et al. 1967), both groups found the results of surgery to yield just over 50% acceptable results. Stewart et al. went on to state that it was the added trauma of surgery and the presence of metal in periarticular locations which directly contributed to stiffness. A review of the publications of these authors and others makes it evident that the techniques of internal fixation then in existence and the implants available were totally inadequate. Sufficient stability could never be achieved to permit early pain-free motion. If motion was permitted, not only did pain inhibit motion and result in stiffness, but displacement and loss of reduction were also very common. To prevent displacement, internal fixation was combined with plaster fixation, and this invariably resulted in permanent stiffness.

The publication of the Swiss AO/ASIF group in 1970 (Wenzel et al. 1970), our own review (Schatzker et al. 1974), and other reviews (Mize et al. 1982; Olerud 1972; Schatzker and Lampert 1979) of results of treatment of major intra-articular injuries utilizing the AO methods and implants indicated strongly that with the new principles, methods, and new implants, stable fixation and early motion after internal fixation was an attainable surgical goal, and that fractures — particularly intra-articular fractures — so treated did amazingly well.

The AO/ASIF methods of open reduction and internal fixation made strong, stable, and lasting fixation possible. Despite early, unprotected mobilization accurate anatomical reduction of the joint and of the metaphyseal fractures could be maintained. Indeed, the patients were so completely free of pain that it was difficult to persuade them not to bear full weight and resume full function before union was complete.

The large number of patients who were treated nonoperatively (Schatzker et al. 1974, 1979) permitted us certain observations which we consider invaluable lessons in articular fracture treatment. Patients whose intra-articular fractures were immobilized in plaster for 1 month or longer ended with permanent marked stiffness of these joints. Patients with similar fractures which were treated by open reduction and internal fixation, but whose joints were subsequently immobilized in plaster, ended with far greater stiffness. Patients whose intra-articular fractures were treated by traction and early motion ended with varying degrees of joint incongruity, but invariably with a much better range of motion. This allowed us to formulate a principle of intra-articular fracture treatment: *Displaced intra-articular fractures which are not treated by open reduction and stable internal fixation should be treated by traction and early motion.*

Fractures which were treated by manipulation and traction often showed persistent displacement of some fragments. At surgery these fragments were always found to be firmly impacted into the metaphyseal cancellous bone and could be dislodged only by direct surgical manipulation. This permitted us to formulate the second principle of treatment: *Intra-articular fragments which do not reduce as a result of closed manipulation and traction are impacted and will not reduce as a result of further manipulation or traction.*

A number of cases of patients with intra-articular fractures which were initially treated closed but eventually operated on led to one further important observation: *Major intra-articular depressions do not fill with fibro-cartilage cartilage to restore joint congruity and instability. If a joint is unstable because of major joint depression, the instability will become permanent unless the fragment is reduced surgically and held in position until union occurs.*

Pauwels (1961) postulated that in a normal joint there is a state of equilibrium between articular cartilage regeneration and articular cartilage destruction. Furthermore, he felt that articular cartilage wear occurred constantly, as a result of stress. As stress is the result of force acting on a specific surface area, i.e., $S = \frac{F}{A}$, it becomes clear that stress can be increased and the equilibrium tipped in favor of joint destruction either by decreasing the surface area of contact (A) or by increasing the force (F), or by both. (F) is increased above its physiologic level by axial overload, the result of a metaphyseal or diaphyseal deformity.

A consideration of the above led us to an inescapable conclusion: *Anatomical reduction of the joint is essential to restore joint congruity and increase the surface area of contact to the maximum possible and metaphyseal and diaphyseal deformity must be corrected to prevent axial overload* (Fig. 2.1).

These are the principles of intra-articular fracture care enunciated by the AO (Müller et al. 1979), and we are in full accord with them. The therapeutic validity of these principles is confirmed by the favorable results of modern operative treatment of intra-articular fractures.

What about articular cartilage damage sustained at the time of injury and the possibility of articular cartilage regeneration? In an elegant experiment, Mitchell and Shepard (1980) studied the effects of the accuracy of reduction and stable fixation. With the aid of histological methods and electron microscopy, they were able to show that anatomic reduction and stable fixation of intra-articular fragments by means of compression resulted in articular cartilage regeneration.

Salter et al. (1980, 1986) studied experimentally and clinically the effects of continuous passive motion on articular cartilage healing and regeneration. They demonstrated very convincingly that

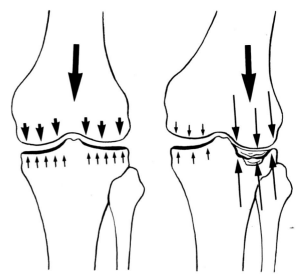

Fig. 2.1. Anatomical reduction of the joint and correction of metaphyseal and diaphyseal deformity greatly reduces the stress on articular cartilage

continuous passive motion stimulated both processes.

These experimental and clinical studies permit us to enunciate the principles of intra-articular fracture treatment as follows:

1. Immobilization of intra-articular fractures results in joint stiffness.
2. Immobilization of articular fractures treated by open reduction and internal fixation results in much greater stiffness.
3. Depressed articular fragments which do not reduce as a result of closed manipulation and traction are impacted, and will not reduce by closed means.
4. Major articular depressions do not fill with fibrocartilage, and the instability which results from their displacement is permanent.
5. Anatomical reduction and stable fixation of articular fragments is necessary to restore joint congruity.
6. Metaphyseal defects must be bone grafted to prevent articular fragment redisplacement.
7. Metaphyseal and diaphyseal displacement must be reduced to prevent joint overload.
8. Immediate motion is necessary to prevent joint stiffness and ensure articular cartilage healing and recovery. This requires stable internal fixation.

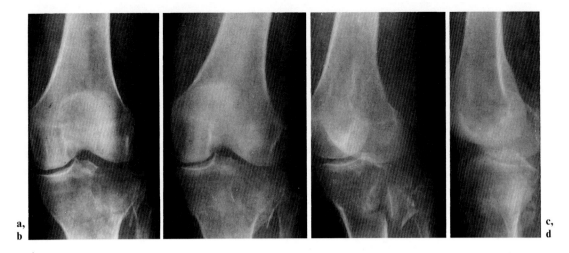

Fig. 2.2a–d. Tibial plateau fracture roentgenograms. a Anteroposterior; b oblique; c oblique; d lateral. Note particularly on the two oblique projections (b and c) the marked improvement in the definition of the lateral plateau comminution and depression

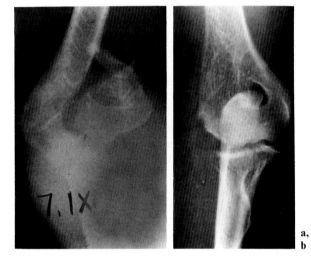

Fig. 2.3. a Anteroposterior roentgenogram of a supracondylar fracture of the humerus. The details of the fracture are almost completely obscured. b Anteroposterior roentgenogram of the opposite, uninvolved elbow to be used as template for preoperative planning

2.1 Clinical Aspects

The clinical aspects of intra-articular fractures are important in the decision-making process regarding the best mode of treatment for a particular injury. We emphasize repeatedly in this book the concept of the personality of the fracture. In order to define the personality, we must know not only such obvious factors as the violence involved in the injury, but also the patient's age, occupation, athletic pursuits, expectations of treatment, and similar details.

2.1.1 Physical Examination

Although radiological examination is indispensable in defining the fracture pattern, it does not shed light on the soft tissue components of the injury. Tenderness over the course of a ligament or its insertion may be the only available clue to a ligament disruption. Similarly, the presence of a neurological deficit, a compartment syndrome, or a vascular lesion is best established by physical examination.

2.1.2 Radiological Evaluation

An anterioposterior and a lateral radiograph are frequently insufficient to define precisely the pattern of injury (Fig. 2.2). We have found that oblique projections, as well as stress X-rays when indicated, add greatly to the definition of an injury. Often intra-articular detail is obscured because of distortion and overlap of fragments (Fig. 2.3).

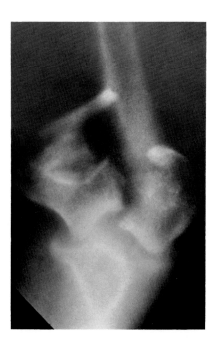

Fig. 2.5. CT scan of a posterior fracture-dislocation of the hip. Note the large intra-articular fragment which was not evident on plain roentgenogram or plain tomography

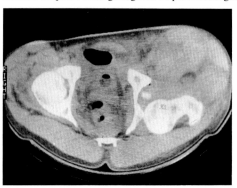

Plain tomography will help in defining the detailed outline of intra-articular and metaphyseal fragments (Fig. 2.4), which will facilitate classification of the injury and determination of its prognosis, and in this way guide its treatment. Computerized axial tomography has been invaluable in some complex fractures such as acetabular injuries, pilon fractures, fractures about the knee, and some shoulder injuries (Fig. 2.5).

2.2 Surgery

2.2.1 Timing

Certain intra-articular injuries, such as ankle and elbow fractures, should be treated as emergencies and operated on as soon as possible. The rapid swelling of a fracture-dislocation of an ankle or of a pilon fracture is the result of a rapidly developing hematoma. Immediate surgery allows the evacuation of such hematomas and the reduction of the distortion of the soft tissues. This vastly improves the circulation and minimizes subsequent swelling. If closure at the end of surgery is difficult because of tissue tension, once the joint is closed we have left the wounds open and have closed them secondarily after the swelling has subsided. This policy has permitted early safe surgery without incurring the price of wound-edge necrosis

or sepsis. We have found that elbow injuries should also be treated as emergencies, not only because of the swelling and possible vascular complications, but also because of the very high incidence of myositis ossificans associated with delays of 4 or 5 days from the time of injury (Fig. 2.6).

We have been delaying surgery of certain intra-articular fractures because of their complexity: among these are difficult supracondylar fractures of the femur, certain tibial plateau fractures, and acetabular fractures. In acetabular fractures, delay has been caused not only by the complexity of the lesion and the time required for its exact definition, but also by associated injuries commonly present and the general condition of the patients. The high incidence of myositis ossificans seen in acetabular fractures operated on through the posterior approach may in part be the result of the delay, as it is in periarticular fractures of the elbow.

2.2.2 Approach and Technique

Once the personality of the fracture is defined by painstaking clinical and radiological investigation, one must carry out a careful preoperative plan of the surgery. This includes a plan of the surgical approach as well as a detailed plan of the internal fixation and any bone grafting required.

The exposure of the joint must be atraumatic, and yet it must be extensive so that all the compo-

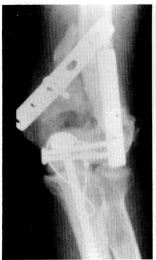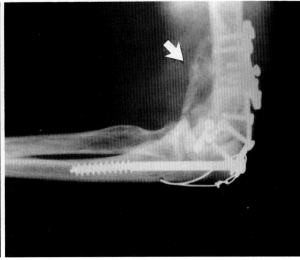

Fig. 2.6. Florid myositis ossificans (*arrow*) particularly in front of the elbow — a frequent complication of delayed surgery about the elbow

nents of the injury can be visualized and become fully accessible to manipulation and fixation. (For detailed descriptions of such exposures, please refer to the chapters on the specific joint fractures.)

The surgical reconstruction of the joint begins with an anatomical reduction of the articular surface. This often requires that depressed portions of the articular cartilage be elevated from their impacted position in the metaphysis. This is best done by elevating the depressed fragments together with the impacted metaphyseal cancellous bone. Once elevated, the fragments must be held provisionally in their reduced positions with Kirschner wires. It is necessary now to bone graft the metaphyseal defect which is invariably created when the articular fragments are disimpacted and elevated. Although some authors have described the use of cortical struts to hold up the articular surface, we prefer autogenous cancellous bone which we compact with a bone punch. This allows good filling of the defects and helps to maintain the articular reduction. Next in order of importance is a careful reduction of the metaphyseal and diaphyseal components of the fracture.

Once the fractures are reduced we secure fixation of the articular components by means of lag screws. The metaphysis must be buttressed to prevent axial overload, and the diaphyseal components must be fixed so that early motion can be started. Prior to closure certain intra-articular structures such as the menisci of the knee should be repaired if torn or peripherally detached. In-substance lesions of the cruciate ligaments are not repaired primarily nor substituted. Such repairs require postoperative immobilization which we like to avoid. The only cruciate lesions we repair

immediately are avulsions of the anterior or posterior cruciate ligament with a piece of bone; these can be fixed with lag screws or wire loops with sufficient stability to allow immediate mobilization. Any other cruciate deficiencies are repaired late if indicated. This policy has allowed us to concentrate on the mobilization of the joints, which we feel is far more important than early anteroposterior stability. This policy does not, however, apply to lateral stability. All collateral ligaments are crefully repaired at the time of the initial surgery; collateral repair does not prevent early mobilization of the joint.

At the end of surgery an atraumatic closure is carried out. It is extremely important to avoid tension of the skin. If at the time of closure the skin cannot be brought together without tension, then, once the joint is closed, we prefer to leave the wound open and carry out a delayed closure in 4 or 5 days, as mentioned above. This policy has allowed us to operate on tense swollen joints without running the risk of wound necrosis and sepsis.

2.3 Postoperative Care

The experiments of Salter et al. (1980) and Mitchell and Shepard (1980) have underlined the importance of early motion. Our clinical experience, as

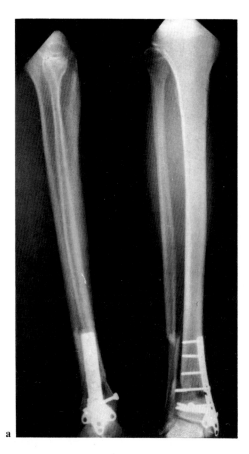

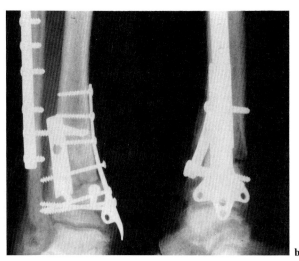

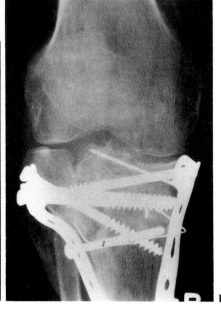

Fig. 2.7. **a** An intra-articular pilon fracture at 6 weeks after surgery. A number of surgical principles have been violated. The fibula was not reduced, the metaphysis was not bone-grafted, and the lesion was not properly buttressed. **b** Note the excellent correction of the deformity achieved by reduction of the fibula, by bone grafting of the metaphyseal defect created once the valgus was corrected, and by proper buttressing of the metaphysis

Fig. 2.8. **a** Serious malreduction of a difficult tibial plateau fracture. **b** Stability was restored by an intra-articular wedge excision of the depressed area. This allowed us to narrow the lateral plateau and reduce the remaining intact portion, which carried the meniscus under the lateral femoral condyle

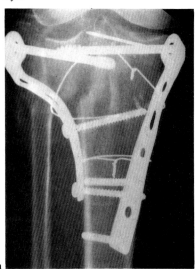

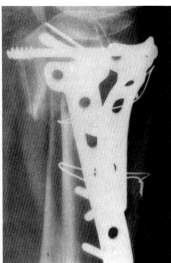

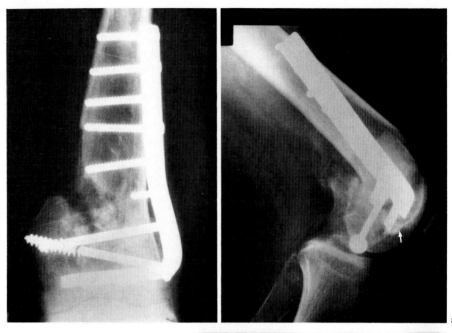

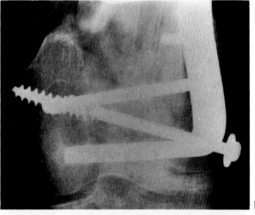

Fig. 2.9. a, b Malunion of the lateral femoral condyle and fracture of the cancellous screw. Note the double contour of the lateral femoral condyle, best seen in **b**. This malunion distorted the intercondylar groove and markedly restricted knee motion. **c** An intra-articular osteotomy was carried out. The excessive fibrocartilage and all callus were carefully excised, recreating the original fracture fragment. This allowed an anatomic reduction of the joint. Note the unorthodox position of a buttress plate on the posterolateral aspects of the distal femoral metaphysis. Anatomical reduction and stable fixation led to an excellent recovery of the joint

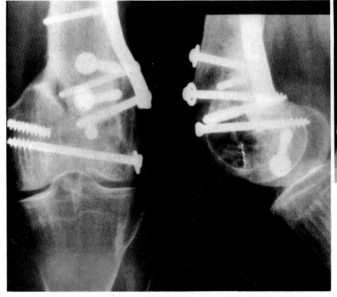

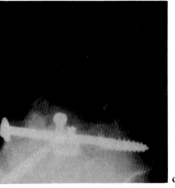

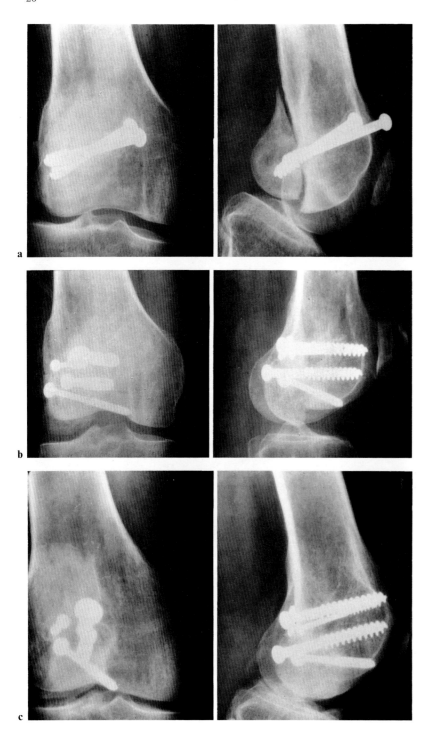

well as that of many other investigators, bears this out. All major intra-articular injuries after their reconstruction are placed on a continous passive motion machine; passive mobilization is started in the recovery room and is continued for 5–7 days. In late joint reconstructions this may be continued for up to 3 or 4 weeks.

One must remember that mobilization and its benefits must be in balance with the degree of stability obtained at the time of surgery. At times, the degree of stability of the internal fixation is insufficient to permit unprotected mobilization. In these instances we have combined the internal fixation with fracture bracing. The fracture brace can be put on in the first day or two without jeopardizing the internal fixation or the care of the wound. Similarly, one must remember that major intra-articular fractures, particularly about the knee, are in at least 25–30% of cases associated with major ligamentous disruptions which must be repaired at the time of the initial surgery. The usual practice is to protect any ligamentous repair in plaster. As we have already pointed out, intra-articular fracture repair combined with plaster immobilization results in an unacceptable degree of stiffness. Therefore we have always managed these combined injuries and repairs by protecting the ligamentous reconstructions by immediate fracture bracing and then carrying on with the usual mobilization on a continuous passive motion machine. Because in-substance cruciate ligament reconstructions require the surgeon to limit the excursion of the knee we have deferred such reconstructions, but have always repaired collateral ligaments and cruciate avulsions with bone. Late cruciate insufficiency has been dealt with when necessary once the joint has been fully rehabilitated. Joint stiffness is one complication which must be avoided at all cost.

2.4 Late Intra-articular Reconstructions

Late intra-articular deformities arise either as result of failed nonoperative treatment, or because of incomplete surgical reduction of the fracture, or because of loss of position due to unstable fixation. Such articular deformities have usually been considered as permanent and not amenable to any surgical reconstruction. We have subjected many such intra-articular deformities to late intra-articular reconstruction, at varying intervals from the time of injury (Figs. 2.7–2.10). This has often required intra-articular osteotomies with meticulous excision of the fibrocartilage from the joint and of the callus from the metaphysis, in order to redefine the original fragments and permit an anatomical reconstruction. We have also treated a number of intra-articular nonunions. The principle followed with these, as with the malunions, has been meticulous reconstruction of the joint, stable fixation of the joint and of the metaphyseal component with bone grafting where necessary, arthrolysis and soft tissue mobilization periarticularly to regain a satisfactory range of motion, and then mobilization of the joint on a continuous passive motion machine. Although we have never managed to achieve a return to a perfectly normal degree of joint function, we have been favorably impressed with the successes attained, and feel that unless there is evidence of seriour post-traumatic arthritis, a late joint reconstruction should be undertaken if it is at all technically feasible. This is preferable to joint arthroplasty or arthrodesis.

References

Charnley J (1961) The closed treatment of common fractures. Livingstone, Edinburgh

Mitchell N, Shepard N (1980) Healing of articular cartilage in intra-articular fractures in rabbits. J Bone Joint Surg 62 A:628–634

Mize RD, Bucholz RW, Grogan DP (1982) Surgical treatment of displaced comminuted fractures of the distal end of the femur. J Bone Joint Surg 64 A:871–879

Müller ME, Allgöwer M, Schneider K, Willenegger H (1979) Manual of internal fixation, 2nd edn. Springer, Berlin Heidelberg New York

Neer C, Graham SA, Shelton ML (1967) Supracondylar fracture of the adult femur. J Bone Joint Surg 49 A:591–613

Olerud S (1972) Operative treatment of supracondylar-condylar fractures of the femur. Technique and results in fifteen cases. J Bone Joint Surg 54 A:1015–1032

Pauwels F (1961) Neue Richtlinien für die operative Behandlung der Coxarthrose. Verh Dtsch Orthop Ges 48:332–366

Salter RB, Simmonds DF, Malcolm BW, Rumble EJ, MacMichael D (1980) The biological effects of continuous passive motion on the healing of full thickness defects in articular cartilage: an experimental investigation in the rabbit. J Bone Joint Surg 62 A:1232–1251

Salter RB, Hamilton HW, Wedge JH, Tile M, Torode IP, O'Driscoll SW, Murnaghan J, Saringer JH (1986) Clinical application of basic research on continuous passive motion for disorders and injuries of synovial joints: a preliminary report of a feasibility study. Techniques Orthopaed I(I):74–91

Schatzker J, Lampert DC (1979) Supracondylar fractures of the femur. Clin Orthop 138:77–83

Schatzker J, Horne G, Waddell J (1974) The Toronto experience with the supracondylar fractures of the femur 1966–1972. Injury 6:113–128

Schatzker J, McBroom R, Bruce D (1979) The tibial plateau fracture: the Toronto experience. Clin Orthop 138:94–104

Stewart M, Sisk D, Wallace SL (1966) Fractures of the distal third of the femur. J Bone Joint Surg 48 A:784–807

Wenzl H, Casey PA, Hébert P, Belin J (1970) Die operative Behandlung der distalen Femurfraktur. AO Bulletin, Bern

3 Open Fractures

J. Schatzker and M. Tile

3.1 Introduction

In spite of the advances made in fracture care and in the prevention of and management of infection, open fractures remain a serious surgical problem. Even now, an open fracture of the tibia with an associated vascular injury results in an amputation in 60% of cases (Lange et al. 1985).

In past decades, open fractures often resulted in the loss of life and/or the loss of limb (Billroth 1866). Tscherne (1984) has described the four major eras in the treatment of open fractures; the era of *life preservation;* the era of *limb preservation;* the era of *avoidance of infection,* and the era of *preservation of function.* In the past two decades, because of advances in fracture care, most of the effort in the management of open fractures has gone into the preservation of function. Prevention of infection and union of the fracture, in the absence of good limb function, is no longer acceptable, except in circumstances where a joint has been destroyed or major muscle or nerve loss has occurred.

The aim of all fracture care is the return of the injured extremity to full function in the shortest possible period of time. In caring for an open fracture the surgeon should aim for no less. Other factors such as major bone loss, muscle injury, or nerve or tendon loss may make this goal unattainable; nevertheless, the goal should be strived for. A recent combined study from the University Hospital in Nottingham, England and Sunnybrook Medical Centre, Toronto, Canada (Beauchamp et al. 1984), showed that this is attainable. In 97 open fractures of the tibial shaft, 89% of the patients achieved excellent functional results.

In this chapter, we will discuss only the general principles of open fracture management. The details of treatment as they apply to particular bones will be found in the chapters dealing with the specific injuries in question.

3.2 Assessment of the Soft Tissue Wound

Many observers have attempted to grade open fractures (Allgöwer 1971; Gustilo and Andersson 1976; Oestern and Tscherne 1984, pp 1–9), but, since all injuries are different, a clear description of each particular injury is more important than a numerical grade. The surgeon must look beyond the skin wound and carefully assess the state of the entire wound including the amount of skin contusion, the apparent damage to subcutaneous tissue, muscle, fascia, vital structures, and bone. In most classifications, a grade I injury is defined as a small puncture would less than 1 cm; however, the location of that puncture wound may be more important than its size. For example, if it is on a subcutaneous border, it may have been caused by a relatively low-energy injury, and therefore may be associated with relatively little muscle damage. However, one must assume that to produce a similar sized wound in an area of thick muscle belly, such as the posterior tibia or the femur, the bone ends must have penetrated a large mass of muscle to reach the skin. Therefore the amount of muscle damage will be far greater (Fig. 17.6). Failure to recognize this fact and consequent failure to resect all the necrotic tissue could lead to grave consequences for the patient, such as gas gangrene, amputation, or even death.

Careful assessment of the wound therefore, and, more importantly, the implications of that wound, are essential to good patient management.

3.3 Classification

In the literature there are several proposed grading systems for open fractures, with widespread acceptance and some overlap.

Allgöwer (1971) described three grades of open fracture: grade I, a small skin wound pierced from within by bone; grade II, a skin wound with skin contusion; grade III, an extensive skin wound with major damage to skin, muscle, and vital structures.

Gustilo and Andersson (1976) used a similar classification, a grade I wound being less than 1 cm, a grade II wound more than 1 cm, and a grade III wound being extensive.

Tscherne (1984) described four grades of soft tissue injury associated with open fracture. In his classification, the size of the skin wound was not important, but the degree of soft tissue damage, the severity of the fracture and the degree of contamination were more important.

The following grading system from Lange et al. (1985) is widely used and is recommended:

Grade I: A skin wound from within, usually less than 1 cm, with little or no skin contusion.

Grade II: a skin wound of more than 1 cm, with skin and soft tissue contusion, but no loss of muscle or bone. A small wound over a major muscle mass should be considered a grade II open fracture.

Grade III: a large, severe, open wound with extensive skin and subcutaneous contusion, muscle crush or loss, and severe periosteal stripping. This grade is divided into three subgrades:

(a) a wound associated with severe bone loss, muscle loss, nerve or tendon injury;
(b) a wound associated with an arterial injury;
(c) a traumatic amputation.

3.4 Management

3.4.1 Decision Making

Many factors must be considered prior to making a final decision as to the method of treatment of any individual open fracture. These factors include general factors such as the age and general medical state of the patient, and the severity of the injury.

The local factors include the extent of the soft tissue wound, the time elapsed between injury and definitive treatment, the fracture configuration, and the presence or absence of major injury to vital structures, especially vascular injuries. All of these factors must be considered and the method of treatment selected must have a favorable risk–benefit ratio for the patient.

3.4.2 Immediate Treatment

After suitable cultures have been taken, the skin wound should be covered with a sterile dressing

Table 3.1. Infection rates of open fractures, with and without continuous sterile covering from accident scene to operating room. (From Tscherne 1984)

	With sterile dressing $n = 16$	Without sterile dressing $n = 77$
Infection rate	5 (4.3%)	15 (19.2%)

as quickly as possible. Once covered, the sterile dressing should not be removed until the patient reaches an operating room for definitive treatment. Tscherne (1984, p. 14) has found a significant increase in the infection rate of open fractures not covered by a continuous sterile bandage from the accident scene to the operating room (Table 3.1).

During resuscitation of the patient, the dressing should not be removed. The patient should be given prophylactic antibiotics, usually a first generation cephalosporin. In grade III injuries we also add an aminoglycoside. Antitetanus prophylaxis must also be given.

3.4.3 Operative Treatment

3.4.3.1 Limb Salvage

The first decision to be made is whether the limb is salvageable or not. This decision will depend upon many factors. If the open fracture is associated with a vascular injury in a polytraumatized individual, amputation may be lifesaving and must be considered, especially in the more distal regions of the extremities. Vascular repair may be a lengthy procedure, greatly prolonging the time a critically ill patient may have to spend under anesthesia. In distal vascular injuries, the chances for a good functioning extremity are remote. In a recent study, 60% of all open tibia fractures associated with a vascular injury eventually required amputation (Lange et al. 1985). Many of the salvaged limbs had poor function. Therefore, if the patient is polytraumatized, the risks of attempting limb salvage may be much greater than the benefit to the patient; the attempt may be costly indeed.

3.4.3.2 Cleansing

The skin should be cleansed with soap and shaved, the bone ends if they protrude through the wound brushed, and the wound irrigated with approximately 12 litres of Ringer's lactate solution. The skin may then be prepared with an antiseptic agent, such as chlorohexadine.

A tourniquet should be applied but not used, unless essential to stop massive bleeding.

3.4.3.3 Débridement

By débridement we mean the removal of all contamination and the meticulous excision of all devitalized tissue. The amount of débridement required depends on the severity of the soft tissue injury. For a grade I injury, the location of the wound will dictate the débridement. If the wound is a small puncture and over a subcutaneous bone, very little extension of the wound is required, since muscle damage is minimal. However, if the puncture wound is over muscle, the wound must be extended sufficiently to reveal all the traumatized tissue, so that an extensive and meticulous débridement can be executed.

All grade II and grade III open wounds must be carefully débrided. Any tight compartments must be decompressed and the muscle viability assessed. The important factors in assessing the viability of muscle include bleeding, contractility, and color. Avulsed ends of muscle, skin, and subcutaneous tissue must be excised.

In grades II and III, the wound must also be extended to allow for easy access to the bone. The exact method of extending the wound will depend on the location of the wound and the decision as to the method of stabilization required. In some circumstances, internal fixation will be performed through the extended wound; in others, a separate wound is preferable for the internal fixation.

If external fixation is to be the method of stabilization, then local extension of the wound will usually suffice.

All small, loose cortical fragments stripped of their muscle attachments should be removed because they are dead. Whether large, structurally important but devitalized fragments of bone are retained depends on their degree of contamination. If severely contaminated, even if they contribute to stability of the fracture, they must be removed.

During the débridement, constant irrigation should be maintained to minimize on the damage to tissue from drying.

3.4.3.4 Choice of Fixation

Once again, decision making must depend upon a favorable risk-benefit ratio for the patient. If the indication for fixation is great, then the risks will be worthwhile.

In open fractures involving joints, or in open epiphyseal plate injuries in children, internal fixation is necessary to maintain reduction and preserve function. The risks of internal fixation are therefore justified. As already mentioned, in open diaphyseal injuries other methods of stabilization, such as an external frame, may be preferable. Other important factors which will lead the surgeon to choose internal fixation are polytrauma in the patient, and fractures associated with a vascular injury.

3.4.3.5 Implant Selection

The selection of an implant for the stabilization of an open fracture depends mainly on the fracture configuration and the extent of the soft tissue injury. If the patient has a *metaphyseal* fracture with or without extension into a joint, open reduction and, if technically possible, internal fixation, using screws and plates, are indicated. The surgical exposure may be achieved by incorporating the laceration in an extended incision or by making a separate incision, leaving at least a 5-cm bridge between the laceration and incision. If the open metaphyseal injury is associated with major bone loss which will require extensive reconstruction, one may use an external fixator across the joint, especially in a grade III wound, as a temporizing measure.

If the open fracture is *diaphyseal,* several methods of management are possible. If the wound is extensive and the fracture configuration allows anatomical reduction without excessive further dissection, we favor open reduction and internal fixation using interfragmental screws and plates, in a grade I or II wound. In a grade III wound, external fixation is indicated. If the open diaphyseal fracture is severely comminuted, and fixation with screws and plates is not possible or desirable, we favor initial external skeletal fixation.

If the wound is small and the fracture an isolated injury and stable after débridement, the limb may be immobilized in plaster or traction or stabilized with an external fixator. Secondary treatment with internal fixation or intramedullary nailing may then be performed at some point between the 1st and 6th week, depending on the condition of the patient and, more specifically, of the soft tissue envelope. As we have already indicated, plaster immobilization and traction are used only under exceptional circumstances. Most often where definitive fixation of a fracture is being delayed in a diaphyseal injury, we favor external skeletal fixation.

Implant selection for open fractures may be summarized as follows:

1. External fixation — for grade III open wounds associated with severe comminution or bone loss in either the metaphysis or diaphysis.
2. Open reduction and internal fixation — for open metaphyseal fractures with or without joint involvement, using interfragmental screws and plates. Also suitable for diaphyseal fractures which can be anatomically reduced because of their configuration, in a grade I or II wound.
3. Combined fixation — minimal internal fixation associated with an external frame for comminuted fractures in grade III wounds, where lag screws are used to improve the stability of the fracture. Here delayed bone grafting is important.
4. Intramedullary nails — not indicated for the primary treatment of open fractures. They may be used secondarily after the wound has been assessed and no sepsis found, usually on the 5th–14th day following trauma.

3.4.3.6 Care of the Soft Tissue Wound

Primary

In most instances, the wound should be left open. This is by far the safest course of action. One can never be certain that devitalized tissue is not left in the wound and closure may precipitate sepsis, even with gas-forming organisms. Therefore, virtually all open fractures should be left open. If possible, sensitive structures such as joints, nerves and tendons should have soft tissue coverage, but the skin wound should be left open. Any extensions of the wound may be closed without tension, but the laceration and any tight portion is left open.

Synthetic skin is being used in some centres and may be of use in massive wounds.

In our opinion, in acute trauma, relaxing incisions and primary flaps should almost never be used, because of the risk of losing the flap.

Table 3.2. Secondary wound care

1. Healing by secondary intent
2. Secondary suture
3. Split skin graft
4. Skin flaps
   (a) local
   (b) regional
   (c) distant
5. Myofascial and myocutaneous flaps
6. Free tissue transfers with microvascular anastomosis (composite graft)

Secondary

First of all, the wound should be covered with a wetting agent, such as glycerol, and an antiseptic. The initial inspection of the wound should be in the operating room between the 2nd and 3rd day after trauma, depending on the potential contamination. A decision as to the appropriate method of skin closure may be made at that time.

The exact method chosen for skin closure will depend upon the wound and the underlying fracture, as well as the method of stabilization (Table 3.2). If there has been *no skin loss,* and if there is no sign of sepsis, the wound can usually be resutured or retaped on the 5th day. Any ragged ends may be left open to heal by secondary intent. If there has been *skin loss* but no underlying muscle loss, a split-thickness skin graft may be applied when the wound is clean with evidence of healthy granulation tissue, between the 5th and 10th postoperative days. In general, if the skin defect is over soft tissue, it is better to close that defect with split-thickness skin grafts than to attempt extensive local, regional, or distant skin flaps.

If there has been skin loss with exposed bone, especially subcutaneous bones, such as the ulna or tibia, a local myofascial flap is the treatment of choice. The exact muscle used will of course depend upon the location. Excellent results have been obtained with this method in the past decade (James and Gruss 1983).

For fractures associated with skin, muscle, or bone loss, a free tissue transfer with microvascular anastomosis may be the most prudent method of treatment. To bridge the bony defect at the same time, one may use either a cancellous bone graft or a composite free vascularized fibular or iliac graft. Which type of bone graft is used depends on a number of factors, with the size of the defect to be bridged being one of the most important determining factors in the choice.

3.4.3.7 Secondary Fracture Care

Early communication between the surgeon and patient is essential. The patient must be told that the primary stabilization is step one in the management of the fracture, that is, it is only the beginning. At the first dressing change, the surgeon must also begin to decide on the follow-up management of the bony injury.

For severely comminuted diaphyseal fractures, if fixed by external skeletal fixation or plating, especially the former, early cancellous bone grafting should be planned. In some of these diaphyseal fractures, the decision may be to remove the external fixator and either convert the fixation immediately to one involving screws and plates, or delay the fixation, keep the limb in traction or a cast, and carry out a delayed intramedullary nailing, usually with a locked nail.

In all open fractures which are treated either by plating or an external fixator, the likelihood of the fracture going on to a delayed union or nonunion is so great that early cancellous bone grafting should be performed, usually between the 10th and 14th days after trauma.

These procedures may be combined with a secondary soft tissue procedure, if necessary.

3.4.3.8 Postoperative Care

The specific follow-up care for each patient should be individualized and will depend on the soft tissue wound, the bony injury and the method of its management. Wherever possible, the patient should be placed in a continuous passive motion machine in the immediate postoperative period. This will allow mobilization of the adjacent joints, but it should only be done if fracture stabilization is adequate. It must be remembered that in open fractures early motion is essential in order to regain function, and should be instituted as soon as the state of the wound permits.

The problems of open fractures specific to the various anatomical regions are dealt with in the chapters dealing with those regions.

3.5 Summary

Open fractures continue to test the decision-making and technical skills of the orthopedic surgeon. The main principles of management in open fractures consist of immediate sterile bandaging of the wound to prevent further contamination followed by cleansing and débridement in the operating room. Where possible, stable fixation of the fracture using either external fixation, open reduction and internal fixation, or combined methods is indicated. The wound should be left open primarily in all cases. Secondary wound inspection in the operating room must be carried out between the 1st and 5th day, depending on the degree of devitalization and contamination. Secondary wound management may be by secondary suture, split-thickness skin graft, flaps, or free tissue transfers.

Secondary cancellous bone grafting is almost always necessary. Where extensive bone loss is present, free bone pedicle transfer may be necessary. The key to the care of an open wound is to observe the fracture closely and change the management as necessary. The commonest and often the most serious error is to attempt definitive care of an open fracture in one step.

References

Allgöwer M (1971) Weichteilprobleme und Infektrisiko der Osteosynthese, Langenbecks Arch Chir 329:1127

Beauchamp CG, Clifford RP, Webb JK, Kellam JF, Tile M (1984) Functional results after immediate internal fixation of open tibial fractures. Paper presented at the Canadian Orthopaedic Association Meeting, Winnipeg, Canada, June 1984

Billroth T (1866) Die allgemeine und chirurgische Pathologie und Therapie in 50 Vorlesungen. Reimer, Berlin

Gustilo B, Andersson JP (1976) Prevention of infection in the treatment of one thousand and twenty-five open fractures of long bones. J Bone Joint Surg 58 A:453

James ETR, Gruss JS (1983) Closure of traumatic and osteomyelitis defects of the lower limb with muscle and musculocutaneous flaps. J Trauma 23:411–419

Lange RH, Bach AW, Hansen ST Jr, Johansen KH (1985) Open tibial fractures with associated vascular injuries: prognosis for limb salvage. J Trauma 25(3):203

Oestern HJ, Tscherne H (1984) Pathophysiology and classification of soft tissue injuries associated with fractures. In: Tscherne H, Gotzen L (eds) Fractures with soft tissue injuries. Springer, Berlin Heidelberg New York, Tokyo, pp 1–9

Tscherne H (1984) The management of open fractures. In: Tscherne H, Gotzen L (eds) Fractures with soft tissue injuries. Springer, Berlin Heidelberg New York Tokyo

Part II
Fractures of the Upper Extremity

4 Fractures of the Proximal Humerus

M. TILE

4.1 Introduction

4.1.1 General Considerations

Fractures of the proximal humerus have for years been relegated to the surgical scrap heap. The majority of these fractures occur in elderly individuals, are stable, and can be successfully treated by judicious neglect. Unfortunately, the same reasoning, and therefore the same treatment, is too often applied to the minority, which occur in young individuals, are unstable, and have a poor prognosis. Surgical nihilism has crept in to influence our management of those cases that do require open reduction. When surgery has been attempted on the proximal humerus, major technical problems have been encountered, such as difficulty with the exposure, osteoporotic bone, excessive comminution, and poor implants, leading to imperfect results. However, by applying the same principles of treatment of this particular fracture as to any other, a logical approach may be developed which will suit all groups of patients.

4.1.2 Anatomy

Codman (1934) recognized that fractures of the proximal humerus may separate into four major fragments (Fig. 4.1). The first fragment is the hu-

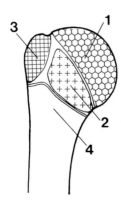

Fig. 4.1. The four major fragments of the proximal humerus. *1*, Humeral head superior to the anatomical neck; *2*, lesser tuberosity; *3*, greater tuberosity; *4*, shaft of the humerus

meral head, consisting of that portion of the humerus superior to the anatomical neck. Since this head fragment is almost completely covered by articular cartilage and devoid of soft tissue attachment, its blood supply is precarious. Therefore, if the head fragment is displaced following injury, avascular necrosis may be the inevitable result.

The second fragment consists of the lesser tuberosity with its attached subscapularis muscle. Avulsion of this fragment may allow undue external rotation of the head in the presence of a humeral neck fracture.

The third fragment is the greater tuberosity with its attached rotator cuff. Isolated avulsions of this fragment are equivalent to rotator cuff avulsions, while those associated with a surgical neck fracture may allow internal rotation of the head fragment.

The fourth fragment is created by a fracture through the surgical neck of the humerus and is the most common fracture in this area. As in other areas of metaphyseal bone, the behavior of this fragment differs according to the type of injury, be it compression, rendering the fracture stable, or shear, rendering it unstable. Also, the presence of ample soft tissue attachment to the large head fragment makes avascular necrosis most unlikely.

These anatomical considerations are of major clinical significance. Fractures of the upper end of the humerus may be compared to those of the upper femur. Fractures through the anatomical neck of the humerus are akin to intracapsular fractures of the femur; that is, they are intracapsular. The fractured fragments are almost entirely covered by articular cartilage and therefore devoid of a blood supply, leading to a high incidence of avascular necrosis for both (Fig. 4.2a, b). Fractures through the surgical neck of the humerus are more akin to intertrochanteric and pertrochanteric fractures of the femur; that is, they are extracapsular, usually with an adequate blood supply and a relatively low incidence of avascular necrosis (Fig. 4.2c, d).

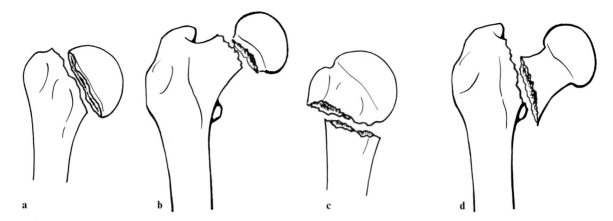

Fig. 4.2a, b. Comparison of the intracapsular anatomical neck fracture of the humerus (**a**) with the intracapsular fracture of the neck of the femur (**b**). Both are almost entirely covered by articular cartilage and therefore devoid of blood supply, resulting in a high incidence of avascular necrosis for both. **c, d** Comparison of the extracapsular surgical neck fracture of the humerus (**c**) with the intertrochanteric extracapsular fracture of the proximal femur (**d**). Since they are extracapsular, the incidence of avascular necrosis is low

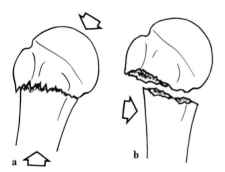

Fig. 4.3a, b. Stable and unstable fractures of the proximal humerus. **a** Typical impacted stable fracture in which the shaft and head move as one unit. **b** An unstable fracture of the proximal humerus, characterized by movement between the shaft and head fragments

4.1.3 Four-Segment Classification

Neer (1970) expanded the anatomical considerations of Codman into a working classification based on the displacement of the fragments. The group of minimally displaced fractures which may be treated by closed means must, in his opinion, have no segment displaced more than 10 mm or angulated more than 45°. He further classified the displaced fractures according to the number of parts fractured, plus the presence of a dislocation. For example, the greater tuberosity fragment may be involved in a two-, three-, or four-part fracture, with or without a dislocation. Neer's classification,

based on a study of 300 cases, has clarified the natural history of these various types. Once it became evident that some types treated by closed means were associated with dismal results, logical decision-making could follow.

4.1.4 Stability

In any classification, consideration should also be given to the stability of a given fracture, as well as to the number of segments involved. Cancellous bone may fail in compression, resulting in a stable impacted fracture, or in tension or shear, resulting in an unstable fracture (Fig. 4.3). These two types of injury behave quite differently. The stable impacted types cause less pain, allowing earlier movement, and heal rapidly. In contrast, the unstable types cause severe pain, precluding early function; in addition, healing is often delayed. Therefore, to consider only the number of fracture segments irrespective of their stability may lead to poor management decisions, usually toward overtreatment. An impacted, stable, relatively painless fracture of the proximal humerus will have a very different outcome than will a fracture with the same number of segments but with inherent instability. Stability must be assessed by a careful clinical as well as a complete radiological investigation.

4.1.5 Surgical Difficulties

If surgery is the answer for some of the unstable fracture types identified as having a poor outcome if treated by nonoperative means, why has it not been universally adopted? The answer is obvious—surgery is not without its own set of problems, such as: (a) osteoporotic bone which greatly reduces the holding power of screws so that they may pull out prior to fracture healing (see

Fig. 4.21); (b) comminution so severe that anatomical reduction may be impossible; (c) avascular necrosis of the humeral head; (d) difficult techniques and imperfect implants. We should not be deterred by these problems, but instead should rise to the challenge in order to improve the results of this difficult injury.

4.2 Classification

Any classification is useful only if it aids the surgeon in the management of a given injury. The proposed classification (Table 4.1), adapted from the previous reports of Codman and Neer, should, if followed, lead the surgeon to logical management based on the natural history of the various fracture types. The two major considerations in this classification are, first, the anatomical features of the fracture, i.e., whether the fracture is through the anatomical neck separating the head fragment (intracapsular) or through the surgical neck (extracapsular), and, second whether the fracture is stable, i.e., the head and shaft are impacted and move together, or unstable.

Table 4.1. Classification of fracture types

1. *Stable*
2. *Unstable*
   A. Minimally displaced
   B. Displaced
      1. *Two-part*
         (a) Lesser tuberosity
         (b) Greater tuberosity
         (c) Surgical neck
         (d) Anatomical neck
      2. *Three-part* — Surgical neck
         (a) Plus lesser tuberosity
         (b) Plus greater tuberosity
      3. *Four-part* — Anatomical neck
         (a) Plus tuberosities
      4. *Fracture-dislocation*
         (a) Two-part   — with greater tuberosity
         (b) Three-part — I. anterior, with
         greater tuberosity
         II. posterior, with lesser tuberosity
         (c) Four-part — I. anterior
         II. posterior
3. *Articular*
   (a) Head impaction — (Hill-Sachs)
   (b) Articular fractures
      1. Humeral head split
      2. Glenoid rim

4.3 Natural History and Surgical Indications

A careful study of the natural history of each of the fracture types in the proposed classification will greatly aid the surgeon in his final decision-making process. Delayed union or nonunion and avascular necrosis are the major complications affecting proximal humeral fractures. By indicating those fractures which are likely to end in a poor result with closed methods, we hope the surgeon will, by deduction, come to open treatment as the preferred alternative. In general, those fractures where open reduction must be considered as a treatment option because of a poor prognosis with nonoperative care are marked in red in Table 4.2.

4.3.1 Stable Fractures

As in other areas of the body, stability must here be considered a relative and not an absolute concept. A stable fracture is one which cannot be displaced by physiological forces. A rigidly impacted fracture of the proximal humerus caused by compressive forces fulfills these criteria, no matter how many fragments may be present. Soft tissue hinges are most likely to be intact, so that avascular necrosis is improbable. Impaction of the cancellous bone allows early pain-free motion and rapid union, both contributing to a good functional result. The natural history of the stable fracture is usually favorable; therefore surgery, except in the most unusual circumstances, is meddlesome and dangerous.

Exceptions to this rule are *stable fractures with unacceptable displacement*, for example, an impacted stable fracture with excessive angulation in a young patient. *Unacceptable* displacement cannot be defined by a number, but can be ascertained only after a careful assessment of all the factors making up the personality of the injury.

4.3.2 Unstable Fractures

The state of the soft tissue envelope will determine the degree of instability present. A grossly unstable fracture will allow the fragments to move independently of each other, as noted in the clinical and radiographic assessment. Instability of the major fragments may result in pain, as well as in delayed union, both contributing to prolonged immobilization and a less than perfect result.

Table 4.2. Fractures of the proximal humerus. Classification and treatment guidelines

	Lesser tuberosity	Greater tuberosity	Surgical neck	Anatomical neck
2 Part				
3 Part				
4 Part				
Fracture dislocation	ant			
	post			
	articular impaction		head impaction	

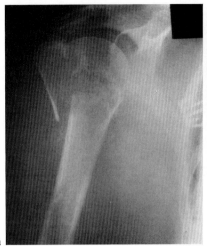 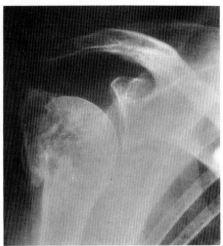

a   b

Displaced fractures of the articular fragment through the anatomical neck often result in avascular necrosis. Thus, the natural history of the unstable proximal injury is markedly different from that of the stable injury and requires a different approach.

4.3.2.1 Minimal Displacement

A minimally displaced fracture usually implies a less violent force and the presence of some soft tissue hinges. Neer (1970) arbitrarily chose less than 1 cm of displacement as indicating some attached soft tissue. This must, of course, be confirmed by clinical examination, often with image intensification. If soft tissue hinges have been retained, the ultimate prognosis is good, no matter how many fragments are present. Vascularity of the head fragment is usually assumed, and surgery is virtually never indicated for this type of injury (Fig. 4.4).

4.3.2.2 Major Displacement

The fractures with major displacement will be considered according to the *anatomical* structures and the *number of segments* involved.

a) Two-Part

Displaced fractures may occur through any of the four segments previously described. The outcome of a single fracture through these segments will vary considerably, depending upon the retained soft tissue envelope.

Lesser Tuberosity. Pure avulsions of the lesser tuberosity are rare and are of little clinical significance. However, an isolated lesser tuberosity frac-

Fig. 4.4a, b. Unstable, minimally displaced three-part fracture of the proximal right humerus in a 67-year-old woman (**a**). Treatment consisted of a sling and a swathe for 3 weeks, until the pain subsided, and then a program of physiotherapy. At 8 weeks (**b**) the fracture is healed in good position. Note the slight inferior subluxation which is almost inevitable in these individuals. When rehabilitation is complete, the inferior subluxation usually reduces spontaneously

ture should always alert the surgeon to the possibility of a *posterior dislocation* of the shoulder, with which it is frequently associated. Unless associated with some other major displaced fragment, closed treatment only is indicated.

Greater Tuberosity. A *displaced* isolated avulsion fracture of the greater tuberosity is indicative of a loss of function of the rotator cuff (Fig. 4.5a). In the two-part pattern, the bony fragment may retract under the acromion, acting as a block to abduction. To correct both the mechanical block and the loss of rotator cuff function, *surgery is mandatory.* We regard the displaced retracted greater tuberosity fracture as an *absolute* indication for surgery.

Greater tuberosity fractures occur more commonly in association with anterior dislocation of the shoulder, and, as will be described in the section on fracture-dislocation, they rarely require open reduction in that particular situation (Fig. 4.5b).

Surgical Neck Fractures. Impacted fractures through the surgical neck are common and usually minimally displaced, thus requiring only closed treatment. However, shearing forces may cause displacement and instability. The large proximal fragment usually has sufficient soft tissue attach-

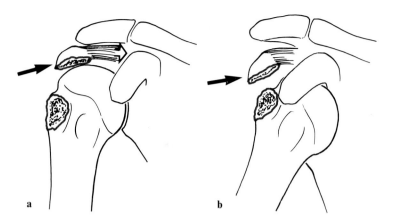

Fig. 4.5a, b. Fracture of the greater tuberosity. a An avulsion-type fracture of the greater tuberosity. This is a true avulsion of the rotator cuff, in which the bone lodges under the acromion and acts as a mechanical block. Surgery is mandatory. b Fracture of the greater tuberosity has occurred at the time of anterior dislocation of the humeral head. In this situation, the tuberosity is in its correct position and does not retract. Therefore, reduction of the dislocation usually leads to an anatomical reduction of the tuberosity to the shaft, and surgery is rarely necessary

ment to ensure the viability of the humeral head. Associated undisplaced fractures into the tuberosities are common, but they do not alter the natural history because the soft tissues are retained. Avascular necrosis is rare, unless the blood supply is destroyed by injudicious surgery; however, union may be delayed because of the gross instability of the main fragments.

These grossly unstable fractures usually occur in young patients with strong cancellous bone and are usually caused by high-energy shearing forces. Severe pain and delayed union will require prolonged immobilization, which may lead to permanent stiffness in spite of lengthy rehabilitation. Open reduction and stable internal fixation, using standard techniques, will immobilize the fracture sufficiently to reduce pain, ensure rapid healing, and allow early motion with improved results. We regard this fracture as a *relative* indication for surgery, especially in young patients with good bone (Fig. 4.6).

Anatomical Neck. Two-part fractures involving the anatomical neck are rare. Since the head segment is covered by articular cartilage, displaced fractures through the anatomical neck are associated with a high incidence of avascular necrosis (see Fig. 4.2a). Because of the instability of the bone fragments, nonunion may also occur. In the two-part anatomical neck fracture with displacement,

surgery should be performed if closed manipulation fails to restore the local anatomy. In such cases, care should be taken to preserve any remaining soft tissue attachments. If compression of the cancellous fracture is achieved by surgery, rapid healing of the cancellous fracture will ensue but avascular necrosis will not be prevented. Some patients may manage reasonably well with an avascular head if the fracture has healed and the head revascularizes in time to prevent collapse.

b) Three-Part

The three-part fracture consists of a large displaced proximal fragment through the surgical neck, associated with an avulsion of either the lesser or greater tuberosity or both. Since the proximal fragment is large, some soft tissue envelope is usually retained. Avulsion of either tuberosity diminishes the blood supply to the humeral head, but avascular necrosis is uncommon, although it occurs with greater incidence than in the two-part surgical neck fracture.

Of much greater clinical significance is the rotatory deformity of the proximal fragment caused by the avulsion of the tuberosities. If the *lesser tuberosity* containing the subscapularis is avulsed, the proximal fragment is externally rotated by the remaining rotator cuff, the supraspinatus, infraspinatus, and teres minor (Fig. 4.7). If the *greater tuberosity* is avulsed, the proximal fragment is internally rotated by the unopposed pull of the subscapularis (Fig. 4.8a). In both instances, the unstable shafts may be driven into the mass of deltoid muscle and may be anterior to the proximal fragment. Poor bone contact will lead to delayed union or nonunion in most cases.

The presence of a round proximal fragment with the appearance of a full moon on the anteroposterior radiograph should alert the astute sur-

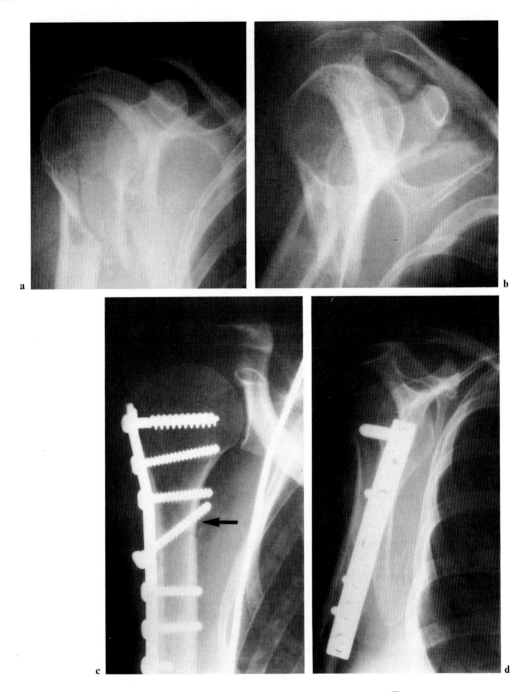

Fig. 4.6a–d. Unstable three-part fracture through the proximal humerus. **a** Anteroposterior and **b** lateral radiographs showing an unstable oblique fracture in the upper humerus with an extension through the greater tuberosity. This fracture occurred when a 33-year-old woman was thrown from a horse and struck a tree. The fracture was grossly unstable on clinical examination, and, in consultation with the patient, treatment consisted of open reduction and internal fixation using a DC plate with a lag screw across the fracture through the plate (**c**, *arrow*; **d**). Excellent stability was obtained. The patient regained full shoulder motion within 10 days of injury

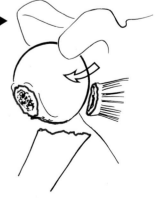

Fig. 4.7. Three-part fracture of the proximal humerus in which the lesser tuberosity is avulsed, allowing the proximal fragment to externally rotate. The radiological appearance of the head is that of a full moon on the anteroposterior view

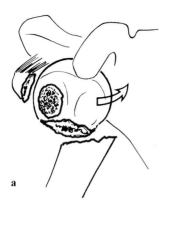

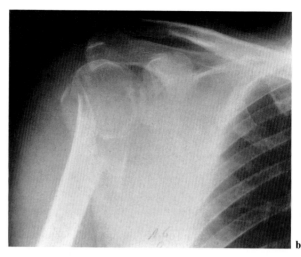

Fig. 4.8. a Three-part fracture of the proximal humerus with avulsion of the greater tuberosity. In this particular case, the remaining attachment of the subscapularis through the lesser tuberosity internally rotates the proximal fragment 90°, again appearing radiographically as a full moon on the anteroposterior view. This is clearly seen in **b**

geon to this injury (Fig. 4.8b). Open reduction and internal fixation should always be performed if delayed union and nonunion are to be prevented.

c) Four-Part

The four-segment fracture is the most difficult to treat and is associated with the poorest results. Added to the problems of the three-part fracture, namely delayed union or nonunion, is avascular necrosis of the humeral head. The pathognomonic feature is the small, crescentic, proximal articular fragment severed from the anatomical neck of the humerus. This fragment may be devoid of all soft tissue, making avascular necrosis a certainty, irrespective of treatment. Occasionally, some capsular attachments may remain; therefore, the presence of a small head fragment does not necessarily doom the head to avascularity.

If the small head fragment is impacted and not acting as a mechanical block to movement, surgery should be avoided, as attempts at open reduction may destroy any remaining blood supply (Figs. 4.9, 4.10). The avulsed abductor mechanism, often in one large fragment consisting of the greater and lesser tuberosities with the intervening long head of biceps tendon, may be replaced without disturbing the impacted head (Fig. 4.11a). If the impacted fragment causes a block to motion during examination of the patient

under anesthesia, then careful open reduction of the fracture is indicated. The technique must be atraumatic, so that any remaining blood supply to the humeral head is not compromised (Fig. 4.11b–e).

If the head fragment is free, it must be reduced to a satisfactory position by either closed or open means, as will be described. A completely free head may have to be discarded during surgery and replaced with a prosthesis; however, in young patients, every effort should be made to retain the head fragment.

d) Fracture-Dislocation

Fracture-dislocations may be considered an extension of the two-, three-, and four-segment classifications. As in our previous discussion, the ultimate prognosis will depend upon the probability of nonunion or avascular necrosis of the fracture. Add to this the problems associated with the dislocation, such as irreducibility of the humeral head or impaction of its articular surface, and one can see why this injury has the worst prognosis of any in this region. In the two- and three-part fracture-dislocations, the proximal fragment is usually of sufficient size to retain capsular attachments, making avascular necrosis uncommon. The retention of at least one tuberosity almost always ensures viability of the humeral head. In the four-part fracture-dislocation, however, the head fragment is usually completely detached and avascular.

Two-Part. The two-part *anterior* fracture-dislocation is associated with an avulsed greater tuberosity (Fig. 4.12a). In older patients with anterior humeral head dislocations, massive tears through the rotator cuff are more common than avulsions

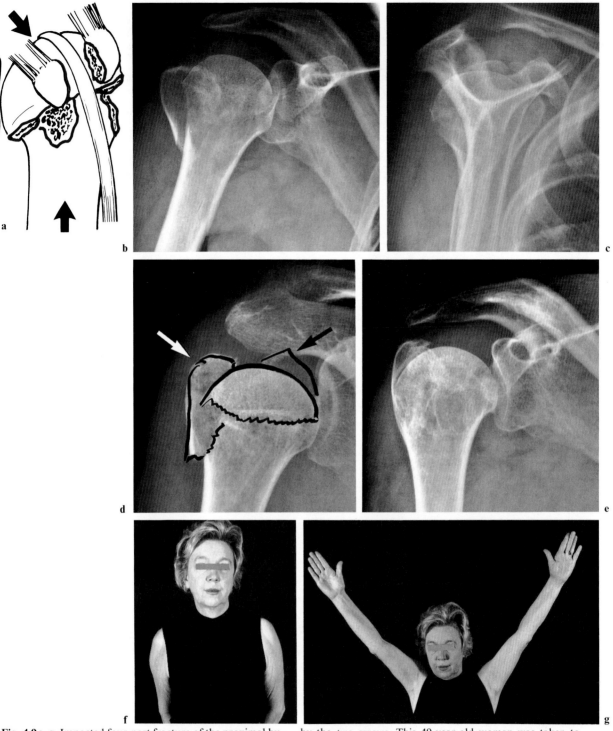

Fig. 4.9a–g. Impacted four-part fracture of the proximal humerus with valgus position of head. **a** Extreme valgus position of the head driven into the soft cancellous bone by the abducted shoulder. Note the avulsion of both the greater and lesser tuberosities, which remain in their normal position. This is clearly seen on the anteroposterior and lateral radiographs (**b**, **c**) and emphasized on the radiograph (**d**). The impacted valgus position of the head is clearly seen, as are the greater and lesser tuberosity avulsions, marked by the *two arrows*. This 49-year-old woman was taken to the operating room and the shoulder manipulated under general anesthesia. Since there was no block to motion and the head and shaft fragments moved together, her injury was treated nonoperatively. At 1 year (**e**) the fracture has united with no evidence of avascular necrosis. The patient's range of motion is almost full (**f**, **g**), and she functions normally

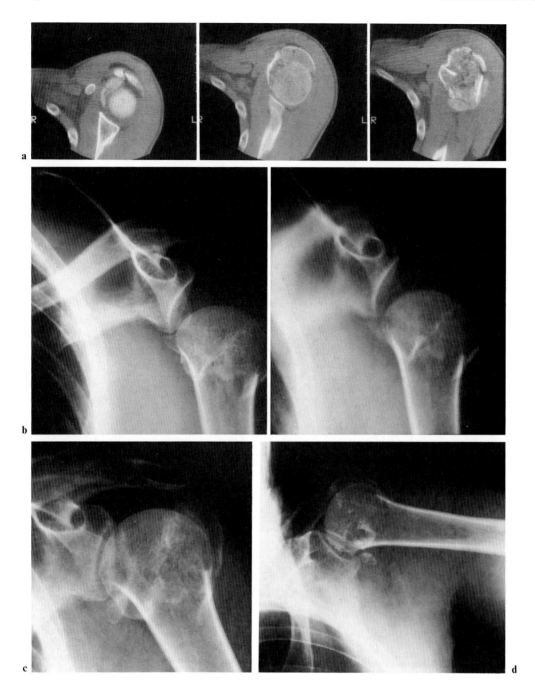

Fig. 4.10 a–d. a Anteroposterior tomograms demonstrating an impacted four-part fracture with the head in marked valgus and inferior subluxation in a 47-year-old orthopedic surgeon. Note the avulsion of the rotator cuff and the valgus position of the head in the CT scans (b). The patient was treated non-operatively and the fracture has united (c, d). Note that the inferior subluxation has corrected and no avascular necrosis is present

of the greater tuberosity and are often overlooked (Fig. 4.12b). Satisfactory reduction is usually achieved by closed means with or without a general anesthetic. In almost all cases, closed reduction with no surgical intervention is indicated. In rare instances, the long head of biceps tendon may act as a block to reduction, causing either irreducibility of the dislocation or persistent displacement of the fracture (Fig. 4.12c). In this situation, open reduction is indicated.

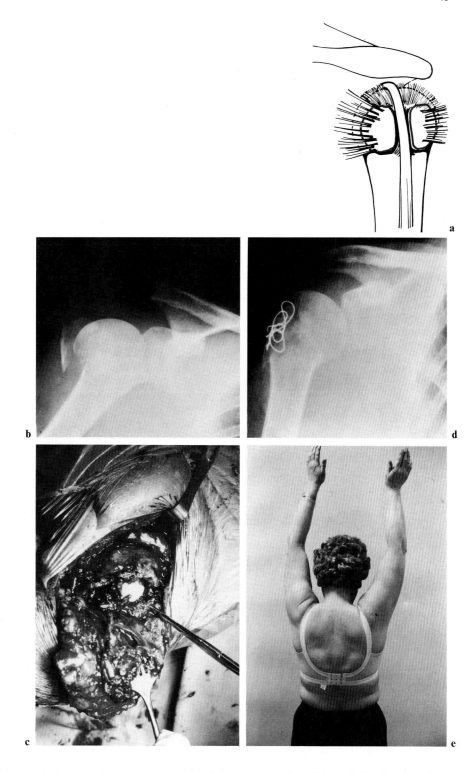

Fig. 4.11. a In a four-part impacted fracture, the rotator cuff is often avulsed as one unit with the biceps tendon intervening. **b** Anteroposterior radiograph of a four-part impacted fracture of the proximal humerus with the head in valgus. **c** Intraoperative photograph showing valgus position of the head. The articular cartilage points superiorly. By very gentle manipulation, using the finger to push the head back into its normal position and allowing the tuberosities to return to their normal site, the anatomy was restored. **d** The tuberosities were wired together and no fixation was used for the head fragment in this case. **e** Final result after 1 year; no avascular necrosis developed. (**b–e** courtesy of Dr. Alexander G. Macdonald, Fredericton, New Brunswick)

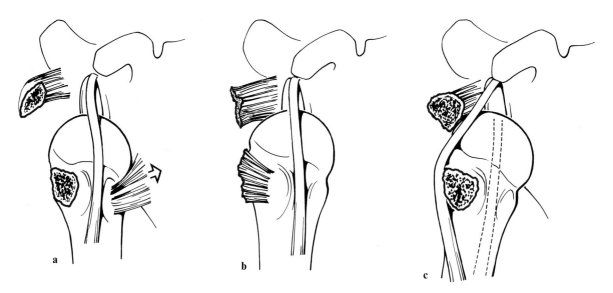

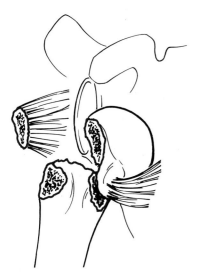

Fig. 4.12a–c. Two-part fracture-dislocations. **a** Two-part anterior fracture-dislocation associated with an avulsed greater tuberosity. **b** Anterior dislocation of the shoulder associated with an avulsion of the rotator cuff. **c** Anterior dislocation of the shoulder with an interposed long head of biceps tendon preventing reduction of the dislocation

Fig. 4.13. Three-part fracture-dislocation. In this anterior dislocation, the humeral head is seen anterior to the glenoid labrum, and the greater tuberosity is avulsed

A two-part *posterior* fracture-dislocation is associated with an avulsed lesser tuberosity. Closed treatment is usually sufficient for this injury.

Three-Part. The major feature of the three-part dislocation is the large proximal fragment created by the fracture of the surgical neck of the humerus (Fig. 4.13). Some capsular tissue is almost always retained on the large head fragment, ensuring its viability. If the head fragment is displaced *anteriorly*, the greater tuberosity is usually fractured, whereas the lesser tuberosity is retained. In the *posterior* fracture-dislocation, the greater tuberosity is usually retained, whereas the lesser is avulsed.

In the three-part fracture-dislocation, closed manipulation with general anesthesia may restore the proximal fragment to an anatomical position. If the proximal fragment cannot be reduced because of soft tissue interposition, then open reduction is mandatory. If gross instability of the fracture remains after closed reduction of the dislocation, then open reduction and internal fixation are desirable. The surgeon must respect the soft tissue attached to the head fragment envelope in order not to destroy the attached soft tissue.

Four-Part. Fracture-dislocations involving the anatomical neck of the humerus propel the small crescentic head fragment inferiorly, anteriorly, (Fig. 4.14a–e) posteriorly, or occasionally intrathoracically (Fig. 4.14f, g). In almost all cases, this small head fragment has no attached soft tissue and will be avascular; therefore, the prognosis must be guarded. Closed manipulation under general anesthesia may restore the head fragment to its normal position. However, in our experience, this is extremely difficult, and anatomic reduction is rarely achieved. Open reduction is usually indicated, but the patient must be informed that avascular necrosis of the humeral head is likely. In young patients, every effort should be made to retain the head fragment; in older patients it is often discarded in favor of a prosthesis.

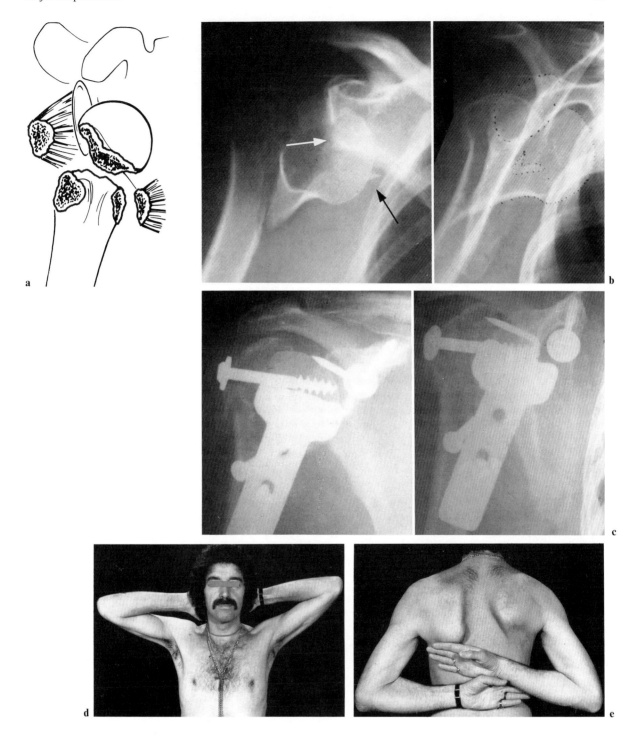

Fig. 4.14a–g. Four-part fracture-dislocations. **a** The head is anteriorly dislocated. Both the lesser and greater tuberosities are avulsed. The humeral head may be attached by a small amount of capsule inferiorly or may be completely devoid of soft tissue attachment. **b** Anteroposterior and lateral radiographs of a four-part anterior fracture-dislocation. The *lower arrow* points to an avulsion from the glenoid labrum, the *upper arrow* to that portion of the glenoid from which the bone was avulsed. Open reduction and internal fixation were performed through an anterior deltopectoral approach. The greater tuberosity was replaced with a lag screw, the major fracture with a lag screw plus T plate, and the glenoid fracture with a screw and staple (**c**). **d** and **e** The result at 18 months, with full movement and no avascular necrosis.

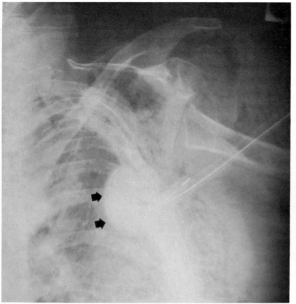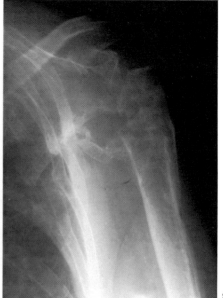

f   g

Fig. 4.14f, g. Intrathoracic fracture-dislocation of the humeral head: **f** Humeral head in the left pleural cavity outlined by the *arrows*; chest drain in place. **g** Appearance after removal of the humeral head, 12 months post-trauma

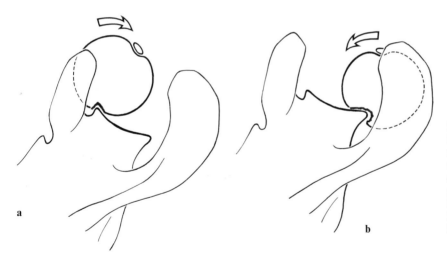

a   b

Fig. 4.15a, b. Impacted articular fractures. Impaction of the articular surface may occur with any type of fracture dislocation. In anterior dislocations (**a**), the impaction of the articular surface occurs posteriorly. In posterior dislocations (**b**), the impaction occurs anteriorly

4.3.3 Articular Fractures

4.3.3.1 Impacted (Hill-Sachs)

Impaction of the articular surface, the so-called Hill-Sachs lesion, may occur with any type of fracture-dislocation. In anterior dislocations the impaction of the articular surface occurs posteriorly, the reverse being true for the posterior dislocation (Fig. 4.15). Very little can be done surgically to restore the normal anatomy, and recurrent dislocation may ensue, to be dealt with secondarily by standard means. In late unreduced fracture-dislocation the defect may be so large that specialized techniques such as insertion of the subscapularis tendon into the anterior defect (McLaughlin 1960) or osteotomy of the humerus or scapular neck for the posterior defect (Müller et al. 1979) may be required to restore stability to the shoulder (Fig. 4.16).

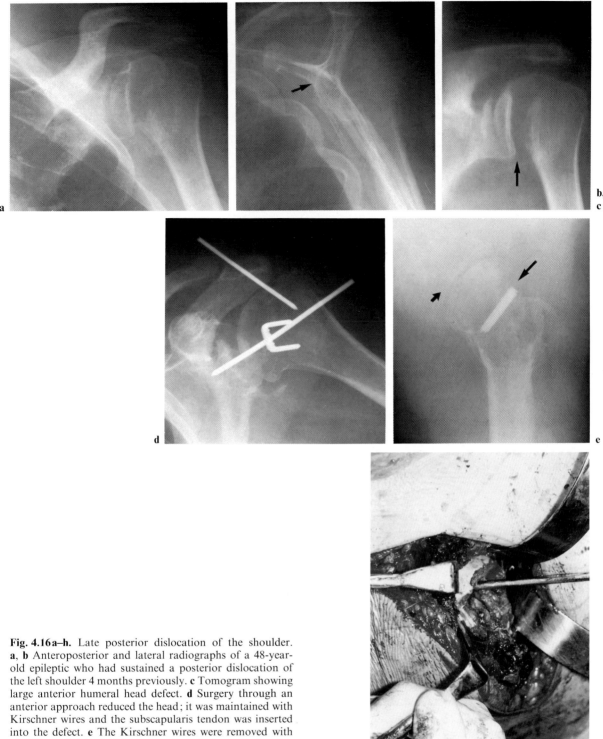

Fig. 4.16a–h. Late posterior dislocation of the shoulder. **a, b** Anteroposterior and lateral radiographs of a 48-year-old epileptic who had sustained a posterior dislocation of the left shoulder 4 months previously. **c** Tomogram showing large anterior humeral head defect. **d** Surgery through an anterior approach reduced the head; it was maintained with Kirschner wires and the subscapularis tendon was inserted into the defect. **e** The Kirschner wires were removed with stability maintained. **f** Intraoperative photograph showing the massive defect.

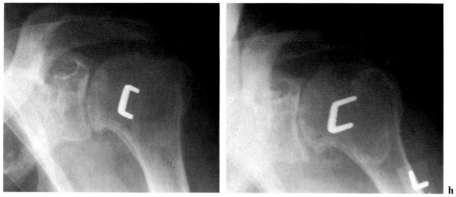

g

h

Fig 4.16g, h The final result: joint narrowing is apparent but function is satisfactory

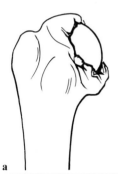

a

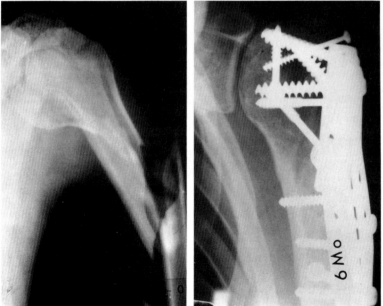

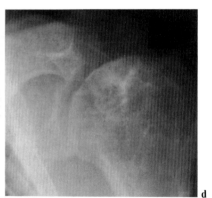

d

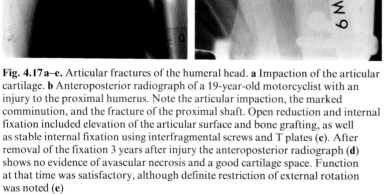

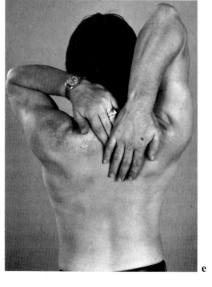

b,
c

e

Fig. 4.17a–e. Articular fractures of the humeral head. **a** Impaction of the articular cartilage. **b** Anteroposterior radiograph of a 19-year-old motorcyclist with an injury to the proximal humerus. Note the articular impaction, the marked comminution, and the fracture of the proximal shaft. Open reduction and internal fixation included elevation of the articular surface and bone grafting, as well as stable internal fixation using interfragmental screws and T plates (**c**). After removal of the fixation 3 years after injury the anteroposterior radiograph (**d**) shows no evidence of avascular necrosis and a good cartilage space. Function at that time was satisfactory, although definite restriction of external rotation was noted (**e**)

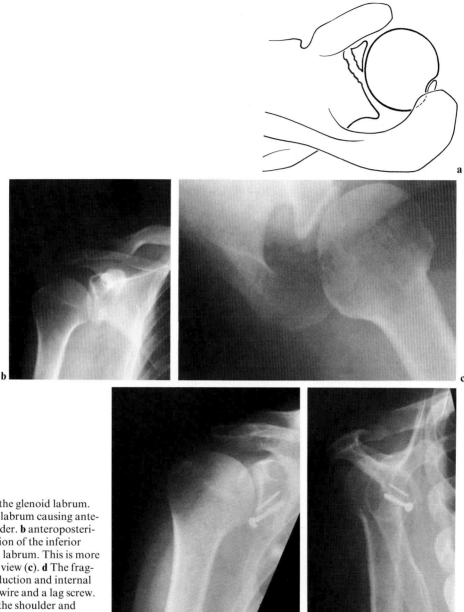

Fig. 4.18a–e. Fractures of the glenoid labrum.
a A fracture of the glenoid labrum causing anterior instability of the shoulder. **b** anteroposterior radiograph shows avulsion of the inferior half of the anterior glenoid labrum. This is more clearly seen on the axillary view (**c**). **d** The fragment was fixed by open reduction and internal fixation using a Kirschner wire and a lag screw. **e** Stability was restored to the shoulder and function was good

4.3.3.2 Humeral Head

As in any other joint, major shearing forces applied to the joint surface may shatter the articular cartilage. The degree of articular damage may vary from small osteochondral fractures to major splits in the humeral head. In this situation, we must revert to basic principles in the management of any joint fracture, i.e., open anatomical reduction and stable fixation, followed by early motion if technically possible (Fig. 4.17). The upper extremity, however, is much more forgiving than the lower

extremity; hence, closed methods may be more prudent than open methods, which could jeopardize the blood supply to the small fragments. These fractures present extremely difficult management problems and require careful analysis before a definitive decision is made.

4.3.3.3 Glenoid Labrum

The usual pathological lesion associated with an anterior dislocation of the shoulder is an avulsion of the glenoid labrum (Bankart lesion) and a posterior impaction fracture of the humeral head (Hill-Sachs lesion). On occasion, the glenoid labrum is avulsed with a small segment of bone which, upon reduction, does not affect the acute stability of the shoulder, but may be associated with recurrent dislocation. Rarely, with anterior dislocation, a large anterior segment of the glenoid is fractured and displaced, rendering the shoulder unstable (Fig. 4.18). This fracture may occur with simple dislocations or with the more complex fracture-dislocations.

If displaced, open reduction and internal fixation are desirable for the following reasons: (a) redisplacement of the shoulder will readily occur with external rotation because of the loss of the anterior portion of the glenoid labrum; (b) since the fragment contains a major portion of the articular surface of the joint, it requires anatomic reduction for optimal results. Closed treatment cannot accomplish this; therefore, operative fixation is *mandatory* when the fragment is large enough to affect the stability of the joint. The opposite lesion may occur with a posterior dislocation; i.e., a large posterior fragment of the glenoid labrum may be fractured and will require operative reduction.

4.4 Management

4.4.1 Assessment

4.4.1.1 Clinical

The first step in logical decision making is a careful clinical and radiological assessment. A painstaking history may indicate the physiological state of the patient, his or her expectations, and the degree of violence involved in the injury. For example, a markedly displaced fracture-dislocation through the proximal humerus of a young patient with normal cancellous bone has a vastly different outlook from that of a fracture-dislocation of similar appearance caused by a simple fall in an elderly individual. Physical examination will determine both the general state of the patient and the local condition of the limb. Complicating factors such as severe soft tissue injury, whether open or closed, and the presence of neurovascular injury will affect the decision to operate and its timing.

Careful manipulation of the limb will often reveal more information about the stability of the fracture than the radiograph. In grossly unstable fractures, the humeral shaft may be easily palpated

in the deltoid muscle mass, moving independently of the proximal fragment.

4.4.1.2 Radiological

Careful radiological assessment is required prior to choosing a definitive treatment method. Standard roentgenograms of this area are often confusing and may be supplemented with tomograms or CT scans (see Fig. 4.11 b). Tomographic investigation will reveal the position and size of the humeral head fragment, the number of segments, and the degree of instability.

Through a careful combination of the clinical and radiological assessments, a proper management scheme for the individual patient will evolve.

4.4.1.3 Examination Under Anesthesia

In most patients, a careful clinical assessment will indicate the degree of instability without the need for a general anesthetic. These individuals may be examined with adequate sedation, their fracture viewed on the image intensifier, and the degree of instability ascertained. With those patients in whom stability cannot be assessed because of severe pain, examination under anesthesia with image intensification will be helpful. The surgeon should be prepared to proceed with immediate definitive surgical management if indicated.

4.4.2 Decision Making

The natural outcome of most stable and minimally displaced unstable proximal humeral fractures is a healed fracture and a satisfactorily functioning extremity. However, unstable fractures or fracture-dislocations have a high probability of delayed union or nonunion, avascular necrosis, irreducibility of the dislocation, and articular cartilage damage. Surgery is indicated where the probability of such complications with closed treatment is high, as previously discussed. The surgeon should assess the *personality* of the injury: this includes the fracture pattern, the condition of the limb, and the patient, as well as his own expertise (the term "personality of the fracture" was first coined by Nicoll (1964) in connection with fractures of the tibia; see Sect. 17.2). These factors are considered in the decision-making algorithm (Fig. 4.19).

4.4.2.1 Stable Fractures

If the clinical and radiological assessment indicates a stable fracture — i.e., the patient can actively

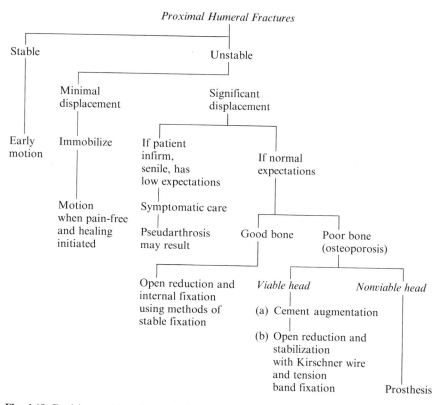

Fig. 4.19. Decision-making algorithm for proximal humeral fracture

move the extremity without pain, and the limb can be moved passively with little pain and no abnormal motion between the shaft and head fragments — the patient should be treated *nonoperatively*. The blood supply to a fractured proximal fragment is often so fragile that ill-advised open reduction will threaten the viability of the humeral head and must be avoided at all costs in stable situations (see Figs. 4.9 and 4.10). The arm may be immobilized in a sling and early motion started immediately. An excellent functional result may be expected in this situation. The only exception to this rule would be a stable fracture with such gross displacement that the function of the extremity would be adversely affected. We agree with Neer that an impacted humeral neck with an adduction deformity of more than 50° would certainly affect the end result, and in rare circumstances this would constitute an indication for open reduction.

4.4.2.2 Unstable Fractures

If the clinical and radiological assessment indicates an unstable fracture, that is, independent motion

is present between the shaft and head fragments, further decision-making will depend upon the degree of displacement and instability present.

a) Minimally Displaced

If the fracture is minimally displaced (cf. Fig. 4.4a, b), no matter how many segments are involved, one might reasonably expect the presence of an intact soft tissue envelope in some portion of the fracture. Examination under image intensification may indicate lack of independent motion between the shaft and the proximal fragment at various degrees of rotation and abduction, confirming the presence of an intact soft tissue envelope. Patients with these fractures have more pain than do patients with a firmly impacted stable fracture; therefore, immobilization is required until sufficient fracture healing has taken place to render the patient pain-free. This is followed by a period of active rehabilitation of the injured limb; this period may vary from 2 to 6 weeks, depending upon the specific fracture. Since most fractures of the proximal humerus fall into the above two types, either the stable or the minimally displaced unsta-

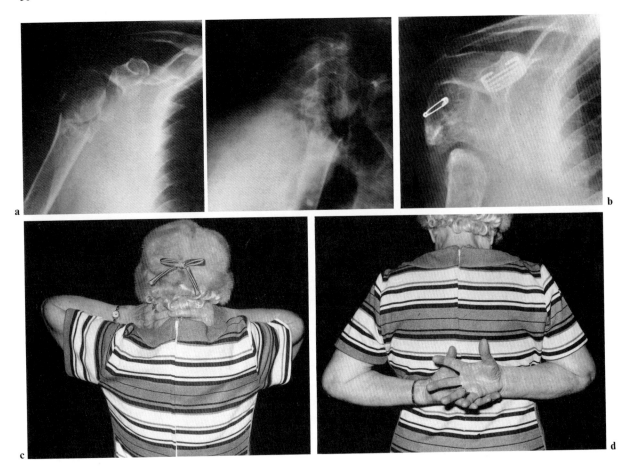

Fig. 4.20a–d. An 82-year-old woman fell and sustained a three-part fracture of the right proximal humerus, seen on the anteroposterior and lateral radiographs in **a**. The patient was treated with a short period of immobilization followed by rehabilitation. At 2 years, a clear pseudoarthrosis is seen on the anteroposterior radiograph (**b**). The patient's function, however, was excellent, with a full range of motion and minimal discomfort (**c, d**). Her major disability was weakness in the right arm

ble fracture, it follows that most fractures of the proximal humerus may be managed by closed means.

b) Displaced

If a careful assessment indicates an unstable fracture or fracture-dislocation, the situation changes markedly. In Sect. 4.3 we discussed in some detail those injuries requiring open reduction. Having determined that the fracture at hand would best be treated by open reduction and stable internal fixation, other factors must now be considered.

Even in the best of circumstances surgery may be difficult; therefore, the stated goal of open reduction — i.e., stable fixation allowing early mo-

tion — may not be realized because of the many technical problems inherent in this area. Therefore, surgery should only be performed in cases where the surgeon is confident of overcoming these difficulties and experienced enough to achieve the stated goal. Of prime importance is *the general state of the patient.*

Poor Patient Expectations. If the patient is infirm, senile, and with low functional expectations, the surgeon should consider nonoperative symptomatic treatment, i.e., *judicious neglect.* Such patients are immobilized in any type of binder or sling for comfort. Between the 4th and 6th week their pain usually subsides. Delayed union and eventually nonunion quickly become apparent in many cases of three- and four-part fractures. With persistence of this nontreatment, the surgeon may be pleasantly surprised at the degree of shoulder function regained by these patients. By 6 months many patients have little pain and a surprisingly good range of motion (Fig. 4.20). They complain of weakness in their extremity and inability to lift heavy objects, but usually carry out their normal daily routine without difficulty. We recommend

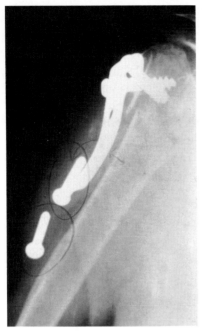

Fig. 4.21. Anteroposterior radiograph taken 4 days following an excellent internal fixation of a four-part proximal humerus fracture in a 79-year-old woman, showing failure of the fixation because of osteoporotic bone, so common in proximal humeral fractures in the elderly

fracture present, but also the physiological state of the bone. It is obvious that this state is not an absolute, i.e., either good or bad, but a spectrum. Assessment of the bone may be difficult; nevertheless, it is extremely important if major errors in technique are to be avoided. Many of these fractures occur in elderly individuals with osteoporotic bone. Standard AO/ASIF techniques will fail because of the poor holding power of the screws in such bone. Therefore, the surgeon might achieve an excellent-looking post-operative radiograph, but he will find that with early motion the screws will often pull out, with disastrous results (Fig. 4.21). Other techniques to be described are preferable in that situation (Figs. 4.22, 4.23).

If the *bone is normal*, i.e., if the state of the skeleton is good enough to ensure the holding power of the screws, anatomical open reduction followed by stable internal fixation is indicated. This may be readily achieved in the two- and three-part configurations, unless comminution or destruction of the articular cartilage is great. Early motion may be instituted and a good result expected (see Fig. 4.14a–e).

In the four-part fracture, the result is more dependent on the state of vascularity of the head fragment, which may compromise the end result. In the young individual, however, we feel that every effort should be made to retain the crescentic head and to institute early rehabilitation. If the ensuing avascular necrosis becomes a major symptomatic problem, secondary prosthetic replacement or shoulder arthrodesis may be performed if necessary.

this *pseudoarthrosis* treatment *only in exceptional circumstances*, such as for the patient with severe physical or mental disease.

Normal Expectations. If our assessment reveals that the patient has expectations for a normally functioning upper extremity, it then becomes necessary to carefully appraise not only the type of

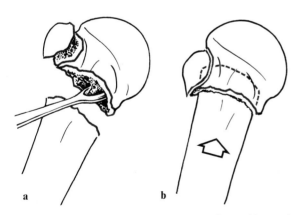

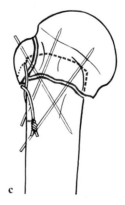

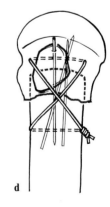

a   b   c   d

Fig. 4.22a–d. Impaction tension band technique of internal fixation. If open reduction is indicated in elderly patients with osteoporosis, the technique will afford good stability. After exposing the fracture, a small portion of soft osteoporotic bone should be curetted from the femoral head and neck (**a**). This will allow impaction of the shaft into the defect so created (**b**). This impaction will restore some stability to the unstable fracture, and the head and shaft can move as a unit. Fixation is achieved with multiple Kirschner wires into the head and shaft, crossing the tuberosities as necessary (**c**). A tension-band wire is then inserted around the Kirschner wires over the inferior portion of the rotator cuff, as shown in **d**

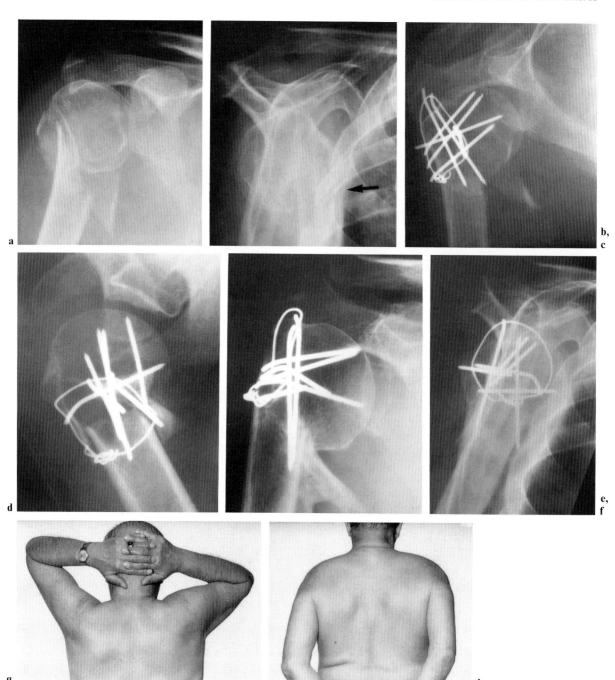

Fig. 4.23a–h. Clinical application of impaction tension band technique. The anteroposterior and lateral radiographs (**a, b**) of this 73-year-old man show the typical moon-shaped head of a three-part unstable fracture of the right proximal humerus. The *arrow* points to the anterior location of the shaft with no contact to the humeral head. The fracture was exposed through a deltopectoral approach. A small amount of bone was curetted and the shaft was impacted and fixed with multiple Kirschner wires and a tension band wire as seen on the postoperative radiographs (**c, d**). At 8 months the radiographs show sound union (**e, f**), and the clinical photographs (**g, h**) show excellent function

If the pre- or intraoperative assessment indicates the presence of *bone so poor* that the holding power of screws would be negligible, other measures must be taken to achieve stability. The surgeon must first determine whether the proximal fragment is viable or not viable. In two- and three-part fractures the head is usually viable, unless the soft tissue is indiscriminately removed by the surgeon. A small crescentic head segment in the four-part fracture is almost always avascular.

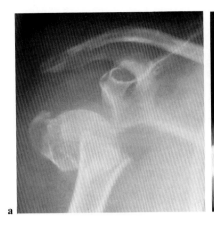
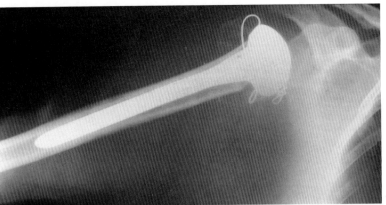

a   b

If the *head fragment is viable*, i.e., if the proximal segment is vascular as in the two- and three-part fractures, but the bone is so poor that it is unlikely that a screw will hold, other options are available. Because the viability of the proximal fragment is not in question, it should *always be retained* and the use of a prosthesis should not be considered. The other options are:

1. *Impaction tension band technique* — By curettage of some cancellous bone from the proximal fragment and impaction of the shaft into that area, stability may be restored to the fracture (Fig. 4.22a, b). Multiple Kirschner wires through the fracture fragments surrounded by a tension band wire will maintain this stable situation (Fig. 4.22c, d; H. Rosen, personal communication). Screws are not used; fixation is dependent upon the multiple Kirschner and tension band wires (Fig. 4.23).
2. *Cement composite fixation* – A second alternative is to use cement in the intramedullary portion of the fracture to improve its stability, or in the predrilled screw holes to improve the holding power of the screws.

If the surgeon has begun a traditional type of open reduction and finds that the screws are not holding in the metaphysis, nuts may be affixed to the cortical screws to increase their holding power. However, in the upper humerus, the major problem is usually poor fixation of the screws in the proximal fragment, for which this technique is obviously unsuitable. The above two alternatives are more suitable for that particular problem.

If the *head is nonviable* — as in a four-part fracture — i.e., if the crescentic fragment is totally avascular and the bone is poor, a unipolar prosthetic replacement should be inserted primarily, great care being taken to restore the function of

Fig. 4.24a, b. Four-part-fracture; treatment by unipolar prosthesis. **a** Anteroposterior radiograph indicating an unstable four-part proximal humerus fracture. A small crescentic head is nonviable. It was replaced with a unipolar Neer-type prosthesis (**b**). Note the rotator cuff reposition with a wire suture

the rotator cuff by carefully reattaching the rotator cuff or the avulsed tuberosities (Fig. 4.24).

4.4.3 Surgical Technique

4.4.3.1 Timing

Since this is an articular or periarticular injury, we prefer to operate immediately, once the decision has been made that surgery is necessary. This will, of course, depend upon the state of the soft tissues and the precise time that the patient is seen following the accident. Surgery should *never* be performed through compromised soft tissues. However, delayed surgery, especially between the 3rd and 7th day after injury, may result in excessive heterotopic ossification and should be avoided if at all possible.

4.4.3.2 Approaches

In most cases, the standard anterior deltopectoral approach will suffice (Henry 1927). Since it is extensile, the incision may be continued distally to expose the entire humeral shaft on its anterolateral surface. The *posterior approach* may be used for irreducible posterior fracture-dislocations but is not indicated for other reconstructive procedures in the area of the shoulder.

a) Incision

The anterior incision should be made along the medial border of the deltoid muscle extending lat-

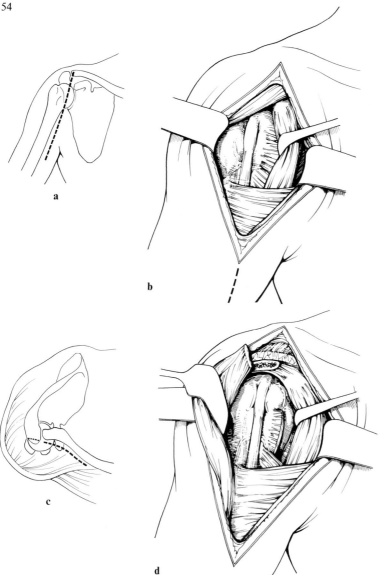

Fig. 4.25 a–d. Anterior approach to the proximal humerus. **a** Anterior incision. **b** Deep dissection in the deltopectoral triangle. Note position of the long head of the biceps muscle. **c** Line of resection of deltoid from clavicle (*heavy dotted line*) and level of acromion osteotomy (*small dotted line*). **d** Increased exposure of the proximal humerus by acromion osteotomy

erally to the humeral shaft (Fig. 4.25 a). The delto-pectoral triangle is identified and the cephalic vein protected. Proximal exposure will depend upon the fracture configuration. If the surgical neck is fractured without extension into the tuberosities, very little deltoid reflection is necessary (Fig. 4.25 b), whereas if greater access to the proximal humerus is required, a more radical removal of the deltoid will be necessary.

The deltoid muscle should be removed from the clavicle by raising an osteoperiosteal flap later-

ally to the acromion. In the three- and four-part configurations, an osteotomy of the acromion, which can be readily reattached with internal fixation, will allow wide access to the proximal humerus (Fig. 4.26 c, d). In our opinion, the advantage gained by this increased exposure far outweighs the potential disadvantage of the deltoid removal and its possible avulsion in the postoperative period. It will also allow the surgeon to work with relative ease on the proximal fragment, so that the vascular soft tissue attachments to that fragment are not further damaged.

b) Reduction

Once easy access has been obtained by reflecting the deltoid, with or without a portion of the acromion, the fracture must be exposed through the disrupted soft tissues. *No* incisions should be made

Fig. 4.26a–c. Atraumatic dissection. **a** Three-part fracture of the proximal humerus. **b** Head fragment being reduced into its normal position with a periosteal elevator. The surgeon's finger is also an excellent reduction tool, and may be more atraumatic. **c** Reduction is complete. Note that the capsular attachment to the proximal fragment has not been interfered with

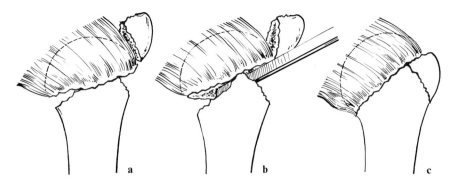

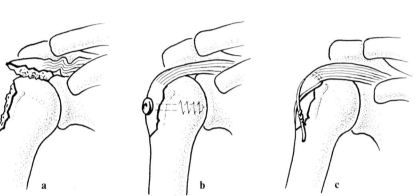

Fig. 4.27. **a** Avulsion fracture of the greater tuberosity with subacromial impingement. Reduction and internal fixation with either cancellous screws (**b**) or a tension band wire (**c**). (From Müller et al. 1979)

through intact soft tissues. No soft tissue should be removed from any of the bony fragments, and only minimal dissection should be performed along the fracture itself. Reduction of the head fragment should be performed atraumatically, especially if the fragment is small (Fig. 4.26). The lesser tuberosity will be found attached to the subscapularis and the rotator cuff to the greater tuberosity. Often, the two are combined as a single fragment, with the long head of the biceps tendon running through it (see Fig. 4.12a).

If the head fragment in the four-part fracture or fracture-dislocation is completely devoid of soft tissue, avascularity, of necessity, must be present; therefore, a decision must be made to retain or discard this avascular humeral head, depending upon the physiological age of the patient.

4.4.3.3 Methods of Internal Fixation

a) Good Bone

If the bone is of normal consistency and will hold a screw, the surgeon may proceed with standard techniques of internal fixation, using lag screws and plates where required.

Tuberosity Fractures. Fractures of the tuberosities are true avulsion fractures; therefore, they require

dynamic compression techniques for stabilization, either by tension band wiring or — in complex fractures — by incorporation of the tuberosity fracture in a tension band plate fixation. Occasionally, cancellous lag screws with washers may be used to achieve stable fixation (Fig. 4.27).

Humeral Neck Fractures. The *choice of implant* will depend upon the fracture pattern. The implants available for the upper humerus are the T plate, the L plate, standard 4.5-mm dynamic compression (DC) plates, the 6.5-mm cancellous screws, both lag and fully threaded, and 4.5-mm cortical screws. In the two-part surgical neck fractures a standard, laterally placed DC plate may be used if there is ample room for two screws proximal to the fracture (Fig. 4.28; see also Fig. 4.6). In the three-part fracture, the DC plate may be supplemented by a tension-band wire, fixing the tuberosity fragments. Two 6.5-mm cancellous screws inserted well into the subchondral area must be used to fix the proximal portion of the plate. These screws should be *fully threaded* to increase their holding power. The use of the DC plate will obviate the need for a T plate placed across the long head of biceps.

If the obliquity of the surgical neck fracture allows, a lag screw should be placed through the

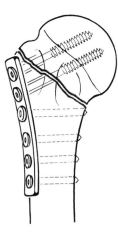

Fig. 4.28. Oblique fracture of the surgical neck fixed with a six-hole DC plate. The two proximal screws are cancellous lag screws compressing the fracture

Fig. 4.29. a Reduction and fixation of a fracture with a T plate. **b** Clinical example of a three-part fracture treated with an interfragmental screw and a long T plate (**c**). (**a** From Müller et al. 1979)

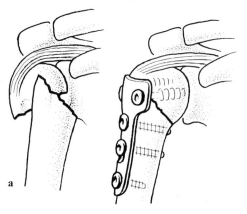

plate across the fracture line. This will greatly enhance the stability of the system (see Fig. 4.6).

In the three- and four-part fracture types, the T or L plates are the implants of choice (Fig. 4.29). If the T plate is chosen, the anterior limb of the T usually crosses the long head of biceps. This can be prevented by the use of the L plate, which allows fixation of the proximal fragment with two large cancellous screws into the proximal fragment and cortical screws into the shaft. The greater tuberosity should be incorporated into the fixation device or, alternatively, may be fixed with tension band wiring.

Either the DC, the T, or the L plate may be applied as a neutralization, buttress, or tension band plate.

The various *fracture types* require different techniques:

1. Transverse or Short Oblique

Surgical Neck — Since these unstable fractures occur in cancellous bone as a result of shearing forces, ideally, the major fragments should be compressed. Transverse or short oblique fractures of the surgical neck are suitable for compression techniques using plates with lag screws across the fracture where possible (Fig. 4.28).

Anatomical Neck — Oblique fractures through the anatomical neck may be compressed by using large cancellous lag screws alone with washers or through a plate (Fig. 4.30).

2. Comminuted or Spiral Fractures

Grossly comminuted or spiral fractures require provisional fixation with Kirschner wires sup-

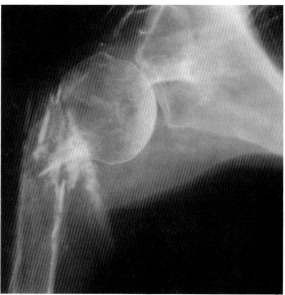

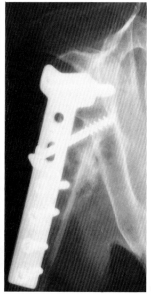

Fig. 4.30a–d. Fixation of anatomical neck fractures. **a** Anatomical neck fractures may be fixed with two screws using washers or through a plate used as a washer. These screws must be lag screws, as depicted. In osteoporotic bone, these screws may not hold and may pull out of the distal fixation. **b** Anteroposterior radiograph of a four-part fracture of the proximal humerus in a 74-year-old woman. The fixation failed, as shown by the radiographs (**c, d**) taken 4 months later. The patient's end result was poor

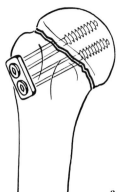

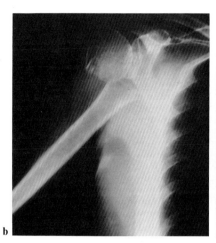

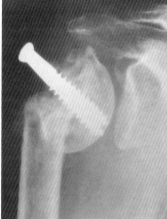

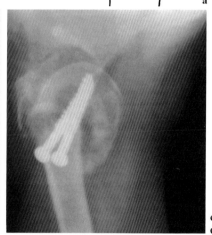

b

c,
d

planted by permanent interfragmental screws. If the fragments are so small that a screw cannot be used, the Kirschner wire should remain as part of the definitive fixation. The fracture must now be stabilized by a neutralization or buttress plate, care being taken to incorporate the avulsed tuberosities, if present, into the system.

3. Articular Fractures

Displaced fractures of the articular surface of the *humeral head* (Fig. 4.18a) should be managed by open anatomical reduction and stable fixation (Fig. 4.18b–e). If the fracture has been impacted, elevation of the fragments will create a gap which must be filled with cancellous bone. Fixation of the joint fragments may be done with lag screws, or occasionally, if they are small, with Kirschner wires. Small avascular fragments should be discarded, as they will usually displace into the joint during rehabilitation and act as loose bodies in the shoulder.

A large anterior or posterior *glenoid rim fracture* affecting joint stability *must* be internally fixed. If the fragment is large enough, it is best fixed with one or two 4.0-mm cancellous lag screws. Occasionally, if the fragment is small, it may be fixed with a staple or with Kirschner wires. Care must be taken that the metal does not penetrate the articular surface — direct visualization of the joint surface is the best way to avoid this complication (Fig. 4.19).

In cases of complex two-, three-, and four-part fracture-dislocations, this glenoid rim fracture should be fixed last, after reconstruction of the other injuries.

b) Poor Bone

Viable Head. Cement Augmentation. Most surgeons develop a rather uneasy feeling during surgery if the cancellous screws in the proximal fragment just keep turning and turning and turning! If only one screw is not holding but the remainder of the fixation is good, then that screw should be removed, low-viscosity cement injected into the

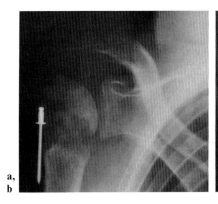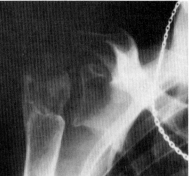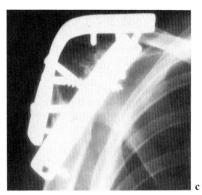

a,
b   c

Fig. 4.31. a Avascular necrosis of a small crescentic head fragment following fracture-dislocation. Seven months later, the fracture has healed but the humeral head has collapsed (**b**). Management of this 22-year-old man was by arthrodesis (**c**)

screw hole, and the screw replaced. This composite type of fixation may reverse a difficult situation. If the entire purchase on the proximal fragment is poor, then low-viscosity cement should be injected into the fracture site as well as into the proximal screw holes to ensure adequate fixation. We have also used this method in other situations where excessive movement may be expected in the postoperative period, for example, in patients with severe tremor due to parkinsonism. On the rare occasion where the proximal fixation is good but the distal fixation poor, nuts may be used on the cortical screws to enhance their fixation.

Impaction and Tension Band Techniques. If the surgeon recognizes preoperatively that the bone is poor and that screws will not hold, a completely different approach is indicated. Under these circumstances, anatomic reduction is not attempted; stability is restored to the fracture by scooping out a portion of the very soft bone in the proximal fragment with a curet and impacting the humeral shaft into the hole so created (Fig. 4.22a, b). This impaction can be done manually by placing the distal fragment into the hole and striking the elbow until impaction occurs. The shaft and head fragments should then move together as one unit, which can be fixed with Kirschner wires (Fig. 4.22c, d). Fine 1.6-mm or 2-mm Kirschner wires are driven across the main fragments with

a power drill; other fragments of bone are similarly fixed. The tuberosity fragments with the attached rotator cuff can also be provisionally fixed with Kirschner wires. A large tension band wire is then inserted around the Kirschner wires in the tuberosities and inserted in the shaft, thereby imparting further stability to the fracture. Stability depends upon the degree of impaction achieved between the shaft and head fragments and upon the tension band wire. Usually, enough stability is obtained to allow early protected motion without fear of the fixation falling apart (Fig. 4.23a–d). Occasionally, cement may be used at the fracture to ensure maintenance of the reduction and to aid in stability.

Nonviable Head. In a four-part fracture or fracture-dislocation through osteoporotic bone the head fragment is usually free and avascular. Often, the bone is so soft that fixation is impossible. Even if fixation were possible, avascular necrosis would certainly ensue, compromising the final result. Under these circumstances, especially in elderly individuals, we suggest a *unipolar prosthetic replacement* (Fig. 4.24). Precise attention to detail, including the correct retroverted position of the prosthetic head and careful restoration of the tuberosity fragments containing the rotator cuff, will give satisfactory results (Neer 1955). We feel that a four-part fracture or fracture-dislocation in an older patient with a totally avascular crescentic head fragment, devoid of all soft tissue, is the *only* indication for primary prosthetic replacement of the humeral head. In younger patients with a nonviable humeral head shoulder arthrodesis may be indicated (Fig. 4.31). This should rarely be done as a primary procedure, since avascular necrosis of the humeral head may be tolerated by the patient.

4.4.3.4 Wound Closure

The deltoid muscle should be reattached with non-absorbable sutures through the attached osteoperiosteal flaps into the clavicle. If the acromion has been osteotomized, nonabsorbable sutures or wire may be used to reattach it. Occasionally, a screw through a predrilled hole may be inserted. The deltoid muscle will then cover the entire fracture complex and the implant. The skin should be closed primarily over suction drains. If the fracture was open, that portion of the skin previously open should be left so and can be dealt with by closure on the 5th day, if clean granulation has appeared.

4.4.3.5 Postoperative Care

a) Early

The early postoperative care will depend upon the surgeon's assessment of the degree of stability present. In the immediate postoperative period, we prefer to immobilize the patient in abduction, either with the use of pillows or with skin traction. If the stability of the fracture is sound, the patient may be taken out of the abducted position on the 2nd postoperative day and allowed pendulum exercises. Active contractions of the deltoid muscle are encouraged if there is no concern about the deltoid resuture. Young patients with anatomic reduction and rigid fixation will rapidly regain full shoulder motion, often to a surprising degree within the first 2 weeks following surgery. If there is concern about the deltoid suture, an abduction splint is applied, the patient being allowed out of the splint for pendulum exercises only. In these circumstances we do not allow active deltoid contraction against resistance until biological healing of the deltoid muscle insertion has occurred, usually within 4–6 weeks.

If the stability of the fracture is in question, the surgeon must use his or her own judgment as to the best method and timing of the rehabilitation process. Pendulum exercises without resistance can usually be carried out with any stable internal fixation, but if the bone is so poor that the fixation is in jeopardy, the patient should be immobilized in an abduction splint until some sign of bone union is noted, usually by the 6th week.

If a prosthetic replacement has been used, the patient is immobilized in abduction in the immediate postoperative period and the abduction splint is used for 4–6 weeks; pendulum and resisted deltoid exercises are allowed during this period.

b) Late

The patient should be followed up carefully for clinical and radiological signs of implant failure, such as lucency around the screws, loss of plate fixation, or movement at the fracture site. If any of these are noticed, it is far better to immobilize the patient in an abduction splint until union has occurred than to persist with early motion, which may result in total loss of the fixation. Reoperation would be more hazardous, because the already porotic bone would be even worse a few weeks after the injury.

References

Codman EA (1934) The shoulder. Rupture of the supraspinatus tendon and other lesions in or about the subacromial bursa. Todd, Boston

Henry AK (1927) Exposure of the long bones and other surgical methods. Wright, Bristol

McLaughlin HL (1960) Recurrent anterior dislocated shoulder. Morbid anatomy. Am J Surg 99:628–632

Müller ME, Allgöwer M, Willenegger H (1979) Manual of internal fixation, 2nd edn. Springer, Berlin Heidelberg New York

Neer CS (1955) Articular replacement for the humeral head. J Bone Joint Surg 37A:215–228

Neer CS (1970) Displaced proximal humeral fractures. I. Classification and evaluation. J Bone Joint Surg 52A:1077–1089

Nicoll E (1964) Fractures of the tibial shaft. A survey of 105 cases. J Bone Joint Surg (Br) 46B:313–381

5 Fractures of the Humerus

J. SCHATZKER

5.1 Introduction

Most fractures of the humerus can be treated successfully by closed means. They unite rapidly. Minor angular and rotational deformities do not result in loss of function, and shoulder and elbow stiffness does not occur. There are circumstances, however, when an open reduction and internal fixation is indicated.

5.2 Indications for Surgery

5.2.1 Failure to Obtain a Satisfactory Reduction

a) Long Spiral Fractures

If displaced with a gap which does not close when rotational alignment is restored (Fig. 5.1), long spiral fractures are almost impossible to reduce because of muscle interposition. If left in good

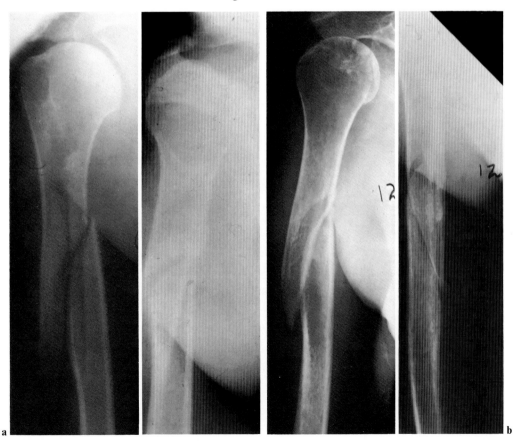

Fig. 5.1. a A long spiral fracture of the humerus. The gap did not close when rotational alignment was restored because of soft tissue interposition. b Complete failure of healing at 3 months

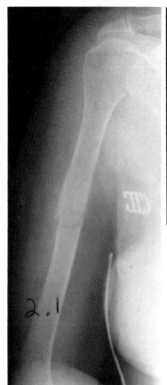

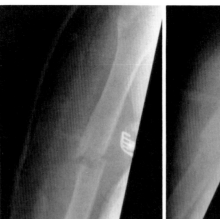

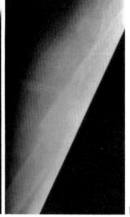

Fig. 5.2. a A transverse fracture of the humerus. Note the slight distraction at the time of the initial X-ray. **b** The same fracture after the application of a sugar tong plaster splint and a sling. The distraction is more marked. **c** The arm was transferred into a cast brace in the hope that active muscle contraction would bring the fracture ends together. The fracture brace could not control the instability of the fracture, and it displaced

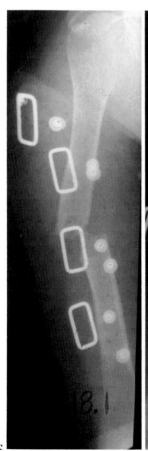

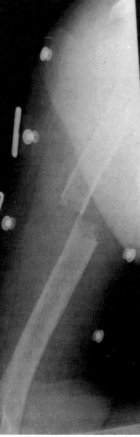

alignment, but with a significant gap between the fracture fragments, these fractures always go on to an atrophic nonunion.

b) Transverse Fractures

Similarly, a transverse fracture which is over-distracted, either as a result of the initial trauma or closed treatment (traction or hanging cast) should be operated upon (Fig. 5.2). Attempts to treat such fractures closed are frustrating to both the patient and the surgeon, first, because the fracture gap cannot be closed by nonoperative means, and second, because alignment is difficult to control. Prolonged immobilization, although frequently employed, is in vain. By the time the clinician finally accepts that nonunion has occurred, some permanent shoulder and elbow stiffness will have become established.

c) Short Oblique Fractures

Short oblique fractures through the distal portion of the shaft just above the olecranon fossa, if displaced, are difficult to reduce and very difficult to maintain in the reduced position. Furthermore, because they are periarticular, prolonged immobilization leads to irreversible elbow stiffness. For

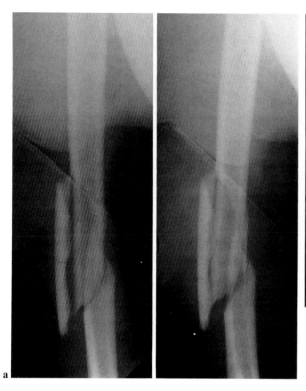
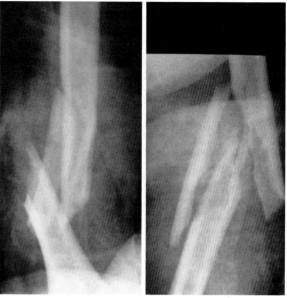

Fig. 5.3. a A comminuted fracture of the humerus in an obese woman with large breasts. Note the initial satisfactory alignment. **b** An attempt to brace the humeral shaft against the bulging breast and chest wall resulted in unacceptable displacement

these reasons, an open reduction and internal fixation is frequently the best form of treatment.

5.2.2 Failure to Maintain Reduction

The "sugar tong" plaster of Paris splint, combined with a Velpeau bandage, is the most effective and most commonly employed method of immobilization of humeral fractures. Very occasionally, we have used a thoracobrachial spica to prevent excessive internal rotation of the fracture. We have found the hanging cast somewhat of an illogical and unsuccessful method. In order for the hanging cast to exert any degree of traction to effect alignment, the patient must remain upright at all times. As soon as the patient lies down, all traction is lost and the cast acts like a lever, causing displacement, since frequently its upper end is at or just above the fracture. Whenever the patient moves while upright, despite the collar and cuff, the cast tends to swing. This not only causes a great deal of pain, but also excessive movement at the fracture. Therefore, we feel that if a fracture cannot be controlled in a sugar tong cast, the hanging long arm cast is not a logical solution.

In the majority of patients, if the arm in the sugar tong cast is bound to the chest wall, the fracture remains reduced, the patient is comfortable, and the fracture unites. However, if a satisfactory position cannot be maintained, then an open reduction and internal fixation is indicated. At times, reduction is lost because of the deformity of the chest wall. This is true in very obese patients and in women with very large breasts (Fig. 5.3). Further manipulative attempts are futile and open reduction and internal fixation should be carried out.

5.2.3 Injuries to the Chest Wall

Patients with coexistent injuries to the chest wall (e.g., rib fractures, flail chest, sucking wound) cannot have the arm bound to the chest wall because it would interfere with ventilation and with care of the chest wall injury.

5.2.4 Bilateral Humeral Fractures

In patients with bilateral fractures, at least one humerus should be stabilized to facilitate self-care. Otherwise, the immobilization results in total disability.

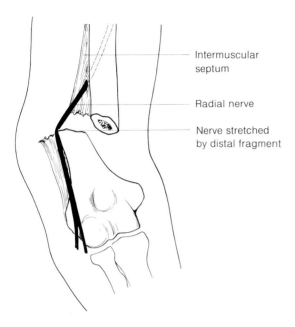

Intermuscular
septum

Radial nerve

Nerve stretched
by distal fragment

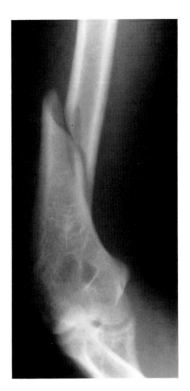

Fig. 5.4. Fracture of the humerus at the junction of the mid and distal thirds (Holstein fracture). Note the lateral displacement of the shaft and the tethering of the nerve by the intermuscular septum

5.2.5 Multiple Injuries

Occasionally, in patients with multiple injuries, open reduction and internal fixation of the humerus is required to facilitate the care and rehabilitation of the patient.

5.2.6 Vascular Lesions

In fractures associated with vascular lesions, the fracture should be stabilized before the vascular repair is executed.

5.2.7 Neurologic Lesions

Fractures of the humeral shaft are at times associated with injury to the radial nerve. The management of the fracture associated with a radial nerve lesion continues to be a controversial issue, with some favoring a delay to see if the radial nerve will recover, and others favoring a policy of immediate exploration, reduction, stabilization of the fracture, and primary nerve repair if the nerve is torn.

The radial nerve is commonly at risk if the fracture is at the junction of the mid and distal thirds of the humeral shaft and particularly if the fracture is associated with lateral displacement of the distal fragment (Fig. 5.4). At this point, the radial nerve emerges from the spiral groove and is tethered as it pierces the intermuscular septum. It cannot yield to the lateral displacement of the distal fragment and is therefore frequently seriously damaged. We feel, therefore, that in the presence of this fracture pattern, immediate exploration is indicated.

If radial nerve function disappears as a fracture is manipulated and reduced, it means that the nerve is caught in the fracture. Spontaneous recovery will not occur if the nerve is not freed and, if one delays the exploration of the nerve, the nerve becomes even more enveloped in the callus of fracture repair. This makes its ultimate exploration very difficult. Therefore, we feel immediate exploration with freeing of the nerve and surgical repair of the fracture is indicated in all instances where radial nerve function is lost as a consequence of closed reduction. In all other closed fractures of the humerus associated with radial nerve lesions, if there are no other indications for surgery, we feel that an observation period of 3 weeks is justifiable. At the end of this time, virtually all neurapraxias will have recovered. Patients with persistent nerve deficit should be explored. If the nerve is in continuity, the lesion is an axonotmesis. Open reduction and internal fixation of the humerus will

Fig. 5.5. a Association of a midshaft fracture of the humerus with a fracture of the olecranon. **b** Internal fixation of both fractures

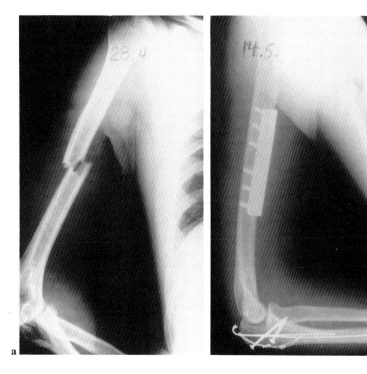

a   b

not hasten neurologic recovery, but the stability of the humerus will hasten functional recovery of the extremity and no harm will have been done. If the lesion is a neurotmesis, a diagnosis which can only be established by early exploration or by the failure of recovery in a suitable period of time, then, if definitive treatment of the nerve has been delayed for 3 months or more, one is faced with the prospect of late nerve reconstruction. This means either a free nerve graft or a shortening osteotomy of the humerus to facilitate an end-to-end suture of the retracted or shortened nerve. Because of the magnitude of this late nerve reconstruction, some surgeons have suggested abandoning the nerve repair in favor of multiple tendon transfer. Instead of condemning the patient to such major reconstructive efforts, we feel it is justifiable to explore a nerve if, at the end of 3–4 weeks, recovery has failed to occur. If the nerve is torn, a primary nerve repair should be carried out after the humerus is reduced and fixed.

5.2.8 Fractures of the Shaft Associated with Intra-articular Fractures

The successful outcome of all intra-articular fractures depends on the anatomic reduction and stable fixation of the fragments, and early motion. Therefore, if a fracture of the humerus either extends into a neighboring joint or is associated with a separate intra-articular fracture of the shoulder or the elbow (Fig. 5.5), then both the shaft and the intra-articular fracture are best managed by an open reduction and internal fixation. This will ensure that the outcome of the intra-articular fracture is not prejudiced by the desire to treat the shaft fracture nonoperatively. There is no adequate method of splinting the shaft and permitting full mobilization of the shoulder and elbow. If the joint were to be kept immobilized after an open reduction and internal fixation, then serious stiffness of the joint would be certain.

5.2.9 Open Fractures of the Humerus

All open fractures, after thorough débridement, require skeletal stability (see Chap. 3).

5.3 Surgical Approaches

We feel that the best approach to the proximal third of the shaft is the standard deltopectoral approach. The more proximal the fracture, the more likely the necessity of detaching the anterior third of the deltoid muscle from the clavicle. In doing this, it is important to preserve both the superficial and deep fascia which invests the deltoid muscle. We no longer leave a cuff of muscle attached to the clavicle to effect a closure because we have found the following method to be more effective. We pass our sutures carefully through both the deep and superficial fascia of the deltoid and then through the fascia of the trapezius muscle at its insertion into the clavicle. As the sutures are tied, the deltoid is drawn snugly up to and over the edge of the clavicle, effecting a strong muscle closure.

In order to protect the resutured portion of the deltoid from avulsion during early mobilization, we insist on passive elevation and abduction for the first 4 weeks. With this regimen, we have not had a single deltoid avulsion. As we extend the incision distally, we approach the insertion of the deltoid. At this point it is important to identify the origin of the brachialis muscle, which blends here with the insertion of the deltoid, because the radial nerve lies a fingerbreadth below and behind the deltoid insertion as it comes forward around the humerus. This is invariably an area where brisk bleeding is encountered as the planes are developed, and the surgeon should be ready to coagulate the bleeding vessels. Further exposure distally is gained by splitting the brachialis muscle down its middle. The lateral half of the muscle is used to protect the radial nerve. By splitting the brachialis, exposure can be extended as far as the elbow joint.

For this part of the approach, we like to have the patient positioned supine with a folded sheet under the scapula to lift the shoulder off the table. This facilitates cleansing of the skin posteriorly and subsequent draping of the shoulder to leave the arm free and fully exposed. The arm is positioned at the patient's side and is supported on an arm board.

It is best to approach the distal third of the humerus posteriorly. For this exposure, the patient is positioned lying on the uninjured side. After draping, which should leave the shoulder and elbow fully exposed, the arm is supported on a rolled sheet and the elbow is flexed. It is extremely advantageous to support the humerus while it is being exposed because it frees an assistant and makes the handling of the fracture fragments much simpler. The triceps aponeurosis is split down the middle or is reflected down as a tongue. The deep head of the triceps is then split in line with its fibers. Care must be taken with the radial nerve in the proximal portion of the incision where it runs within the muscle.

5.4 Surgical Methods of Stable Fixation

5.4.1 Biomechanical Considerations

The cortex of the humerus splinters very easily. Therefore, even long spiral fractures must be protected after lag screw fixation with a neutralization plate, and one must never rely on screw fixation alone. Furthermore, to prevent longitudinal fissuring whenever the humerus is plated, one should use the broad plate. The screw holes in these broad plates are staggered. This increases the distance between successive screws and decreases the likelihood of fissuring the bone longitudinally.

In patients with a normal elbow the posterior cortex is under tension (Müller et al. 1970). If the patient has a stiff elbow, the anterior cortex becomes the one under tension (Weber and Čech 1976). This would mean that in patients with a mobile elbow, the "compression" or tension band plates should be applied posteriorly, and in patients with a stiff elbow, anteriorly.

Because the radial nerve lies in the spiral groove posteriorly, the posterior surgical approach to the mid-diaphysis is more difficult and the radial nerve is at great risk of injury. For this reason, we prefer Henry's anterior approach to the upper and mid-diaphysis (Henry 1959) and apply the plates most commonly to the anterolateral surface of the bone. Because the humerus is not a weight-bearing bone and is not subjected to forces as great as those acting on the femur or the tibia, this biomechanical infringement has not resulted in any failures of fixation.

Fractures of the distal third should be plated posteriorly. There are four reasons for this. The humerus is flat posteriorly and it is easier to apply the broad plate to that surface. It is much easier to insert the most distal screws from the posterior approach because one is not close to the cubital fossa with all its converging soft tissue structures, which create a very tight envelope and make anterolateral or anterior screw insertion difficult and hazardous. If applied posteriorly, the plate can also reach further distally without compromising elbow flexion. Furthermore, a distal diaphyseal fracture of the humerus lends itself at times to stabilization with two semitubular plates (Fig. 5.6) or two 3.5-mm DC plates. This greatly increases the stability of fixation in this difficult transition zone of the humeral shaft.

When exposing the distal third of the humerus posteriorly, the surgeon must remember that the radial nerve will be close to the upper end of the

Fig. 5.6. a A single plate failed to provide adequate stability and the fracture went on to nonunion. **b** In the metaphysis, we can use two plates without running the risk of stress shielding. Thus, two shorter and thinner plates (semitubular) applied to the rounded posteromedial and posterolateral edge have provided significant stability

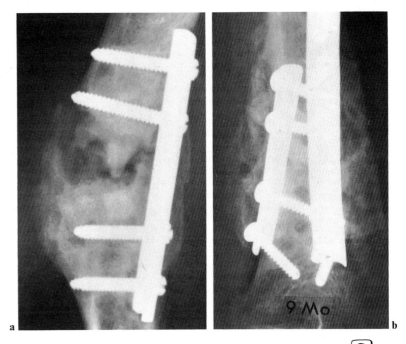

exposure. It may have to be isolated and protected. If the exposure approaches the elbow, then the ulnar nerve has to be isolated and protected as it passes behind the medial epicondyle.

With the exception of the supracondylar area, where the small fragment 3.5-mm cortex screws, 4.0-mm cancellous screws, and the corresponding plates find their application, the 4.5-mm large fragment screws and the corresponding plates should be used for fixation of the humeral shaft. As already emphasized, the broad plates should be used on the diaphysis to prevent longitudinal fissuring of the bone. One might make an exception in an extremely small individual with very slender bone and use the narrow 4.5-mm DC plate. The 3.5-mm DC plates should be used only in the supracondylar area (Fig. 5.7). In the proximal portion of the shaft, where the bone flares to meet the metaphysis, the cortex is very thin and very difficult to tap. If one inadvertently allows the tap to wander, it can easily miss the hole in the far cortex and then either strip the thread in the near cortex or break out a segment of bone from the opposite cortex. One must exercise great care to prevent this complication.

As already emphasized, even in long oblique or spiral fractures, lag screws must not be used alone to secure internal fixation (Fig. 5.8). The lag screw is the most efficient means of securing interfragmental compression, and as such it is the principal means of securing a stable fracture interface and structural continuity of fragments. However,

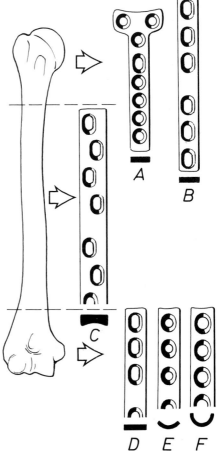

Fig. 5.7. The different plates and their place on the humerus: *A* T plate; *B* narrow 4.5-mm DC plate; *C* broad 4.5-mm DC plate; *D* 3.5-mm DC plate; *E* 1/one-third tubular plate (3.5-mm screws); *F* semitubular plate (4.5-mm screws)

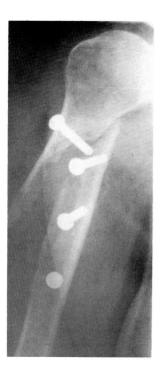

Fig. 5.8. Even in a long spiral fracture, lag screws alone cannot provide adequate stability

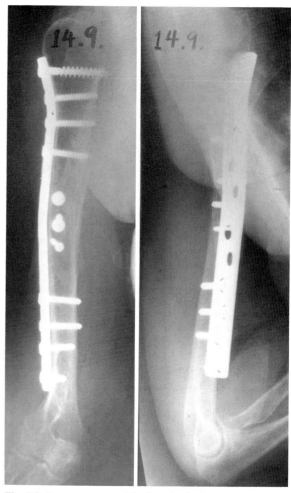

Fig. 5.9. Lag screws provide the principal means of achieving interfragmental compression and, in this way, structural continuity. The neutralization plate protects the stability achieved by means of lag screws

mechanically, such fixation is not sufficiently strong to withstand the forces of bending shear and torque. Therefore, the lag screw fixation must be protected with a neutralization plate (Fig. 5.9).

Transverse or short oblique fractures are stabilized by means of axial compression. The stability of the fixation is greatly enhanced if a lag screw is passed through the plate and across the fractures. If technically, because of the configuration of the fracture, the lag screw cannot be passed through the plate, it should still be inserted across the fracture to improve the stability of the fixation (Fig. 5.10). In the distal third of the humerus, there is only a small portion of the brachialis muscle which separates the radial nerve from the plate applied to the anterolateral surface of the bone. In some patients, the nerve has been left in direct contact with the plate. We have not observed any damage to the nerve, either early or late, as a result of this. The relationship of the nerve to the plate and, in particular, where it crosses the plate in relationship to the screw holes, should be carefully recorded in the operative note. This will protect the nerve from damage at the time of plate removal if this becomes necessary.

For stable fixation of the humerus, one must have screw purchase in the cortex in six places on each side of the fracture. This means that the shortest plate one can safely use on the humerus is a six- to seven-hole plate. With osteoporosis, one must increase the number of screws on each

side of the fracture and use a longer plate. The fixation on each side of the fracture must be equally strong. Therefore, as one approaches the metaphysis, either two plates are used or else specially shaped buttress plates which permit the insertion of a greater number of screws through a shorter segment of the plate.

Intramedullary splintage, either with a nail or Rush rods, has virtually no place in the treatment of acute humeral fractures. Not only can the nail or Rush rod or the Küntscher nail easily lead to damage and stiffness of the shoulder joint because of interference with the rotator cuff, but they also fail to provide sufficient stability. We have used Hackethal retrograde stacked pinning for undisplaced pathologic fractures of the mid-diaphysis (Fig. 5.11). Because the point of entry is distal above the olecranon fossa, no problems arose with

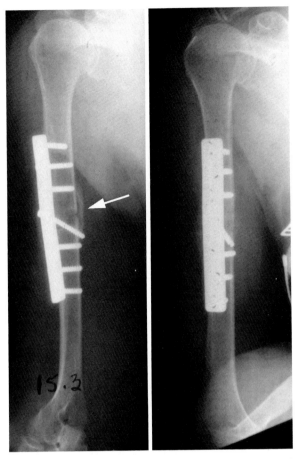

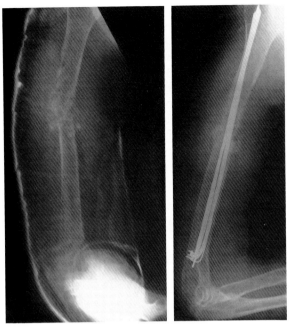

Fig. 5.11. Hackethal stacked intramedullary pinning of the humerus

Fig. 5.10. Lag screw used to increase the stability achieved by means of a tension band plate

shoulder stiffness and, with early mobilization, we have avoided triceps adhesions and elbow stiffness. Three or four precontoured 3-mm Steinmann pins are stacked to fill the medullary canal. Because they flare out in the proximal metaphysis, they provide sufficient rotational stability to allow movement. The fixation they provide in bending is elastic and similar in principle to Ender's nailing of the femur. Intramedullary fixation is also preferable if there are multiple metastatic deposits scattered throughout the shaft.

In displaced pathologic fractures, we have found the so-called composite type of fixation of methyl methacrylate and plating to be most reliable (Fig. 5.12). The fracture is reduced before any attempt is made to evacuate the tumor mass. A plate is then contoured, applied to the anterolateral surface of the bone, and fixed with one or two screws proximally and distally. In pathologic fractures, because of the frequent destruction of cortex and osteoporosis, one must use longer plates than in nonpathologic fractures. One must

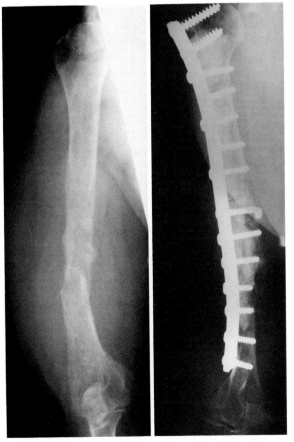

Fig. 5.12. Composite fixation (plate and methyl methacrylate cement) of a pathologic fracture of the humerus

also exercise care that the plate does not stop at or near a metastatic deposit. Once the bone is provisionally stabilized, a window is cut to permit the introduction of a curette and methyl methacrylate. This window should bridge both fragments and encompass at least three or four screw holes on each side of the metastatic deposit, but it should not extend to the end of the plate. Once the window is cut, all of the tumor is evacuated with curettage and suction. The screw holes are than predrilled, measured, tapped, and the screws prepared in the order of insertion. Methyl methacrylate bone cement is then mixed and, while in the early doughy stage, rapidly pushed into the prepared trough and defect. Before the cement sets, the screws are rapidly screwed in and finally snugged up once the methyl methacrylate has polymerized.

5.5 Postoperative Regimen

Following surgery, it is best to immobilize the arm on a posterior plaster splint with the elbow in almost full extension and suspend it for 24–48 h from an intravenous drip pole to minimize postoperative edema. The patient is allowed up for meals and to the toilet. Suction drains are removed in 24–36 h, depending on the amount of drainage. The wound is inspected daily. If healing is progressing satisfactorily without any complicating features such as hematoma or sepsis, active mobilization is started on the 2nd or 3rd postoperative day.

If the fixation is stable, apart from minor wound discomfort, mobilization is painless. The cooperative patient will carry out active mobilization exercises as instructed and will not require a formal program of rehabilitation. The anxious or less well motivated individual requires supervision, but strict instructions must be issued to the physiotherapist not to carry out joint manipulations or resisted exercises lest the fixation be lost from mechanical overload.

The surgeon is the only individual able to judge accurately the stability of any fixation because only the surgeon knows how well each screw held as it was tightened in bone. If the fixation be judged unstable, then of course this program of early mobilization has to be modified and the extremity protected.

In cases of early failure of the fixation, either in the early postoperative period or during the phase of fracture healing, a surgical revision of the fixation should be undertaken if it is technically feasible. It is important to recognize modes of failure.

Early failure, the result of mechanical overload, either because of inadequate primary fixation or because of the patient overloading the fixation, should be revised surgically to a stable internal fixation.

If failure of fixation is recognized at, say, 6 weeks or later, it is important to differentiate instability in the presence of an irritation callus from instability without an irritation callus, which displays a widening fracture gap, halo around the screws, periosteal reaction at the plate ends, and resorption of cortex deep to the plate. In the former, with an evident irritation callus, protection of the extremity from load by immobilizing it in a cast will usually result in the irritation callus changing to a fixation callus with healing of the fracture. In the latter, with evidence of failure but no callus, further immobilization and protection are of no avail. Surgical revision must be executed. Stable fixation has to be achieved by revising the existing internal fixation. Usually it is also necessary to bone graft to promote union.

Fractures of the humerus are usually solidly united in 3 months. If union should be delayed but the fixation remain stable, unlike in the lower weight-bearing extremity, where failure of the plate would be almost certain, in the upper extremity we can afford to wait for consolidation to occur. Clearly the patient would be completely symptom-free and the only clue to the delayed union would be radiologic.

5.6 Removal of Internal Fixation

Plates should be removed only if they give rise to symptoms. In removing plates from the humerus, one must always remember the proximity of the radial nerve to the plate and the danger of leaving the patient with a radial nerve palsy. Following plate removal, the patient should abstain from heavy lifting for a period of 6–8 weeks.

References

Henry K (1959) Extensile exposure. Livingstone, Edinburgh, p 25
Müller ME, Allgöwer M, Willenegger H (1970) Manual of internal fixation, 1st edn. Springer, Berlin Heidelberg New York, p 121
Weber BG, Čech O (1976) Pseudoarthrosis. Huber, Bern, p 109

6 Fractures of the Distal End of the Humerus

J. Schatzker

6.1 Introduction

Fractures of the distal end of the humerus fall into two categories: the simple epicondylar and condylar fractures, and the difficult supracondylar fractures. The former, although sometimes part of a more complex injury, such as dislocation of the elbow, are relatively easy to treat and usually have a good prognosis. They will be discussed first. We will then in the remaining part of the chapter discuss supracondylar fractures, which continue to be a difficult and controversial problem. Although we will indicate, for the benefit of those who wish to refer to the *Manual of Internal Fixation* (Müller et al. 1979), the designation of each fracture in accordance with the AO classification (Fig. 6.1), we are not entirely in accord with this classification of fractures about the elbow. We feel that a classification of fractures should group fractures which have similar problems in treatment and a similar prognosis. The fate of fractures about the elbow is determined by the anatomical part involved, by the degree of displacement, and by the degree of comminution. We see little merit in grouping the extra-articular epicondylar fracture (A_1) together with the difficult supracondylar A_2 and A_3 fractures or the grouping of the condylar B_1 or B_2 fracture with the coronal osteochondral fractures B_3 of which a capitellar fracture is a good example. All three are intra-articular, but that is the only feature which B_3 shares with B_1 and $B_2 \cdot B_3$ differs in the mechanism of injury, in the treatment, and in the prognosis. We feel, therefore, that from a prognostic point of view, it is more prudent to classify fractures about the elbow as simple or complex, discussing each type separately, since each has its distinguishing features worthy of mention. Similarly, the supracondylar fractures and those with extension into the joint will be grouped together because they share the mechanism of injury, anatomical features, surgical exposures, methods of internal fixation, and prognosis. The individual differences of this group may be expressed by isolating these fractures into subtypes.

6.2 Simple Fractures

6.2.1 Fractures of the Epicondyles

6.2.1.1 Fractures of the Lateral Epicondyle

An avulsion fracture of the lateral epicondyle is an extremely rare injury in the adult. It may occur as part of a posterolateral or posterior dislocation of the elbow. In the latter case, it is frequently associated with a fracture of the medial epicondyle. In the child where the lateral epicondyle is avulsed with varying portions of the capitellum, it may turn on itself through 180°, turn the fracture surface outward, and go on to nonunion and deformity. This complication is not seen in the adult. When the elbow is reduced, the epicondylar fragment reduces and heals in place, usually by bone, although occasionally by fibrous tissue.

6.2.1.2 Fractures of the Medial Epicondyle (A_1)

This fracture is most common in children, but may be seen in the adult either as a result of a direct injury or as an avulsion. The fragment may vary in size, displacement, and degree of comminution. If small and undisplaced, it does not require surgical treatment. If displaced and caught in the joint, as may occur in the reduction of a lateral dislocation of the elbow, it has to be reduced surgically and fixed in place. This is best done with a small 4.0-mm cancellous screw. If the fragment is comminuted, only suture to the adjacent soft tissues may be possible. Occasionally, the fragment may be quite large and displaced. Whenever displaced or comminuted, it should be openly reduced and stabilized by internal fixation to prevent the onset

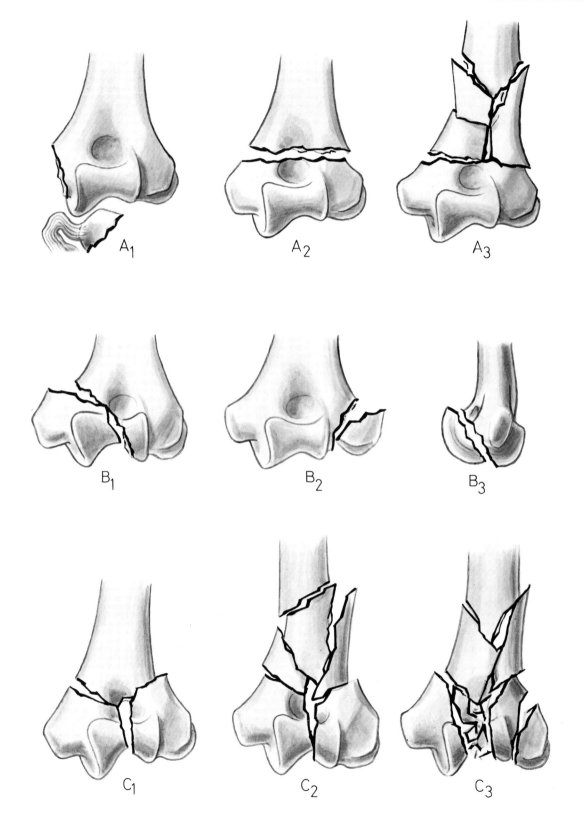

Fig. 6.1. The AO classification of fractures of the distal end
of the humerus. (From Müller et al. 1979, p. 177)

of ulnar palsy. The approach is medial. The ulnar nerve must be identified and protected before the reduction is attempted. Anterior transposition of the nerve may be necessary if the nerve comes to rest on bony irregularities or the internal fixation.

6.2.1.3 Fractures of the Lateral Condyle (B₂)

This fracture is comparable to the fracture of the lateral condyle in children. It is always larger than it appears on X-ray. In our experience, it always extends medially and involves part of the trochlea. It is a major intra-articular fracture and must be accurately reduced and fixed to ensure preservation of normal joint function (Fig. 6.2).

The approach is lateral. We prefer two small 4.0-mm cancellous screws for fixation. We favor internal fixation, even if the initial displacement is minimal, because we feel that early motion is essential to prevent stiffness. If the fracture is not stabilized, early motion could lead to displacement, with dire consequences.

6.2.1.4 Fractures of the Capitellum (B₃)

The capitellum is the smooth, rounded, knob-like portion of the lateral condyle, covered with articular cartilage only on its anterior and inferior surfaces. The head of the radius rotates on its anterior

surface when the elbow is in flexion and on its inferior surface when the elbow is in extension.

We have seen fractures of the capitellum more commonly as part of comminuted supracondylar fractures than as isolated injuries. As an isolated injury, the fracture occurs as a result of the head of the radius being forcibly driven against the capitellum with the elbow in some degree of flexion, or from a direct blow to the elbow when it is fully flexed (Alvarez et al. 1975). When fractured, the capitellum becomes a free intra-articular osteochondral body and is always displaced anterosuperiorly into the radial fossa. We feel that this fracture requires special mention because closed manipulation always fails (Keon-Cohen 1966; Alvarez et al. 1975) and because attempts at internal fixation of the isolated fragment have given poor results. The recommended treatment of an isolated fracture of the capitellum is excision of the fragment (Alvarez et al. 1975).

When we have encountered this fracture as part of a supracondylar fracture, we have visualized it in every instance through a posterior approach combined with an osteotomy of the olecranon. Reduction is difficult to maintain because the fragment tends to slide upward out of view. It has to be held in place with a small hook while it is provisionally fixed with a small Kirschner wire (Fig. 6.3). Definitive fixation is then executed with small 4.0-mm cancellous screws introduced from back to front. The fixation is always difficult because the fragment is small and is subjected to considerable shearing forces which tend to displace it. In isolated fractures of the capitellum if the fragment is small, it should be excised. If it is suffi-

Fig. 6.2a, b. Fracture of the lateral condyle extending medially to involve the trochlea. Secure fixation is accomplished with two lag screws

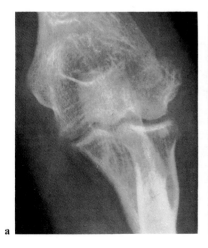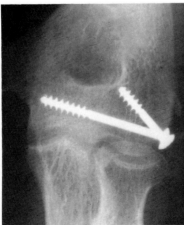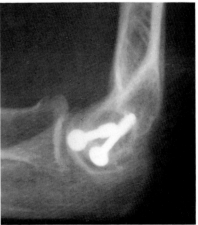

a   b

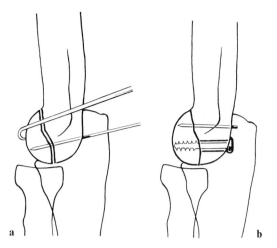

Fig. 6.3a, b. Steps in the open reduction and internal fixation of a fracture of the capitellum

ciently large to allow for stable fixation as described previously, then we prefer to fix it. The exposure is lateral with the fixation from the posterior aspect.

6.3 Complex Fractures

6.3.1 Supracondylar Fractures

6.3.1.1 Natural History

Stiffness and pain of the elbow are the results of failure of treatment. Varus or valgus deformity, frequently seen following improperly treated supracondylar fractures in children, is not as significant a problem in the adult as is stiffness, although these deformities are not uncommon.

In order to prevent stiffness, all periarticular and intra-articular fractures require early active motion. Prolonged plaster immobilization leads to irreversible joint stiffness. Traction, although it affords some degree of immobilization and pain relief, and although it permits early active motion, does so only within a limited arc of movement. Furthermore, although traction may improve the position of displaced intra-articular fragments, it almost never leads to the accurate joint reduction required for the return of normal function.

Early attempts at open reduction and internal fixation relied on screws, Kirschner wires, and occasionally on plates for stability (Fig. 6.4). Although the radiological appearance of the fracture was frequently improved, the need for postoperative plaster immobilization, which was carried out

for 3–6 weeks or longer, resulted in a considerable degree of elbow stiffness. Internal fixation without the use of compression was not stable. Attempts at early active movement resulted not only in an increased incidence of malunion or nonunion, but also in stiffness. The patients felt severe pain because of instability and were unable to execute the required range of movement.

Passive manipulation of these fractures rarely improved the result and was sometimes disastrous because it led to myositis ossificans which permanently marred the result. Controversy continued and, whereas most surgeons were opposed to any form of surgical intervention (Keon-Cohen 1966; Riseborough and Radin 1969), others championed the operative approach (Bickel and Perry 1963; Miller 1964). The opponents of surgical intervention felt that the results of internal fixation were extremely bad (Keon-Cohen 1966) and that stiffness was the result of surgical dissection, necessary for the exposure of all components of the fracture and insertion of the internal fixation. Inability to achieve a reasonable reduction by manipulation and traction was considered to be the only indication for an open reduction and internal fixation.

The champions of the surgical approach have clearly outlined the disadvantages of closed treatment. Manipulation and traction often fail to restore perfect joint alignment. Thus, the patient not only faces stiffness, but pain from joint incongruity and post-traumatic osteoarthritis. Traction is often required for 4–6 weeks before sufficient stability is gained to permit guarded mobilization. Traction may not be possible: (a) because the patient may not tolerate the imposed supine position because of age or temperament; or (b) because of associated injuries which demand mobilization. Furthermore, traction may have to be discontinued because the anticipated satisfactory reduction is not obtained. Unfortunately, this decision is often reached at an inopportune time for an open reduction. Because of delay, the fragments will have usually become matted together by callus, softened by disuse and hyperemia, and the joint will have become stiff because of the trauma and inactivity.

The advocates of surgical treatment (Bickel and Perry 1963; Miller 1964) have further pointed out the following. In the displaced fracture, an anatomical reduction of the joint can be obtained only by operative means. Furthermore, in the absence of any inherent stability of the bony fragments, the reduction can only be maintained by internal fixation. Open reduction and internal fixation has-

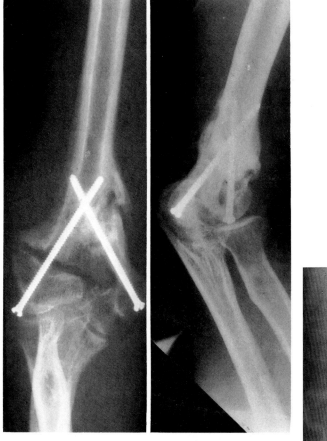

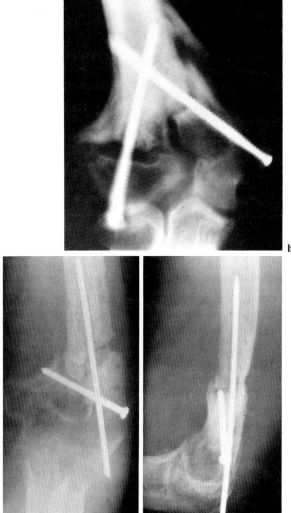

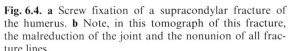

Fig. 6.4. a Screw fixation of a supracondylar fracture of the humerus. **b** Note, in this tomograph of this fracture, the malreduction of the joint and the nonunion of all fracture lines.
c In another patient, the threaded Compere wire failed to provide adequate stability and the supracondylar fracture went on to nonunion

ten ambulation of the patient and active motion of the elbow.

The development by the AO group of stable internal fixation, utilizing compression as the keystone of stability, and the development of new implants and operative techniques have greatly increased the scope of surgery for the supracondylar fracture. Of particular help in the treatment have been the small cortex and cancellous screws, the one-third tubular plates, the small DC plates, and the small reconstruction plates. They have made it possible to achieve the goals of internal fixation, namely, stable fixation and early motion.

6.3.1.2 Factors Influencing Decisions in Treatment

Our own experience strongly supports the view of those who have championed surgery as the method of treatment of this fracture. We are of the opinion that accurate anatomical reconstruction of the joint surfaces, stable internal fixation, and early active motion are the only means available to ensure a patient with this fracture a return of function as close to normal as possible. Surgery, however, is not always possible nor advisable. Surgeons must carefully evaluate all factors before deciding on a course of treatment. Technique must not triumph over reason. We stress repeatedly throughout this book the concept of the "personality of the fracture" as a guide in decision mak-

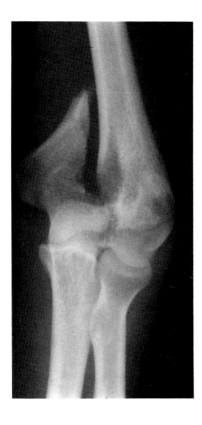

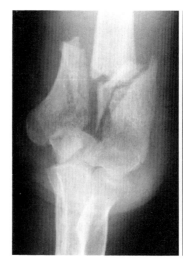
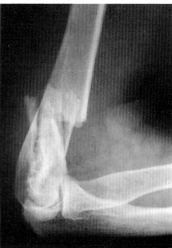

Fig. 6.6. Supracondylar fracture (C_3) in an elderly osteoporotic woman. Note the severe degree of comminution

◄   Fig. 6.5. Supracondylar fracture in a young man (C_1). There is no comminution

ing. This is perhaps nowhere as important as in the evaluation of an intra-articular fracture. The factors which limit success are the degree of comminution, the degree of joint involvement, and osteoporosis.

Age and Osteoporosis

The typical mechanism which leads to the so-called Y or T supracondylar fracture is a fall on the point of the elbow. But how different these injuries are in a young, healthy man (Fig. 6.5) and in an elderly, frail, and osteoporotic woman (Fig. 6.6)! The weakest link in any correctly executed internal fixation is the bone. If the bone is fragile and osteoporotic, the surgeon may have difficulty in securing a satisfactory purchase for any screws. Thus, the first factor to be determined is the patient's age. This will not only shed some light on the expected degree of osteoporosis, but may modify the goals of treatment. Clearly, the goals will be different for a young, athletic man and for a retired octogenarian.

Type of Fracture

The next factor to be determined is the type of fracture. The supracondylar fracture A_2 and A_3

(see Fig. 6.1) may pose difficulties, particularly if the distal fragment is small or if the supracondylar segment is badly comminuted. These difficulties, however, are greatly overshadowed by the difficulties posed by a comminuted articular surface.

Degree of Displacement

An undisplaced fracture may not require surgery. Displacement, particularly of the joint fragments, is clearly an indication for an open reduction. Displacement is also an index of the ease of reduction and the degree of devitalization. Considerable displacement is usually the result of high-velocity force which not only drives the fragments apart in an explosive fashion, but strips them of their soft tissue attachment and blood supply. Devitalization prolongs the healing process. Therefore, such a fracture would be more prone to failure of its internal fixation, yet the displacement makes open reduction almost mandatory.

Degree of Comminution and Joint Involvement

The supracondylar fracture A_2 and A_3 (see Fig. 6.1) may pose difficulties with internal fixation, particularly if the distal fragment is small or if the supracondylar segment is badly commi-

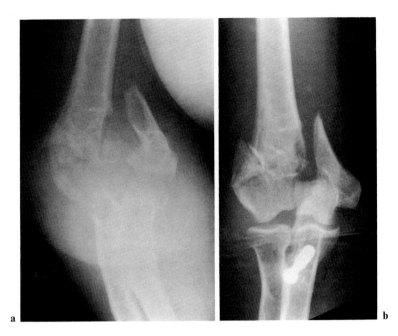

a   b

nuted. These difficulties, however, are greatly overshadowed by the almost insurmountable problems of the severely compressed and comminuted articular surface of a C_3 fracture (Riseborough and Radin 1969).

It is most important to evaluate the degree of joint comminution before embarking on surgery. The displacement of the fragments may be such that it is impossible to interpret the radiograph. In these cases, we have found it very useful to obtain our radiograph while the patient is under anesthesia and traction is applied to the elbow (Fig. 6.7). This may restore sufficient alignment to make an analysis possible.

In our experience, the only major contraindications to surgery have been severe osteoporosis and advanced age. We have found all too frequently at the time of surgery that a radiograph of an osteoporotic humerus with an intra-articular fracture did not give an accurate indication of the degree of comminution, particularly of the joint. The multiplicity of the fragments, their small size, and the poor holding power of the bone have been the chief causes of less than satisfactory results. In younger patients, we have achieved our treatment goals, but we would like to offer a word of caution about the C_3 fracture. The tremendous comminution and compression of the articular surface and of the subjacent bone leads at times to irreconstructible conditions of the articulation. These fractures are examples of extremes of violence and extremes of intra-articular injury where

Fig. 6.7. a Before application of traction. **b** After application of traction: the pattern of the fracture becomes discernible. The screw in the ulna served for temporary preoperative overhead traction

the return of any degree of useful function can be judged as satisfactory because the results are usually poor. In dealing with these fractures it is particularly important to evaluate carefully whether the trochlea can be reconstructed.

If the trochlea can be reconstructed, then a useful degree of function can be anticipated, which is better than what can be achieved by closed treatment. If the trochlea is beyond the scope of surgical reconstruction, then traction with early motion is preferable to the failure of an ill-advised surgical attempt.

There are certain situations where the decision to operate must be made on considerations other than the fracture.

6.3.1.3 Indications for Surgery

Open Fracture

We feel that, in addition to débridement, the single most important prophylactic measure in preventing sepsis is stable internal fixation. The surgeon who carries out a débridement and then secures immobilization, either in a cast or traction, in order to execute a delayed open reduction should sepsis have been prevented, compromises the only chance the patient may have to regain good function. We are not advocating extremes of exposure with further devitalization of fragments, nor are we advocating massive internal fixation, but feel that a successful joint reconstruction can only be achieved early. The amount of internal fixation used should be sufficient to provide initial stability. Mechanical overload and failure as a result of movement may destroy such marginal fixation, but we would rather revise a failed internal fixation in a patient with mobile soft tissues and a mobile joint free of sepsis than face a stiff joint and a scarred soft tissue envelope or an unstable joint which has become infected. Recent evidence has destroyed the notion that the presence of metal raises the incidence of sepsis. That was true if fixation was unstable. Even if disaster should strike and sepsis develops, one is in a far better position to treat this complication in the presence of stable internal fixation. These techniques apply, of course, only if there is a soft tissue envelope and a joint which has not been totally deformed and destroyed. If the soft tissue injury is severe, we advocate reduction and fixation of the articular component and then bridging of the elbow with an external fixator to provide immobilization, and allow for easy access and care of the soft tissue. Once the soft tissues have healed, one can evaluate what further reconstruction is possible.

Vascular Injury

The fibers of the brachial muscle are the only protection afforded the brachial artery from the jagged and sharp ends of the thin and flared portion of the distal humerus. Thus, it is not surprising that vascular injuries, particularly in children, are not rare. We feel that if a vascular injury is present, surgical stabilization of the skeleton is demanded in order to safeguard the surgical repair of the vascular lesion.

Associated Fracture

An associated fracture of the humerus or radius and ulna demands surgical stabilization of all fractures to safeguard the function of the elbow (see Chap. 9).

Associated Injuries

The care of associated injuries such as chest injuries or other fractures (e.g., femur, pelvis) may demand an upright and mobile patient and may make surgical stabilization of the supracondylar fracture advisable.

6.3.1.4 Surgical Treatment

Timing of Surgery

The supracondylar fracture is a complex intra-articular injury which requires very careful evaluation, preparation for surgery, and surgical execution. Unfortunately, one rarely has the luxury of time. Supracondylar fractures frequently require emergency surgery because of an associated vascular lesion, or an open fracture. Even if not faced with an emergency, we do not like to delay unduly because the elbow tends to swell rapidly which may severely compromise the soft tissue closure following an internal fixation. Furthermore, a delay of even 5 days has been associated with a disturbingly high incidence of myositis ossificans. Therefore, we favor carrying out open reduction and internal fixation as soon as possible. If the elbow is too swollen to permit closure of the soft tissues without tension, we insert a few approximating sutures and leave the wound open to carry out a secondary closure once the swelling has subsided.

In patients who are to be treated by closed means, we insert a cancellous screw into the volar aspect of the olecranon at the level of the coronoid process and suspend the patient's arm in overhead traction (Fig. 6.8). The advantage of the cancellous screw is the great ease of insertion and the avoidance of all danger to the ulnar nerve, which can be pierced by a Kirschner wire inserted into the olecranon for traction. Mobilization of the elbow can be started while it is still in traction. Once the fracture becomes "sticky" (i.e., deformable, but not displaceable), we transfer the extremity to a cast brace.

Diagnosis

The case history is important because it sheds light on the mechanism of injury and on the forces involved. It also tips the surgeon off about associated vascular or neurologic injuries, which so commonly accompany this fracture. The physical examination discloses a swollen, painful elbow which the patient holds protectively and refuses to move. Physical examination will serve little in delineating the exact pattern of the fracture, but it is invaluable in the evaluation of an associated vascular injury, compartment syndrome, or an associated neurological complication.

The radiological examination is the only method available which will give a detailed picture of the fracture. It is important to remember that, de-

Fig. 6.8. Olecranon screw used for overhead traction

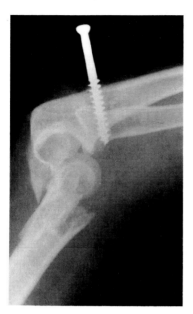

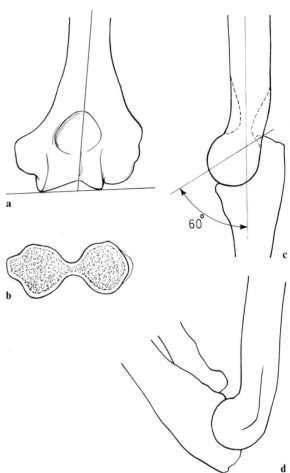

Fig. 6.9 a–d. The distal end of the humerus. **a** Note the distribution of the articular cartilage. The posterior aspect of the capitellum has no articular cartilage. Note also the downward projection of the trochlea, responsible for the carrying angle. **b** The distal humerus in cross section at the level of the fossa olecrani. The two columns of bone on either side of the fossa are dense and strong and offer a good hold for screws. **c** With the elbow in extension, the tip of the olecranon lodges in the olecranon fossa. If the fossa is blocked by a screw or plate, extension of the elbow is impossible. **d** Note also the 60° anterior angulation of the articular portion of the humerus. This forward angulation makes it difficult to apply a plate to the radial aspect of the distal end of the humerus

spite this, a patient with a vascular compromise must not be sent off to the radiology, department. If a pulse does not return following gentle realignment, the patient must be taken to the operating room as an emergency and any radiological assessment, including angiography, should be executed while the patient is prepared for surgery.

At times, the elbow is so distorted that it is impossible to make out the definition of the fracture fragments. Tomography is very helpful, particularly in evaluating the comminution, but if the distortion is great, we have found it very useful to obtain an X-ray with the patient under anesthesia while traction is applied to the forearm with the elbow in extension. This often results in sufficient reduction to make possible the identification of the fragments and of the fracture pattern (see Fig. 6.7).

Classification

Although we continue to use the AO classification of these fractures (see Fig. 6.1), we do so with reservations we have already mentioned. We would like to reiterate that epicondylar and condylar fractures are sustained by a different mechanism to supracondylar fractures, are relatively simple to treat, and have a good prognosis. The supracondylar A_2 and A_3 fractures and the supracondylar intra-articular fracture C_1, C_2, and C_3 pose common problems which relate to the fracture and to the anatomical region. They share methods of treatment and prognosis, and therefore should be considered together.

Surgical Anatomy of the Distal Humerus

The distal end of the humerus is flattened, expanded transversely, and rounded at the end (Fig. 6.9). The rounded end of the condyle presents articular and nonarticular surfaces. The articular portion forms the elbow joint and articulates with the radius and ulna. The lateral convex surface of the condyle is the capitellum, which is covered on its anterior and inferior surfaces with articular cartilage. It articulates with the head of the

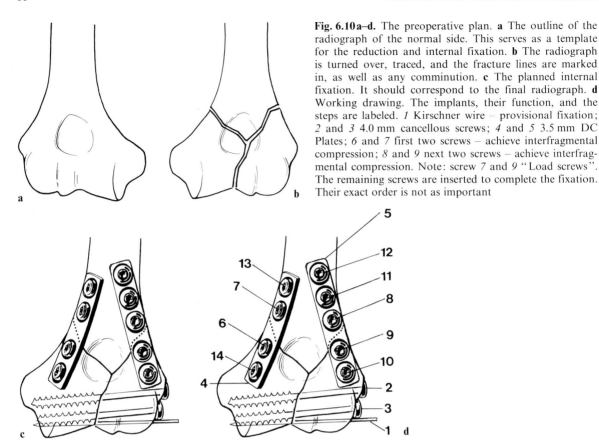

Fig. 6.10a–d. The preoperative plan. **a** The outline of the radiograph of the normal side. This serves as a template for the reduction and internal fixation. **b** The radiograph is turned over, traced, and the fracture lines are marked in, as well as any comminution. **c** The planned internal fixation. It should correspond to the final radiograph. **d** Working drawing. The implants, their function, and the steps are labeled. *1* Kirschner wire – provisional fixation; *2* and *3* 4.0 mm cancellous screws; *4* and *5* 3.5 mm DC Plates; *6* and *7* first two screws – achieve interfragmental compression; *8* and *9* next two screws – achieve interfragmental compression. Note: screw *7* and *9* "Load screws". The remaining screws are inserted to complete the fixation. Their exact order is not as important

radius. The fact that the posterior surface is nonarticular is important in the fixation of the fractures of the capitellum, since lag screws can be inserted from back to front through the nonarticular surface without interfering with the joint (see Fig. 6.3).

The trochlea is medial, larger, pulley-shaped, and completely covered with articular cartilage. It articulates with the trochlear notch of the ulna. When the elbow is extended (Fig. 6.9c), the inferior and posterior aspects of the trochlea are in contact with the ulna and the tip of the olecranon lodges within the olecranon fossa. When the elbow is flexed, the trochlear notch of the ulna rolls on to the anterior aspect of the trochlea and the coronoid process rests in the coronoid fossa and the radial head in the radial fossa. The downward projection on the medial side of the trochlea is responsible for the physiological valgus tendency of the elbow in full extension. This valgus tendency is referred to as the carrying angle and is approximately 170° (Fig. 6.9a).

The portion of the humerus immediately above the trochlea is hollowed out and, as indicated, anteriorly forms the coronoid fossa and posteriorly the olecranon fossa. The two fossae share a common floor which in some individuals may be absent and be represented by a hole. The two columns of bone on either side of the fossa (Fig. 6.9b) are dense and strong and very important in the internal fixation of a supracondylar fracture (Müller et al. 1965); they are the only portions of bone in this region into which screws can be inserted, since the olecranon and coronoid fossa must not be obstructed in any way. The medial epicondyle forms an extension of the medial column medially. It is grooved on the posterior aspect by the ulnar nerve. When the ulnar nerve is lifted out of its groove and transposed to the front, the medial epicondyle becomes a very useful portion of bone for the insertion of screws.

Planning the Surgical Procedure

A simple fracture requires little planning. By contrast, a complex fracture requires a very careful fracture analysis and careful planning of the internal fixation (Fig. 6.10). It is extremely helpful to obtain an anteroposterior radiograph of the normal elbow, to serve as a template of the distal humerus (Fig. 6.10a). We turn the radiograph over and trace the outline of the normal distal

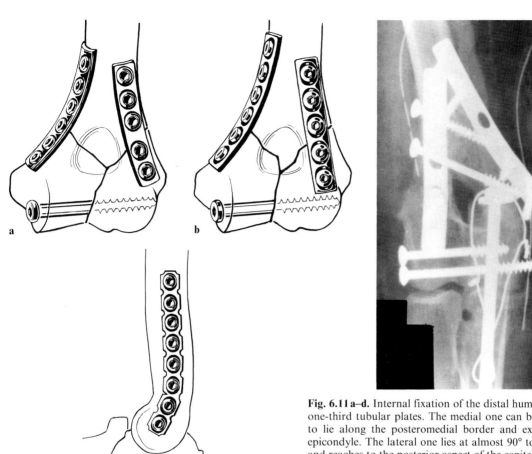

Fig. 6.11 a–d. Internal fixation of the distal humerus. **a** Two one-third tubular plates. The medial one can be contoured to lie along the posteromedial border and extend to the epicondyle. The lateral one lies at almost 90° to the medial and reaches to the posterior aspect of the capitellum. **b** Two 3.5-mm DC plates are applied, one medially and one laterally. Because the DC plates are flatter, the medial one comes to lie more posteriorly in the plane of the medial epicondyle. **c** The 3.5-mm reconstruction plate, because of its notching, can be bent forward; thus, it is best suited if a plate is to be applied laterally and reach as far as the lateral condyle. **d** Note in this post operative X-ray the two lag screws used to stabilize the oblique fracture line between the medial epicondylar and condylar fragment and the shaft. Whenever possible lag screws should be used to achieve primary stability. The plates function then in addition to their tension band effect as neutralization plates

humerus on tracing paper. Since both the fractured elbow and the normal elbow are radiographed at the same distance from the X-ray tube, the magnification is the same. It is now possible, with the aid of the anteroposterior radiograph of the fractured elbow, to mark in the fracture lines on the tracing (Fig. 6.10 b). It is important to draw in the comminution as well as any bone defects which exist. We are now in a position to plan the internal fixation.

The reconstruction of an intra-articular fracture always begins with the reconstruction of the joint. One should decide whether the trochlear and capitellar fragments will be lagged together with a malleolar screw or two small 4.0-mm cancellous screws. If a defect exists in the articular surface, it is wrong to lag the fragments together because this narrows the hinge and makes the elbow joint incongruous. In such a case, one should plan to

fix the condylar fragments with a 4.5-mm cortical screw. Both fragments are tapped. The cortical screw then acts as a fixation screw rather than as a lag screw and maintains the fragments the correct distance apart (see Fig. 6.1).

Once the joint is reconstructed, the fixation of the supracondylar fracture should be planned. The first rule to be kept in mind is that no piece of internal fixation must encroach on the olecranon fossa, because this would permanently block extension. The second is that screws alone cannot achieve stable fixation of the supracondylar fracture. The diaphyseal segment should be assessed

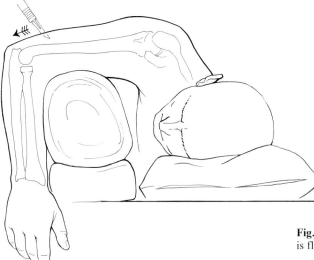

Fig. 6.12. The lateral position of the patient. The elbow is flexed. The weight of the forearm applies traction

to see whether there are fragments which should be reduced and lagged together. This is an important step because it increases the stability of the fixation and reduces the number of fragments to deal with, which makes reduction easier. It is important to mark on the drawing the exact position and direction of the lag screws. Frequently, it is advantageous to predrill a gliding hole or a thread hole before the reduction is carried out. If possible, the supracondylar fracture is fixed with two one-third tubular or two 3.5-mm DC plates. If this appears impossible, then we try to apply a plate along the lateral border of the shaft with the last screw of the plate opposite the condylar fragment (Fig. 6.11). We use the 3.5-mm reconstruction plate for this purpose because it is easier to contour in order to accommodate the anterior angulation of the distal epiphysis. The last screw through the plate must go into the condyles and may even be used to lag them together. One must remember, however, that the longitudinal axis of the lateral condyle makes a 60° angle with the longitudinal axis of the shaft. The plate must, therefore, be angled forward or an extension deformity of the distal fragment will result (see Fig. 6.9c).

Thus, the final working drawing (Fig. 6.10d) will have marked on it all the screws and plates, their function, and the order of insertion. The time spent on preoperative planning gives the surgeon that much more time to spend on the internal fixation, ensures thorough familiarity with the individual fracture, and will vastly improve the quality of the internal fixation and thus the final result.

Positioning and Draping the Patient

The positioning of the patient will be determined by the habitus of the patient and any associated injuries. We prefer to position the patient lying on the side opposite the involved extremity (Fig. 6.12). This position automatically exposes the posterior aspect of the elbow and allows a direct, unobstructed surgical approach. The elbow must be free to be flexed through a full range which is extremely important in the surgical exposure and reduction of the fracture. With the patient lying on the uninjured side, the force of gravity maintains traction on the forearm and keeps it in the correct position throughout surgery. This releases an assistant who would otherwise be required to hold the forearm in a position indicated by the surgeon. As the assistant tires, the arm begins to wander and the exposure, and at times even the reduction, can be lost. This can lead to a great deal of unnecessary tension and frustration and may adversely affect the outcome of surgery. With the patient in the lateral decubitus position the position of the elbow and forearm is adjusted simply by placing a rolled-up sheet under the forearm and elbow and shifting it as required.

We wish to stress that particularly the patient with an associated vascular lesion must not be positioned prone. This obstructs the access to the anterior arm and cubital fossa and makes vascular repair impossible. With the patient lying on the uninjured side, one has easy access to the front and back of the elbow. Two surgical incisions are

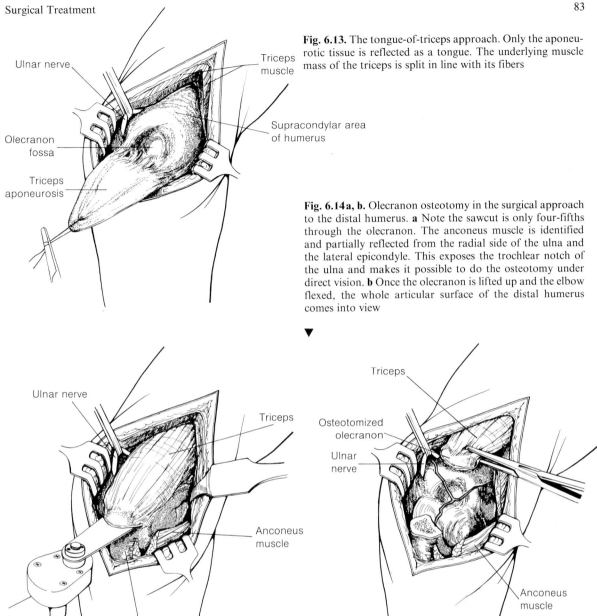

Fig. 6.13. The tongue-of-triceps approach. Only the aponeurotic tissue is reflected as a tongue. The underlying muscle mass of the triceps is split in line with its fibers

Fig. 6.14a, b. Olecranon osteotomy in the surgical approach to the distal humerus. **a** Note the sawcut is only four-fifths through the olecranon. The anconeus muscle is identified and partially reflected from the radial side of the ulna and the lateral epicondyle. This exposes the trochlear notch of the ulna and makes it possible to do the osteotomy under direct vision. **b** Once the olecranon is lifted up and the elbow flexed, the whole articular surface of the distal humerus comes into view

necessary if a vascular repair has to be done. It is impossible to deal adequately with a supracondylar fracture from in front or through one or two side incisions.

Draping

An assistant should apply traction to the upper extremity and hold it with the elbow in extension while the surgeon scrubs it from the axilla to the wrist. The upper extremity is then draped free to allow for free manipulation and full unobstructed flexion and extension of the elbow.

Tourniquet

Where feasible, we prefer to use a tourniquet on all intra-articular fractures. This decreases bleeding, allows better visualization of the intra-articular components, and leads to a more accurate reconstruction of the joint.

Surgical Exposure of the Distal Humerus

The surgical exposures for simple fractures of the distal humerus have already been discussed (see p. 66). We shall concern ourselves now with the surgical exposure of complex supracondylar fractures. As suggested by our preferred positioning of the patient, we favor the posterior approach. Fractures which do not involve the joint are approached through the tongue-of-triceps approach as described by Van Gorder (1940). Fractures which involve the joint are approached through a transverse osteotomy of the olecranon as described by Cassebaum (1952).

The skin incision is begun posteriorly in the center of the distal arm and is extended distally on the medial side of the olecranon to a point 4–5 fingerbreadths distal to the point of the olecranon. The incision should not cross the tip of the olecranon as it might lead to a painful scar. We prefer the incision on the medial side for two reasons. First, it is cosmetically less apparent, and, second, it allows ready exposure of the ulnar nerve. If the olecranon is not esteotomized, we make an effort to preserve the olecranon bursa.

The first step in the posterior approach is the isolation and protection of the ulnar nerve. Normally, it is readily found and easily palpated in the groove posterior to the medial epicondyle. The distorted skeleton and swollen ecchymotic soft tissues can make isolation of the ulnar nerve difficult. However, it must be found and protected, for it is easily injured. At times, it is easier to isolate it more proximally and trace it distally through the distorted tissues.

In the tongue-of-triceps approach (Fig. 6.13) a tongue of the triceps aponeurosis is developed with the apex proximally and the base at the olecranon. It is then turned down and the remaining fibers of the triceps are split and elevated with a periostial elevator. The muscle masses are retracted medially and laterally and held with Hohmann retractors. One must be very careful on the lateral side in positioning the tip of the retractor because it can easily be placed around the radial nerve anteriorly and inadvertently damage the nerve.

If the fracture extends into the joint, we favor the transolecranon approach (Fig. 6.14). The olecranon is exposed, and the anconeus muscle is partially lifted from the radial side of the ulna to expose the lateral edge of the trochlear fossa. A 3.2-mm drill hole is made in the center of the olecranon and is directed along the long axis of the ulna. This hole is tapped with the large cancellous tap for subsequent insertion of a cancellous screw. With the articular margin in sight medially and laterally, a transverse cut is made with an oscillating saw in the olecranon opposite the deepest point of the trochlear fossa. The cut is extended through four-fifths of the olecranon. A broad osteotome is then inserted into the cut and the olecranon is pried apart. Thus, the osteotomy is completed by fracturing through the subchondral bone. This leads to irregular bony spicules in the subchondral bone which are used at the end of the procedure as a guide to reduction. The sawing also results in about 1 mm loss of bone. If one were to cut right through, one could damage the articular cartilage and have a 1-mm loss of the articular surface.

The olecranon is separated medially and laterally and is lifted proximally, together with the triceps muscle, which is dissected free from the underlying bone. Hohmann retractors aid in the exposure. The same care must be exercised on the lateral side in inserting the Hohmann retractor. On the medial side, care must be taken, of course, not to injure the ulnar nerve. The exposure of the joint can be further increased by flexion of the elbow. This gives a full and unobstructed view of the joint and allows reduction and fixation of all the fragments.

At the end of the procedure, the olecranon is lagged in place with a large cancellous screw. The predrilling and tapping of the hole ensures an anatomical reduction. The lag screw fixation alone is not adequate and must be protected with a tension band wire which is passed deep to the triceps tendon (see p. 93).

Technique of Reduction and Internal Fixation of a Supracondylar Fracture

In dealing with an intra-articular fracture, one should always begin with the reconstruction of the joint. It is important to expose the joint, evaluate the comminution, and decide which is the major and best preserved fragment. The small articular fragments should not be discarded and care should be taken in the exposure not to allow any significant fragment to fall out. The only time a segment of the articulation might be discarded and replaced by a cancellous graft is when that portion is completely crushed and comminuted. Once all the frag-

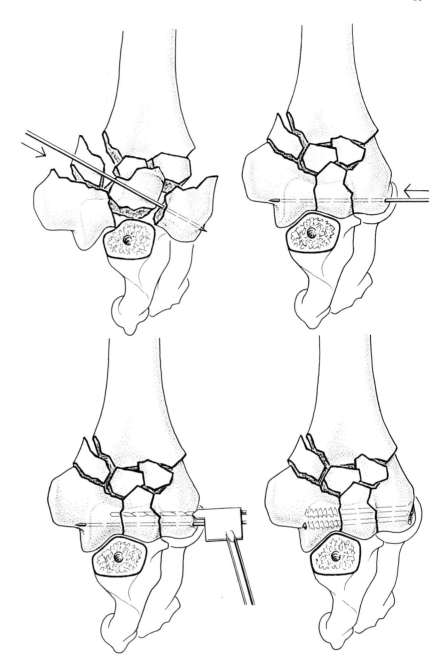

Fig. 6.15. The technique of open reduction and internal fixation of the supracondylar fracture. (Modified from Heim and Pfeiffer 1972)

ments are identified, it is important to compare the findings with the sketched plan of the operation. The fragments should be carefully manipulated, rotated, and aligned until one is certain of their exact fit and of the steps in the reduction. The most important step in the procedure is a meticulous reconstruction of the trochlea. The trochlea forms the hinge of the elbow, and if it is not anatomically reconstructed, the elbow will be incongruous and the result correspondingly poor.

The fragments should be provisionally fixed with Kirschner wires. Depending on the size of the fragments involved, we use either 0.5-mm or 1.0-mm Kirschner wires for the provisional fixation. These wires must be inserted with a power drill. A hand drill wobbles too much and can frequently result in the loss of a difficult reduction.

The insertion of the first 1.0-mm Kirschner wire is crucial because it will serve as a guide to the internal fixation of the condylar fragments. One should decide which is the major articular fragment. Preferably, one should select the radial fragment, because it is better to insert the lag screws in a radioulnar direction since this offers less chance of damage to the ulnar nerve later when the metal is removed. However, if the radial fragment is too small or comminuted, one begins with the ulnar fragment. The first Kirschner wire must be drilled through the center of the fragment, equidistant from the anterior and posterior articular cartilage but low enough to permit the insertion of a screw above it (Fig. 6.15).

Once the first wire is drilled through, the articular fragments are carefully reduced and, if necessary, kept in place with fine 0.5-mm Kirschner wires. The first Kirschner wire is now drilled in a retrograde fashion into the other major condylar fragment and, if possible, through any other major intervening articular fragment. The pointed 2.0-mm three-hole drill guide is now slipped over the Kirschner wire which serves not only as the major provisional fixation of the articular fragments, but also as a guide for the drilling of the hole for the first lag screw. After the 2.0-mm hole is drilled and tapped, the 4.0-mm small cancellous screw is inserted as a lag screw for fixation of the fragments. One must be extremely careful and preserve the width of the trochlea. If a defect is present, one must fix the condylar fragments with a 4.5-mm cortical screw which is inserted as a fixation screw. This means that all the fragments are tapped. When the screw is inserted, no compression results and the trochlea is not narrowed. The gap between the condylar fragments is filled with a cancellous bone graft.

Once the joint is reconstructed, one proceeds to the fixation of the supracondylar fracture. As already described on p. 81, the diaphyseal segment should be assessed, and if any major fragments can be lagged to the shaft, this should be done before one attempts to fix the supracondylar fracture itself. This is an important step in the procedure. The lag screw fixation of comminuted fragments will increase the stability of the fixation and will reduce the number of fragments to deal with. This makes the reduction easier.

The first rule to be kept in mind is that no piece of internal fixation may encroach on the olecranon fossa or coronoid fossa because it would block extension or flexion respectively. The second rule is that crossed lag screws or threaded pins cannot achieve stable fixation of the supracondylar fracture. The supracondylar fracture should be reduced and held provisionally with Kirschner wires while the reduction is checked, the situation again compared with the preoperative plan, and the final fixation decided upon.

If possible, we prefer to fix the supracondylar fracture with two 3.5-mm DC plates, or occasionally, in very small bones, with one-third tubular plates, which must be carefully positioned and contoured to fit the medial and lateral ridges on either side of the olecranon fossa (see Fig. 6.11). Clearly, in a simple fracture without comminution, these two plates should be inserted as compression plates, which will greatly enhance the stability of the fixation. If comminution exists, these plates will function as buttress plates or neutralization plates where they protect a lag screw fixation. The plates have to reach the diaphysis, or, if the fracture pattern is such that it is impossible to fix it with two plates, then we resort to one plate which is best carefully contoured and applied along the lateral border of the humerus (see Fig. 6.11 c), in such a way that the lowermost one or two screw holes will permit insertion of one or two screws into the condylar fragment. This plate should be either a 3.5-mm reconstruction plate or a regular DC plate. The choice will clearly depend on the length of plate required as well as on the segment of humerus involved. If the plate is designed to fix the lower diaphysis, then it should be stronger and we would favor the 4.5-mm DC or reconstruction plate. The choice of plate must, of course, also be governed by the size of the patient. In applying this side plate, one must remember the anterior angulation of the lateral condyle. If difficulty is encountered with the lateral late, particularly because of the angulation, then the plate can be applied medially and extended over the epicondyle which is in line with the shaft axis (see Fig. 6.11 b, c).

Postoperative Care

The elbow is splinted in approximately 120°–130° extension on a well-padded posterior plaster slab and suspended for elevation for the first 24–36 h from an overhead bar or pole. On the 2nd day, we remove the suction drain, and on the 3rd or 4th day, we remove the splint and the dressing and examine the wound. If no complications are found, active flexion–extension exercises are begun.

Early active movement is essential if function is to be regained. If the internal fixation is such that external protection and immobilization are required, then all the advantages of surgery will be lost. The only person who can accurately assess the stability of the internal fixation is the surgeon. A radiograph projects the configuration of the internal fixation, but only the surgeon can attest to the quality of the bone and to the holding power of the screws. At times, despite proper judgement and care, one is left with an internal fixation which must be protected or mechanical overload with failure is certain. Under these circumstances, we have made use of cast bracing. This has permitted early, active mobilization with a certain degree of protection of an otherwise tenuous fixation. We feel that plaster of Paris fixation, recommended for 3 weeks or longer by some, is almost certain to become associated with a serious degree of stiffness.

We have found hydrotherapy a useful adjunct in the active mobilization of joints. Under no circumstances should passive manipulation be employed. It robs the patient of the protective sensory feedback and may lead to a ripping apart of the internal fixation. It may also lead to a rapid onset of myositis ossificans which can lead to irreversible stiffness. If, in the course of active mobilization, the patient develops local pain, redness, and swelling, and one can be certain that these are manifestations of instability rather than sepsis, then immobilization must be instituted until some degree of biological stability has been achieved. We have made use of continuous passive motion machines in the postoperative treatment of supracondylar fractures and have found the recovery period to be shorter, the mobilization less painful, and the recovery of movement more rapid. The machine is started while the patient is still under anesthesia and motion continued without any lengthy interruptions for the 1st week. We have found the Mobilimb (Toronto Medical Corporation) particularly useful because it is portable and allows patient mobilization. After the 1st week, the patient is treated in the same manner as the patient who began with early active mobilization. In comparing the two groups of patients, we feel that postoperative mobilization with the aid of a continuous passive motion machine is preferable. The patients are more comfortable, the edema subsides more rapidly, and the range of motion in the joint returns more quickly. In addition, there is the beneficial effect of continuous passive motion on the healing of articular cartilage (Salter et al. 1980).

References

Alvarez E, Patel MR, Nimberg G, Pearlman HS (1975) Fractures of the capitelum humeri. J Bone Joint Surg 57A:1093–1096

Bickel WE, Perry RE (1963) Comminuted fracture of the distal humerus. JAMA 184:553–557

Cassebaum WH (1952) Operative treatment of T and Y fractures of the lower end of the humerus. Am J Surg 83:265–270

Heim U, Pfeiffer KM (1972) Periphere Osteosynthesen. Springer, Berlin Heidelberg New York

Keon-Cohen BT (1966) Fractures of the elbow. J Bone Joint Surg 48A:1623–1639

Miller WE (1964) Comminuted fractures of the distal end of the humerus in the adult. J Bone Joint Surg 46A:644–657

Müller ME, Allgöwer M, Willenegger H (1965) Technique of internal fixation of fractures. Springer, Berlin Heidelberg New York, p 196, fig 210

Müller ME, Allgöwer M, Schneider R, Willenegger H (1979) Manual of Internal Fixation, 2nd edn. Springer, Berlin Heidelberg New York

Riseborough EJ, Radin EL (1969) Intercondylar fractures of the humerus in the adult. J Bone Joint Surg 51A:130–141

Salter RB, Simmonds DF, Malcolm BW, Rumble EJ, MacMichael D (1980) The biological effects of continuous passive motion on the healing of full thickness defects in articular cartilage: an experimental investigation in the rabbit. J Bone Joint Surg 62A:1232–1251

Van Gorder GW (1940) Surgical approach in supracondylar "T" fractures of the humerus requiring open reduction. J Bone Joint Surg 22:278–292

7 Fractures of the Olecranon

J. Schatzker

7.1 Introduction

A fracture of the olecranon with displacement represents a disruption of the triceps mechanism and, as a consequence, the loss of active extension of the elbow. The necessity for surgical repair has been appreciated since Lord Lister attempted an open reduction and suture of the olecranon (Keon-Cohen 1966). The methods of surgical repair have varied. Some authors have advocated excision of the fragment or fragments with repair of the triceps aponeurosis (Keon-Cohen 1966). Others have advocated the fixation of the fragment with intramedullary nails, screws, or plates (Weseley et al. 1976). As indications became more clearly defined, resection of the proximal fragment and reattachment of the triceps tendon to the distal fragment was reserved for the elderly patient in whom the fracture was proximal to the middle of the trochlear notch (Rowe 1965). Younger patients were subjected to an open reduction and an attempt was made to stabilize the fragments, either with a through-and-through loop of wire (Fig. 7.1) or with a long intramedullary lag screw (Fig. 7.2).

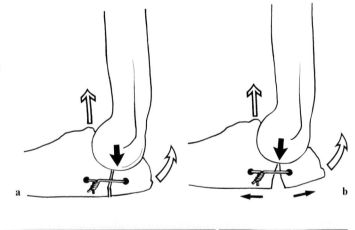

Fig. 7.1 a, b. A wire loop inserted through the substance of the olecranon (**a**) is unable to resist the pull of the triceps and brachialis muscles against the intact trochlea (**b**). Gaping of the fracture with varying degrees of displacement, despite protection in a cast, is the usual outcome

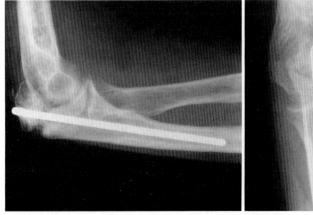

Fig. 7.2. A Rush rod or an intramedullary screw is also unable to resist the pull of the triceps and brachialis muscles. Note the displacement of the olecranon

If the olecranon fragment was small, excision usually resulted in a stable elbow with a satisfactory range of motion. If the fragment was large, it became increasingly more difficult to preserve an adequate cuff of the triceps aponeurosis to effect a repair. If the fragment involved more than 50% of the articular surface, instability of the elbow followed resection. Instability was a serious problem because it compromised function, and therefore excision was abandoned as a form of treatment for any but the smallest of fragments.

The methods of internal fixation with either the wire loop, intramedullary Rush rod, or an intramedullary lag screw did not provide sufficient stability to allow early motion. The joint had to be immobilized until union occurred. Despite plaster of Paris immobilization, the triceps pull was frequently sufficient to cause displacement (Fig. 7.2). Typically, the fracture gaped dorsally, and frequently some separation of the fragments occurred, which led to gaps in the articular surface and to joint incongruity.

The duration of immobilization and the associated joint disorganization frequently led to varying losses in the range of flexion and extension. The dorsal gaping with displacement of the proximal fragment blocked full extension. Therefore, the loss of extension was often more severe than the loss of flexion. Because the elbow is not a weight-bearing joint and it does not transmit such great forces as does the knee joint, incongruity does not result rapidly in post-traumatic osteoarthritis. However, if the patient is called upon to perform heavy work requiring elbow flexion and extension against resistance, then progression of the osteoarthritis and an increase in pain and disability are to be expected.

In 1965, the AO group published the *Technique of Internal Fixation of Fractures* (Müller et al. 1965), which introduced *tension band wiring* as the most effective method of internal fixation of olecranon fractures. Their experiments showed tension band wiring to be six times stronger than any other fixation technique. It was possible, therefore, if one used this technique, to forego the application of a plaster fixation and begin active movement soon after surgery. At 4–6 weeks, the olecranon fracture was usually sufficiently healed to allow the patient full function. The rate of malunion or nonunion was extremely low, as was the degree of residual disability.

7.2 Methods of Evaluation and Guides to Treatment

The indication for surgery is an olecranon fracture with displacement which represents a disruption of the triceps mechanism and loss of active extension of the elbow. If the fracture is undisplaced, the surgeon must determine whether the triceps aponeurosis is intact or not. With an intact triceps aponeurosis, a patient is able to extend the elbow against gravity without causing any displacement of the fragments. Such a fracture is stable, will not displace under the influence of physiological forces, and requires only symptomatic treatment. If any doubt exists as to the continuity of the triceps aponeurosis, the elbow should be examined with the aid of an X-ray image intensifier. Any degree of displacement on full flexion signifies damage to the triceps aponeurosis.

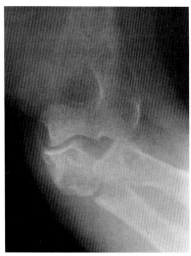 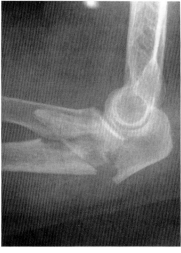

Fig. 7.3. A fracture of the olecranon with displacement. Note in this example, the associated disruption of the elbow joint with subluxation

The diagnosis is simple. Typically, the patient gives a history of having fallen and of not being able to use the elbow. The olecranon is very painful, swollen, and bruised. The exact diagnosis is established on an appropriate anteroposterior and lateral radiograph (Fig. 7.3). The anteroposterior view is more useful for an overall examination of the elbow to exclude other injuries: the olecranon itself is obscured in this view. The lateral projection gives a clear view of the olecranon. If one has doubts as to the degree of comminution or articular surface depression, one should request lateral tomograms to obtain an accurate definition of the fracture.

7.3 Classification

7.3.1 Intra-articular Fractures

7.3.1.1 Transverse

The simple fracture occurs at the deepest point of the trochlear notch (Fig. 7.4). It is an avulsion fracture and results from a sudden pull of both the triceps and brachialis muscles. It may also result from a direct fall on the olecranon itself.

Complex

Fractures which result from a direct force, such as a fall, frequently have comminution and depression of the articular surface (Fig. 7.5).

7.3.1.2 Oblique

This fracture usually results from a hyperextension injury of the elbow. It begins at the midpoint of the trochlear notch and runs distally (Fig. 7.6).

7.3.1.3 Comminuted Fractures and Associated Injuries

These fractures are the result of a high-velocity direct injury to the elbow, such as might result from a considerable fall directly on the elbow. The fracture lines are variable, but certain features must be distinguished.

1. Fractures of the Coronoid Process

Small fractures of the coronoid process itself are unimportant. If the fragment is large, it represents the distal articular surface of the trochlear notch and cannot be neglected, because of resultant instability of the elbow in extension (Fig. 7.7).

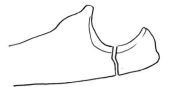

Fig. 7.4. A transverse fracture of the olecranon

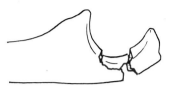

Fig. 7.5. A complex transverse fracture. Note the impaction of the central portion of the articular surface. This fragment is frequently difficult to reduce and, because of its position, difficult to fix. Once the fragment is disimpacted, a hole is left which may occasionally have to be bone grafted

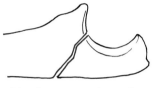

Fig. 7.6. An oblique fracture of the olecranon — the result of hyperextension

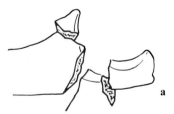

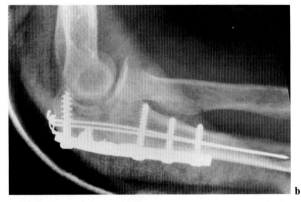

Fig. 7.7. a Severe comminution. Note also the fracture of the coronoid process. Such a comminuted fracture requires a neutralization plate which can also act as a tension band. b A comminuted fracture of the olecranon fixed with a plate, Kirschner wires, and a tension band wire

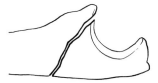

Fig. 7.8. A fracture of the olecranon which is distal to the midpoint of the trochlear notch. If not comminuted, such an oblique fracture should be first stabilized with one or two lag screws. Kirschner wires are not enough for lateral support. To overcome varus/valgus instability and resistance to torque, these distal fractures, even if fixed with lag screws, should be fixed with a plate. Semitubular plates are not strong enough to resist torsional forces. One should use the 3.5-mm DC plates to stabilize these fractures

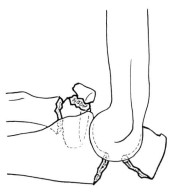

Fig. 7.9. A fracture of the olecranon associated with a fracture of the radial head. These fractures are frequently associated with a rupture of the medial collateral ligament of the elbow. The elbow remains unstable until the olecranon fracture is fixed, the medial collateral ligament repaired, and the radial head either reduced and fixed with screws or replaced with a prosthesis. Resection of the radial head will result in valgus subluxation of the elbow

2. Distal Extent of the Fracture

If the fracture extends distally past the midpoint of the trochlear notch (Fig. 7.8), it no longer represents only a disruption of the triceps mechanism. It compromises the stability of the elbow in withstanding varus or valgus forces.

3. Fracture or Dislocation of the Radial Head

An associated fracture of the radial head signifies a dislocation of the elbow and is usually associated with a disruption of the medial collateral ligament (Fig. 7.9). It implies ligamentous instability of the elbow which may not be corrected by reduction of the fracture and repair of the ligament. The radial head has to be reduced and fixed or replaced by a prosthesis.

7.3.2 Extra-articular Fractures

7.3.2.1 Avulsion Fracture of the Tip

Avulsion fractures of a small part of the tip of the olecranon with the attached triceps tendon result in the same loss of function as a transverse fracture of the olecranon. The mechanism of injury is probably the same.

7.4 Surgical Treatment

7.4.1 Positioning the Patient

The patient should be positioned either prone or lying on the uninjured side. This position automatically exposes the posterior aspect of the elbow and allows a direct unobstructed surgical approach. The elbow is free to be flexed or extended. The force of gravity maintains traction on the forearm and keeps it in the correct position throughout surgery. This releases an assistant who would otherwise be required to hold the forearm of a supine patient in a position indicated by the surgeon. With the patient lying on the uninjured side or prone, the position of the forearm is adjusted simply by placing a rolled-up sheet under the forearm as required (see p. 82).

7.4.2 Draping

The surgical scrub should extend from the level of the tourniquet, which is applied as high as possible on the arm, to the wrist. The extremity must be draped free to allow for unobstructed flexion and extension of the elbow.

7.4.3 Tourniquet

We prever to use a tourniquet on all intra-articular fractures. It reduces bleeding, allows better visualization of the intra-articular components, and leads to a more accurate reconstruction of the joint.

7.4.4 Surgical Exposure

The incision is begun posteriorly in the middle of the supracondylar area of the humerus and is extended distally on the medial side of the olecranon to a point three or four fingerbreadths distal to the fracture. The incision should not cross the

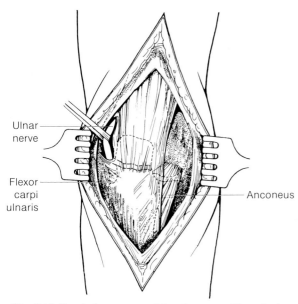

Ulnar nerve

Flexor carpi ulnaris

Anconeus

Fig. 7.10. Surgical exposure of the olecranon. Note the isolated and protected ulnar nerve which dips into the tunnel of the flexor carpi ulnaris muscle next to the fracture. To visualize the joint, one must reflect the fibers of the flexor carpi ulnaris and the anconeus muscles

point of the olecranon as it might lead to a painful scar. We prefer the incision on the medial side of the olecranon for two reasons. First, it is cosmetically more pleasing because it is less apparent. Second, we feel that the ulnar nerve should be identified and protected during the surgical exposure and reduction (Fig. 7.10). If the incision is radial, it is more difficult to expose the ulnar nerve and follow it distally without undermining a considerable flap. The olecranon bursa is incised and no effort is made to protect it. If the fracture is exposed with the elbow flexed it usually gapes, which facilitates the identification of the fracture lines without undue stripping of the flexor carpi ulnaris muscle from the medial side of the olecranon. The fracture and the articular surface should be exposed through the fracture by increasing the deformity of the proximal fragment. If the fracture is comminuted, but particularly if the joint surface is depressed, it is necessary to visualize the articular surface to check the accuracy of the reduction. This cannot be done safely from the medial side because of the ulnar nerve and because of the attachment of the deltoid ligament. Good exposure of the joint can be obtained from the lateral side by detaching some of the fibers of the anconeus muscle from the radial side of the ulna (Fig. 7.10).

7.4.5 Techniques of Reduction and Internal Fixation

7.4.5.1 Transverse Fractures

The reduction of the olecranon fracture is easiest with the elbow in extension, which relaxes the pull of the triceps muscle. Once carefully reduced, the fracture should be held reduced with a towel clip-like reduction clamp. Two Kirschner wires are then inserted. These must be parallel to one another in the direction of the long axis of the ulna. A common error is to cross them, but this holds the fracture apart and prevents compression. Another common error is to angle them anteriorly and exit them through the anterior cortex near the coronoid process, where they may damage vital structures. If they are angled too far anteriorly, they may enter the joint. Correct insertion of the wires is greatly eased if the elbow is slightly flexed and if the cortex of the olecranon is predrilled with a 2.0-mm drill bit. The Kirschner wires should be 1.6 mm in diameter. If they are any thicker, they are too difficult to bend. They should be inserted with a power drill with the help of a telescoping wire guide. One should aim parallel to the subcutaneous border of the ulna. These wires are important because they are an internal splint which prevents rotation and lateral displacement.

The wire for the tension band is inserted through a 2.0-mm drill hole which is drilled distally, approximately the same distance from the fracture as the tip of the olecranon. The drill hole must be deep to the subcutaneous cortex of the ulna. If it is too superficial, the wire will cut out. The wire for the tension band should be 1.0–1.2 mm in diameter and should be made of stainless steel which is sufficiently ductile to permit twisting.

The tension band wire must pass deep to the triceps tendon and be just proximal to the two Kirschner wires. We have found a gauge 14 or 16 needle a great help in passing the wire correctly deep to the triceps tendon. If the wire is passed deep to the tendon without support of the two Kirschner wires, one runs the risk of triceps rupture.

B.G. Weber (circa 1972, personal communication) advises that before the figure eight tension band is tightened, two loops should be made to allow simultaneous twisting and tightening of both limbs of the figure eight, to ensure uniform compression on both sides of the fracture. The two loops are not absolutely essential as long as one makes sure that the wire is straightened out and pulled very tight before it is placed under tension by twisting. Once tension is applied, the wire binds and will not slide in bone. If the wire is not pulled tight and straightened before it is tightened, it may straighten after the internal fixation is completed, and thus lengthen, which loosens the tension band and leads to failure of the fixation. The tension band should be tightened in full extension to effect a slight overreduction of the fracture, which will disappear as the elbow is flexed. This ensures dynamic compression on the whole fracture surface.

As the tension band is tightened, a slight gap in the articular surface is created, and the only part of the bone under constant axial compression is the posterior cortex and some adjacent cancellous bone. This is the only part which heals by primary bone healing. The remainder of the fracture is subjected to changing degrees of compression because the compression rises when the elbow is flexed and falls when it is extended. This flux in the degree of compression was seen in an experimental investigation to result in the central and subchondral areas of the fracture healing by endochondral ossification. The articular defect heals by the formation of fibrocartilage (Schatzker 1971).

With tension band fixation, flexion of the elbow increases the axial compression. This is fortunate because it increases the stability of the reduction and fixation, while with lag screw fixation or loop cerclage wiring, flexion causes displacement because of the unopposed pull of the triceps. Fractures of the olecranon fixed with a tension band wire should not be splinted in extension, therefore, but should be allowed early active flexion since this actually increases compression and stability. A further advantage of tension band fixation is that it can be employed successfully in osteoporotic bone since its strength does not depend on the holding power of a screw in the bone. Its strength is determined by the resistance of the bone to the cutting out of the wire where it traverses the ulnar cortex and by the stability and resistance of the two parallel Kirschner wires which support the tension band wire deep to the triceps tendon.

7.4.5.2 Transverse Fractures with Joint Depression

The transverse fracture with comminution and joint depression requires special attention (see Fig. 7.5). The articular fragment which is depressed and driven into the underlying cancellous bone represents a separate piece of bone with a disrupted blood supply. If it is large and left unre-duced, joint incongruity and instability result. Therefore, it must be elevated in a manner similar to that described for the tibial plateau (see Sect. 16.4.5). The resultant defect must be bone grafted. The graft, together with the axial compression, will aid in preventing redisplacement. Occasionally, it may also be possible to splint it in position with one of the two axial Kirschner wires. At the end of the procedure, the Kirschner wires are bent, cut to length, and the free ends are driven into the bone, which further increases the stability of the fixation and hinders the wires from backing out.

7.4.5.3 Oblique Fractures

The oblique fracture is reduced in the same way as a transverse fracture. The stability of the fixation can be greatly increased if a lag screw is inserted at right angles to the fracture line. The internal fixation then follows as described previously, with the two Kirschner wires and a tension band wire. In this instance, the tension band wire can be viewed as a neutralization wire, protecting the compression and fixation achieved with the lag screw. If the fixation with the lag screw is secure, the Kirschner wires can be omitted; the tension band wire alone will be enough. If the fracture is distal, one should use a plate for fixation instead of a wire (see Fig. 7.7b).

7.4.5.4 Comminuted Fractures

These fractures, the result of high-velocity injury, are frequently complex and may pose great difficulties when reduction and fixation are attempted. The reduction should commence distally and proceed toward the joint. Thus, if there is a butterfly fragment distal to the coronoid process, an attempt should be made to reduce it and fix it with a lag screw before one proceeds with the reduction of the joint surface. The articular surface of the distal fragment must be clearly visualized. Frequently, this can only be achieved if the proximal and distal fragments are widely separated.

The fracture of the coronoid, if significant in size, should be reduced first, and held provisionally with small bone-holding forceps or a Kirschner wire while it is fixed with a lag screw passed up through the posterior cortex of the ulna. The reduction and fixation of this fragment is important if stability of the elbow in extension is to be restored. The remaining fragments are then reduced and fixed one to the other by whatever means is most suitable. Once reduced, the olecranon is then splinted by the insertion of the two axial Kirschner wires.

If the fracture extends past the coronoid process, it can no longer be viewed as an isolated fracture of the olecranon subjected only to the pull of the triceps. Once the fracture involves the whole trochlear notch of the ulna and extends distal to the coronoid process it becomes subjected to considerable torque and valgus/varus stress and the simple Kirschner wires and tension band fixation are no longer enough. For such fractures, we like to combine the Kirschner wire and tension band fixation with a plate which is applied along the posterior cortex of the ulna and olecranon (see Fig. 7.1 b). This plate protects the fracture from the varus/valgus and torsional stresses. Occasionally, we resort to the use of a plate even if the fracture does not extend distal to the coronoid process, but is very comminuted so that no continuity exists in the posterior cortex. In such a case, as a tension band is tightened, the fragments tend to telescope, and the reduction might be lost and the joint become deformed. For such fractures, we use a plate which buttresses the fragments and helps maintain their relative position. We have found the small 3.5-mm DC plate very useful for this purpose. A semitubular plate is not to be used because it is too weak and tends to break.

7.5 Postoperative Care

Suction drains are used to prevent hematoma formation. These are removed after the first 24–36 h. The olecranon is held at 90° flexion on a padded posterior plaster splint for the first 2–3 days. The splint is then removed and the wound carefully inspected. If no complications exist, the patient is encouraged to begin active flexion-extension exercises which continue until a full range of movement is regained. The fractures, if uncomplicated, are usually healed in 6 weeks. At this point, full unprotected use of the extremity can be resumed. Comminuted fractures, particularly those with extension into the diaphysis of the ulna and those with devitalized bone fragments, require a longer time for consolidation and must be protected from overload to prevent implant failure with malunion or nonunion. More recently, we have used continuous passive motion (CPM) machines to mobilize olecranon fractures and have found them here, as with other intra-articular fractures, to be most useful and preferable to other methods. With the CPM machine, mobilization is begun immediately and is continued for the first 4–7 days. The more comminuted the fracture and the more extensive the associated bony and soft tissue injuries, the longer the time required for CPM.

References

Keon-Cohen BT (1966) Fractures of the elbow. J Bone Joint Surg 48A:1623–1639

Müller ME, Allgöwer M, Willenegger H (1965) Technique of internal fixation of fractures. Springer, Berlin Heidelberg New York

Rowe CR (1965) Management of fractures in elderly patients. J Bone Joint Surg 47A:1043–1059

Schatzker J (1971) Fixation of olecranon fractures in dogs. J Bone Joint Surg 53B:158

Weseley MS, Barenfeld PA, Risenstein AL (1976) The use of the Zuelzer hook plate in fixation of olecranon fractures. J Bone Joint Surg 58A:859–862

8 Fractures of the Radial Head

J. SCHATZKER

8.1 Introduction

The goal of treatment of fractures of the radial head is the preservation of elbow flexion and extension as well as pronation and supination of the forearm.

8.2 Mechanism of Injury

The vast majority of fractures of the radial head are sustained in a fall onto the outstretched hand. The force of the fall is transmitted through the radius to the elbow, where the head of the radius is driven against the capitellum. Thus, the damage may not only be to the radial head, but also to the capitellum. Occasionally, the radial head may fracture as a result of a valgus force to the elbow, when the injury may also become complicated by a fracture of the olecranon. In these complex injuries, one must not forget the medial collateral ligament of the elbow, which is frequently torn. The rupture of the collateral ligament on one side and the fracture of the radial head on the other render the elbow joint completely unstable.

8.3 Guides to Treatment

Considerable confusion continues to exist on how best to treat fractures of the radial head. Much of the confusion has been caused by an attempt to treat the radiograph rather than the patient. Some have advocated excision of the radial head if the fracture involved more than one-ninth of the circumference, while others with equal dogmatism felt that it should be one-sixth, and some that it should be one-third. Some surgeons, guided by the experience that not only is the fragment always bigger than suggested by the radiograph but also that the damage to the radial head, in the form

of comminution and articular depression, is always greater than anticipated, have gone so far as to advocate: "When in doubt, operate" and excise (Keon-Cohen 1966).

Since the goal of treatment is the preservation of function, the treatment must be directed to preserving motion at the elbow. Permanent loss of motion occurs either as a result of a bony block caused by a displaced piece or pieces of bone, or by capsular and pericapsular scarring. Early movement is the only measure available to prevent capsular and pericapsular scarring. Loss of movement due to a bony block can be corrected only by removal of the block. Thus, we feel that once the diagnosis of a displaced fracture of the radial head has been established radiologically, the surgeon must establish beyond doubt whether a bony block to movement exists or not.

An intra-articular fracture is invariably associated with varying degrees of hemarthrosis. The distended joint is painful and the patient is reluctant to attempt any active movement or permit any passive manipulation. Considerable relief of pain is gained by aspiration of the hemarthrosis and infiltration of the joint with a local anesthetic, such as 2% xylocaine. The advantage of local anesthesia is that once the joint becomes relatively painless it is possible to determine whether there is a bony block to motion or not. If no block to motion is present, then early active motion is to be encouraged. We have treated displaced fractures in this fashion, regardless of their radiological appearance. The results have been gratifying, and despite incongruity of the articulation between the radial head and the capitellum, post-traumatic osteoarthritis has not developed. Loose intra-articular fragments and fractures with a block to motion under anesthesia, however, constitute an indication for surgery.

Excision of the radial head is not advisable. Studies by Pennal and Barrington (T. Barrington, personal communication) have demonstrated that in those who make heavy demands on their wrist

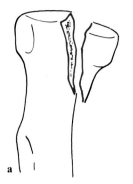
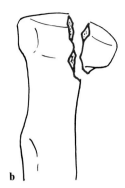
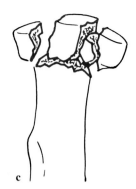

Fig. 8.1. a A wedge fracture. In this fracture, a part of the head remains intact. Fixation is simple with two 2.7-mm cortical screws used here as lag screws. The heads are recessed below the level of the articular cartilage. b An impaction fracture. Here again, a part of the head remains intact. The fracture fragments may be single, but more often there is some comminution. The fragments are tilted and the bone beneath them crushed or impacted. There may also be a transverse fracture across the neck. c A severely comminuted fracture. There are many fracture fragments, usually with significant displacement

and elbow, such as manual workers, excision of the radial head is followed by proximal migration of the radius. This leads to inferior radioulnar joint disturbance with pain and weakness of the wrist.

Radiographs of a fractured radial head are difficult to interpret and are often misleading. An accurate assessment of the fracture is only possible at the time of surgery. One is then able to determine whether open reduction and internal fixation of the radial head are feasible or whether the radial head should be excised. We do not believe in partial excision of the head because the results have been uniformly less satisfactory than after excision of the whole head.

8.4 Surgical Treatment

We consider the following to be indications for surgery: major loose intra-articular fragments, displaced fractures which under anesthesia can be demonstrated to constitute a block to motion, and displaced fractures of the radial head associated with fractures of the olecranon or with rupture of the ulnar collateral ligament, or with both.

Although one might contemplate excision of the radial head as definitive treatment for a comminuted fracture if such a fracture is in isolation, one cannot consider it as an option if the fracture of the radial head is associated with rupture of the ulnar collateral ligament. A repair of the ulnar collateral ligament will not render the elbow stable if the radial head is missing. Therefore, under these circumstances, one can either perform an open reduction and internal fixation of the radial head fracture or excise the head and replace it with a prosthesis which will act as a spacer and stabilize the joint. We feel that preservation of the radial head is preferable to excision. The decision whether an open reduction and fixation is feasible has to be based, as in all other fractures, on the personality of the fracture. In evaluating radial head fractures, we recognize three types.

8.4.1 Classification

Type I: wedge fracture. The fracture consists of a simple wedge fragment which may be displaced or undisplaced (Fig. 8.1 a).

Type II: impaction fracture. In this fracture pattern, part of the head and neck remain intact. The portion involved in the fracture is tilted and impacted, with the amount of comminution being variable (Fig. 8.1 b).

Type III: severely comminuted fracture. The hallmark of this fracture is that no portion of the head or neck remains in continuity and that the comminution is very severe (Fig. 8.1 c).

Severely comminuted fractures are irreconstructible. Here the decision rests, if a block to motion exists, between simple excision or excision and prosthetic replacement. In the other two fracture patterns, if there is an indication for surgery because of a block to motion, the decision between excision and reduction and fixation has to be made on the basis of the personality of the fracture. As already stated, in the younger patient, we prefer reduction and fixation to excision.

8.4.2 Positioning and Draping the Patient

The patient is positioned supine. The limb is prepared from the axilla to the wrist and is draped free to permit pronation and supination of the forearm. The procedure is performed under tourniquet control.

8.4.3 Surgical Exposure

The approach is lateral. The incision begins at the lateral epicondyle and is extended just distal to the radial head. The common extensor muscle is split along the line of its fibers in line with the skin incision. Care must be taken to stay posterior to the radial nerve which crosses just in front to enter the substance of the supinator muscle, approximately 2 cm distal to the radial head. The incision must therefore not extend distally below the annular ligament. Furthermore, if damage to

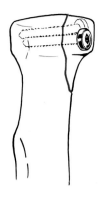

Fig. 8.2. The fixation of a wedge fracture is simple. Two 2.7-mm cortical screws are used as lag screws. The heads of the screws are recessed below the level of the articular cartilage

the nerve is to be avoided, retraction must be gentle and, if difficulty in visualization of the joint is encountered, it is best to release the lateral collateral ligament with an attached piece of the lateral epicondyle. At the close of the procedure the continuity of the collateral ligament is reestablished by screwing the osteotomized piece of bone back into place. The capsule is opened laterally

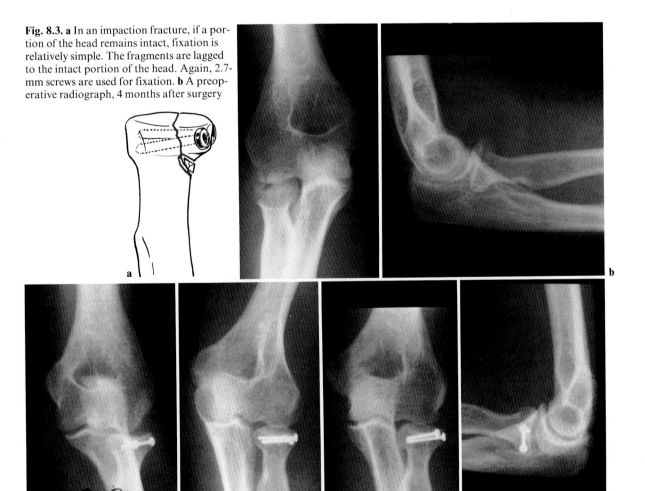

Fig. 8.3. a In an impaction fracture, if a portion of the head remains intact, fixation is relatively simple. The fragments are lagged to the intact portion of the head. Again, 2.7-mm screws are used for fixation. **b** A preoperative radiograph, 4 months after surgery

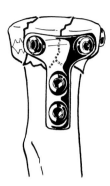

Fig. 8.4. If there is a transverse fracture of the neck, fixation of the head must be supplemented with a plate. The mini T plate must be carefully contoured and positioned in such a way as not to interfere with the radioulnar articulation in pronation or supination

and the radial head is visualized. Pronation and supination permit different portions of the head to be brought into direct vision. Another useful approach is dorsal. Exposure of the radial head and neck is achieved by detachment of the anconeus muscle from the ulna and the lateral epicondyle. This gives a better exposure of the medial portion of the head and of the radioulnar articulation.

8.4.4 Techniques of Reduction and Internal Fixation

8.4.4.1 Comminuted Fractures

The type III severely comminuted fracture in which there is no continuity of the head and neck cannot be reduced and fixed. The head is therefore excised. The decision whether a prosthetic replacement is carried out must be made individually. We feel that the only absolute indication for prosthetic replacement of the radial head is a dislocation of the elbow with rupture of the medial collat-

Fig. 8.5. Small, free, comminuted fragments can be reduced and fixed with lag screws. Because of their small size, they revascularize without collapse. **a** Note the displacement of the fragment. It blocked flexion of the elbow. **b** Six months after reduction and fixation

eral ligament, with or without an associated fracture of the olecranon. The prosthesis is required to act as a spacer and prevent valgus displacement and possible redislocation, even if a direct repair of the medial collateral ligament is carried out.

8.4.4.2 Wedge Fractures

These type I fractures are easily reduced and fixed with a lag screw. We have found the 2.7-mm cortical screw best for fixation of these fractures. If the screw is inserted through the articular cartilage of the head, it should be recessed below the articular surface (Fig. 8.2).

8.4.4.3 Impaction Fractures

These type II fractures, the commonest type, fall in complexity between type I and type III. The fragments are tilted, depressed, and impacted. Whether reduction and fixation is possible depends on the degree of comminution. If only one or two fragments are present, reduction is usually possible. The fragments should be elevated, provisionally fixed with a Kirschner wire, and then lagged to the remaining portion of the head and neck with one or two 2.7-mm screws as in type I. Since the injury is usually the result of a valgus force with the forearm in supination, the medial portion of the head and neck is usually intact (Figs. 8.3, 8.4, 8.5). Occasionally, the central comminution may be such that compression with a lag screw would narrow and distort the head. In such cases, cortical screws should be used for fixation. To accomplish this, all fragments should be drilled with the 2.0-mm drill bit and tapped with the 2.7-mm tap.

8.4.5 Postoperative Care

Suction drainage is used for the first 24 h. Stable fixation eliminates bone pain and makes it safe

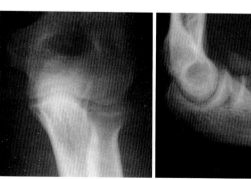
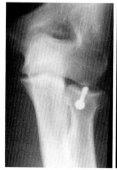
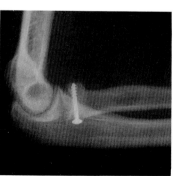

a   b

and possible to begin early active flexion-extension and pronation-supination exercises. We immobilize the elbow at 90° in a padded posterior splint. On the 2nd or 3rd day, the dressings are removed and, if no complications exist, active mobilization exercises are started. We discourage the use of a sling because it maintains the elbow in flexion. Pronation, supination, and flexion usually return almost to normal without much difficulty. The last 10°–15° of extension are very difficult to regain in both groups of patients, no matter what form of treatment is used. As with all intraarticular fractures more recently we have been using CPM during the postoperative phase.

Reference

Keon-Cohen BT (1966) Fractures of the elbow. J Bone Joint Surg 48A:1623–1639

9 Fractures of the Radius and Ulna

M. Tile

9.1 Introduction

Fractures of the forearm present unique management problems. In these particular diaphyseal fractures, perhaps more than any others, the combination of skeletal stability with mobility of the extremity is necessary to produce excellent functional results. The ASIF system of stable internal fixation is admirably suited to this end; therefore, it is not surprising that the use of this system in diaphyseal fractures of the radius and ulna has revolutionized their management and improved the end results.

9.2 Natural History

9.2.1 Closed Treatment

For many years, surgeons have grappled with the difficulty of restoring early function to the fractured forearm. Early authors recommended closed reduction followed by lengthy plaster immobilization, but the deficiencies of this method were soon recognized. Malunion and nonunion were frequent complications with resultant poor functional results.

Böhler (1936) recognized that to maintain skeletal length, continuous traction was often required. He recommended Kirschner wires inserted above and below the fracture and held by a plaster cast to achieve this goal; however, the results were not significantly improved. Perhaps the most severe indictment of the closed method was made by Hughston (1957), reporting 92% unsatisfactory functional results in the treatment of 41 isolated, displaced radial shaft fractures (Galeazzi type). Therefore, even Charnley (1961), in his classic treatise "Closed Treatment of Common Fractures", strongly recommended operative treatment of forearm fractures.

9.2.2 Open Treatment

Early attempts at enhancing the functional results by open reduction and internal fixation did little to improve the situation, but they represented pioneering efforts. Unstable fixation with inadequate and poorly applied plates required long-term plaster immobilization, again compromising the final results. In spite of the necessary cast immobilization, which resulted in some stiffness of the injured extremity, the nonunion rate remained significantly high. This was particularly evident in the report of Knight and Purvis (1949).

Smith and Sage (1957) attempted to change this outlook by the development of specialized intramedullary devices, with improved results, but their nonunion rate was unacceptably high. Intramedullary devices cannot restore the most important rotatory stability to the injured forearm. Also, they tend to straighten the normal dorsoradial bow of the radius and are therefore not well suited to this injury.

9.2.3 AO/ASIF Techniques

Major improvements in the results of this injury awaited the development of advanced techniques. Danis (1947) is generally credited with initiating the era of compression plates. The introduction of AO implants and the strict adherence to AO principles have changed the outlook dramatically. Stable internal fixation using these proven techniques has eliminated most external casts and splints; this, in turn, has led to markedly improved functional results for the patient, depending on the degree of soft tissue injury. Malunion should be eliminated with use of the proper technique and nonunion should almost disappear, further enhancing the results. Most recent surveys have indicated a nonunion rate of less than 5%. Even if nonunion does develop, the final result should not be compromised, since these patients, free of all external casts and splints, can maintain full function of the extremity during this period.

Lack of recognition of the important biological and biomechanical principles of modern techniques of internal fixation is the most common cause of failure. In our first 60 consecutive cases in which this method was used prior to obtaining the sophisticated skills later possessed, we achieved 90% excellent functional results (Tile and Petrie 1969). All our failures were technical, as were those of Anderson et al. (1975), who achieved union rates of 97.9% for the radius and 96.3% for the ulna, with excellent functional results. These results and those of others are a far cry from those reported only a decade earlier, when the usual scenario for the fractured forearm was an open reduction with imperfect fixation, requiring the use of a plaster cast for a minimum of 8–12 weeks. Even then, a nonunion rate for one or the other bone of 20% or more was expected.

9.3 Management

9.3.1 Principles

To achieve excellent results, anatomical reduction and stable fixation are required. The forearm fracture requires anatomical reduction for the following reasons: (a) restoration of normal radial and ulnar length will prevent subluxation of either the proximal or distal radioulnar joint and will re-establish length to the muscles controlling that most beautiful tactile instrument of the body, the hand; and (b) restoration of rotational alignment is essential for normal pronation-supination function of the forearm. The restoration of the normal dorsoradial bow of the radius is essential to maintain this rotatory function — again, difficult to achieve with intramedullary devices. Therefore, intramedullary devices are not suited for the treatment of forearm fractures and should rarely be used, if ever.

Anatomical reduction and stable internal fixation with plates will reduce pain and allow early soft tissue rehabilitation, without the use of external splints or casts. Rapid restoration of both hand and forearm function is assured by the use of plates, either as a tension band, axially compressing the fracture, or as a neutralization plate with prior interfragmental compression.

In summary, the forearm fracture, whether of one or both bones, more than any other diaphyseal fracture in the body, requires open anatomical re-duction with stable fixation, preferably with plates, for optimal functional results.

9.3.2 Indications for Surgery

As stressed in other chapters in this book, the indications for surgery in this type of fracture are dependent upon a knowledge of the natural history of the fracture combined with an assessment of its personality. *The natural history of the forearm fracture, under almost all circumstances, is so uncertain when treated by means other than anatomical open reduction, stable fixation with plates, and early motion of the extremity, that this treatment alone can be recommended in almost all of the cases described below.*

9.3.2.1 Fractures of Both Bones

For reasons previously discussed, displaced fractures of both radius and ulna should be treated by open reduction, stable internal fixation, and early motion.

9.3.2.2 Fracture of One Bone

a) Fractures of the Shaft of the Radius
or the Ulna with Radioulnar Subluxation
(Galeazzi or Monteggia Fractures)

Displaced single-bone fractures of the radius or ulna, if treated nonoperatively, have a notoriously poor outcome. Displacement at the fracture site is always accompanied by displacement at the corresponding radioulnar joint, whether proximal or distal. Reduction must be *absolutely anatomical* or subluxation of that radioulnar joint will remain, with significant functional loss. Therefore, the displaced fracture of the radial shaft with distal radioulnar subluxation (Galeazzi fracture; see Fig. 9.9b–e) and the displaced fracture of the ulnar shaft with proximal radioulnar subluxation (Monteggia fracture) constitute *absolute indications for surgery.*

b) Isolated Fracture of the Ulna

The management of this fracture, usually caused by a direct blow and not associated with a proximal radial head dislocation, has been a subject of controversy. Even with minimal displacement and prolonged immobilization in a plaster cast, union may be delayed (Fig. 9.1). Proximal ulnar fractures are the most dangerous, as they are subjected to a greater torque and may bow. Therefore,

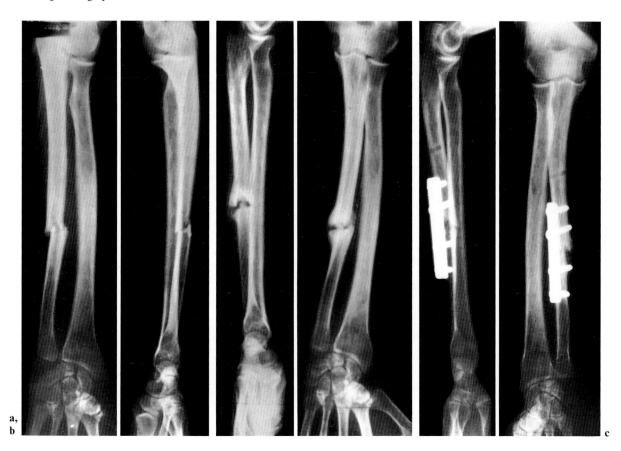

a,
b

c

to obviate these problems, surgery may be indicated for this seemingly innocuous fracture.

Recent reports by Sarmiento et al. (1975) and others dispute this, indicating universally good functional results with a simple below-elbow splint. We feel that most of these fractures, if relatively undisplaced, may be treated with casts or splints with the expectation of a good result (Fig. 9.2). However, in certain instances, open reduction and internal fixation may be preferable to prolonged splinting for the patient. In these cases, the patient should share in the decision-making process, after being informed of the advantages and disadvantages of each method (Fig. 9.3).

9.3.2.3 Open Fracture of the Forearm

Open fractures of the forearm require open reduction and internal fixation, for the same reasons as closed fractures do. Early restoration of mobility and function is even more important in these cases, so stability must be restored early. Some surgeons delay internal fixation for several days, but we prefer to fix the fracture at the time of

Fig. 9.1 a–c. Isolated fracture of the ulna — nonoperative **a** Anteroposterior and lateral radiographs of an isolated fracture of the ulna caused by a direct blow. No injury to the elbow or wrist is apparent. **b** After 24 weeks of immobilization in plaster, the radiograph shows nonunion requiring internal fixation (**c**)

the original cleansing and débridement, having noted no difference in the rate of sepsis or the complications in those so treated, where careful open wound management was maintained (Moed 1986).

9.3.3 Timing of Surgery

Since surgery is usually indicated for all displaced forearm fractures, we prefer to proceed with it as soon as possible following injury.

Early surgery is desirable but not essential. The advantages of early surgery are both technical and functional. One of the technical advantages is ease of reduction prior to shortening of the bone ends, which ensures the anatomical reduction so necessary in this fracture. Also, evacuation of the hema-

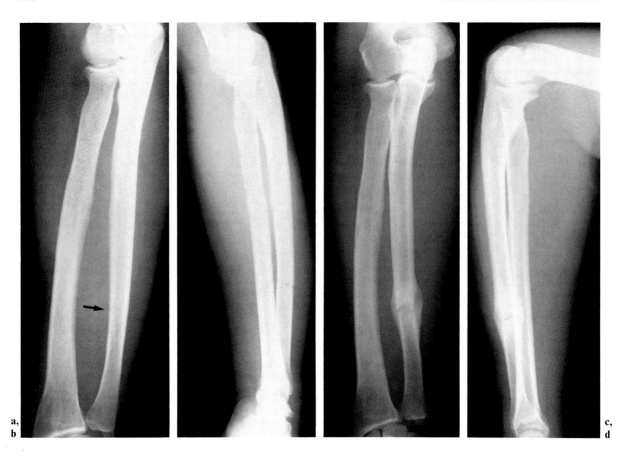

a,
b

c,
d

Fig. 9.2. a, b Anteroposterior and lateral radiographs of a 45-year-old man with an isolated undisplaced fracture of the ulna. After immobilization in a functional forearm brace for 16 weeks, the anteroposterior and lateral radiographs (c, d) show massive callus formation and bony union

toma, stable fixation of the fracture, and wound drainage allow the patient to move the hand and forearm early, thus eliminating the period of immobilization necessary if surgery is delayed, and aiding early functional recovery.

Surgery may be delayed by general factors, such as the poor state of the polytraumatized patient, in whom other musculoskeletal or visceral injuries have greater priority. Delay may also be necessary if the patient arrives late and the state of the soft tissues would compromise the surgery — for example, if fracture blisters are already present. Under these circumstances, the surgery should be performed at the earliest appropriate time.

We dispute the contention by Smith and Sage (1957) and others that delayed surgery will ensure union more often than immediate surgery, as measured by the formation of increased callus at the

fracture site. Without arguing the biological merits of delayed surgery, we feel that the present methods of internal fixation are so good that the possible added help of delayed surgery is not required. It would be difficult to improve on the present excellent results — namely 97%–98% union — by delaying surgery. The technical difficulties of reduction and the delay of functional recovery far outweigh any theoretical benefits in fracture healing.

Fig. 9.3a–h. Isolated fracture of the ulna — operative management. The anteroposterior and lateral radiographs (a, b) illustrate an isolated fracture in the distal third of the ulna in a 27-year-old urology resident. After discussing the options with the patient, it was elected to perform an open reduction and internal fixation using an interfragmental compression screw and a neutralization plate, as shown in the immediate postoperative radiographs (c, d). At 16 weeks, primary bone union is seen (e, f). The patient required no postoperative immobilization and returned to his internship within 2 weeks. The implants were removed 24 months after injury (g, h). The patient's functional result is excellent

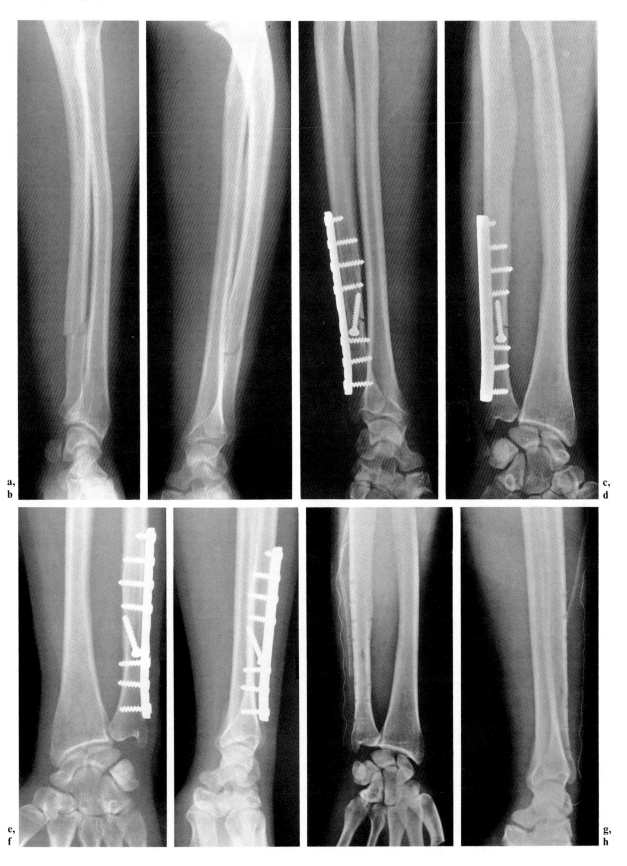

a,
b

c,
d

e,
f

g,
h

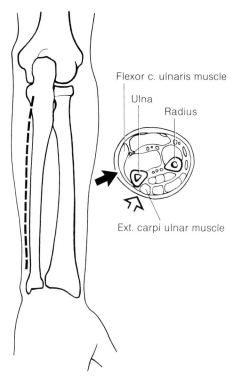

Fig. 9.4. Skin incision for a fracture of the ulna should never be made over the bone itself but always over soft tissue. This is true for all subcutaneous bones. The cross-sectional illustration indicates the approach between the flexor and extensor carpi ulnaris muscles

9.3.4 Surgical Technique

9.3.4.1 Preliminary Considerations

a) Positioning the Patient

We prefer the prone position for fractures of the ulna or fractures of both bones. The arm is placed on an arm board with the shoulder at 90°, allowing the ulna to be approached by pronation and the radius by supination. The same can be achieved by placing the patient in the lateral position with the arm on an arm board. This position is more suitable than the prone position for regional block anesthesia and for obese patients. In isolated fractures of the radius, the supine position may be used.

b) Tourniquet

We prefer a tourniquet in closed fractures to ensure a bloodless field, which reduces the operating time. In open fractures, however, the tourniquet should be in place but not used unless necessary to stop the oozing, which prevents proper identifi-

cation of the soft tissue structures such as nerves and vessels, increasing the difficulty of anatomical reduction of the fracture.

9.3.4.2 Surgical Approaches

a) Ulna

The approach to the ulna is relatively simple (Fig. 9.4). The ulna is a subcutaneous bone and is easily exposed throughout its length. However, as with other subcutaneous bones, the basic principle of making the skin incision over muscle rather than over bone must be followed. Therefore, we recommend an incision just off the subcutaneous border of the ulna, either on its anterior or posterior aspect, depending on which approach is used for the radius. The correct incision should allow the widest possible bridge between the ulnar and radial incision.

The direct approach to the bone is between the flexor carpi ulnaris and the extensor carpi ulnaris muscles. Periosteal stripping should be kept to a minimum, and all bone fragments with attached soft tissue should be handled carefully, to preserve that soft tissue and maintain bone viability.

b) Radius

Anterior Approach (Henry). There are several standard approaches to the radius. We prefer the anterior, as described by Henry (Fig. 9.5), especially in the proximal and distal thirds, for the following reasons:

1. The approach is extensile, allowing the surgeon to expose the radius from the elbow to the wrist. It is the only approach that allows a major reconstruction of the radius throughout its length.

2. In the upper third, the radial nerve is well protected by the supinator muscle belly during the primary operation. Of even greater importance is the relative safety of the radial nerve in secondary operations such as plate removal.

3. For plate application, this approach is ideally suited to the flat anterior surface of the lower third of the radius. Consideration of tensile versus compressive forces in plate application is not as important in the upper extremity as in the lower extremity; therefore, even on the curved upper and middle thirds of the radius, application on the anterior or anterolateral surface will not compromise the final results.

4. The technique is relatively easy if precise attention to detail is followed. Remember, an upper-third radial fracture in close proximity to the el-

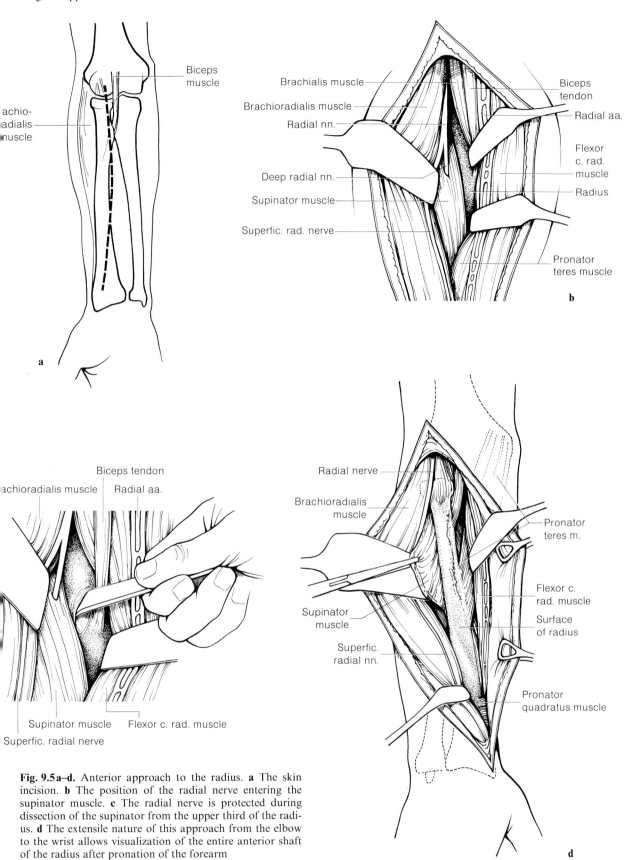

Biceps muscle

achio-
adialis
muscle

Brachialis muscle
Brachioradialis muscle
Radial nn.

Deep radial nn.
Supinator muscle
Superfic. rad. nerve

Biceps tendon
Radial aa.
Flexor c. rad. muscle
Radius
Pronator teres muscle

a

b

achioradialis muscle | Biceps tendon | Radial aa.

Supinator muscle   Flexor c. rad. muscle
Superfic. radial nerve

Radial nerve
Brachioradialis muscle
Supinator muscle
Superfic. radial nn.

Pronator teres m.
Flexor c. rad. muscle
Surface of radius
Pronator quadratus muscle

d

Fig. 9.5a–d. Anterior approach to the radius. **a** The skin incision. **b** The position of the radial nerve entering the supinator muscle. **c** The radial nerve is protected during dissection of the supinator from the upper third of the radius. **d** The extensile nature of this approach from the elbow to the wrist allows visualization of the entire anterior shaft of the radius after pronation of the forearm

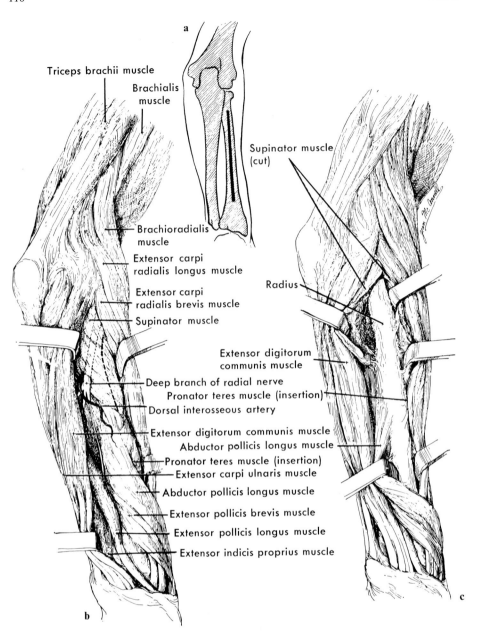

Fig. 9.6a–c. The posterior (Thompson) approach to the proximal middle third of the posterior surface of the radius. **a** Skin incision. **b** Relationship of supinator muscle to the deep branch of the radial nerve at the proximal third of radius. **c** Completed approach. (Reproduced by permission from: A.H. Crenshaw, "Surgical Approaches," in Edmondson and Crenshaw (eds.), *Campbell's Operative Orthopaedics*, 6th edn., St. Louis 1980, The C.V. Mosby Co.)

bow joint requires a generous incision, extending proximal to the anterior elbow crease. Otherwise, the surgeon will be working in a small "hole" and may damage the important neural structures in the area.

Posterior Approaches. The posterior approach of Thompson (Thompson 1918; Fig. 9.6) is especially suitable for the middle third of the radius, and we occasionally use this. However, it is not suitable for distal-third radial fractures because the posterolateral application of the plate may interfere with the outcropping tendons to the thumb, disturbing their function. Fractures of the upper third of the radius and ulna may also be approached by the Boyd technique (Boyd 1940; Fig. 9.7). Care must be taken in this approach to avoid injury to the radial nerve; therefore, it cannot be recommended for routine use.

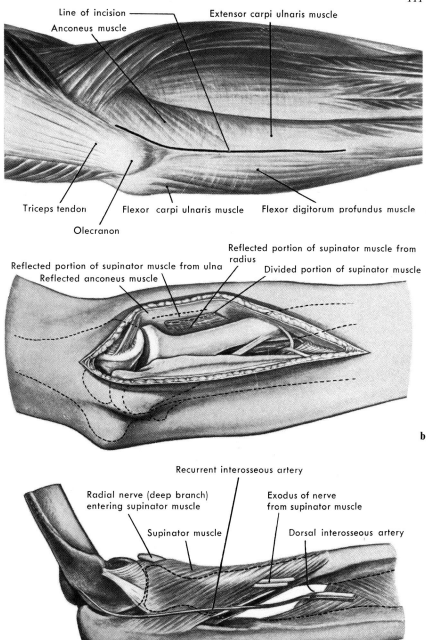

Line of incision

Anconeus muscle

Extensor carpi ulnaris muscle

Triceps tendon

Olecranon

Flexor carpi ulnaris muscle   Flexor digitorum profundus muscle   **a**

Reflected portion of supinator muscle from ulna
Reflected anconeus muscle

Reflected portion of supinator muscle from radius

Divided portion of supinator muscle

b

Recurrent interosseous artery

Radial nerve (deep branch) entering supinator muscle

Supinator muscle

Exodus of nerve from supinator muscle

Dorsal interosseous artery

c

9.3.4.3 Technique of Fracture Fixation

a) Principles of Stable Fixation

As previously indicated, to obtain maximum function the surgeon must achieve anatomical reduction and stable internal fixation. Stable internal fixation may be achieved by internal splinting with intramedullary devices or by compression. In the lower extremity, especially the femur, intramedullary fixation is a mainstay of treatment. However, in the forearm, intramedullary devices *do not con-*

Fig. 9.7a–c. The Boyd approach to the proximal third of the ulna and proximal fourth of the radius. **a** Skin incision. **b** Approach has been completed. **c** Relation of the deep branch of the radial nerve to the superficial and deep parts of the supinator muscle. (Reproduced by permission from: A.H. Crenshaw, "Surgical Approaches," in Edmondson and Crenshaw (eds.), *Campbell's Operative Orthopaedics,* 6th edn., St. Louis 1980, The C.V. Mosby Co.)

trol rotational stability and should therefore rarely be used (Fig. 9.8). Therefore, *compression*, with interfragmental screws or plates under tension, is the method of choice.

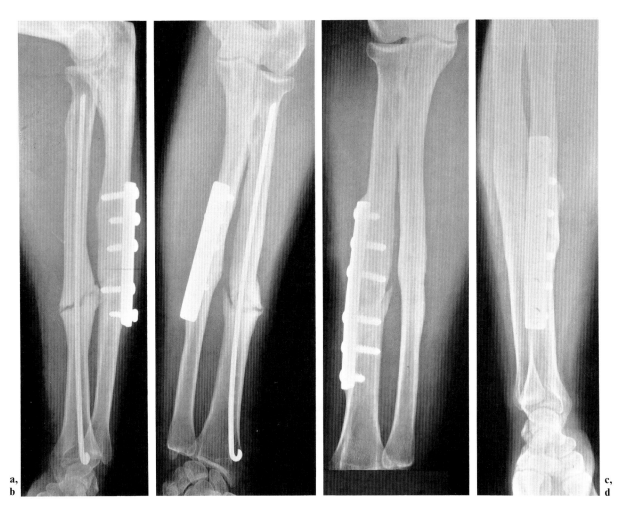

a,
b
c,
d

Fig. 9.8a–d. Intermedullary splinting of the radius. **a** Lateral and **b** anteroposterior radiographs at 9 months following open reduction and internal fixation of a fracture of both bones of the forearm. The ulna has been plated and has healed, although the distal screw in the plate is loose. The radius was treated with a Rush intermedullary rod and has not united. As this time, the patient had pain on movement and tenderness at the site. The rod was removed and a six-hole DC plate applied to this hypertrophic nonunion; the ulnar plate was removed at the same time. **c, d** Complete bony union 1 year after the second operative procedure

b) Methods by Fracture Type

Transverse or Short Oblique Fractures. If the fracture of the radius or ulna is either transverse or short and oblique, a plate under tension may be used to compress the fracture; that is, the plate is under tension, the fracture under compression. In the forearm, where exposure is often limited, *dynamic compression (DC) plates* should be used wherever possible, making the tension device unnecessary.

The application of a plate under tension in a transverse fracture, if carried out correctly, will afford compression to the fracture, thereby stabilizing it and allowing early motion (Fig. 9.9). The same is true of the short oblique fracture. However, in all cases where the obliquity of the fracture allows, a lag screw should be inserted through the plate across the fracture to increase rotational stability (Fig. 9.10).

Spiral or Comminuted Fractures. For spiral or comminuted fractures, interfragmental compression with lag screws is the keystone of treatment (Fig. 9.11). After anatomical reduction has been achieved, stability in such a fracture is best obtained by lag screws conferring compression to the fragments. These lag screws are the building blocks of all internal fixation. They should be used with appropriate techniques to completely stabilize the fracture and compress all the major fragments where possible.

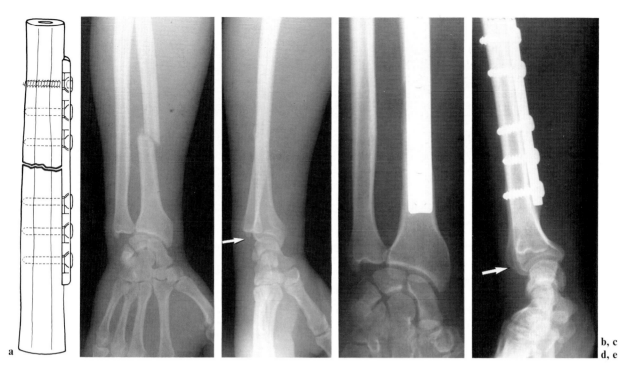

Fig. 9.9a–e. Fixation of a transverse fracture with a dynamic compression (DC) plate. **a** Application of a six-hole DC plate to a fracture of the radius or ulna. **b** Anteroposterior and **c** lateral radiographs of a 21-year-old man with a dis-placed fracture of the radius and a subluxation of the distal radioulnar joint (*arrow*). **d, e** Osteosynthesis of this transverse fracture at 1 year. Primary bone union is complete, the functional result excellent

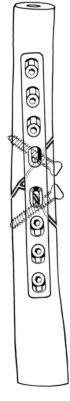

Fig. 9.10. Application of a lag screw through the plate and across an oblique fracture wherever possible, to increase the strength of the fixation

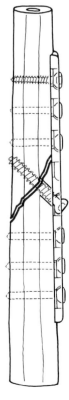

Fig. 9.11. Fixation of a forearm fracture with a butterfly. Following anatomical reduction, the butterfly is secured with interfragmental compression using lag screws. A neutralization plate is then applied

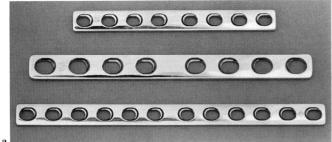

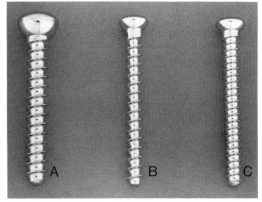

Once interfragmental compression has been achieved, a neutralization plate must be applied to protect the stability of the fracture (Fig. 9.11). Wherever possible, lag screws should be used through the plate and across any of the fracture lines, either in the spiral fracture or in the comminuted fracture, to increase the stability of the system.

c) Implant Selection

The choice of implant will depend upon the size of the bone. For large adult men we prefer the large, 4.5-mm DC plate on both the radius and the ulna. A six-hole plate is the preferred implant, allowing at least five cortices to be fixed on either side of the fracture; however, the length of the plate will ultimately depend on the degree of comminution present. The greater the degree of comminution, the greater should be the length of the plate, in order to achieve adequate fixation of the plate and prevent early mechanical overload and failure.

For smaller individuals, such as most adult women, the 3.5-mm, or small, DC plate is the implant of choice. These 3.5-mm plates may be used in any patient only if the warning below is heeded.

The 3.5-mm DC plates are not only smaller in width and thickness, but also shorter than their counterparts in the larger DC series; for example, an eight-hole large DC plate is 135 mm long, whereas an eight-hole small DC plate is only 97 mm long, as shown in Fig. 9.12a. Also, the 3.5-mm DC screw has less holding power; therefore, more screws are required to achieve stable fixation (Fig. 9.12b). A new 3.5-mm cortical screw has recently been introduced and is recommended for use with the 3.5-mm DC plate in the forearm. The holding power of the screw is increased by a larger shank (2.7 mm) and more threads per length. The instrumentation is characterized by a

Fig. 9.12. a An eight-hole 3.5-mm DC plate, an eight-hole 4.5-mm DC plate, and a 12-hole 3.5-mm DC plate. Note that the length of the 12-hole 3.5-mm plate is approximately equal to that of the eight-hole 4.5-mm DC plate, whereas the eight-hole 3.5-mm DC plate is much shorter. **b** A 4.5-mm cortical screw (*A*), a 3.5-mm cancellous screw (*B*), and the new 3.5-mm cortical screw (*C*)

new 2.5-mm drill. All of the instrumentation has a bronze coloration.

In those instances where small DC plates are chosen, one must be certain that the plate has sufficient length to neutralize the bending forces present and allow firm and rigid immobilization of the fracture. In tall individuals for whom the small 3.5-mm DC plate is chosen, an eight- to twelve-hole plate is essential, allowing for the fixation of a minimum of seven cortices on each side of the fracture. This will provide adequate holding of the plate for a sufficient length of time to allow both early motion of the extremity and sound union of the fracture. Use of the wrong implant may prejudice an otherwise excellent open reduction, as shown in Fig. 9.13, and lead to early failure of the osteosynthesis.

d) Site of Plate Application

The ulnar plate is applied to the medial border (Fig. 9.14). Occasionally, removal of bony irregularities from this surface will aid in the placement of the plate.

The radial plate application will depend on the surgeon's choice of incision. Since we favor the anterior approach, the radial plate is applied ideally to the flat surface of the lower third of that bone. Through this same anterior approach the plate may be fixed to the anterior or lateral surface of the middle third and the anterior surface of the upper third. Occasionally, difficulty may be encountered in applying the plate laterally through

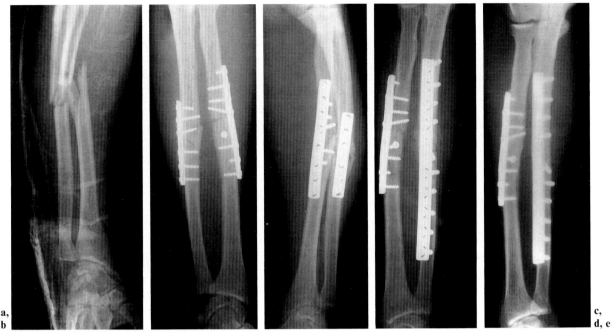

a,
b

c,
d, e

Fig. 9.13a–e. A short 3.5-mm DC plate on the ulna, resulting in failure. **a** Anteroposterior radiograph of a forearm
fracture in a tall 21-year-old man. The radius was fixed
with an eight-hole 3.5-mm DC plate and an interfragmental
compression screw. The ulna was fixed with a six-hole
3.5-mm DC plate, with no fixation in the butterfly fragment.
Note the short plate compared with the relatively long ulna,
allowing a long lever-arm effect. **b** Displacement of the fracture at 10 weeks. **c** Marked limitation of pronation-supination ensued in spite of plaster immobilization. At that time,
further surgery on the ulna allowed anatomical reduction
and application of a twelve-hole 3.5-mm DC plate (**d**). No
immobilization was necessary; good forearm rotation returned. **e** The final result at 18 months

the anterior incision. If posterior approaches are
preferred, especially in the middle third of the radius, the plates are fixed to the lateral or dorsolateral
surfaces.

e) Bone Grafts

Bone grafts are indicated when anatomical reduction has not been achieved due to comminution,
or when bone loss is a factor.

Comminution. If an anatomical reduction cannot
be achieved because of severe comminution, the
stability of the system may be jeopardized. Under
these circumstances, the race between implant failure and bone union is loaded against bone union.
Judicious use of cancellous bone grafts will ensure
rapid union prior to implant failure in almost all
cases and is therefore highly recommended. The
bone graft must not be placed along lacerations

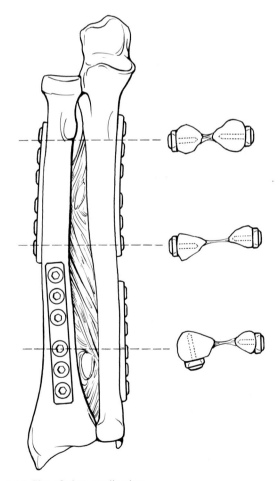

Fig. 9.14. Site of plate application

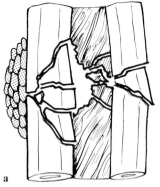

Fig. 9.15a–e. Bone grafts to forearm. **a** The graft should be placed on the surface of the bone opposite the interosseous membrane, which is usually torn, to prevent cross-union. **b** Anteroposterior and **c** lateral radiographs of a 39-year-old police officer who was struck by a bullet and sustained a fracture of his radius. Initial treatment was débridement, open wound treatment, and fixation with pins and plaster. Upon referral at 12 weeks the pins were removed, and after wound healing, a plate was applied to the anterior surface of the radius. **d, e** A massive cancellous bone graft allowed sound union of this fracture and a good functional result

a

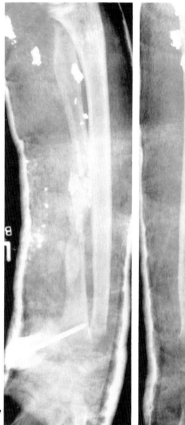
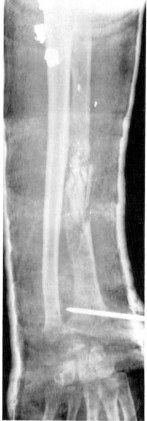
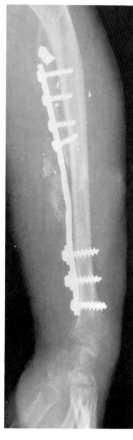
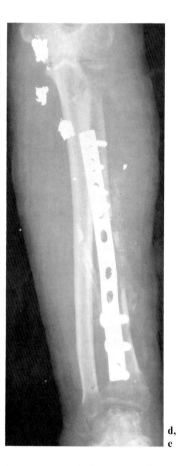

b,
c

d,
e

in the interosseous membrane, as this may favor a cross-union; it should be placed at sites distant from that membrane, to fill all gaps in the bone and to bridge the fracture (Fig. 9.15a).

Bone Loss. Cancellous grafting is especially indicated if there has been significant bone loss in open fractures. In these instances we prefer internal fixation with a plate to bridge the gap and the use of a cancellous bone graft, usually applied on the 5th to 7th day into a granulating wound, to ensure union (Fig. 9.15b–e).

On rare occasions, however, an external frame may be used. This method may be applied to the forearm, but it is not recommended, except for comminuted fractures of the distal end of the radius and contaminated open fractures with or without sepsis. If external fixation is used as the definitive treatment in diaphyseal fractures, bone grafting should be used to minimize the risk of nonunion.

f) Wound Closure

Skin closure must be carried out using a meticulous atraumatic technique and with no tension. Suction drainage will reduce hematoma formation and is always used postoperatively, where possible.

Not infrequently, in fractures of both bones of the forearm, swelling of the forearm muscles makes closure of one incision without tension difficult. *Under these circumstances, we do not hesitate to leave a portion of one wound open, even if it leaves a part of the implant exposed.* This has been so frequent in our practice that we now inform the patients preoperatively that they may require a secondary closure of one wound. The ulnar wound, located so close to the subcutaneous border, should always be closed. *The radial wound, over soft tissues, may be safely left open throughout a portion of its length, since careful placement of the metal implant will bury it under a muscle cover.* With early functional rehabilitation, the swelling rapidly disappears from the arm, and it is usually a simple matter to close the wound on the 5th to the 7th postoperative day with sterile tapes or fine sutures. Open treatment of the tense wound prevents necrosis secondary to pressure, prevents sepsis, and has little deleterious cosmetic effect.

Postoperative Care. If, at the end of the procedure, the surgeon feels that anatomical reduction with stable fixation has been accomplished, then early functional rehabilitation should be started. A bulky bandage is applied to the forearm with no plaster cast, and the patient is allowed to move elbow, wrist, and fingers in the immediate postoperative period. In the first 48 h the arm is elevated on a pillow or a stockinette support and suspended from an intravenous drip pole. The support is removed for elbow and wrist exercises. With stable fixation only soft tissue pain is present, and this quickly disappears from the wound area, making early restoration of function the rule. Even in those instances where one wound cannot be closed this program should be instituted, since exercise will reduce swelling and allow early secondary closure.

If the surgeon is concerned with the stability of one or both bones because of comminution or poor bone quality, then the bulky postoperative dressing may be removed on the 7th day and replaced with a small functional forearm splint, as described by Sarmiento et al. (1975). This will allow early motion and still afford protection to the internal fixation.

If the fixation is deemed to be stable, the patient should be encouraged to use the arm for all reasonable activities, but should not, prior to evidence of bony union, take part in sporting activities or do any heavy lifting. The patient should be seen at regular intervals, usually monthly, and follow-up radiographs should be taken. With stable internal fixation, the precise time of bone union is difficult to determine. If no untoward radiographic signs of failure are present, such as irritation callus, bone resorption at the fracture site, or loosening of the screws, and if no clinical signs of failure such as inflammation and pain appear, one may assume that healing is proceeding normally. Radiographic evidence of the fracture line disappearing with no evidence of irritation callus is a positive indication of union. The average time for union to occur will be 8–12 weeks, with delays often arising in markedly comminuted fractures requiring bone grafts. Once union has occurred, the patient is encouraged to resume his or her normal life style.

9.4 Special Considerations

9.4.1 Fractures of Both Bones of the Forearm

Definitive fixation of either fracture should not be carried out prior to the provisional stabilization of both. If either the radius or the ulna is firmly and rigidly fixed before careful reduction of the other fracture, reduction may prove impossible (Fig. 9.16a). Therefore, we usually provisionally expose and fix the fracture that appears simpler, either by location — as for example, the ulna rather than the radius — or by its nature — e.g., the transverse or oblique as opposed to the comminuted. Once the first fracture has been carefully exposed using small Hohmann retractors and provisionally fixed with a plate held in place by small reduction or Verbrugge clamps, the other bone is exposed and provisionally fixed in a similar manner (Fig. 9.16b). At this time the surgeon may proceed with definitive fixation of the fracture.

9.4.2 Fractures of One Bone

9.4.2.1 Fractures of the Radius with Distal Radioulnar Subluxation (Galeazzi)

Displaced fractures of the radius associated with some disruption of the distal radioulnar joint (Fig. 9.17) should be treated by open anatomical reduction and stable fixation (see Fig. 9.9b–e). This will restore the length of the radius, which in turn ensures the accurate reduction of the distal radioulnar joint, provided proper rotation has been restored. In most cases, no specific treatment is required for this distal injury. If a fracture has

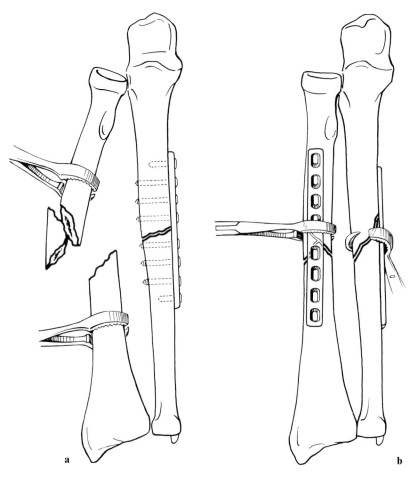

Fig. 9.16. a Fixation of one bone, in this case the ulna, will prevent reduction of the other. **b** Reduction of both bones prior to firm fixation is essential to prevent this intraoperative complication

occurred through the distal ulna, either through its styloid or distal portion, open reduction and screw fixation in that area will serve to stabilize the distal injury. In most cases, however, the injury occurs through soft tissue, and if the anatomy of the radius is restored by proper open reduction and stable internal fixation, the soft tissues of the distal radioulnar joint will usually heal without major functional impairment. The approach, techniques, and implants are as previously described for radial fractures.

Primary wound closure for a solitary radial fracture is usually easy to accomplish and open wound care is rarely required, except for an open fracture.

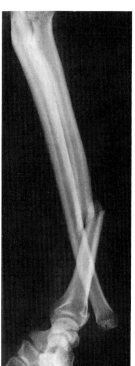

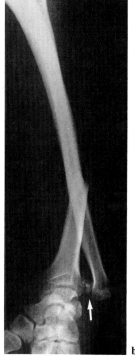

Fig. 9.17a, b. Anteroposterior and lateral radiographs of a fracture of the radius with a distal radioulnar subluxation. Note the small intra-articular fracture from the distal ulna (*arrow*). Open reduction and internal fixation of this fracture are essential

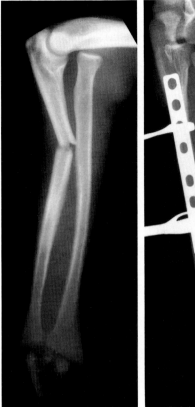
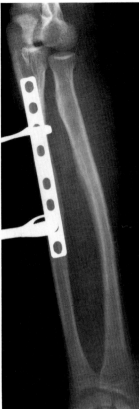
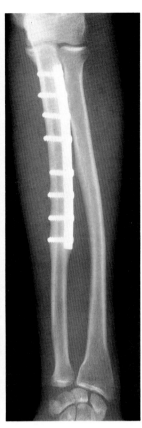

a

b,
c

If stability has been achieved in the radius, the postoperative program consists of a large bulky dressing on the forearm with elevation for the first 48 h and immediate encouragement of elbow, wrist, and hand motion. Patients may be moderately uncomfortable with a wrist injury, but we have not found the use of postoperative splinting to be necessary in most cases.

However, if the distal radioulnar joint is unstable following fixation of the radial fracture, the forearm should be immobilized in supination for 6 weeks.

9.4.2.2 Fractures of the Ulna

a) With Associated Radioulnar Dislocation (Monteggia)

Fractures of the ulna with associated radial head dislocations must be fixed by open anatomical reduction and stable internal fixation to achieve satisfactory results (Fig. 9.18). If the ulna is not anatomically reduced, the radial head will remain in a subluxed position (Fig. 9.19).

In most cases, following anatomical reduction and stable fixation of the ulna, the radial head will anatomically reduce and remain stable (Ta-

Fig. 9.18a–c. Fracture of the ulna with dislocation of the proximal radioulnar joint (Monteggia fracture). **a** Radiograph showing a displaced fracture of the ulna with a dislocated radial head. **b** Intraoperative radiograph showing anatomical reduction of the ulna with perfect position of the radial head. **c** At 1 year, sound primary bone union is seen following application of an eight-hole 3.5-mm DC plate. Note the perfect position of the radial head. Function in this 22-year-old engineering student was excellent. An injury to the radial nerve at the time of injury recovered in 3 months with no operative intervention to the nerve

ble 9.1). Therefore, following fixation of the ulna by techniques and implants already described, the surgeon should immediately examine elbow function. Using the image intensifier while the patient is under general anesthetic, he should determine the position of stability for the radial head. If the radial head is stable in all positions, then the postoperative program consists of early active motion of the extremity with no external splints.

If the radial head is unstable in various degrees of rotation or extension but stable at 90° of flexion, this usually indicates a malreduced ulna (Fig. 9.19). Either the ulnar length has not been restored or the rotation is not anatomical. The only logical method of dealing with this problem

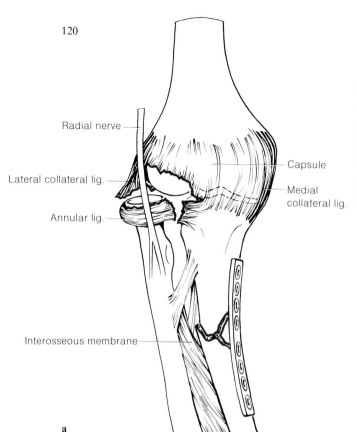

Radial nerve

Lateral collateral lig.

Annular lig.

Interosseous membrane

Capsule

Medial collateral lig.

a

Fig. 9.19a–e. Malreduction of the ulna, causing continuing subluxation of the radial head. **a** A fracture of the ulna plated in a valgus position. The radial head remains subluxated. **b** Radiograph of a comminuted fracture of the ulna with a displaced radial head. **c** An open reduction and internal fixation of the ulnar fracture resulted in a valgus position, in spite of interfragmental screws and a neutralization plate. Note the subluxation of the head of the radius of the small *arrow*. **d** The fracture was allowed to heal with persistent subluxation of the radial head (*arrow*). **e** Lateral view of the ulnar fracture and its flexed position. The patient had continuing pain in his elbow joint

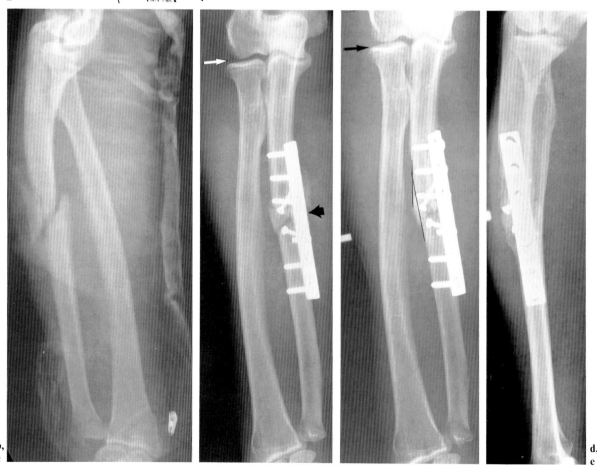

b, c

d, e

Table 9.1. Treatment of a Monteggia fracture

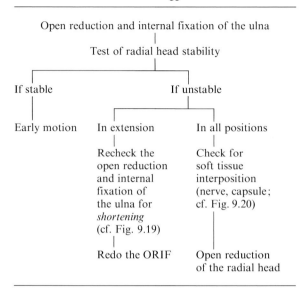

Open reduction and internal fixation of the ulna
|
Test of radial head stability

If stable → Early motion

If unstable:
- In extension → Recheck the open reduction and internal fixation of the ulna for *shortening* (cf. Fig. 9.19) → Redo the ORIF
- In all positions → Check for soft tissue interposition (nerve, capsule; cf. Fig. 9.20) → Open reduction of the radial head

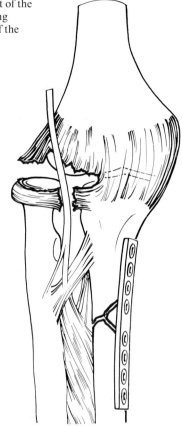

Fig. 9.20. Entrapment of the radial nerve preventing complete reduction of the radial head

is to take apart the ulnar fixation, start again, and ensure an anatomical reduction. The radioulnar subluxation should reduce fully and be stable in all positions. Occasionally, if concern continues, a cast brace to limit extension in the postoperative period may be used.

If, however, the radial head cannot be reduced or is grossly unstable in all positions except extreme flexion, then a direct operative approach should be made to the radial head to remove any soft tissue interposition — usually a torn annular ligament, but occasionally the radial nerve (Fig. 9.20). The radial head may be approached by extending the ulnar incision proximally toward the lateral epicondyle of the humerus. This posterior approach, reflecting the anconeus and extensor muscle origins anterolaterally, is safe, as it protects the radial nerve. After adequate exposure, the soft tissue interposition must be removed and the radial head reduced. After repair of the annular ligament, the stability of the radial head may be checked under direct vision, and if it is stable, early motion may be instituted, with or without a cast brace.

Gross instability of the radial head occurs in less than 10% of Monteggia fractures, so those instances requiring an open approach to the elbow are relatively few. However, Monteggia fractures have shown a greater tendency to result in permanent elbow stiffness than any other forearm fracture, as may be expected. Proper reduction of the ulna to restore proximal radioulnar stability and perhaps, in the future, the use of continuous pas-

sive motion in the immediate postoperative period may improve these functional results.

b) With Fracture of the Radial Head

In rare instances, a fracture of the shaft of the ulna may be associated with a fracture-dislocation of the radial head. Under these circumstances, the fragments of the radial head may act as a block to pronation and supination and may also prevent stabilization of the proximal radioulnar joint. Therefore, it is almost mandatory to open the elbow joint in this situation and inspect the fracture. If a single fragment is involved, it should be replaced with a lag screw to restore stability of the radial head. If the fracture is grossly comminuted, the only alternative method of treatment available is excision of the radial head and, if necessary, replacement with a Silastic or metal radial-head spacer to maintain the stability of the radius until soft tissue healing has occurred (Fig. 9.21).

In summary, the Monteggia fracture is a most challenging forearm injury for the surgeon. Stable anatomical fixation will restore ulnar length. A careful appraisal of the proximal radioulnar joint

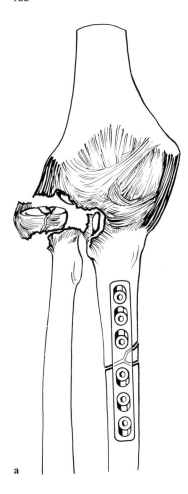

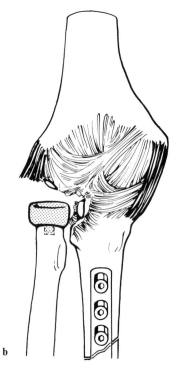

Fig. 9.21 a, b. Fracture of the proximal ulna with fracture of the radial head and neck. a A proximal ulnar fracture with a fracture of the radial neck with intra-articular extension. If the fracture of the radial head is comminuted, the ulnar fracture should be fixed internally and the radial head excised, and if unstable, it should be replaced with a radial head prosthesis (b)

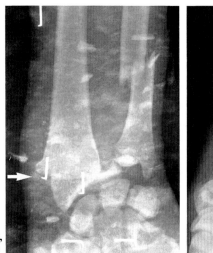

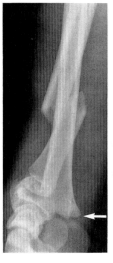

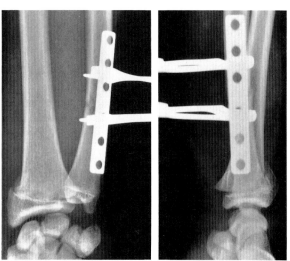

Fig. 9.22 a–l (continue see p. 123). Fracture of the ulna with distal periarticular radial fracture.
a Anteroposterior b lateral radiographs of a fracture of the distal ulna and an epiphyseal separation of the distal radius in a 16-year-old boy. c, d Intraoperative radiographs indicating the dorsal displacement of the radial epiphysis, even with anatomical reduction of the ulna. e, f The ulnar fracture was fixed with the distal radial epiphysis displaced 30°.

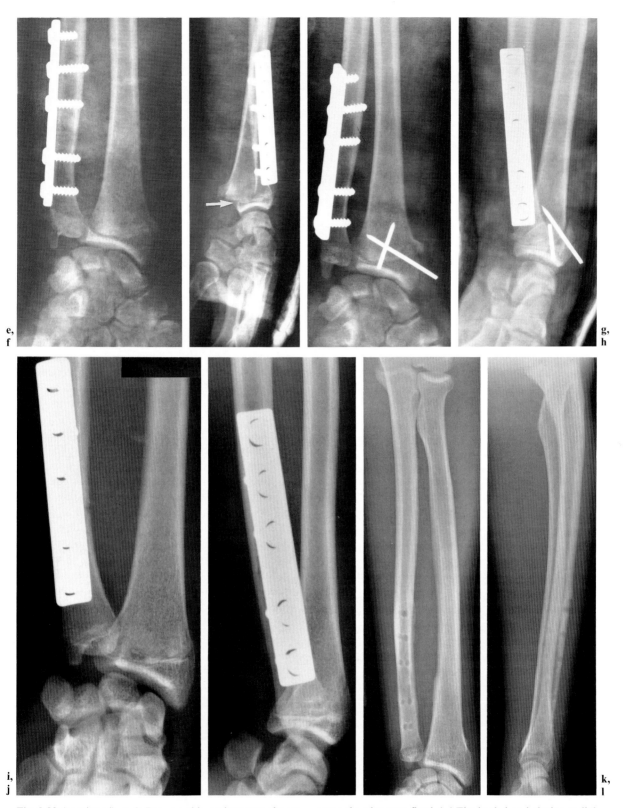

Fig. 9.22 (continued). **g, h** Because this patient was almost at the end of his growth, the position was deemed inadequate and an open reduction and internal fixation using Kirschner wires was performed. Reduction was difficult be-cause the ulna was fixed. **i, j** The healed and closing radial epiphysis and union of the ulnar fracture. **k, l** At 2 years the ulnar plate was removed. Note the anatomical reduction of the radius and ulna. At this time, function was excellent

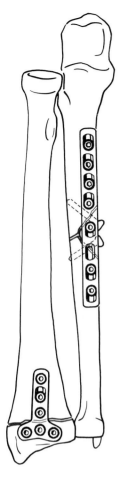

Fig. 9.23. Use of a buttress plate on the distal radius

will aid the surgeon in choosing the most appropriate technique for dealing with the injury and will allow a program of early functional rehabilitation.

c) With Distal Periarticular Radius Fracture

Fractures of the shaft of the ulna associated with distal radial epiphyseal fractures are relatively uncommon, but difficult to manage when they occur. The ulnar shaft fracture does not usually pose a major problem and should be treated as previously indicated. However, the distal radial metaphyseal fracture is often comminuted, unstable, and difficult to fix. If stable fixation of the radius is not achieved, early motion cannot be started, and problems of wrist stiffness and shortening of the radius are common (Fig. 9.22).

Therefore, the distal fracture of the radius requires careful evaluation. If the fracture is not grossly comminuted and the surgeon feels that internal fixation is possible, then this is the ideal treatment. The preferred appliance is the small buttress plate (Fig. 9.23).

In many circumstances, however, the fracture of the distal end of the radius is too grossly comminuted to support a buttress plate. In such cases we favor the use of an external fixation device to maintain continuous traction of the fracture while healing progresses, usually for a period of 6–8 weeks (Fig. 9.24).

The postoperative program for these individuals will, of course, vary with the ability of the surgeon to achieve stability of the distal radial fracture. Motion of the elbow and the fingers should always be encouraged. It is only the wrist function that may be compromised in this situation.

9.4.3 Fractures of the Forearm in Adolescents

Most forearm fractures in children should be managed by closed means, whereas almost all such fractures in adults require open treatment. Remodeling of a bone following a fracture in a child is dependent on several factors, including the proximity of the fracture to the joint, the direction of deformity, and the age of the patient. The greatest correction is possible in fractures close to the joint with deformities in the line of joint motion, for example, dorsal angulation in the radius; also, the younger the child, the greater the potential for remodeling.

A diaphyseal forearm fracture is distant from the joint, and the greatest deformity is often rotatory; therefore, there is little chance of complete remodeling in children approaching adolescence. The presence of an open epiphysis will not guarantee a good result by closed means. The surgeon must assess the growth potential of the patient, as in scoliosis management. If growth is unlikely to result in adequate remodeling in the time remaining, then open reduction and internal fixation should be performed.

Most girls over the age of ten and most boys over the age of twelve are better treated by internal fixation to ensure a perfect functional result — allowances being made, of course, for individual differences.

9.4.4 Open Fractures of the Forearm

The indications for open reduction in the forearm are so strong that we do not vary our technique for an open fracture. The general principles in the management of all open fractures apply. Careful cleansing and débridement are mandatory. Once

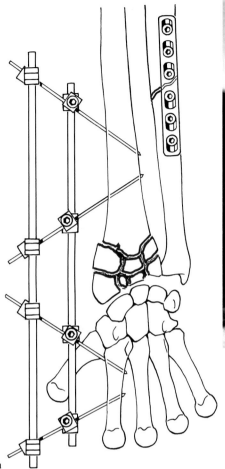

a

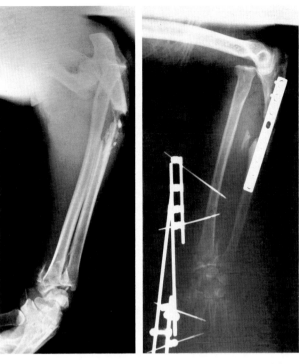

b,
c

Fig. 9.24a–c. Fracture of the ulna with a comminuted fracture of the distal radius. **a** Open reduction and internal fixation of the ulnar fracture, with external skeletal fixation of the distal radial fracture. **b** Severe comminution of the distal radius, with bone loss and severe comminution of the proximal ulnar fracture. **c** The distal radius shows a satisfactory reduction with external skeletal fixation. Note, however, that the malreduction of the ulna with shortening has allowed the radial head to displace anteriorly. Note also the fracture in the radial head. Further surgery was required to lengthen the ulna, correct the flexion deformity, and allow stabilization of the radial head

these have been achieved, we proceed immediately to open anatomical reduction and internal fixation. We feel that the advantages of early stable fixation in the open forearm fracture greatly outweigh the theoretical disadvantages. If exemplary soft tissue management is carried out there is no increased risk of sepsis. However, the importance of the soft tissue management cannot be overemphasized. If the wound is small, careful assessment of the soft tissues is required in order to choose the appropriate approach. After stabilization of the fracture, the surgical incisions should be closed but the small puncture wound left open.

If the wound is large, with varying degrees of skin and soft tissue loss, we again proceed with the necessary fracture stabilization as soon as possible (Fig. 9.25). Careful preoperative planning is essential so that, wherever possible, the metal implant is buried under viable muscle. The skin is left open and covered with a gauze dressing to prevent drying. The patient is returned to the operating room on the 3rd to the 5th postoperative day and the wound inspected.

If there has been no skin loss, and the wound is clean and granulating at that time, wound closure using fine sutures or sterile strips is effected over suction drainage. If the wound is not suitable for resuturing it is left to granulate by secondary intention or covered by a split-thickness skin graft when it is ready.

If skin was lost at the time of injury, closure may be carried out by split-thickness grafting or other techniques, depending on the depth and extent of the wound. A healthy layer of granulating tissue must, of course, have covered the wound before a skin grafting procedure can be attempted.

In cases with bone loss we prefer to delay the bone-grafting procedure until the first or second

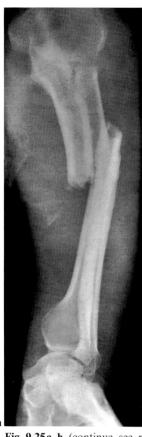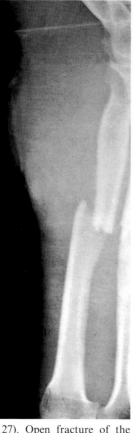

Fig. 9.25a–h (continue see p. 127). Open fracture of the forearm.
a Anteroposterior and **b** lateral radiographs of a 51-year-old man who caught his hand in a garbage incinerator, causing a major soft tissue avulsion and fractures of both bones of the forearm.

dressing change, between the 5th and 10th days post trauma. At that time, only cancellous bone graft may be inserted through the open wound, if it is clean and granulating. No cortical bone must be used, as it does not resist infection well. Again, as previously discussed, if there is no skin loss the wound is closed over suction drainage, but if there is skin loss and a layer of granulating tissue has appeared, the appropriate cover can be used, as outlined above. Occasionally, with complex bone and deep soft tissue muscle loss, a free myocutaneous-osseous flap may be indicated. With or without skin closure, early functional rehabilitation is started. If the fracture fixation is firm, finger and wrist motion is started within 48 h. If a gap exists at the fracture site, or the degree of comminution prejudices the stability of the system, then a simple functional forearm splint will be sufficient to allow early motion.

We have used these techniques even in the face of grossly contaminated wounds with few ill effects; other authors have had similar experiences (Moed 1986).

In summary, we feel that the management of open fractures of the forearm should consist of the following principles:

– Careful cleansing of the soft tissues and bone
– Antitetanus and antibiotic treatment, instituted immediately
– Careful cleansing and débridement of the soft tissues in the operating room
– Anatomical open reduction and stable fixation of the fractures
– Open management of the soft tissues, with the metal implants buried under muscle where possible
– Secondary skin closure or skin grafting where indicated and secondary bone grafting where necessary
– With major muscle loss, complex myocutaneous or composite myocutaneous-osseous free flaps
– Early functional rehabilitation of the extremity

9.5 Complications

9.5.1 Radioulnar Synostosis

This unfortunate complication may occur with 1%–8% of fractures of the forearm, and may greatly distress both the patient and the surgeon. Among our first 60 reported cases we had two examples (Tile and Petrie 1969). Anderson et al. (1975) reported an incidence of 1.2%, Teipner and Mast (1980), 4.8%. Botting (1970) reported ten cases from the Birmingham Accident Hospital but gave no incidence. This complication may occur with any method of treatment, but it is more common in severely comminuted or open fractures and more common with open reduction. We believe that delayed open treatment of a forearm fracture increases the risk of synostosis considerably. Seven of Botting's ten cases had delay of internal fixation, and this was also true in the Teipner and Mast series. One of our two cases had delayed open reduction (Fig. 9.26); in the other, an unusual case of "wrenched" elbow, synostosis was perhaps unavoidable, considering the magnitude of the injury (Fig. 9.27). To avoid this complication, we recommend immediate primary surgery for the fractures, with great care being taken to refrain from placing bone-graft material around the disrupted interosseous membrane. Any bone graft should be placed as far from that membrane as possible.

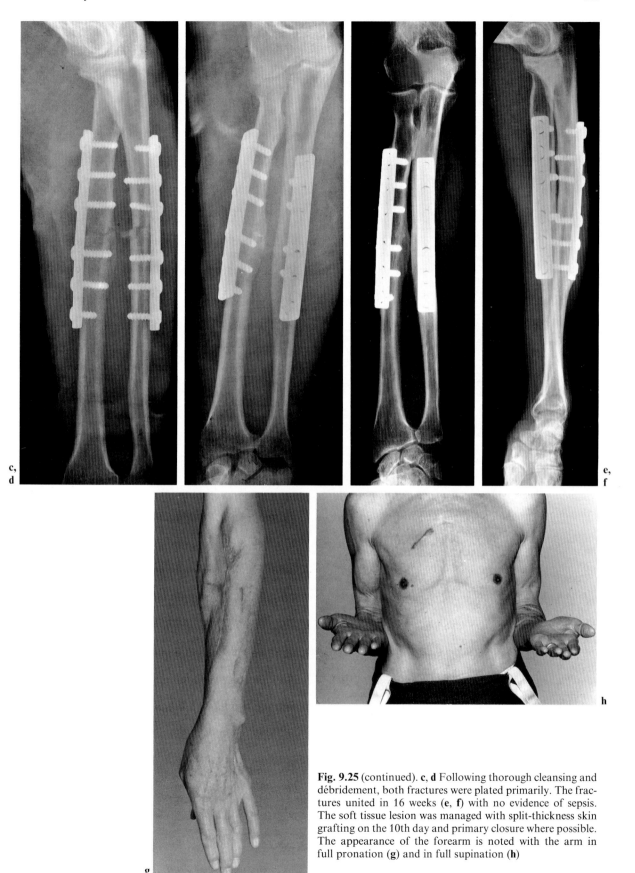

Fig. 9.25 (continued). **c, d** Following thorough cleansing and débridement, both fractures were plated primarily. The fractures united in 16 weeks (**e, f**) with no evidence of sepsis. The soft tissue lesion was managed with split-thickness skin grafting on the 10th day and primary closure where possible. The appearance of the forearm is noted with the arm in full pronation (**g**) and in full supination (**h**)

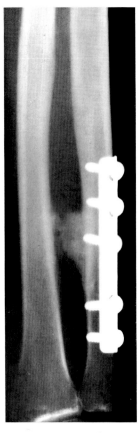

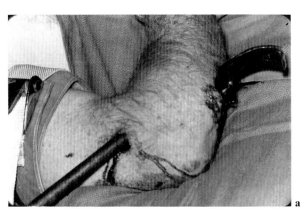

Fig. 9.27a–c. Cross-union due to open injury. A workman's ▶ arm was impaled by a flying wrench, shown in the clinical photograph (a) and the radiograph (b). After removal of the wrench, both bones were plated (c). A solid cross-union developed. (Courtesy of Dr. Glen A. McDonald)

Fig. 9.26. Cross-union. Anteroposterior radiograph of a 39-year-old man with an isolated fracture of the ulna treated with a five-hole plate. No bone graft was used. Note the massive cross-union developing 24 weeks following injury

9.5.2 Stress Fracture

Stress fractures may occur at the ends of either plate. The use of a single screw through the proximal and distal hole may reduce this incidence by allowing a more gradual stress distribution.

9.5.3 Refracture and Plate Removal

We cannot be dogmatic about the question of plate removal in the forearm following bone union. In general, *we do not routinely remove plates from upper extremities*. We suggest removal in young individuals, or in patients who have some pain, especially due to the subcutaneous ulnar plate, or to the lower screw of the radial plate, which often interferes with the function of the extensor pollicis longus muscle. *The plates should never be removed until the cortex has returned to a normal radiographic appearance — in general, a minimum of 2 years following injury*. Early removal of the plate has resulted in many refractures, which are most embarrassing to the surgeon and most difficult for the patient. If a plate is to be removed, the patient should be immobilized in a functional forearm splint for a 6-week period. This will help to reduce the number of refractures but will not completely prevent them.

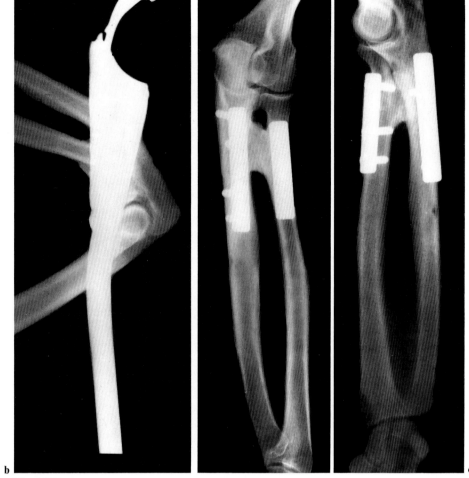

b

Fig. 9.27 b, c

c

References

Anderson LD, Sish TD, Tooms RE, Park WI (1975) Compression plate fixation in acute diaphyseal fractures of the radius and ulna. J Bone Joint Surg 57-A:287–297

Böhler J (1936) Treatment of fractures. Wright, Bristol, p 421

Botting TD (1970) Post-traumatic radioulna cross-union. J Trauma 1:16–24

Boyd HB (1940) Surgical exposure of the ulna and proximal third of the radius through one incision. Surg Gynecol Obstet 71:86

Charnley J (1961) Closed treatment of common fractures, 3rd edn. Livingstone, Edinburgh

Danis R (1947) Théorie et pratique de l'ostéosynthèse. Masson, Paris

Hughston JD (1957) Fractures of the distal radial shaft, mistakes in management. J Bone Joint Surg 39-A:249–264

Knight RA, Purvis GD (1949) Fractures of both bones of the forearm in adults. J Bone Joint Surg 31-A:755–764

Moed BR, Kellom JF, Foster RJ, Tile M, Hansen ST Jr (1986) Immediate internal fixation of open fractures of the diaphysis of the forearm. J Bone Joint Surg [Am] 68(4):1008–1017

Sarmiento A, Cooper JS, Sinclair WF (1975) Forearm fractures. J Bone Joint Surg 57A:297–304

Smith H, Sage FP (1957) Medullary fixation of forearm fractures. J Bone Joint Surg 39-A:91–98

Teipner WA, Mast JW (1980) Internal fixation of forearm diaphyseal fractures: double plating versus single compression (tension-band) plating — a comparative study. Orthop Clin North Am 3:381–91

Thompson JE (1918) Anatomical methods of approach in operations on the long bones of the extremities. Ann jSurg 68:309

Tile M, Petrie D (1969) Fractures of the radius and ulna. J Bone Joint Surg 51-B:193

Part III
Fractures of the Pelvis and Acetabulum

10 Fractures of the Pelvis

M. TILE

10.1 Introduction

In the past decade, traumatic disruption of the pelvic ring has become a major focus of orthopedic interest. Previously, conventional orthopedic wisdom held that surviving patients with disruptions of the pelvic ring recovered well clinically from their musculoskeletal injury. However, the literature on pelvic trauma was mostly concerned with life-threatening problems and paid scant at-

tention to the late musculoskeletal problems reported in a handful of articles published prior to 1980. In spite of the clinical impressions that most patients do well, some authors have suggested otherwise.

Holdsworth (1948) reported on 50 pelvic fractures and indicated that of the 27 patients with a sacroiliac dislocation, 15 had significant pain and were unable to work, whereas those with a sacral or iliac fracture had more satisfactory re-

Fig. 10.1. a Anteroposterior radiograph of a 19-year-old woman with a relatively undisplaced stable fracture of the pelvis involving the left sacrum and all four pubic rami. With simple bed rest the fractures healed in excellent position with no permanent disability. Compare this to the anteroposterior radiograph (b) of a 21-year-old male who sustained a crush injury to the pelvis. The degree of instability of this fracture was not recognized. This patient was also treated with bed rest while his extremity fractures were tended. c Anteroposterior radiograph showing his final result. Note the marked shortening, as indicated by the *two upper arrows*, and the severe rotatory deformity of the right hemipelvis. Note also the extremely high position of the right ischial tuberosity, which made sitting almost impossible (*lower arrow*). Comparison of these two cases is like comparing apples to oranges or chalk to cheese

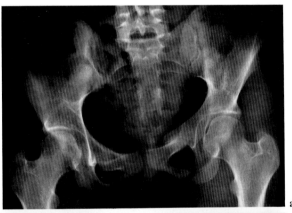

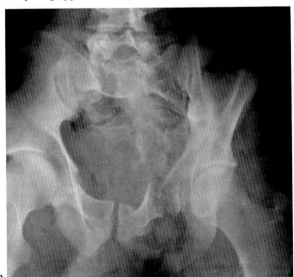

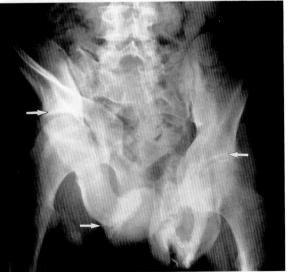

sults. Pennal and Sutherland (1959), in a large, unpublished study of 359 cases, further suggested that patients with unstable vertical shear injuries had many late complications. Slätis and Huittinen (1972), and Monahan and Taylor (1975) both confirmed the significant percentage of late musculoskeletal problems.

In reading the literature, one must determine the case mix for each series, otherwise the conclusions may be erroneous. Pelvic fractures must be classified according to their degree of instability or severity. If a series contains a large number of stable, inconsequential fractures, the overall results with simple treatment will be excellent, whereas if it contains a high percentage of displaced, unstable pelvic disruptions, the results with simple treatment will be quite different (Fig. 10.1). Therefore, in reading the literature, we must be certain that we are not comparing apples with oranges or chalk with cheese.

10.2 Natural History

In an attempt to further elucidate the incidence and severity of the early and late musculoskeletal complications of this injury, we undertook a clinical study in association with R. Lifeso, D. Dickinson, and R. McBroom (Dickinson et al. 1982). The purpose of this study was to place the management of this injury in perspective by determining which pelvic fractures had the poorest prognosis. With the current trend to internal fixation of the pelvis, a study of the natural history of this injury is even more important, in order to place that trend in perspective, for without a knowledge of the natural history, logical decision making becomes impossible. The results of our review of 248 cases are shown in Tables 10.1–10.5.

In this study, every patient was recalled, personally interviewed, examined, and radiographed using the inlet, outlet, and anteroposterior views. The conclusions may be summarized as follows:

1. *Stable* injuries gave few major long-term problems. Pain, if present, was usually mild or moderate.
2. By contrast, patients with *unstable* pelvic disruptions had many problems at review. Approximately 30% of this group had continuing pain, including 3% with nonunion of the posterior complex, and 5% with malunion, defined as having a greater than 2.5-cm leg length discrepancy. Also, 5% had permanent nerve dam-

Table 10.1. Comparison of Series A and Series B Patients[a]. (From Tile 1984)

	Series A 148 Cases	Series B 100 Cases
1. Age (range)	34.2 yr (15–81)	30.9 yr (14–85)
2. Sex		
Male	91	55
Female	57	45
3. Injury types		
Motor vehicle accidents	89 (60%)	81
Fall	17 (11.5%)	11
Crush	34 (23%)	4
Miscellaneous	8 (5.5%)	4
4. Workmen's Compensation Board	43 (29%)	5
5. Associated injuries		
CNS	31 (21%)	38
Chest	19 (13%)	15
Gastrointestinal	10 (6.6%)	20
Genitourinary		
Bladder	17 (11%)	8
Urethra	6 (4%)	4
Nerve	12 (8%)	3
Musculoskeletal	63 (43%)	10
6. Follow-up average	60 mo	2 yr

[a] In Tables 10.1–10.5, series A is a group of 148 cases of pelvic fracture managed in Toronto teaching hospitals and in nonteaching hospitals in Ontario, retrospectively reviewed; series B consists of the first 100 cases of pelvic fracture treated at the Sunnybrook Medical Center, Toronto, prospectively reviewed

Table 10.2. Factors resulting in unsatisfactory results. (From Tile 1984)

	Series A: 37/148	Series B: 35/100
Pain	37	32
Leg length discrepancy >2 cm	7	2
Nonunion	5	3
Permanent nerve damage	9	3
Urethral symptoms	5	1
Deaths		17

age, and 3% continuing urethral problems following urethral rupture.

The pain, when present, usually arose from the posterior sacroiliac joint area or from the lower lumbar spine. Computed tomography (CT) has shown lumbar spine involvement in significant numbers of patients with pelvic disruption. The pain in these cases was more severe, and usually

Table 10.3. Pain (moderate and severe). (From Tile 1984)

	Series A: 148 Cases				Series B: 100 Cases			
	No.	Nil	Moderate	Severe	No.	Nil	Moderate	Severe
Incidence	53 (36%)	–	–	–	35	–	–	–
Location								
Posterior	47 (32%)	–	–	–	32	–	–	–
Anterior	6 (4%)				3			
Severity								
Anteroposterior								
Compression	23	14	8	1	6	3	3	
Lateral compression	86	47	35	4	69	53	16	
Unstable (shear)	9	4	2	3	25	9	13	3
Total	118[a]	65	45	8	100	65	32	3

[a] Thirty cases with major acetabular involvement were not considered in this total

Table 10.4. Leg length discrepancy (malunion). (From Tile 1984)

Amount (cm)	Series A (%)	Series B (%)
0	64	68
0–1	19.5	19
1–2	11.5	11
>2	5	2

associated with an unreduced sacroiliac dislocation or a nonunion.

In summary, the natural history of pelvic trauma depends on the degree of violence, the type of injury, the method of treatment, and the presence or absence of complications such as a urethral tear, permanent nerve damage, malunion, malreduction of the sacroiliac joint, or nonunion. The unstable vertical shear injury results in a significant number of permanent problems resulting in posterior pain.

Therefore, it is obvious that most of our energies should be directed to the management of the unstable vertical shear injury, especially if the sacroiliac joint is dislocated or subluxated, since more stable injuries achieve good to excellent results when managed by simple means, as will be described.

10.3 Pelvic Biomechanics

In order to better understand our proposed classification and rationale of management, some knowledge of pelvic biomechanics is essential.

10.3.1 Ring Structure of the Pelvis

Firstly, the pelvis is a true ring structure. It is self-evident that if the ring is broken in one area and displaced, then there must be a fracture or dislocation in another portion of the ring. Thus, the vast literature describing anterior or posterior pelvic fractures suggesting that they appear in isolation is misleading. Gertzbein and Chenoweth (1977), in a series of patients with *undisplaced* anterior

Table 10.5. Results by fracture type. (From Tile 1984)

	Series A: 148 Cases					Series B: 100 Cases				
	Total No.	Satisfactory		Unsatisfactory		Total No.	Satisfactory		Unsatisfactory	
		No.	%	No.	%		No.	%	No.	%
Anteroposterior compression	23	18	78	5	22	6	3	50	3	50
Lateral compression	114	79	69	35	31	69	53	77	16	23
Unstable (shear)	9	5	56	4	44	25	9	36	16	64

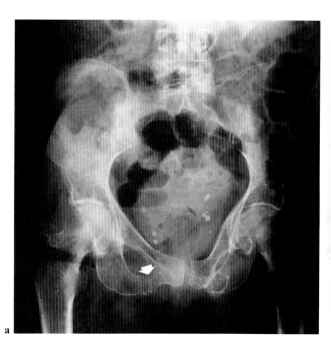

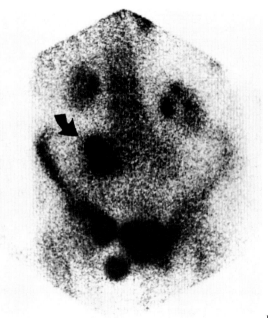

a

b

Fig. 10.2. a Radiograph of a patient with an apparently undisplaced fracture of the inferior and superior pubic ramus on the right side (*white arrow*). No lesion is seen posteriorly. The deformity of the left hemipelvis represents a mal-union of an old left acetabular fracture. **b** Technetium polyphosphate bone scan of the same patient clearly showing the increased uptake of the superior and inferior pubic ramus fracture anteriorly, but also a massive increased uptake at the right sacroiliac joint, indicating a posterior lesion (*black arrow*). (From Tile 1984; courtesy of Dr. S.D. Gertzbein)

pelvic fractures noted that a technetium polyphosphate bone scan of the posterior sacroiliac complex gave a positive reading in every case, indicating the definite presence of a posterior lesion (Fig. 10.2). This was further confirmed in the recent publication of Bucholz (1981), in which posterior lesions at autopsy were found in all patients with pelvic trauma even when the radiograph had revealed only an anterior lesion.

The anterior pelvic lesion may be through the symphysis pubis or through the pubic rami unilaterally or bilaterally. A symphysis disruption may also occur with pubic rami fractures. The posterior lesion may be a fracture of the ilium, often in the coronal plane, a dislocation or fracture-dislocation of the sacroiliac joint, or a fracture through the sacrum (Fig. 10.3). The commonest lesion is a sacral fracture followed by a combined injury, that is, a fracture dislocation of the sacroiliac joint, usually with a portion of the ilium remaining attached to the main sacral fragment.

Of greater importance than the site of the posterior lesion is the degree of displacement of the posterior sacroiliac complex. This can best be seen on the inlet radiograph showing posterior displacement of the so-called sacrogluteal line (Fig. 10.4) and is best confirmed by CT scan. Therefore, the posterior lesion, although present, may be undisplaced and have intact posterior ligaments, often associated with a sacral crush, or may be displaced with a major ligamentous disruption of the posterior pelvic complex (Fig. 10.5).

10.3.2 Stability of the Pelvis

This leads us to a discussion of pelvic stability. Stability may be defined as the ability of the pelvis to withstand physiological forces without significant displacement. It is obvious that pelvic stability is dependent not only on the bony structures but also on the strong ligamentous structures binding together the three bones of the pelvis, that is, the two innominate bones and the sacrum. If one removes these ligamentous structures, the pelvis falls into its three component parts.

The stability of the pelvic ring depends upon the integrity of the posterior weight-bearing sacroiliac complex (Fig. 10.6). The major posterior ligaments are the sacroiliac, the sacrotuberous, and the sacrospinous.

The intricate posterior sacroiliac complex is a masterly biomechanical structure able to with-

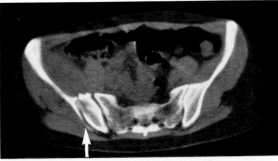

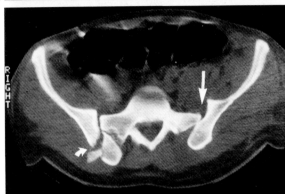

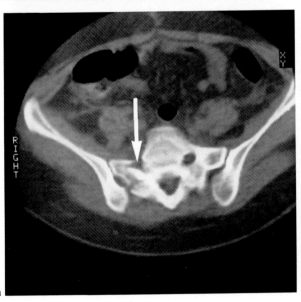

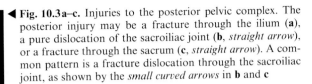

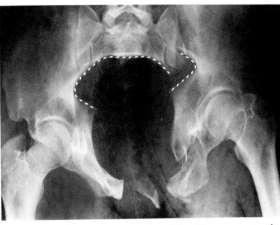

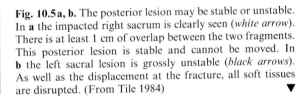

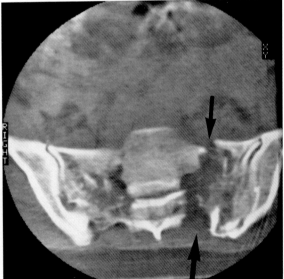

◀ **Fig. 10.3a–c.** Injuries to the posterior pelvic complex. The posterior injury may be a fracture through the ilium (**a**), a pure dislocation of the sacroiliac joint (**b**, *straight arrow*), or a fracture through the sacrum (**c**, *straight arrow*). A common pattern is a fracture dislocation through the sacroiliac joint, as shown by the *small curved arrows* in **b** and **c**

Fig. 10.4. The *dotted line* on the *right* side represents the sacrogluteal line on this inlet view of the pelvis. Any break in the continuity of this line, as shown on the *left* side, represents displacement of the posterior complex, an ominous prognostic indicator. (From Tile 1984)

Fig. 10.5a, b. The posterior lesion may be stable or unstable. In **a** the impacted right sacrum is clearly seen (*white arrow*). There is at least 1 cm of overlap between the two fragments. This posterior lesion is stable and cannot be moved. In **b** the left sacral lesion is grossly unstable (*black arrows*). As well as the displacement at the fracture, all soft tissues are disrupted. (From Tile 1984) ▼

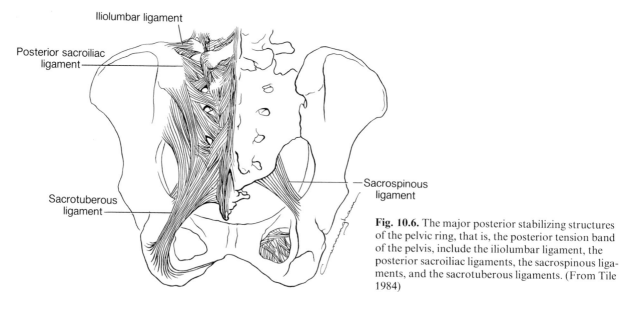

Iliolumbar ligament

Posterior sacroiliac ligament

Sacrospinous ligament

Sacrotuberous ligament

Fig. 10.6. The major posterior stabilizing structures of the pelvic ring, that is, the posterior tension band of the pelvis, include the iliolumbar ligament, the posterior sacroiliac ligaments, the sacrospinous ligaments, and the sacrotuberous ligaments. (From Tile 1984)

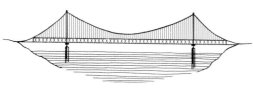

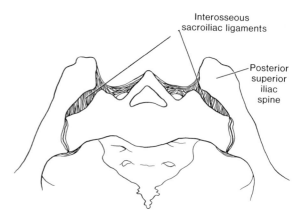

Interosseous sacroiliac ligaments

Posterior superior iliac spine

Fig. 10.7. The suspension bridge-like appearance of the ligaments binding the posterior sacroiliac complex. Note the vertical direction of the interosseous posterior sacroiliac ligaments. Noted by Grant to be the strongest in the body, as well as the transverse component acting as the suspension, joining the pillars, represented by the posterior superior iliac spines, to the sacrum. (From Tile 1984)

stand the transference of the weight-bearing forces from the spine to the lower extremities. The ligaments have a major role as posterior stabilizers because the sacrum, contrary to what is expected, does not form the shape of a keystone in a Roman arch but is quite the reverse. Therefore, the strong posterior sacroiliac interosseous ligaments have been described as the strongest in the body, maintaining the sacrum in its normal position in the pelvic ring. Also, the iliolumbar ligaments join the transverse processes of L5 to the iliac crest, and the intervening transverse fibers of the interosseous sacroiliac ligaments further enhance the suspensory mechanism. The entire complex looks and functions like a suspension bridge (Fig. 10.7).

The strong sacrospinous ligament, with fibers running transversely from the lateral edge of the

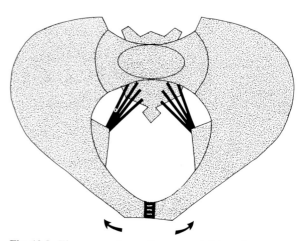

Fig. 10.8. The sacrospinous ligaments, joining the sacrum to the ischial spines, resist external rotatory forces (*arrows*). (From Tile 1984)

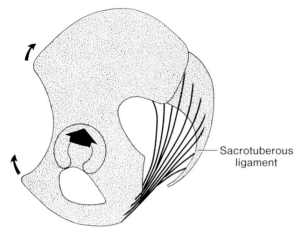

Fig. 10.9. The sacrotuberous ligament, joining the sacrum to the ischial tuberosity, resists a shearing rotatory force (*arrows*). (From Tile 1984)

sacrum to the ischial spine, resists external rotation of the pelvic ring (Fig. 10.8). The complex sacrotuberous ligament arises from most of the sacroiliac complex posterior to the sacrospinous ligament and extends to the ischial tuberosity. This strong ligament, positioned in the vertical plane, resists vertical shearing forces applied to the hemipelvis (Fig. 10.9). Therefore, these two supplementary ligaments, the sacrospinous and sacrotuberous, placed at 90° to each other, are well adapted to resist the two major forces acting upon the pelvis, that is, external rotation and vertical shear. In this way, they supplement the posterior sacroiliac ligaments.

The anterior sacroiliac ligaments are flat and strong and resist external rotation and shearing forces, although they do not have the strength of the posterior ligaments.

10.3.3 Types of Injurious Forces Acting on the Pelvis

Most forces acting upon the pelvis are either: (a) external rotation, (b) internal rotation (lateral compression), or (c) shearing forces in the vertical plane. In the complex high-energy trauma seen in our society, some forces defy description, but, in general, the above are the three major force vectors acting upon the pelvic ring.

External rotation forces occur with a direct blow to the posterior superior spine or by forced external rotation through the hip joints unilaterally or bilaterally. This force usually produces an open book type injury, that is, the symphysis pubis disrupts, and as further force is applied, the sacrospinous ligament and the anterior ligaments of the sacroiliac joint may also open (Fig. 10.10).

The force of internal rotation or lateral compression may be transmitted by a direct blow to the iliac crest, often causing an upward rotation of the hemipelvis or the so-called bucket-handle fracture, or through the femoral head, often causing an ipsilateral injury (Fig. 10.11).

Shearing forces in the vertical plane cross the main trabecular pattern of the posterior sacroiliac complex, whereas a lateral compressive force causes impaction of the cancellous bone and usually allows retention of the ligament integrity. Shear-

Fig. 10.10. a A direct blow to the posterior superior iliac spines will cause the symphysis pubis to spring open. **b** External rotation of the femora or direct compression against the anterior superior spines will also cause springing of the symphysis pubis. (From Tile 1984)

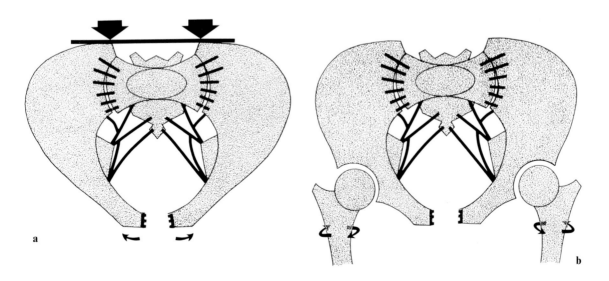

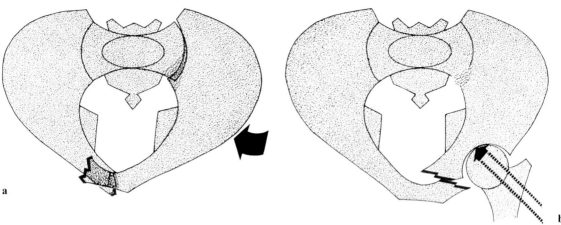

Fig. 10.11. a A lateral compressive force directed against the iliac crest will cause the hemipelvis to rotate internally, crushing the anterior sacrum and displacing the anterior pubic rami. **b** Lateral compression injury may also be caused by a direct force against the greater trochanter. In that situa-tion the femoral head acts as a battering ram, dividing the pubic rami as shown, often through the anterior column of the acetabulum. The ipsilateral sacroiliac complex is also crushed in this injury. (From Tile 1984)

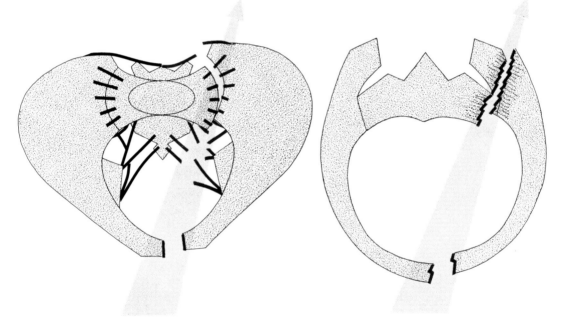

Fig. 10.12. A shearing force (*arrows*) crosses perpendicular to the main trabecular pattern of the posterior pelvic complex in the vertical plane. These forces cause marked displacement of bone and gross disruption of the soft tissues, resulting in major pelvic instability. (From Tile 1984)

ing forces cause marked displacement of bone and gross disruption of the soft tissue structures (Fig. 10.12). Continuation of these forces beyond the yield strength of the soft tissues produces an unstable pelvic ring with major anterior and poste-rior displacement. No finite point is reached with these shearing forces; therefore, the entire hemi-pelvis may be avulsed from the body, occasionally resulting in a traumatic hindquarter amputation.

10.4 Classification

By combining the two concepts of stability and force direction, a meaningful classification may be developed to aid in patient management (Ta-ble 10.6). Fractures of the pelvis may be divided into three types: stable, unstable, or miscellaneous, the miscellaneous group being further divided into fractures with a complex pattern, those associated

Table 10.6. Classification of disruptions of the pelvic ring

1. Stable
2. Unstable
3. Miscellaneous
    – Complex
    – Associated acetabular disruption
    – Bilateral sacroiliac dislocation with intact anterior arch

Table 10.7. Open book injuries

External rotation
No vertical displacement

Stage I	– Symphysis open < 2.5 cm
Stage II	– Symphysis open > 2.5 cm
Stage III	– Symphysis open > 2.5 cm with peroneal wound

with acetabular fractures, and those involving bilateral sacroiliac dislocation with an intact anterior arch.

The two major types, however, are injuries that are stable and those that are unstable. It must be understood, however, that the concept of stability must be considered not as black and white but various shades of gray. Therefore, various types of pelvic ring disruption will fall at various points along a stability scale, depending on their precise pathoanatomy. As will be described in the next section, the best way of determining the stability of the pelvic ring is by physical examination and radiographic assessment.

By definition, *unstable means instability in the vertical plane,* that is, vertical displacement is possible because of the bony or ligamentous disruption of the posterior sacroiliac complex.

The stable injuries are of two varieties: the open book or anteroposterior compression injury, caused by external rotation, and the lateral compression injury, caused by internal rotation. It should be remembered that the open book injury

caused by an external rotatory force is unstable in external rotation, whereas the lateral compression injury is unstable in internal rotation, but neither is unstable in the vertical plane unless a shearing force is also added, disrupting the posterior ligamentous structures. Also, it is self-evident that unstable pelvic injuries may be produced by any force vector which overcomes the yield strength of the soft tissues.

10.4.1 Stable Fractures

10.4.1.1 Open Book (Anteroposterior Compression) Fractures

External rotatory forces applied to the pelvis cause a disruption of the symphysis pubis. The anterior lesion, however, may also be an avulsion fracture of the pubis adjacent to the symphysis or a fracture through the pubic rami. However, the symphysis avulsion or disruption is much more common. Several stages of the open book injury are recognized (Table 10.7).

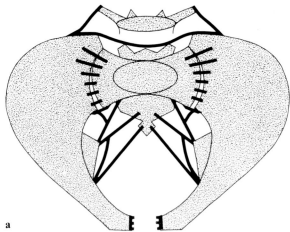

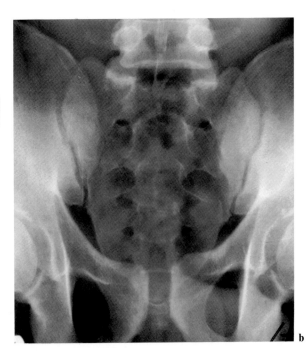

Fig. 10.13a, b. Stage I of an open book injury is a disruption of the symphysis pubis only with no involvement of the sacroiliac joints (**a**). The patient in **b** a hockey player who sustained a direct blow to the posterior sacroiliac area bilaterally, noted immediate pain anteriorly at the symphysis pubis. His radiograph indicates a symphysis pubis separation of 1.5 cm with no opening of the sacroiliac joints posteriorly. (From Tile 1984)

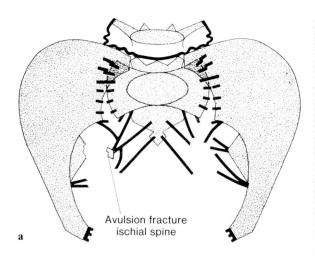

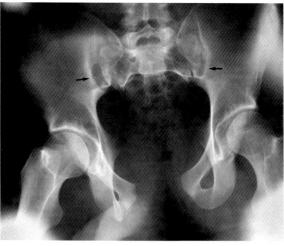

Fig. 10.14a, b. Stage II open book injury. **a** In this diagram, note that the symphysis pubis has disrupted more than 2.5 cm. If that occurs, the sacrospinous ligaments tear or an equivalent avulsion of the adjacent sacrum or ischial spine occurs, as well as an avulsion of the anterior sacroiliac ligaments, causing a wide anterior opening of the sacroiliac joints. However, pelvic stability is maintained by the intact posterior ligamentous structures, indicated by the *black lines*. The end point is reached when the posterior iliac spines abut against the sacrum. **b** A typical radiograph showing the disruption of the symphysis pubis and the markedly widened sacroiliac joints anteriorly (*arrows*). (From Tile 1984)

a) Stage I

Opening of the symphysis pubis less than 2.5 cm permits stability to be retained in the pelvic ring, a situation not dissimilar to that observed during delivery of a baby. In the rare traumatic injury, the sacrospinous and anterior sacroiliac ligaments remain intact (Fig. 10.13). Therefore, a CT scan will show no opening of the sacroiliac joints.

b) Stage II

Continuation of the external rotatory force will reach a finite end point when the "book" opens to the extent that the posterior iliac spines abut upon the sacrum. In this particular circumstance, the sacrospinous ligaments and the anterior sacroiliac ligaments are torn but the strong posterior sacroiliac ligaments remain intact (Fig. 10.14). Therefore, this injury is unstable in external rotation, but as long as the force does not continue beyond the yield strength of the posterior ligaments, stability can be returned to the pelvic ring by internal rotation.

It is extremely important to realize that the external rotatory force may in fact continue beyond the yield strength of the posterior ligament, causing a complete avulsion of the hemipelvis. This is no longer an open book configuration but is now an unstable fracture of the worst variety (Fig. 10.15). In fact, as previously indicated, a

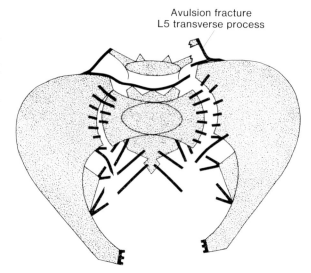

Fig. 10.15. The presence of a symphysis disruption does not imply a stable configuration; in fact, most symphysis disruptions are associated with unstable posterior lesions, as shown. Note the telltale avulsion fracture of the L5 transverse process, indicating instability and posterior displacement of this fracture. (From Tile 1984)

complete traumatic hemipelvectomy may ensue. Therefore, the presence of a symphysis disruption does not always imply an open book fracture. Careful assessment is required to be certain that vertical instability is not also present.

c) Stage III

The stage III injury consists of a symphysis disruption as well as involvement of the pelvic soft tissues such as the vagina, the urethra, the bladder, or the rectum.

d) Atypical Varieties

Atypical varieties of open book fracture may occur with fractures anteriorly through the pubic rami unilaterally or bilaterally or posteriorly through the ilium rather than through the sacroiliac joints.

10.4.1.2 Lateral Compression Fractures

There are several types of lateral compression injury depending upon the site of the anterior and posterior lesion (Table 10.8). The anterior and posterior lesion may be on the same side or ipsilateral (type I) or they may be on opposite sides, producing the so-called bucket-handle type of injury (type II). The bucket-handle injury may be of one of two types: (a) a contralateral lesion anteriorly and posteriorly or (b) a four-pillar or straddle frac-

Table 10.8. Lateral compression (internal rotation) injuries

Type I:	Ipsilateral – Both rami fractured – Locked symphysis – Superior ramus fractured with symphysis disruption
Type II:	Bucket-Handle – Contralateral – Four-pillar

ture of all four rami in front with a posterior injury.

a) Type I: Ipsilateral

The ipsilateral fractures are of three types: a fracture of both rami anteriorly, a locked symphysis, or an atypical type of fracture through the superior ramus often involving the anterior column of the acetabulum, with disruption through the symphysis pubis.

Fractures of Both Rami. An internal rotation force applied to the ilium or, more commonly, a direct

Fig. 10.16a–c. Stable lateral compression fracture, type I: Ipsilateral. The diagram (**a**) shows a typical ipsilateral type of lateral compression injury. Note the anterior crush to the sacrum and the overlap of the pubic rami. In this particular case there is posterior disruption, but stability is afforded by the crush in the sacrum. The force necessary to produce this seemingly minimally displaced fracture is often underestimated because of the elastic recoil of the pelvis. This fracture, barely perceptible in the inlet radiograph (**b**, *arrow*), was obviously grossly displaced at the moment of injury, since the bladder was pulled back into it, as shown in the cystogram (**c**, *arrow*). (From Tile 1984)

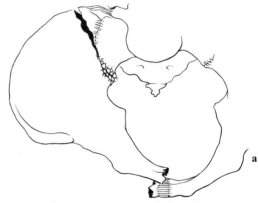

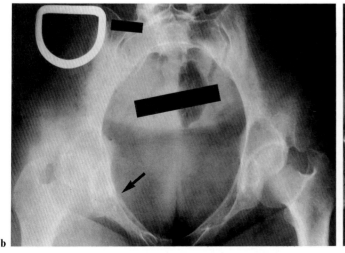

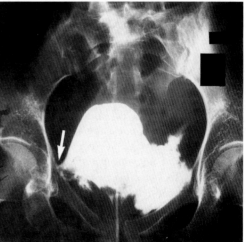

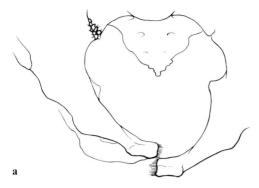

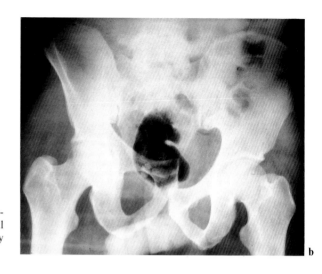

Fig. 10.17 a, b. Locked symphysis. **a** Diagram and **b** antero-posterior radiograph showing an unusual type of lateral compression injury where the symphysis becomes firmly locked anteriorly. (From Tile 1984)

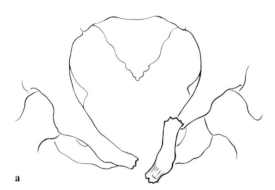

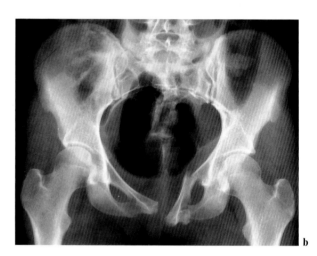

Fig. 10.18. a A variant of the type I injury often seen in young women. The lateral compressive force fractures the superior ramus, often through the anterior column of the acetabulum. Continuing lateral compression rotates the distal fragment through the symphysis pubis, thereby disrupting it. This distal fragment assumes a vertical position and may impinge on the perineum as demonstrated in the anteroposterior radiograph (**b**) From Tile 1984)

blow to the greater trochanter may cause a typical lateral compression or internal rotation fracture of the hemipelvis. The superior and inferior rami break, then a crush may occur anteriorly at the sacroiliac joint but, commonly, the posterior ligamentous structures do not disrupt (Fig. 10.16a). The entire hemipelvis may be forced across to the opposite side, thereby rupturing the bladder or blood vessels within the pelvis. The elastic recoil of the tissues may deceive the examiner and the fracture appear undisplaced in the radiograph. However, the radiographs in Fig. 10.16b, c show the bladder being drawn back into the fracture site by the recoiling pelvis.

Locked Symphysis. This rare injury is a form of ipsilateral lateral compression type. As the hemipelvis internally rotates, the symphysis disrupts and locks, making reduction extremely difficult (Fig. 10.17).

Atypical Variety. We have identified an atypical variety of lateral compression injury often seen in young females. As the hemipelvis migrates internally, the symphysis disrupts and a fracture occurs through the superior ramus, often involving the anterior column of the acetabulum distally. With continued internal rotation, the superior ramus migrates inferiorly and posteriorly into the perineum (Fig. 10.18).

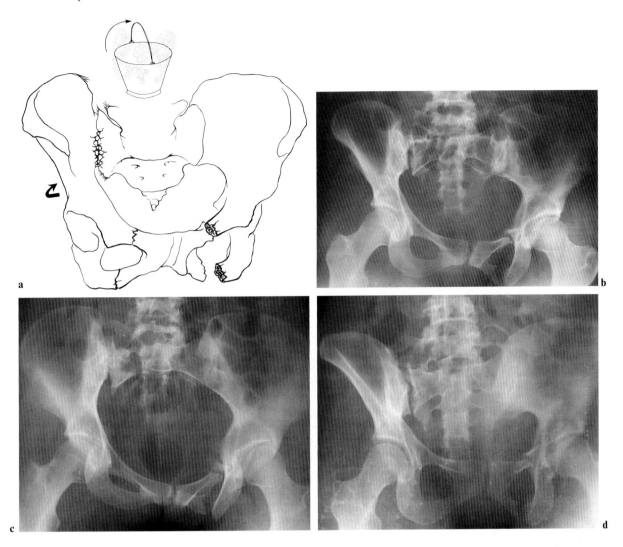

b) Type II: Bucket-Handle

The bucket-handle type of injury is usually caused by a direct blow to the pelvis. The anterior fracture may be on the opposite side to the posterior lesion (contralateral type) or all four rami may fracture anteriorly. Another combination might be a symphysis disruption with two rami fractures.

This injury has particular characteristics that may seem confusing. The affected hemipelvis rotates anteriorly and superiorly like the handle of a bucket (Fig. 10.19). Therefore, even if the posterior structures are relatively intact, the patient may have a major leg length discrepancy. Very often, the posterior structures are firmly impacted, the deformity being clearly noted on physical examination. Reducing these fractures and thereby the leg length discrepancy requires derotation of the hemipelvis rather than pure traction in the vertical plane.

Fig. 10.19. The diagram (**a**) demonstrates a typical type II lateral compression injury, characterized by compression of the posterior sacroiliac complex associated with a straddle or butterfly fracture of the four pubic rami anteriorly. The anteroposterior (**b**), inlet (**c**), and outlet (**d**) views of this 19-year-old woman show this classic lesion with upward rotation and impaction of the right hemipelvis. Even under general anesthesia, this hemipelvis could not be moved on the third day following injury, indicating severe posterior impaction

With continued internal rotation, the posterior structures may yield, producing some instability. However, the anterior sacroiliac crush is usually so stable that reduction is difficult.

This is akin to the situation with a vertebral fracture, where the vertebral body may be crushed by flexion forces but the posterior spinous ligament has ruptured. An excellent example of this is shown in Fig. 10.20a. The original radiograph

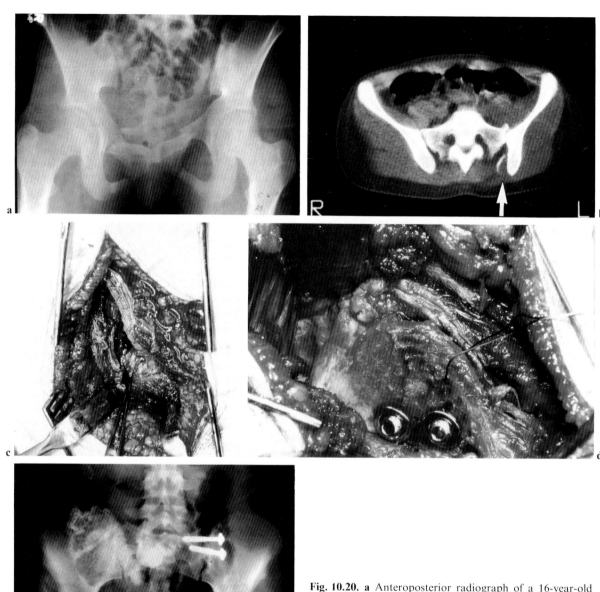

Fig. 10.20. a Anteroposterior radiograph of a 16-year-old girl with a type II bucket-handle fracture. The fracture involves all four pubic rami and the left sacroiliac joint. b CT clearly outlines the essential features of this fracture. Note the anterior crush of the sacrum, the internal rotation of the left hemipelvis and, in this case, the avulsion of the iliac apophysis which had not yet fused to the ilium (*arrow*). c Clinical appearance at surgery of this apophysis avulsion (outlined by the probe, *arrow*). d Appearance after reduction and fixation with two lag screws crossing the sacroiliac joint. e Postoperative radiographic appearance

of this 16-year-old girl shows the internal rotation of the left hemipelvis and the posterior impaction. All four rami are broken anteriorly and the leg length discrepancy is seen. The CT scan (Fig. 10.20b) again shows the left hemipelvis to be internally rotated and the anterior portion of the sacroiliac joint crushed. Posteriorly, the arrow points to the avulsion of the posterior iliac apophysis (Fig. 10.20b, c). At surgery, the apophysis was clearly avulsed but the posterior sacroiliac ligaments completely intact. After posterior reduction of the fracture and fixation by two screws, the pelvis is anatomically reduced (Fig. 10.20d, e).

10.4.2 Unstable Fractures

An unstable pelvic disruption implies a rupture of the pelvic floor including the posterior structures as well as the sacrospinous and sacrotuberous ligaments (Fig. 10.21). The unstable injury may be unilateral, affecting one posterior iliac complex, or may be bilateral, affecting both. Telltale radiographic signs of instability include avulsion of the transverse process of the L5 vertebra or of either attachment of the sacrospinous ligament (Fig. 10.22). The CT scan shows the radio-

graphic appearance of the unstable posterior complex better than the plane radiograph and should be obtained in all cases.

A comparison of the CT scans (Fig. 10.23) shows clearly the difference between the impacted stable posterior complex and the grossly unstable complex of the vertical shear injury.

10.4.3 Miscellaneous Types of Fracture

a) Complex

Many severe types of fracture dislocation of the pelvis defy precise classification because of the complex forces causing the injury. In these cases, the pelvic ring may be disrupted in a very bizarre

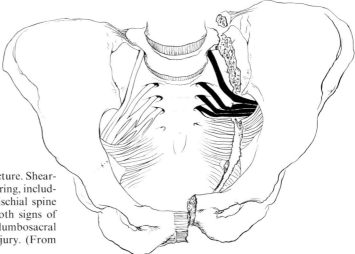

Fig. 10.21. Unilateral unstable vertical shear fracture. Shearing forces cause massive disruption of the pelvic ring, including the pelvic floor. Note the avulsion of the ischial spine and the tip of the transverse process of L5, both signs of pelvic instability. Note also the stretch of the lumbosacral plexus, commonly injured in this pattern of injury. (From Tile 1984)

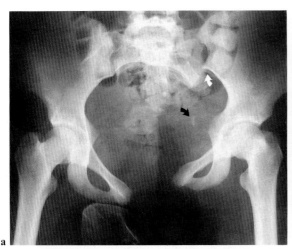

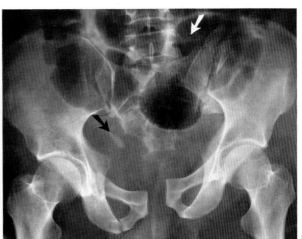

Fig. 10.22a, b. Telltale signs of instability: **a** an avulsion of the ischial spine (*black arrow*) and posterior displacement of the ilium (*white arrow*); **b** avulsion of the sacral end of the sacrospinous ligament (*black arrow*) and the tip of the transverse process of L5 on the opposite side (*white arrow*) in this bilateral injury. (From Tile 1984)

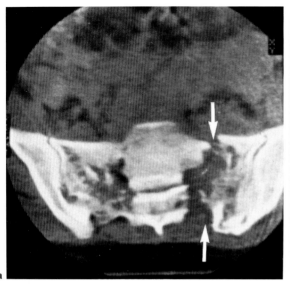
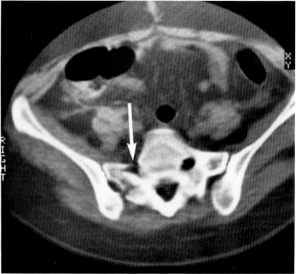

a   b

Fig. 10.23. a CT scan showing marked disruption and instability of the left sacrum as a result of a shearing force.
b CT scan showing impaction of the right sacrum from
a lateral compression injury. This young woman sustained
an acetabular fracture as well, confirming the mechanism
of injury. Note the marked over-riding of the sacral fragments on the fractured side as compared to the normal
left side. Impaction was so rigid that no abnormal movement of the hemipelvis was detected on physical examination with image intensification. (From Tile 1984)

fashion. Because of the high-energy forces involved, the pelvic ring is usually unstable.

b) Bilateral Sacroiliac Dislocation with an Intact Anterior Arch

This unusual injury is usually caused by hyperflex-
ion of the legs (for example, two of our cases were
in young women who were crushed in the hyper-
flexed position under a horse which reared and
fell backwards). In this particular situation, the
anterior complex remains intact but both sacroiliac joints dislocate posteriorly.

c) Pelvic Disruptions Associated with Acetabular Fractures

If a pelvic ring disruption is associated with an
acetabular fracture, the prognosis will clearly
change and will be more dependent upon the acetabular component than upon the pelvic ring disruption. These complex injuries are relatively common. CT scanning of acetabular fractures has indicated a significant number of sacroiliac injuries
and pelvic ring disruptions associated with acetabular fractures.

10.5 Management of the Pelvic Disruption

Management of the severely polytraumatized patient with a pelvic fracture may be considered
under the following four headings: Assessment,
resuscitation, provisional stabilization, and definitive stabilization.

10.5.1 Assessment

10.5.1.1 General Assessment

It is beyond the scope of this chapter to detail
the general assessment of the polytraumatized patient. Suffice it to say that a polytraumatized patient with a pelvic fracture represents a therapeutic
challenge to the treating surgeon because the mortality rate remains at approximately 10%. The necessity of a planned treatment protocol for the
polytraumatized patient cannot be overemphasized. The patient must have immediate appropriate treatment from the time of injury until stabilization in an appropriate intensive care unit. The
central theme of system management during resuscitation is *simultaneous* rather than *sequential* care.
We recommend the treatment protocol of the
American College of Surgeons in the Advanced
Trauma Life Support (ATLS) Program (Aprahamian et al. 1981).

In the primary survey, problems involving the
airway, bleeding (shock), and the central nervous
system have the highest priority. Immediate lifesaving resuscitation, therefore, must be directed
to both the airway and the presence of shock. In

pelvic trauma, shock may be profound due to ret-roperitoneal arterial or venous hemorrhage.

The secondary survey following the primary re-suscitation includes further examination of the air-way, bleeding, the central nervous system, the di-gestive system, the excretory system, and, finally, the fracture. For further study in the management of polytrauma patients refer to the excellent mono-graph on this subject by the American College of Surgeons mentioned above.

10.5.1.2 *Specific Musculoskeletal Assessment*

For the management of the musculoskeletal injury, assessment is directed to the determination of the stability of the pelvic ring.

a) Clinical

As in all areas of clinical medicine, an accurate history is essential; patients who have sustained a high-energy injury from motor vehicle trauma or falls from a height are much more likely to have an unstable pelvic injury than those who have sustained low-energy trauma.

The physical examination is at least as impor-tant as the radiographs in determining pelvic sta-bility. The essence of the physical examination is to inspect the patient for major bruising or bleed-ing from the urethral meatus, vagina, or rectum. If these latter two areas are not carefully inspected, occult lacerations may be overlooked, with dire consequences, since these lacerations always mean an *open* fracture of the pelvis.

Determination of pelvic stability can simply be done by applying one's hands to the anterior supe-rior spine and moving the affected hemipelvis (Fig. 10.24a). Open book injuries are maximally externally rotated and can be closed by compres-sion of both anterior iliac spines. Lateral compres-sion injuries are usually in an anatomical recoiled position unless they have been impacted. Further internal rotation by compression of the iliac crests will displace the fracture. Finally, by applying one hand to the pelvic iliac crest and using the other to apply traction to the leg, displacement in the vertical plane can usually easily be diagnosed (Fig. 10.24b). If possible, these manipulations should be done under image intensification to veri-fy the type of displacement and whether displace-ment in the vertical plane is present.

b) Radiographic

Plain Radiographs. As a routine in the acute situa-tion, a single anteroposterior radiograph as com-

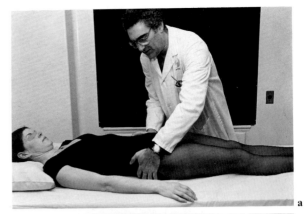

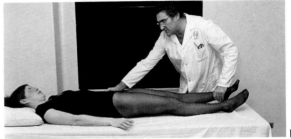

Fig. 10.24. a Direct palpation of the iliac crest will reveal crepitus or abnormal motion, which, if present, is the best indicator of instability of the pelvis. **b** With one arm control-ling the injured hemipelvis and the second arm applying traction, one can again determine the amount of instability present. (From Tile 1984)

monly used in most trauma centers is usually suffi-cient to determine the presence or absence of pelvic ring instability. Although this radiograph will suf-fice in the acute injury during the resuscitative phase, a single anteroposterior radiograph may be misleading. Therefore, for accurate assessment of pelvic ring displacement, an inlet and an outlet view should be added (Fig. 10.25). The inlet view, taken by directing the X-ray beam 60° from the head to the mid-pelvis, is the best radiographic view to demonstrate posterior displacement. The outlet view, taken by directing the X-ray beam from the foot of the patient to the symphysis at an angle of 45°, demonstrates superior or inferior migration of the hemipelvis.

CT Scan. The CT scan is the best single investiga-tive tool for determining pelvic instability, since the sacroiliac area is best visualized by this tech-nique. Stable impacted fractures of the sacrum can be clearly differentiated from grossly unstable ones by this method (Fig. 10.3, 10.5).

Careful clinical and radiographic assessment will allow the surgeon to determine the personality of the pelvic injury, that is, whether the musculo-

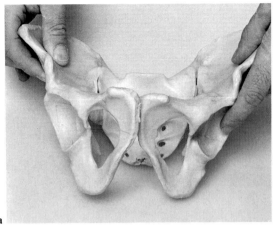 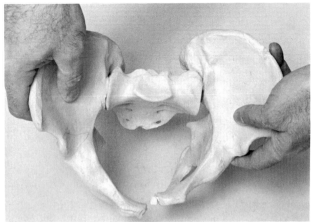

a   b

Fig. 10.25. When placed in the anteroposterior plane (**a**), the skeleton appears intact, when in fact, as shown in **b**, the left hemipelvis is displaced posteriorly. Therefore, the anteroposterior radiograph of the pelvis may be misleading and the inlet view is the best view for determining posterior displacement. (From Tile 1984)

Table 10.9. Management of pelvic hemorrhage

1. General (ATLS protocol)
2. Pneumatic antishock garment (PASG)
3. Fracture stabilization
4. Embolization
5. Surgical control

skeletal injury is more to the stable or to the unstable end of the stability scale. Patients with an unstable pelvic disruption are at much greater general risk than those with a stable pelvis. In our first prospective study of 100 patients, 12 of the 15 mortalities were in this unstable group (McMurtry et al. 1980). Their blood transfusion requirements were three times greater (15.5 units to 5.5 units), their injury severity score was 37 as against 29, and their overall complication rate was three times higher.

Since retroperitoneal and retropelvic hemorrhage is the major complication of pelvic trauma, we will direct our attention briefly to this matter (Table 10.9).

Patients suffering this complication require *massive fluid replacement,* as outlined by the American College of Surgeons' ATLS protocol. Early management of shock should include the *pneumatic antishock garment* (PASG). The advantages and disadvantages of the PASG are listed in Table 10.10. In our opinion, the advantages outweigh the disadvantages, the only notable disadvantage being restriction of access to the abdomen. The garment must not be precipitously released. During gradual release of the garment, the blood pressure must be carefully monitored. Any drop greater than 10 mm Hg in the systolic blood pressure is a contraindication to further deflation. Other guidelines of importance include inflation

Table 10.10. Pneumatic antishock garment. (From Tile 1984)

Advantages	Disadvantages
1. Simple 2. Rapid 3. Reversible 4. Splints fractures 5. Accessible and available 6. Safe	1. Decreased visibility of abdomen and lower extremities 2. Decreased access to abdomen and lower extremities 3. Complication of abuse 4. Exacerbation of congestive heart failure (congestive cardiac failure is an absolute contraindication to the use of PASG) 5. Decreased vital capacity 6. Compartment syndrome

of the legs prior to the abdominal portion and reversing that order during deflation.

Fracture stabilization belongs in the resuscitative phase of management. There is a growing body of evidence to suggest that the application of a simple anterior external frame will reduce retropelvic venous and bony bleeding to the extent that other intervention is rarely required. Therefore, pelvic stabilization should be performed early. We are presently designing a pelvic clamp which can be applied in the emergency room with or without direct skeletal fixation. It is hoped that this will

reduce mortality by allowing the volume of the
pelvis to decrease to its normal size, thereby restoring the tamponade effect of the bony pelvis and
helping to stop the venous bleeding. The precise
method for early fracture stabilization will be discussed in the next section.

We have found *embolization* of the pelvic vessels to be of little overall value in the management
of these patients. In our trauma unit, we have narrowed its use to those patients who are bleeding
mainly from a small-bore artery such as the obturator or the superior gluteal arteries. It is of little
value in the hemodynamically unstable patient
with massive bleeding from the major vessels of
the internal iliac system, because the emboli cannot control this type of hemorrhage, and the patient may die during the attempt. It is also, of
course, of no value in venous or bony bleeding.

Small-bore artery bleeding may be assumed if,
although the patient can be well controlled using
the above methods of fluid replacement, pneumatic antishock garment, and fracture stabilization, he or she goes back into a shocked state each
time the fluid is slowed down. In those circumstances, after hemodynamic stability has been
achieved, the patient is moved to the vascular
suite, an arteriogram performed, and if a small-
bore artery is lacerated, it is embolized with Gelfoam (Upjohn Pharmaceutic Co.) or other embolic
material.

Direct surgical control is rarely indicated and
usually unsuccessful. The main indications for
open surgery are the open pelvic fracture and major vessel injury leading to a patient in extremis
from hypovolemic shock.

Very high mortality rates have been reported
with open pelvic fractures (Richardson et al.
1982). However, the type of open pelvic injury,
be it posterior or peroneal, is of great prognostic
significance, and all open pelvic fractures cannot
therefore be lumped together. It must be recognized that some pelvic fractures are really traumatic hemipelvectomies, and, rarely, completing
the hemipelvectomy may be *lifesaving* (Lipkowitz
et al. 1982).

If a patient is in extremis (that is, with a blood
pressure of under 60 mm Hg with no response to
fluid replacement), urgent methods must be
adopted in order to save time. If thoracic and abdominal bleeding are ruled out, then retroperitoneal bleeding must be assumed. Laparotomy followed by aortic clamping may buy time while appropriate methods of hemostasis and vessel repair
are applied.

10.5.3 Provisional Stabilization

Provisional stabilization is required only for those
fractures that potentially increase the volume of
the pelvis, that is, the wide open book injury or
the unstable pelvic fracture. It is rarely required
for lateral compression injuries, which make up
60% of the total number of pelvic disruptions.

As previously stated, we are introducing a pelvic clamp which can be applied in the emergency
department which may alleviate the need for an
immediate external fixator. Otherwise, to achieve
provisional fixation, a simple anterior external fixator should be applied as a matter of urgency.
The anterior frame will reduce the volume of the
pelvis, thereby reducing venous and bony bleeding.
An added beneficial effect is a major reduction
in pain and the ability to induce the upright position in order to better ventilate the patient in the
intensive care unit. Since such patients are usually
extremely ill, we believe that a simple configuration will suffice—two pins percutaneously placed
in each ilium at approximately 45° to each other,
one in the anterior superior spine and one in the
iliac tubercle, joined by an anterior rectangular
configuration (Fig. 10.26).

Biomechanical studies performed in our laboratory and elsewhere have shown that simple frames
can give good stability in the open book fracture
(Fig. 10.27). However, in the unstable pelvic disruption, even the most elaborate frames cannot

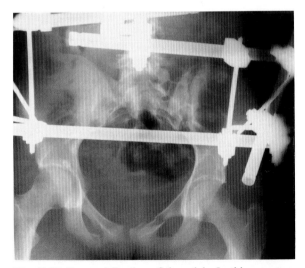

Fig. 10.26. External fixation of the pelvis. In this case, two
pins at 45° to each other were placed in each hemipelvis
and joined by a rectangular configuration of the frame.
Note that the left sacroiliac joint still shows slight opening
and posterior displacement, but the general alignment of
the pelvis is good

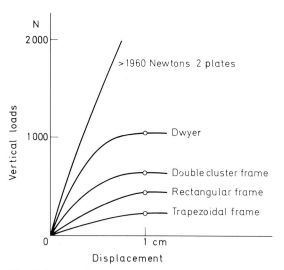

Fig. 10.27. Results of the biomechanical tests in the typical anteroposterior (open book) type injury, produced in the laboratory by division of the symphysis pubis and anterior sacroiliac ligaments. The posterior tension band of the pelvis was intact. Of the external frames, the double cluster frame was best, the trapezoidal the weakest. Since 1 kg equals approximately 10 N, both the rectangular and double cluster frames gave suitable stable fixation for this type of injury. (Adapted from Tile 1984)

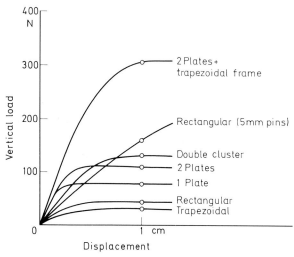

Fig. 10.28. Biomechanical results of the unstable vertical shear injury, produced by complete division of the symphysis pubis anteriorly and a fracture of the ilium posteriorly, as well as division of the sacrospinous and sacrotuberous ligaments. Note now that the vertical axis is measured in hundreds of newtons as compared to thousands in the stable configuration (compare with Fig. 10.27). A 100-N load is equal to approximately 10 kg. From this graph, one can see that all forms of anterior fixation fail under 20 kg of load when used on an unstable vertical shear type pelvic disruption. The best frame tested was one anchored on 5-mm pins, with a rectangular configuration and two side bars for triangulation. (Adapted from Tile 1984)

fully stabilize the pelvic ring if the patient is to be ambulated (Fig. 10.28). In our opinion, sophisticated frames requiring dissection to the anterior inferior spine are contraindicated in the acute resuscitation period. They have some biomechanical advantage, but this advantage is so slight that the added risk of the operative procedure is not worth taking. We have also seen two cases of pins placed in the hip joint with secondary sepsis and destruction of the joint.

In the hemodynamically unstable patient, open reduction and internal fixation of the pelvic ring injury is contraindicated. However, if the patient is hemodynamically stable, some centers favor early internal fixation of the disrupted pelvis if a clear indication for surgery exists. At the moment, this method cannot be recommended for general use, but should be carefully monitored on an experimental basis by those centers proposing it.

10.5.4 Definitive Stabilization

Definitive stabilization of the musculoskeletal injury depends upon a precise diagnosis of the fracture configuration. No matter what the configuration, if the pelvic ring is stable and undisplaced or minimally displaced, symptomatic treatment only is necessary. Patients with this injury may be mobilized quickly and the pelvic fracture, that is, the musculoskeletal injury, largely ignored.

However, displaced fractures of the pelvic ring require close scrutiny, as outlined below.

10.5.4.1 Stable Fractures

a) Open Book (Anteroposterior Compression) Fractures

Type I. In the type I open book fracture, with the symphysis pubis open less than 2.5 cm, no specific treatment is indicated. Patients with this injury usually have no posterior disruption and have intact sacrospinous ligaments (Fig. 10.13). Therefore, the situation is somewhat akin to the stretching of the symphysis pubis that takes place during pregnancy. With simple symptomatic treatment, that is, bed rest until comfortable, healing is usually adequate and few patients complain of any symptoms.

Type II. If the symphysis pubis is open more than 2.5 cm (Fig. 10.14), several options are available to the surgeon.

External Fixation. We prefer stabilization of the pelvis with a simple *anterior external frame* as described above (Fig. 10.26). The pins should remain in place for approximately 6–8 weeks; the frame should then be loosened and radiographs taken under stress to see whether healing has occurred and there is stability across the symphysis. If healing is adequate, the pins are removed at this stage. If not, the anterior frame is reattached for a further 4-week period.

With no vertical displacement possible, the patients may be quickly ambulated.

Reduction is best obtained in the lateral position or in the supine position with both legs fully internally rotated.

Internal Fixation. If the patient has a visceral injury necessitating a paramedian midline or Pfannenstiel incision, internal fixation using a 4.5-mm plate will restore stability. This should be done immediately after the abdominal procedure prior to closure of the skin. In this instance a double plate, recommended for symphysis fixation of unstable fractures, is unnecessary, since the open book fracture is inherently stable.

Spica or Sling. The patient with an open book fracture may also be treated with either a hip spica with both legs internally rotated or in a pelvic sling. These two methods are better suited to children and adolescents than to adults and we much prefer external fixation as definitive treatment for this fracture configuration.

b) Lateral Compression Fractures

Lateral compression fractures are usually stable, therefore surgical stabilization is rarely required; it is called for only if reduction is necessary to correct malalignment or leg length discrepancy. Since these injuries often result in an impacted posterior complex and a relatively stable pelvis, disimpaction and reduction should only be done if the clinical state of the patient warrants it. This will

Fig. 10.29 a–c. Stable lateral compression injury (type I). **a** Anteroposterior X-ray of a 16-year-old girl with a stable lateral compression injury. Note the fracture in the left ilium (*arrow*) and all four pubic rami. **b** Cystogram of the same patient showing a ruptured bladder. **c** Final result at one year was excellent. Treatment consisted of eight weeks of complete bed rest followed by ambulation with partial weight bearing for a further 4 weeks. Note that all fractures are healed and the position is good

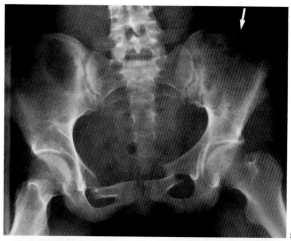

a

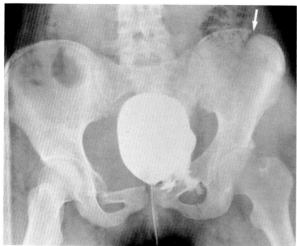

b

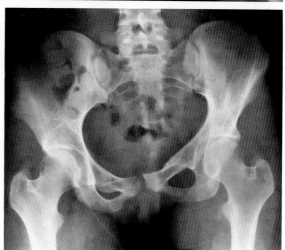

c

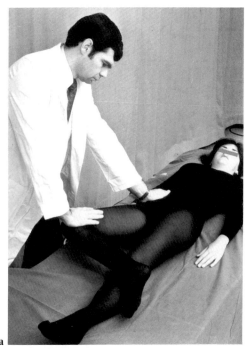

a

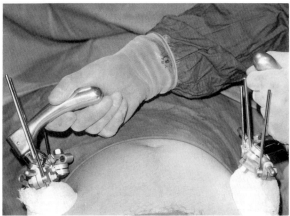

b

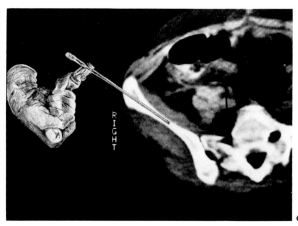

c

Fig. 10.30. a Closed reduction of a lateral compression type injury is performed by external rotation of the hip with the knee flexed and direct pressure on the hemipelvis, as shown. **b** The type of leverage one can obtain by placing handles on the crossbars of the external fixation device to allow for both internal and external rotation of the unstable hemipelvis. **c** Diagrammatic representation on a CT scan indicating the type of direct leverage one can obtain on the affected hemipelvis. (From Tile 1984)

vary with the age of the patient, the general medical state, the degree of rotation of the hemipelvis, and the amount of leg length discrepancy. In a young individual, a leg length discrepancy of more than 2.5 cm would be an indication to reduce the lateral compression injury. This is especially true in bucket-handle injuries. *However, we must stress again that the vast majority of lateral compression injuries may be treated with bed rest alone and do not require any external or internal fixation* (Fig. 10.29).

If reduction is desirable for the above reasons, it may be effected manually with external rotation (Fig. 10.30a) or with the aid of external skeletal pins placed in the hemipelvis (Fig. 10.30b, c). By placing a handle on the cross rod and applying

an external rotation force, the bucket-handle fracture may be reduced by derotation externally and posteriorly, allowing disimpaction of the posterior complex. In some instances, reduction is impossible and the surgeon must decide whether open reduction, the only remaining option is necessary.

If external skeletal pins have been used to help with reduction, a simple rectangular anterior frame should be applied at the end of the maneuver to hold the hemipelvis in the external rotated position.

Internal fixation of a lateral compression injury is rarely indicated except in the atypical type with bony protrusion into the perineum, especially in females. In that particular case, a short Pfannenstiel incision will allow derotation of the superior

Fig. 10.31. The original radiograph (**a**) demonstrates the rotated superior ramus of the left pubis through a disrupted symphysis pubis. Since the posterior complex is stable, open reduction and internal fixation with a threaded Steinman pin restored stability (**b**). Union occurred quickly, and the pin was removed at 6 weeks (**c**). (From Tile 1984)

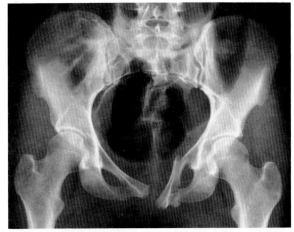

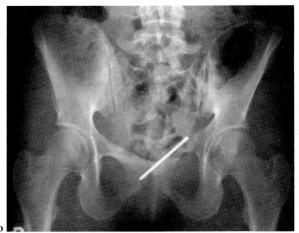

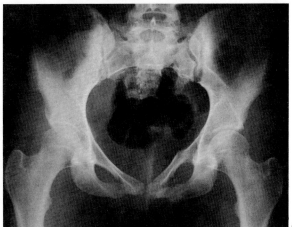

ramus and fixation with a threaded pin is ample (Fig. 10.31). The pin may be removed at 6 weeks in the stable configuration.

Warning: Pelvic slings, are *contraindicated* in lateral compression and unstable vertical shear injuries since they will cause further major displacement (Fig. 10.32).

10.5.4.2 Unstable Fractures

In unstable shear fractures, simple anterior frames will not be adequate for definitive management, as an attempt to ambulate the patient will often result in redisplacement (Fig. 10.33). Therefore, the two options open to the surgeon are either the addition of femoral supracondylar skeletal traction or internal fixation.

a) Skeletal Traction with External Fixation

Isolated, unstable shear injuries may be safely and adequately managed by the addition of a supracondylar femoral traction pin to a pelvis stabilized with an anterior external frame (Fig. 10.34). In our

clinical review, patients managed in this fashion, especially those with fractures of the sacrum, fracture dislocations of the sacroiliac joint, or fractures of the ilium had satisfactory long-term results. Redisplacement, if it occurred, was minimal and rarely clinically significant. Since internal fixation of the posterior pelvic complex is fraught with many complications, it is far safer for the general orthopedist to manage pelvic trauma, especially isolated pelvic trauma, in this manner, than attempt ill-advised open reductions.

The traction must be maintained for 8–12 weeks and the patient monitored with anteroposterior and inlet radiographs as well as CT scans where indicated. A major problem in the past has been too early ambulation of these patients, who require a longer period of recumbency to allow for sound bony union.

b) Open Reduction and Internal Fixation

Internal fixation of the pelvis, especially the posterior sacroiliac complex, was virtually unreported

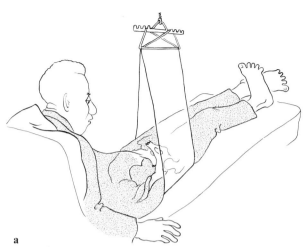

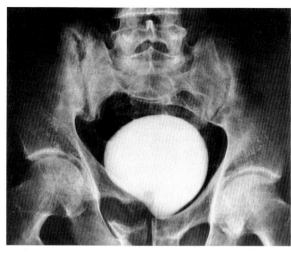

Fig. 10.32. a Pelvic slings are illogical in patients with lateral compression or unstable injuries as they will recreate the original force and cause displacement. **b** Note the amount of persistent displacement and impingement on the bladder. Note also that the superior ramus is ununited, as is the fracture through the sacrum. (From Tile 1984)

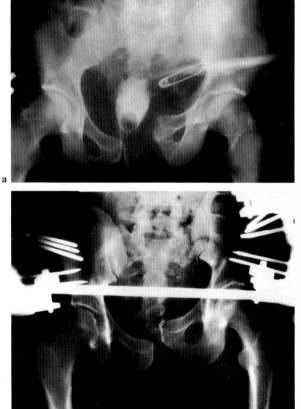

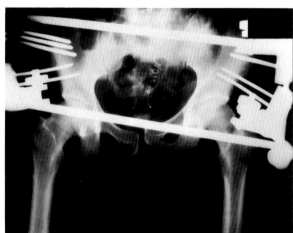

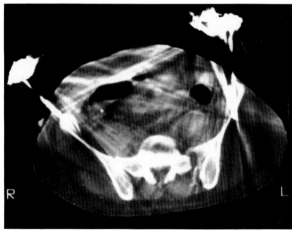

Fig. 10.33. a Anteroposterior cystogram showing an unstable fracture of the pelvic ring including a symphysis disruption and fracture through the left sacrum. Treatment consisted of a double cluster frame. The postreduction radiograph (**b**) shows adequate position. After ambulation, however, redisplacement occurred, as shown on the radiograph (**c**) and CT (**d**). Anterior frames do not afford sufficient stability to allow early ambulation in unstable pelvic ring disruptions. (Case courtesy of Ronald E. Rosenthal, MD, Long Island, New York)

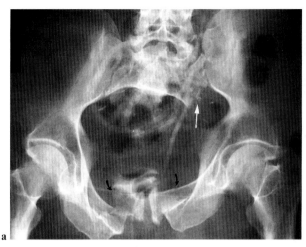
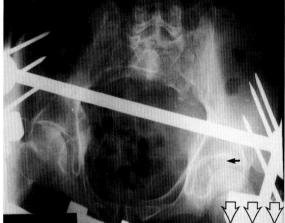
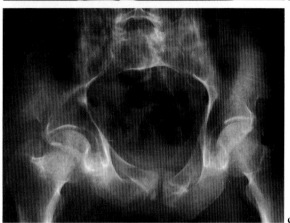

Fig. 10.34 a–c. Unstable pelvic disruption treatment with external frame and traction. **a** Anteroposterior intravenous pyelogram of a 59-year-old man who sustained a grossly unstable pelvic ring disruption in a motor vehicle accident. The *white arrow* indicates the marked disruption of the left sacrum with posterior displacement of 2.5 cm, causing an injury to the lumbosacral nerve plexus. The two *black arrows* show the avulsion of the rectus abdominus muscle anteriorly through the symphysis. **b** Restoration of alignment was possible with an anterior frame and 30 lb (about 13.5 kg) of supracondylar traction on the left leg (*broad arrows*). Note the distraction of the left hip joint (*black arrow*). **c** Final result showing healing of all fractures and adequate restoration of the pelvic ring. The clinical result was good except for a permanent nerve damage in the left leg. (From Tile 1984)

prior to 1980, with almost no literature on this subject except for sporadic case reports. There are reports of plating and wiring of the anterior symphysis complex but few of the posterior complex. The past 5 years have brought an epidemic of internal fixation of the pelvis and we must examine whether this is justified or not. We have seen from out study of the natural history of pelvic fractures that the stable injuries, which comprise 60%–65% of the total number of cases, have almost no indication for internal fixation. For unstable disruptions, many patients can be safely and adequately managed by external fixation and skeletal traction. Therefore, posterior internal fixation of the pelvis should be done infrequently and only in cases showing significant indications (Table 10.11).

Advantages and Disadvantages. The *advantages* of pelvic internal fixation are as follows:

1. Anatomical reduction and stable fixation would allow easier pain-free nursing of the polytraumatized patient since excellent stability may

Table 10.11. Indications for open reduction and internal fixation of the pelvis

A. Anterior internal fixation:
   1. Symphysis disruption (if laparotomy is being performed)
   2. Displaced fracture in the perineum
   3. Associated anterior column acetabular fracture

B. Posterior internal fixation:
   1. Unreduced posterior complex (especially sacroiliac dislocation)
   2. Polytraumatized patient with an unstable pelvic ring fracture as in B.1
   3. Open posterior fracture (not perineum)
   4. Associated posterior column acetabular fracture

be restored to the pelvic ring, as shown on the accompanying bar graph (Fig. 10.35).

2. Modern techniques of internal fixation (especially compression) wound be useful on the large cancellous surfaces of the pelvis to avoid malunion and nonunion.

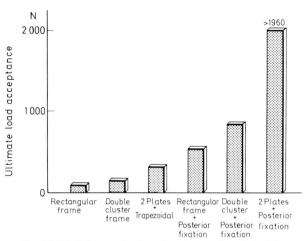

Fig. 10.35. A bar graft depicting the results of the biomechanical testing again shows the superior stability afforded the pelvis by posterior fixation in the unstable vertical shear injury. (Adapted from Tile 1984)

The *disadvantages* include:

1. *Loss of tamponade and the possibility of massive hemorrhage.* The superior gluteal artery is commonly injured during pelvic trauma (it may be reinjured during surgical exploration), but the injury may be unrecognized because the artery may clot. With the massive blood transfusions required in these patients, the clotting mechanism may be defective on the 5th–10th postoperative day when surgical exploration is performed. Reinjury to the artery during exposure of the fracture may result in massive hemorrhage.

2. *Sepsis.* Posterior incisions in the acute trauma situation have resulted in an unacceptably high rate of skin necrosis. Even without posterior incisions, we have seen skin breakdown in many of our patients with severe unstable vertical shear injuries (Fig. 10.38). At surgery, the gluteus maxi-

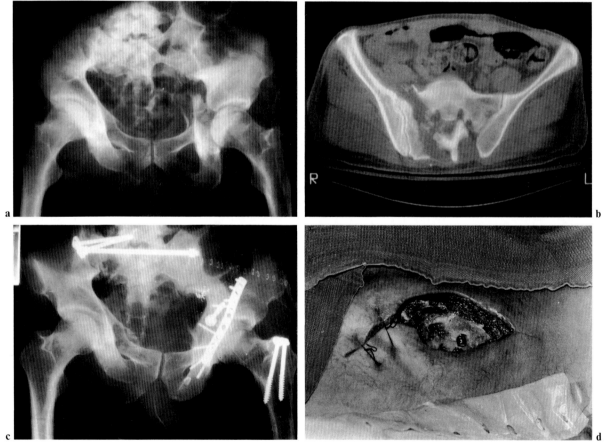

Fig. 10.36. a Anteroposterior radiograph showing a fractured left acetabulum and right sacrum taken 5 weeks following injury. The disruption of the right sacrum is better seen on the CT (**b**). **c** The left acetabular fracture was openly reduced and internally fixed, as was the right sacroiliac joint, with two screws and a sacral bar. At the time of surgery,

the gluteus maximus muscle was completely avulsed from its insertion on the ilium. The skin was avascular, and the underlying muscle fibrous and atrophied. The wound edges necrosed, but the patient refused further surgery and eventually the entire wound was covered with granulation tissue (**d**)

mus muscle is often torn from its insertion leaving no underlying fascia to nourish the skin. Skin breakdown has been frequent in spite of meticulous technique, adequate nutrition, and preoperative antibiotics (Fig. 10.36).

3. *Neurological damage.* We have now seen seven cases of neurological damage caused by screws entering the first sacral foramen or the spinal canal. These injuries have occurred in patients previously neurologically normal (Fig. 10.37). The insertion of screws posteriorly across the sacroiliac joint must be precise in order to avoid that complication.

Indications. The indications for open reduction and internal fixation of the pelvis are listed in Table 10.11.

Anterior Internal Fixation

1. Symphysis disruption. If the patient has a disrupted symphysis pubis and the general surgeons, urologists, or trauma surgeons are proceeding with a laparotomy or exploration of the bladder, then plating the symphysis pubis in a reduced position will greatly simplify the management of the case. If the fracture pattern is a stable open book variety, a short 2- or 4-hole plate can be placed on the superior surface of the symphysis pubis to restore stability. If the symphysis pubis disruption is part of an unstable pelvic ring pattern, then double plating to prevent displacement in the vertical and anteroposterior planes is preferable (Fig. 10.38). When combined with an external frame, stability will be restored, as shown in the accompanying bar graph (Fig. 10.35). However, plates should not be used in the presence of fecal contamination or the proposed use of a suprapubic tube; in that situation, use external fixation.

2. Displaced fracture in the perineum (see Fig. 10.18). In the atypical type of lateral compression injury, with rotation of the superior pubic ramus through the symphysis into the perineum, a limited Pfannenstiel approach, derotation of the fragment, and fixation with a threaded pin will maintain the fracture until healing has been completed, usually a period of 6 weeks for this stable fracture.

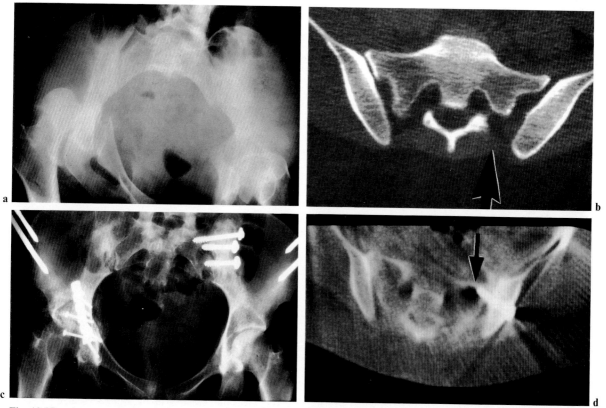

Fig. 10.37. a Anteroposterior radiograph showing a fracture dislocation of the right hip as well as a dislocation of the left sacroiliac joint, better seen on the CT (**b**, *arrow*). Treatment consisted of open reduction and internal fixation of the right acetabular fracture, internal fixation of the left sacroiliac joint and an anterior frame. Note the position of the screws (**c**). **d** Postoperative CT showing the tip of the screw in the first sacral foramen (*arrow*)

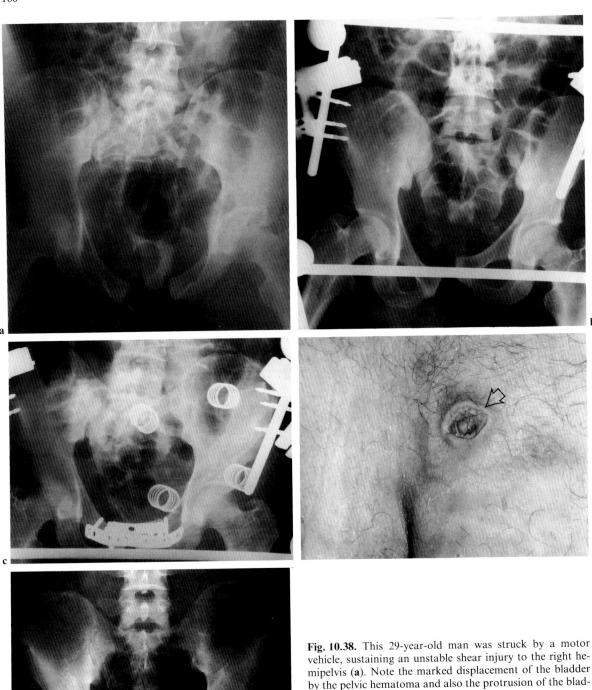

Fig. 10.38. This 29-year-old man was struck by a motor vehicle, sustaining an unstable shear injury to the right hemipelvis (**a**). Note the marked displacement of the bladder by the pelvic hematoma and also the protrusion of the bladder through the symphysis on this intravenous pyelogram. Application of an external skeletal fixator (**b**) restored only partial stability. Note the deformity of the right hemipelvis with the fixator in place. Stability was restored by dual plating of the symphysis pubis (**c**). Ten days following injury, he spontaneously drained a large hematoma on the right sacroiliac joint (**d**), indicating the marked soft tissue lesion of the posterior ligamentous complex. His final result was good with sound healing of the right sacroiliac joint and no displacement of the pelvic ring (**e**). (From Tile 1984)

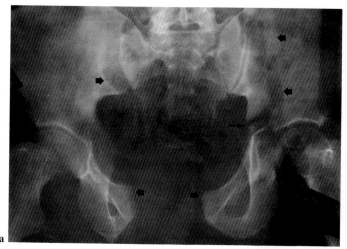
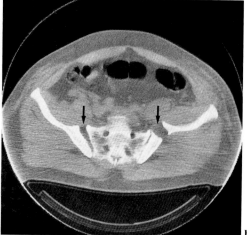
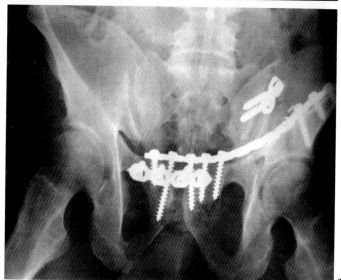

Fig. 10.39. a Anteroposterior radiograph demonstrating a left acetabular fracture associated with a pelvic ring disruption. Note the left acetabular fracture (*long arrow*) and the massive symphysis pubis disruption associated with a fracture of the left ilium and an anterior opening of the right sacroiliac joint, a variation of an open book fracture (*short arrows*). The open right sacroiliac joint and left iliac fracture are best seen on the CT (**b**). Open reduction and internal fixation was performed through an ilioinguinal approach with fixation as shown in **c**. (From Tile 1984)

3. Associated anterior acetabular fracture: If a fracture of the anterior column of the acetabulum or a transverse fracture is associated with a symphysis disruption, a displaced sacroiliac joint, or a fracture in the ilium, an ilioinguinal approach can be used to fix both components of the fracture, as shown in Fig. 10.39. This case represents an unusual configuration of an open book injury with a massive symphysis disruption, an anterior opening of the right sacroiliac joint and an external rotation injury to the left ilium extending into the anterior column of the acetabulum with major displacement. This fracture was approached through an ilioinguinal incision and all components fixed as shown.

Posterior

If the pubic rami are fractured, then anterior fixation is impractical. Therefore, if an approach is to be made to the pelvis, it should be posterior. The indications for a posterior pelvic fixation are as follows:

1. *Malreduction of the posterior sacroiliac complex:* In some instances, closed reduction of the posterior sacroiliac complex will be unsatisfactory, especially in cases of pure sacroiliac dislocation, which frequently result in chronic sacroiliac pain. However, there may be instances where the fracture itself cannot be reduced, thus requiring open reduction, as shown in Fig. 10.40. In that particular case, the patient was injured in a collision between a motor bike and a motor vehicle. Note the external rotation of the left hemipelvis. This unusual injury caused by an external rotatory force on the left hemipelvis has fractured the ilium and driven the iliac portion of the sacroiliac joint anteriorly until it rested on the front of the sacrum.

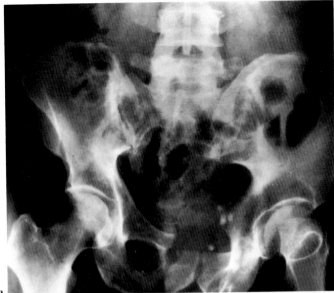

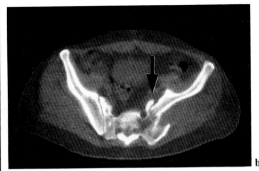

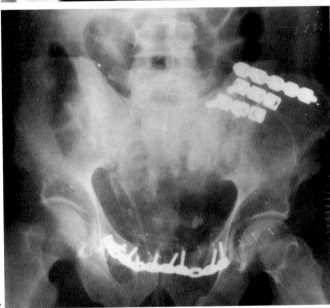

Fig. 10.40. a Anteroposterior radiograph of an unstable pelvic ring disruption. The injury looks relatively innocuous; however, note that the left hemipelvis is externally rotated approximately 45° compared to the right. The left hemipelvis shows an iliac oblique view, the right an anteroposterior view. This is more clearly seen on the CT (b). Note that the hemipelvis anterior to the iliac fracture has rotated externally and has compressed into the sacrum (*arrow*). The patient had a lumbosacral nerve plexus injury. The pelvis failed to unite, and 7 months after the original injury, because of severe pain, a combined anterior and posterior approach was employed and resulted in reduction of the pelvis and fixation as shown in c. Stability was restored and the final result is good

The lumbosacral plexus was injured but gradually recovered, except for the fifth nerve root which was permanently damaged. When seen at 6 months following injury, the left hemipelvis was externally rotated 45° and the fracture dislocation was not united. The patient had significant pain on sitting or standing. All four rami were fractured anteriorly, the right ones being ununited but the left united. Utilizing two teams of surgeons with the patient in the right lateral position, the sacroiliac joint was approached from both the inside and the outside of the pelvis. The fracture could not be reduced until the left anterior pubic rami fractures, which were healed, were osteotomized. At that point, the left hemipelvis could be reduced and held with three anterior plates placed across the sacroiliac joint. One long anterior plate across the symphysis pubis and the rami fractures fixed the anterior complex.

2. *Polytrauma:* Current surgical wisdom requires polytraumatized patients to be nursed in the upright position to improve chest ventilation. If the pelvic fracture is so unstable that this becomes impossible, then open reduction may aid in the post-trauma care of the patient. Since stabilization with an anterior external frame will usual-

ly allow nursing in the upright position for the first few days, when this position is often lifesaving, this indication would be relative rather than absolute.

3. *Open posterior fracture:* In those uncommon instances when the posterior sacroiliac complex is disrupted and the posterior skin has been lacerated from within, the same principles applied to other open fractures can be applied here. With the wound already open, the surgeon should take the opportunity to stabilize the posterior complex in a manner described later in this chapter. In those instances, the wound may be left open and closed secondarily.

However, if the open wound is in the perineum, then all forms of internal fixation are contraindicated. Both the rectum and the vagina must be examined carefully for lacerations to rule out occult open fractures of the pelvis. Open fractures into the perineum are dangerous injuries and result in a high mortality rate. Treatment for the open pelvic fracture should include cleansing and careful débridement of the wound followed by open wound care. The fracture should be stabilized in the first instance with an external skeletal frame. Both bowel and bladder diversion with a colostomy and cystostomy are essential.

4. *Associated posterior acetabular fractures:* Transverse or posterior fractures of the acetabulum associated with pelvic ring disruption are also an indication in some instances for posterior fixation of the pelvic ring and acetabulum. This requires careful decision making and preoperative planning. The acetabular fracture cannot be reduced anatomically until the pelvic portion is reduced.

10.5.4.3 Surgical Techniques

a) General Aspects

Timing

In general, we prefer to wait with pelvic open reduction until the patient's general state has improved, which is usually between the 5th and the 7th post-trauma day. During this initial period, relative stability is maintained with the external fixator.

Exceptions to this rule are instances when a laparotomy or bladder exploration has been carried out, so that the symphysis is already exposed; it should then be internally fixed primarily. Secondly, in the rare instance of a vascular injury to the femoral artery necessitating vascular repair,

associated with a pelvic factor, the incisions may be carefully planned with the vascular surgeon to allow stabilization of the anterior pubic rami.

As previously mentioned, a posterior open fracture may also be a rare indication for immediate open reduction and internal fixation.

Antibiotics

Prophylactic antibiotics are routinely given for these major operative procedures. A first-generation cephalosporin is given intravenously just prior to surgery and continued for 48 h or longer if necessary.

b) Implants

Plates. Because of the difficulty in contouring the standard plates in the several directions required, we recommend the 3.5-mm and 4.5-mm reconstruction plates for pelvic fixation (see, e.g., Figs. 10.39, 11.35). These plates can be contoured in two planes and are most useful. In general, the 3.5-mm plates are used on most women and smaller men and the 4.5-mm plates on larger men. Preshaped reconstruction plates are available for the anterior column fractures.

Screws. The 3.5-mm fully threaded cancellous screws and the 6.5-mm fully threaded cancellous screws are essential components of the fixation system, as well as all the standard lag screws in the two sizes (4.0 mm and 6.5 mm). Screws of exceptional length, up to 120 mm, are required in the pelvis.

Instruments. Since reduction of the pelvic fragments is the most difficult part of the operation, special pelvic clamps are essential. These include the pointed fracture reduction clamps and the large pelvic reduction clamps held in place with two screws (see Fig. 11.33). Other specialized pelvic reduction clamps are also available. We also find the flexible drills and taps as well as the universal screwdriver to be essential for pelvic open reduction and internal fixation. This allows one to work around corners, especially necessary when working on anterior fixation of the symphysis pubis in obese individuals.

c) Anterior Pelvic Fixation

Symphysis Pubis Fixation

Surgical Approach. If the abdomen is already open through a midline or paramedian incision, then the symphysis can be simply fixed through that

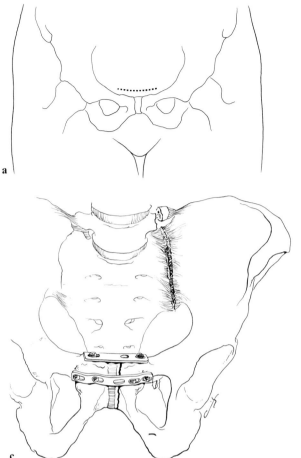

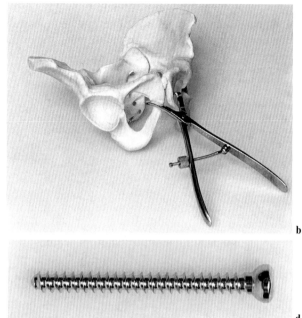

Fig. 10.41. a Open reduction of the symphysis pubis is done through a Pfannenstiel incision. **b** A large fracture reduction clamp is inserted around the medial border of both obturator foramina. Closure of the clamp will easily restore the anatomy of the symphysis pubis. **c** Fixation is secured, using two 4.5-mm dynamic compression plates placed at right angles to each other. **d** Fully threaded cancellous screws should be used to anchor the plates to the soft bone of the symphysis. (From Tile 1984)

approach. If no incision has been made and the symphysis is being approached primarily, the Pfannenstiel incision transversely offers excellent visualization (Fig. 10.41). In the acute case, the rectus abdominis muscle has usually been avulsed and dissection is easy. The surgeon must stay on the skeletal plane to avoid injury to the bladder and urethra.

Reduction. Reduction of the symphysis is usually easy in the acute case. The medial aspect of the obturator foramen should be exposed and the fracture reduction clamp inserted through the foramen (Fig. 10.41 b). Reduction should be anatomical. Care must be taken to avoid catching the bladder or urethra in the symphysis when closing the clamp.

Internal Fixation. In the stable open book configuration, a simple two- or four-hole 3.5-mm or 4.5-mm reconstruction plate applied to the superior surface of the symphysis will afford excellent stability. An external frame is not essential in this particular injury.

In the symphysis disruption associated with an unstable pelvic disruption, we favor a double plate technique (Fig. 10.41 c). A two-hole plate, usually 4.5 mm, is fixed to the superior surface of the symphysis with two 6.5-mm cancellous screws (Fig. 10.41 d) immediately adjacent to the symphysis pubis. To avoid displacement in the vertical plane, an anterior plate, usually a 3.5-mm reconstruction plate in a female or a 4.5-mm one in a male, fixed with the appropriate screws and applied anteriorly will often offer increased stability. Restoration of this anterior tension band will allow the previously inserted anterior frame to compress the posterior complex by externally rotating the hemipelvis at the time the clamps are closed. Good stability may be obtained and the patient may assume the upright position.

Pubic Rami Fractures

Although technically possible, we have not favored direct fixation of the pubic rami. If the fractures are laterally placed, the major dissection of an ilioinguinal approach, often bilateral, would be required to fix these fractures. If fractures of the pubic rami are associated with a posterior pelvic disruption, we feel that it would be more prudent to approach the pelvis posteriorly, since restoration of stability in that location is far superior to anterior fixation. Therefore, we see very few indications for fixation of the pubic rami.

Posterior Pelvic Fixation

The posterior sacroiliac complex may be approached anterior or posterior to the sacroiliac joint. Decision making for either approach is in a state of flux at this time but, in general, the following guidelines may be given. Firstly, the complication rate for posterior incisions in the post-traumatic period is high. In our series, the incidence of wound breakdown from skin necrosis was unacceptable, especially in patients with a crush injury. The posterior skin is often in a precarious state and spontaneously breaks down even without surgery because of the avulsion of the underlying gluteus maximus fascia. Therefore, there is a growing trend toward anterior fixation of the sacroiliac complex. It is of historical interest that our mentor, George Pennal, from whom we learned a great deal about pelvic disruption, originally approached the sacroiliac joint anteriorly, but because of poor fixation methods using staples, abandoned the approach. With the use of plates anteriorly, stability can be restored. This more physiological approach is now being advocated with greater frequency.

Therefore, we favor the anterior approach for fixation of sacroiliac dislocations and some fracture dislocations and the posterior approach for some iliac fractures and sacral crush.

d) Anterior Fixation of the Sacroiliac Joint

Surgical Approach. A long incision is made from the posterior portion of the iliac crest to beyond the anterior superior spine. The iliac crest is exposed and the iliacus muscle swept by subperiosteal dissection posteriorly to expose the sacroiliac joint including the ala of the sacrum (Fig. 10.42a). If further exposure is required, the incision may be extended distally as for the iliofemoral or Smith-Petersen approach to the hip joint. The greater sciatic notch should be clearly exposed to protect the sciatic nerve.

The L5 nerve root exits from the intervertebral foramen between L5 and S1 and crosses the L5–S1 disc to the ala of the sacrum, where it joins the

S1 nerve root as it exits from the S1 foramen (Fig. 10.42b, c). These nerves are in jeopardy in this approach and care must be taken not to injure them either by pointed reduction clamps or by plates that are longer than one screw on the sacral portion.

This technique is not suitable to fractures of the sacrum because of the proximity to the nerves; therefore, it can only be used in sacroiliac dislocations or fractures of the ilium. Reduction may be difficult, and is aided by longitudinal traction and pointed fracture clamps in the anterior superior spine of the ilium pulling anteriorly. The reduction should be checked anteriorly at the greater sciatic notch.

Two two- or three-hole 4.5-mm plates held by 6.5-mm fully threaded cancellous screws afford excellent fixation. A slight over-contouring of the plate will aid in reduction, since tightening the lateral screw will tend to anteriorly reduce the ilium (Fig. 10.42d–e). A rectangular external frame will supplement the posterior fixation if no fixation is present at the symphysis. The wound should be drained and closed.

If the patient is young and good stability has been attained, the upright position may be assumed, but weight bearing should be restricted until healing progresses, a period of approximately 6 weeks.

e) Posterior Fixation of the Sacroiliac Joint

As noted previously, the posterior approach to the sacroiliac joint is safe and straight-forward but the risk of complications such as wound breakdown and nerve damage are significant, and it should therefore be approached with considerable caution. The indications include an unreduced sacral crush, sacroiliac dislocation, and fracture-dislocation. Since no clear indications exist at this time for favoring either the anterior or the posterior approach to the sacroiliac joint, the surgeon's choice of approach can often be guided by personal preference.

Surgical Approach. The incision should be longitudinal just lateral to the posterior superior iliac spine over the belly of the gluteus maximus muscle (Fig. 10.43a). One should always avoid the subcutaneous border of any bone, especially in this area. The incision is opened to the posterior superior spine and iliac crest area. The gluteus maximus muscle, which is often avulsed, is further dissected by the subperiosteal route to expose the superior gluteal notch. The sciatic nerve must be protected

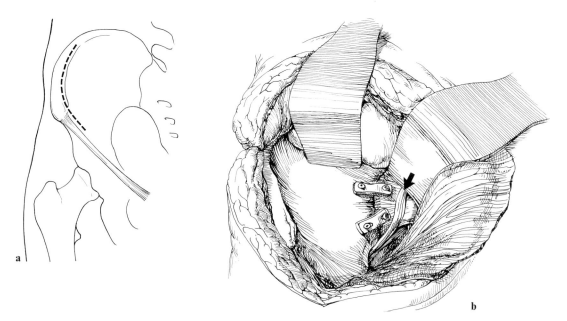

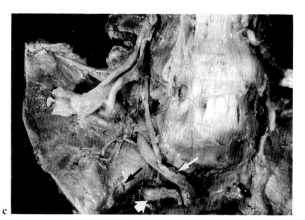

Fig. 10.42 a–e. Anterior fixation of the sacroiliac joint. **a** Incision just medial to the iliac crest. **b** Subperiosteal dissection of the iliacus muscle will expose the sacroiliac joint. Note the proximity of the L5 nerve root (*arrow*), which when joined by the S1 nerve exiting through the S1 foramen becomes the sciatic nerve which leaves the pelvis through the greater sciatic notch, as shown. **c** Anatomical dissection showing the relationship of the L5 nerve root to the sacroiliac joint. The L5 nerve root (*small white arrow*) is seen crossing the ala of the sacrum and joining with the S1 nerve root exiting the first sacral foramen (*broad white arrow*). The sacroiliac joint is outlined by the *black arrow*. **d** Inlet view showing an unstable right hemipelvis with posterior displacement of the right sacroiliac joint and disruption of the symphysis. **e** Fixation of the right sacroiliac joint with two anterior plates and a single plate on the symphysis pubis

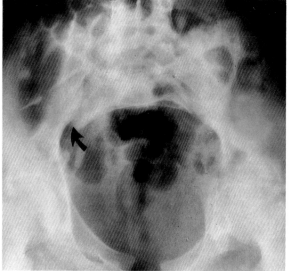

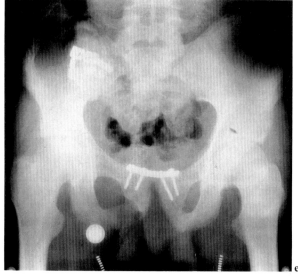

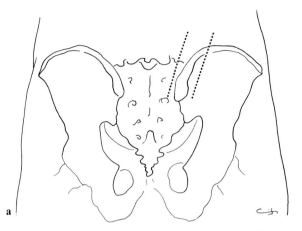

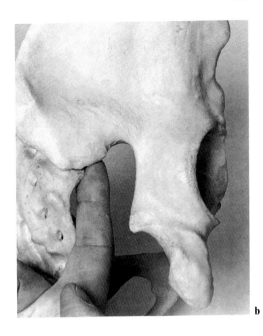

Fig. 10.43a, b. Posterior pelvic fixation. **a** The skin incision should be made just lateral or just medial to the posterior superior spine, depending on whether the fracture is in the ilium or the sacrum. **b** The reduction should be assessed by placing the finger around the distal end of the sacroiliac joint in the region of the greater sciatic notch. (From Tile 1984)

as it exits through the notch. In the unstable fracture for which this incision is indicated, the examining finger can be placed through the notch to explore the anterior aspect of the sacrum (Fig. 10.43b). Anatomical reduction can be verified only by this maneuver. *Image intensification is most desirable,* especially if screws are to be used across the sacroiliac joint and one is to avoid the sacral foramina.

f) Techniques

Fractures of the Ilium: Screw and Plate Fixation. Posterior fractures of the ilium or fracture dislocations of the sacroiliac joint are best fixed with standard techniques of open reduction of the fracture and primary internal fixation with lag screws across the fracture, followed by the application of a 4.5-mm or 3.5-mm reconstruction plate, as a neutralization plate. Usually two plates are required to prevent displacement (Fig. 10.44).

Sacroiliac Dislocations: Screw Fixation. Screw fixation across the sacroiliac joint affords excellent fixation. The screws can be used alone or through a small plate as a washer, especially in older individuals. The technique of placement of these screws must be precise, otherwise, damage to the cauda equina by penetration of the spinal canal or to the S1 foramen will be unacceptably common. If this technique is to be used, *image intensification is essential in two planes.*

The superior screw should be placed in the ala of the sacrum and across into the area of the S1

body. A 2-mm Kirschner wire should be inserted first and checked on the image intensifier to confirm the position. Across the sacroiliac joint, 6.5-mm cancellous lag screws over washers must be used (Fig. 10.47).

In a sacroiliac dislocation, a length of 40–45 mm will suffice. However, for a sacral fracture or sacral nonunion, the screw must penetrate the S1 body to cross the fracture line. In those circumstances, longer screws of 60–70 mm must be used, and therefore the position of the screw is critical. The surgeon must have his finger over the top of the iliac crest and on the ala of the sacrum as a guide and the drill and guide wire must be inserted under image intensification (Fig. 10.45).

The second screw, again using image intensification, should be inserted distal to the S1 foramen. To avoid the nerve within the foramen, the final screw can be placed distal to the S1 foramen, although in this area it is extremely difficult because of the thinness of the bone. The foramen can be seen on the image intensifier or may be seen directly by posterior disruption and dissection. Often two screws may be placed proximally and one distally. It is essential that the surgeon embarking on this technique learn it in a manual skills laboratory prior to inserting these screws into a patient.

Sacral Crush: Sacral Bars Fixation. In the acute sacral crush requiring open reduction through a posterior approach, the use of sacral bars is safe and adequate. Since the device does not penetrate

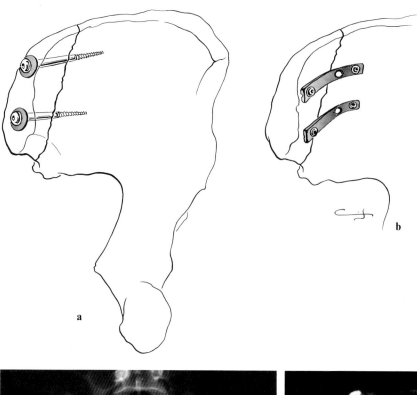

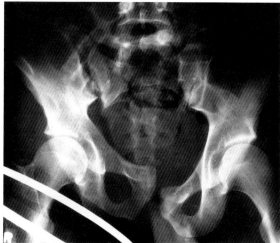

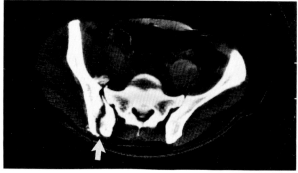

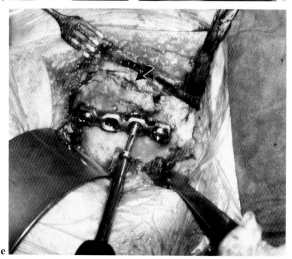

Fig. 10.44. a The use of lag screws to fix a fracture of the ilium. b The use of plates to fix the posterior ilium. c Antero-posterior radiograph showing a fracture through the ilium. d CT scan of same patient. e 4.5-mm reconstruction plate fixing the anatomically reduced fracture in the coronal plane. Note the lag screw fixation being used to compress this fracture. (From Tile 1984)

Fig. 10.45. The position of the drill for insertion of a screw across the sacroiliac joint. Note the surgeon's finger over the iliac crest on the ala of the sacrum to direct the drill. This procedure is best carried out under image intensification

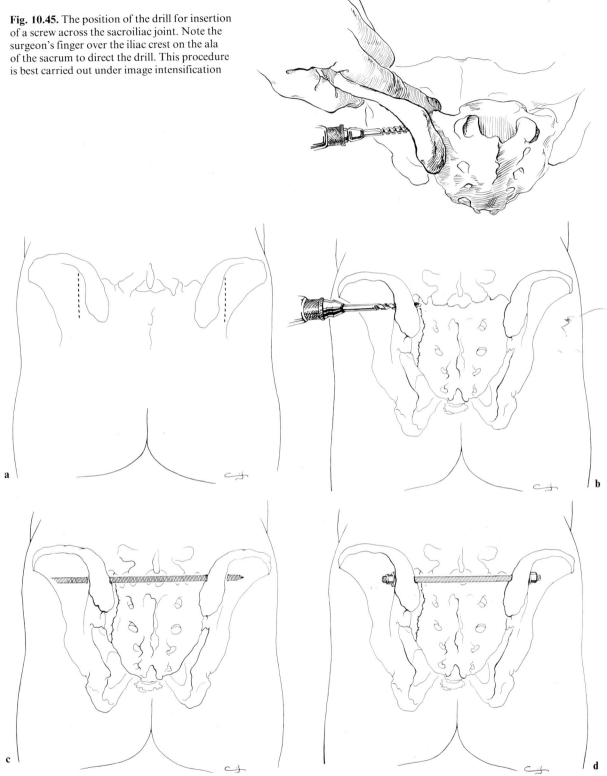

Fig. 10.46a–g. Sacral bar posterior fixation. Two slightly curved, vertically placed incisions are made just lateral to the posterior superior spines (**a**). After reduction of the fracture-dislocation, Kirschner wires are placed across the sacroiliac joint as provisional stabilization. The posterior iliac crest in the region of the posterior spine is predrilled with a 0.25-inch (6.4-mm) drill bit to provide a gliding hole (**b**).

A second hole is predrilled for the second bar. The sacral bar is then inserted posterior to the sacrum and the sharp trochar point driven into the opposite posterior iliac spine (**c**). A standard washer is used to prevent sinking of the sacral rod nut into the bone. Then the nuts are tightened, compressing the sacroiliac joint or the sacral fracture (**d**).

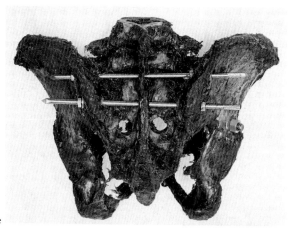

e

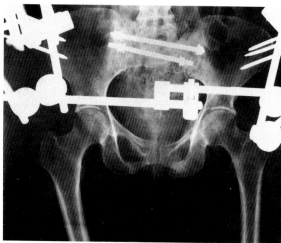

f

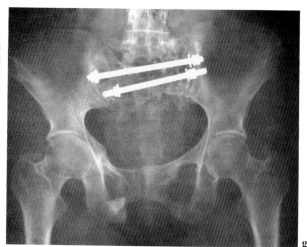

g

Fig. 10.46 (continued). **e** shows the two sacral bars in place on a cadaveric specimen. The tips of the bars should of course be cut short so as not to interfere with the posterior soft tissues. **f** is an anteroposterior radiograph of a case of pelvic disruption in a 32-year-old female, showing the two sacral bars stabilizing the posterior lesion and an anterior frame, the anterior lesion. The final result after healing of the fracture and removal of the anterior frame is shown in **g**. (From Tile 1984)

the sacrum, the neural elements are not at risk. The insertion of two sacral bars will restore excellent stability to the posterior complex, as shown in Fig. 10.46. The addition of the anterior frame will complete the stabilization.

The incision on the side of injury is the same as previously mentioned, just lateral to the posterior superior iliac spine. The posterior spine is exposed, a gliding hole made, and the threaded sacral bar driven through until it hits the opposite posterior iliac spine. The sharp point on the sacral bar is driven through the posterior spine until it emerges on the outer table of the iliac crest. Washers and nuts are inserted and the bars cut off flush at the nut. A second bar is inserted distally. An absolute contraindication is a fracture in the posterior superior spine area. If none exists, good compression may be obtained for the sacral crush without fear of damaging the neural elements. We favor this approach for the acute sacral crush, where necessary.

Bilateral Sacroiliac Injuries. In bilateral injuries, the sacral bars cannot be used unless supplemented with screw fixation into the sacrum on at least one side to prevent posterior displacement of the entire complex.

10.5.4.4 Postoperative Care

Postoperative care depends entirely on the quality of the bone and the quality of the fixation. If the bone quality is good and fixation is stable anteriorly and posteriorly, ambulation with crutches is possible. However, in most cases, a period of postoperative traction is prudent and may prevent late displacement.

Nonunion

Since nonunion of the pelvis is not a rare event, occurring in 3% of cases, the above techniques may prove valuable in the management of these difficult problems. The surgeon must be familiar

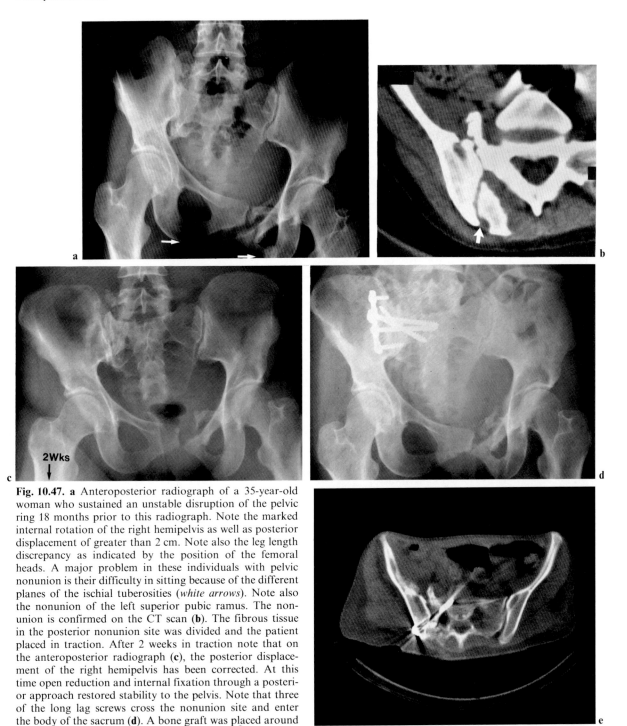

Fig. 10.47. a Anteroposterior radiograph of a 35-year-old woman who sustained an unstable disruption of the pelvic ring 18 months prior to this radiograph. Note the marked internal rotation of the right hemipelvis as well as posterior displacement of greater than 2 cm. Note also the leg length discrepancy as indicated by the position of the femoral heads. A major problem in these individuals with pelvic nonunion is their difficulty in sitting because of the different planes of the ischial tuberosities (*white arrows*). Note also the nonunion of the left superior pubic ramus. The nonunion is confirmed on the CT scan (**b**). The fibrous tissue in the posterior nonunion site was divided and the patient placed in traction. After 2 weeks in traction note that on the anteroposterior radiograph (**c**), the posterior displacement of the right hemipelvis has been corrected. At this time open reduction and internal fixation through a posterior approach restored stability to the pelvis. Note that three of the long lag screws cross the nonunion site and enter the body of the sacrum (**d**). A bone graft was placed around the nonunion, which subsequently healed. The appearance in the CT scan after healing is shown in **e**

with all of the above techniques before embarking on the management of a nonunion, especially in the malreduced position. These complex problems require individualization and careful preoperative planning. Posterior iliac osteotomies may be re-quired to correct vertical displacement. If major amounts of correction are necessary (more than 2.5 cm), we favor a staged procedure. The first operative procedure should include freeing up of the nonunion and corrective osteotomies posteriorly or anteriorly, as required. The patient should then be placed in supracondylar skeletal traction with a weight of 30–40 lb (14–18 kg) applied to the limb. With the patient awake, correction can be monitored radiographically. Problems with the sciatic nerve may be detected because the patient is awake. At 2–3 weeks following the primary operation, a secondary procedure to stabilize the pelvis may be performed (Fig. 10.47). Occasionally, the large double cobra plate or a long contoured DC plate may be helpful for these difficult cases.

10.6 Summary

Disruption of the pelvic ring is a serious injury with a significant mortality. Early management is directed to the essentials of polytrauma care. Complications of this injury are many, including massive hemorrhage, rupture of a hollow viscus, especially bladder, urethra and small bowel, and open wounds in the perineum. As the general aspects of the injury are dealt with, the musculoskeletal injury should not be forgotten but should be managed concurrently with the other injuries. The trauma or orthopedic surgeon must carefully plan the early management to include stabilization of the pelvic fracture. A knowledge of the fracture types is essential for logical decision making.

The role of *external* skeletal fixation may be lifesaving in provisional fixation of the unstable pelvic disruption. It should be applied quickly and simply. External skeletal fixation may also be used as definitive treatment in the stable open book (anteroposterior compression) fracture, in the occasional lateral compression injury which requires reduction by external rotation, and in the unstable pelvic disruption in association with supracondylar skeletal traction or open reduction and internal fixation.

The role of *internal* fixation is not as clear, since most cases of pelvic disruption will do well using simpler traction methods. However, some indications do exist for fixation of the symphysis pubis

anteriorly, and of the sacroiliac complex posteriorly from either the anterior or posterior approach to that joint. We favor the anterior approach to the sacroiliac joint for sacroiliac dislocations and iliac fractures, and the posterior approach for sacral fractures and some fracture dislocations of the sacroiliac joint. For sacral disruptions, we favor the insertion of two sacral bars posteriorly, for sacroiliac dislocations, anterior plating, and for iliac fractures, standard techniques of lag screw fixation with plates.

Above all, these fractures occur in very ill polytraumatized patients and are often extremely complex. Therefore, management must be individualized and cannot be doctrinaire.

References

Aprahamian C, Carrico CJ, Collicott PE et al. (1981) Advanced trauma life support course. Committee on Trauma, American College of Surgeons
Bucholz RW (1981) The pathological anatomy of Malgaigne fracture dislocations of the pelvis. J Bone Joint Surg 63A(1):400–404
Dickinson D, Lifeso R, McBroom R, Tile M (1982) Disruptions of the pelvic ring. J Bone Joint Surg 64B(5):635
Gertzbein SD, Chenoweth DR (1977) Occult injuries of the pelvic ring. Clin Orthop 128:202–207
Holdsworth FW (1948) Dislocation and fracture dislocations of the pelvis. J Bone Joint Surg 30B:461–466
Lipkowitz G, Phillips T, Coren C, Spero C, Glassberg K, Velcek FT (1982) Hemipelvectomy: a lifesaving operation in severe open pelvic injury in childhood. J Trauma 25 (9):823–827
McMurtry R, Walton D, Dickinson D, Kellam J, Tile M (1980) Pelvic disruption in the polytraumatized patient: a management protocol. Clin Orthop 151:22–30
Monahan PR, Taylor RG (1975) Dislocation and fracture dislocation of the pelvis. Injury 6(4):325–333
Pennal GF, Sutherland GO (1959) The use of external fixation. Paper presented at the Canadian Orthopaedic Association annual meeting
Richardson JD, Harty J, Amin M et al. (1982) Open pelvic fractures. J Trauma 22(7):533–538
Slätis P, Huittinen VM (1972) Double vertical fractures of the pelvis: a report on 163 patients. Acta Chir Scand 138:799–807
Tile M (1984) Fractures of the pelvis and acetabulum. Williams and Wilkins, Baltimore

11 Fractures of the Acetabulum

M. TILE

11.1 Introduction

Fractures of the acetabulum are relatively uncommon, but because they involve a major weight-bearing joint in the lower extremity, they assume great clinical importance. The principle of management for this fracture is as for any other displaced lower extremity intra-articular fracture, namely, that anatomical reduction is essential for good long-term function of the hip joint. In some cases, anatomical reduction may be obtained by closed means, but more often, open reduction followed by stable internal fixation allowing early active or passive motion will be required. In the past, the achievement of this ideal, that is anatomical reduction, has been difficult because of technical problems such as those caused by complicated anatomy, difficulty with surgical exposure, severe comminution in many cases, and major associated injuries. Permanent disability was reported to be high, whether open or closed methods were used.

11.1.1 Natural History

A search of the early literature on this subject may seem confusing because it is based on broad generalizations made by lumping all acetabular fractures together. It is important when reading this literature to remember that it is not the overall results that are important, since they may reflect a high proportion of inconsequential fractures. If one is making broad generalizations based on a number of acetabular fractures, a knowledge of the case mix of the series becomes essential. If a large percentage of the cases are of the type shown in Fig. 11.1a, then one would expect good results from simple closed treatment. On the other hand, if the majority of cases are like the one in Fig. 11.1b, poor results may be expected from closed treatment. Therefore, it is essential when reading the literature to separate the apples from the oranges, that is, to compare only similar fracture types (Fig. 11.1c).

For example, in the article by Rowe and Lowell (1961), closed methods using traction were recommended as the treatment of choice for acetabular fractures. However, close scrutiny of this paper describing 93 fractures in 90 patients revealed a large number of inconsequential fractures in older individuals with expected good results. However, in examining the high-energy injuries, 26 involved the superior weight-bearing dome of the acetabulum. When anatomical reduction was obtained, 13 of 16 had a good result, but when anatomical reduction of the dome fragment was not obtained, ten out of ten had a poor result. Of the posterior wall fractures, of which there were 17, closed management led to poor results in six out of nine cases, whereas open management led to good results in eight out of eight cases. The undisplaced fractures and the medial wall fractures in elderly individuals without protrusio gave satisfactory results with closed means. Thus, the conclusion from this early series should have been that high-energy injury involving the posterior wall or the superior weight-bearing dome were best treated by open reduction and internal fixation, if the anatomy could not be restored by closed means.

Judet et al. (1964) reached a similar conclusion. They recommended open reduction and internal fixation for all displaced acetabular fractures and proposed a classification of these fractures based on the pattern of injury.

Pennal et al. (1980), reporting on 103 fractures of the acetabulum, indicated that of those with a poor reduction, 72% had clinical and radiographic osteoarthritis at 5-year follow-up, whereas of those with a good reduction, only 30% had such changes. Although the incidence of osteoarthritis in those with a good reduction in this series may seem high, the severity of the arthritis was much less and the incidence less than half of those with a poor result.

Letournel (1980) reported on 350 fractures of the acetabulum with very good results in 75%, good results in 8%, and poor results in 17%. Of

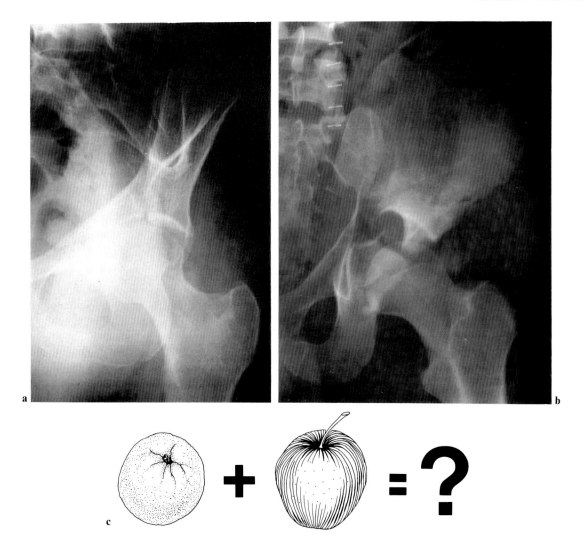

Fig. 11.1 a–c. Comparing the undisplaced acetabular fracture (**a**) to the grossly displaced comminuted acetabular fracture associated with a pelvic ring disruption (**b**) is like comparing an orange to an apple (**c**). (From Tile 1984)

the 74% of the patients with an anatomically reduced hip joint, 90% had a good result. Of the 26% imperfectly reduced, only 55% had a good result if some incongruity remained, only 11% if a degree of protrusio remained, and only 9% if there were major technical failures.

In a recent review of our own case material (Tile et al. 1985), 227 charts were reviewed. Ninety-five cases of minor trauma were eliminated because displacement was less than 5 mm at the joint. Thus, all inconsequential fractures were removed from this series. Only two of those 95 had any difficulty with their hip at review. There were 13 deaths, eight in the post-trauma period, all in

older individuals between 59 and 88 years of age, and five with subsequent trauma, a frequent finding in such a series. Fifteen cases were lost to follow-up, two were treated at nine and twelve months and thereby eliminated from the series, leaving a series of 102 cases. At review, all patients were recalled, personally examined by one of the authors, and standard radiographs taken. Our findings mirrored those in the literature. Excellent results could be attained if anatomical reduction was achieved and complications avoided.

Thus, the literature is not confusing and, if fractures of a similar type and severity are compared, makes the following statement with surprising unanimity: *joint congruity is essential for good long-term function.* Joint congruity must be assessed by strict radiographic means, including CT, and must cover all the essential parts of the acetabulum, including the anterior column, the superior weight-bearing portion, and the posterior column. Failure

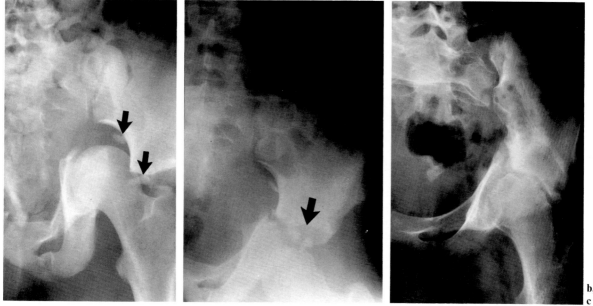

Fig. 11.2a–c. Anteroposterior radiograph (**a**) of the left hip of a 17-year-old girl demonstrating a transverse fracture of the left acetabulum through the dome with a central dislocation of the hip. The two *arrows* in **a** point to loose bony fragments. Following closed reduction (**b**), the two bony fragments have been retained within the joint (*arrow*). In spite of traction, reduction is inadequate, with bony fragments in the joint and incongruity between the femoral head and acetabulum. Definitive treatment consisted of traction until the fracture healed. Her result at 18 months is shown in **c**. Note the severe narrowing and erosions on the superior weight-bearing margin of the femoral head. The patient's clinical result was poor. She had a 60° flexion deformity with continuous pain and required an arthrodesis. (From Tile 1984)

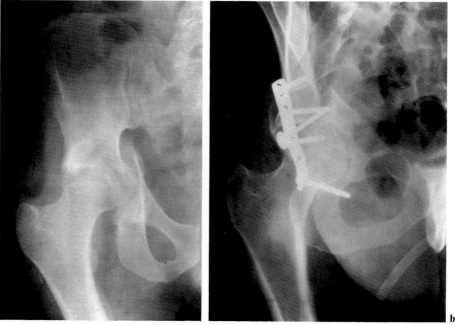

Fig. 11.3. a Radiograph of a 59-year-old man with a transverse fracture of the acetabulum associated with a posterior wall fracture. **b** Postoperative radiograph of the same patient showing a plate placed on the posterior column and one screw in the posterior wall. Note, however, that the fracture is unreduced, the femoral head is subluxated anteriorly, and there is no interfragmental compression between the major fragments of the transverse fracture. This incongruous reduction resulted in a total hip arthroplasty 2 years following the acetabular fracture

to recognize incongruity caused by displacement of the columns, comminution, or articular impaction will result in early destruction of the hip joint (Fig. 11.2).

If closed reduction fails to achieve congruity, then open reduction is essential, but open reduction and internal fixation will only improve the results if anatomical reduction is achieved and operative complications are avoided. Failure to obtain an anatomical reduction in the patient shown in Fig. 11.3 resulted in an early total hip arthroplasty. Note that the plate is on the posterior column; however, the head is displaced anteriorly and the anterior column remains unreduced as on the preoperative radiograph. The basic tenet of fracture care, that is, interfragmental compression of the major fragments, has been forgotten, with the predictable result.

Surgery on this injury is extremely demanding and requires adequate resources, both human and material. A minimum of two qualified assistants and a complete surgical armamentarium including specialized pelvic equipment is essential. Therefore, the natural history of an acetabular fracture may be summarized as follows: if the joint is stable and congruous following reduction, and if complications are avoided, a satisfactory result may be

expected; but if the joint is incongruous, joint destruction will ensue. The major factors affecting the prognosis are as follows:

1. The degree of initial displacement
2. The damage to the superior weight-bearing surface of the acetabulum
3. The degree of hip joint instability caused by a posterior wall fracture
4. The adequacy of reduction, either open or closed
5. The late complications of
   - avascular necrosis of the femoral head
   - heterotopic ossification
   - chondrolysis
   - sciatic or femoral nerve injury

11.1.2 Surgical Anatomy

One must be adept at three-dimensional conceptualization to master the complex anatomy of the acetabulum. From its lateral aspect, the acetabulum is cradled by the arms of an inverted Y (Fig. 11.4a, b). The posterior column is strong and triangular, with extremely thick bone at the greater sciatic notch. The medial surface forms the posterior aspect of the quadrilateral plate.

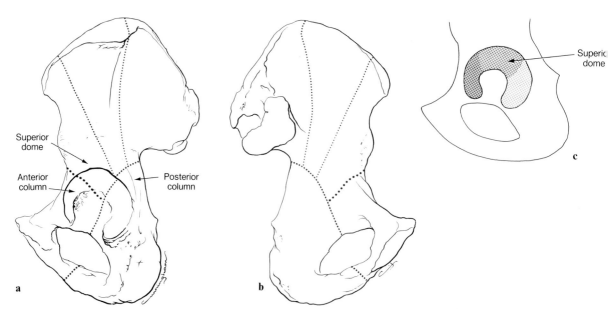

Fig. 11.4. a Lateral aspect of the hemipelvis and acetabulum. The posterior column is characterized by the dense bone at the greater sciatic notch and follows the *dotted line* distally through the center of the acetabulum, the obturator foramen, and the inferior pubic ramus. The anterior column extends from the iliac crest to the symphysis pubis and includes the entire anterior wall of the acetabulum. Fractures involving the anterior column commonly exit below the anterior inferior iliac spine as shown by the *heavy dotted line*. **b** The hemipelvis from its medial aspect. The area between the posterior column and the heavy dotted line, representing a fracture through the anterior column, is often considered the superior dome fragment, represented by the *middle portion* (**c**). (From Tile 1984)

The anterior column extends from the symphysis pubis to the iliac crest. Fractures of the anterior column may comprise any portion of the column. Most commonly, the anterior column fracture exits below the anterior inferior iliac spine. Inspection of the lateral aspect of the acetabulum will indicate the important articular fractures, especially in the weight-bearing dome area (Fig. 11.4c). This area, although vague anatomically, has great clinical significance, since fractures of this area left unreduced will inevitably result in post-traumatic arthritis of the hip joint.

11.1.3 Mechanism of Injury

The pathological anatomy of the fracture depends on the position of the femoral head at the moment of impact (Fig. 11.5). The femoral head acts as a hammer against the acetabulum producing the injury. There are two basic mechanisms of injury: first, those caused by a direct blow on the acetabulum and, second, the so-called dashboard injury, in which the flexed knee joint strikes the dashboard, driving the femur posteriorly on the acetabulum. A blow directly upon the greater trochanter usually causes a transverse type acetabular fracture, depending on the degree of abduction and rotation of the femoral head, whereas the dashboard injury causes a posterior wall or posterior column fracture or fracture-dislocation of the hip joint.

In general, the externally rotated hip causes injuries to the anterior column, the internally rotated hip to the posterior column; the abducted hip

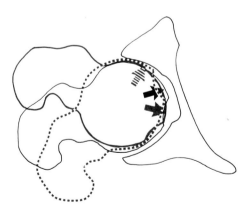

Fig. 11.5. The type of acetabular fracture will depend upon the position of the femoral head at the moment of impact. If externally rotated (*striped arrow*) the anterior column will be involved; if internally rotated (*solid arrow*) the posterior column will be involved. (From Tile 1984)

causes a low transverse fracture, the adducted hip a high transverse fracture.

11.2 Assessment

For logical decision making, a precise diagnosis is imperative, so careful assessment of the patient is essential.

11.2.1 Clinical

The general patient profile is of great importance in decision making. Older individuals have poor bone, reducing the holding power of screws and making anatomical open reduction much more difficult. Therefore, with severely comminuted fractures in older people, other options such as traction, followed by total hip arthroplasty if necessary, are more advisable than for younger patients. Thus, the age and general medical state of the patient are important, as well as the assessment of other major injuries in the polytraumatized patient, especially those involving the affected limb, such as fractures of the femur or neurovascular injuries.

11.2.2 Radiological Assessment

The radiological assessment should include the following:

11.2.2.1 Special Radiographs of the Pelvis

These should include the anteroposterior view, the inlet view, and the outlet view (see p. 149). This will allow an overview of any other injuries in the pelvic ring.

11.2.2.2 Specific Acetabular Views

Anteroposterior. It is essential that the surgeon treating these difficult fractures become completely familiar with the anatomical landmarks as seen on these particular views of the acetabulum. These landmarks include the iliopectineal line denoting the limit of the anterior column, the ilioischial line denoting the limit of the posterior column, the anterior lip of the acetabulum, the posterior lip of the acetabulum, and the line depicting the superior weight-bearing surface of the acetabulum, ending in the medial teardrop (Fig. 11.6a, b). The anteroposterior view of the hip shows all of these landmarks clearly (Fig. 11.6c).

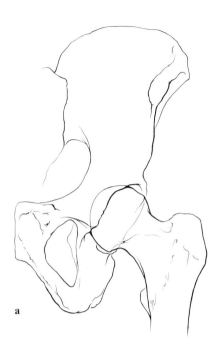

a

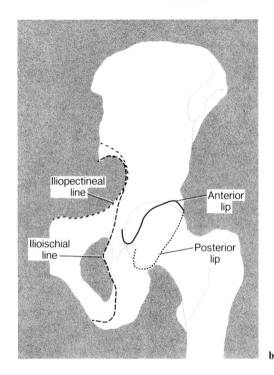

Iliopectineal line

Anterior lip

Ilioischial line

Posterior lip

b

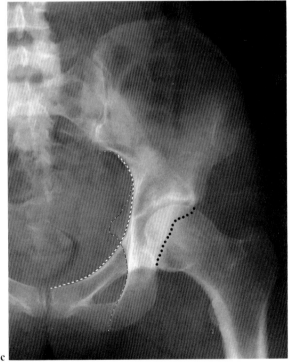

c

Fig. 11.6. a The anatomical landmarks seen on the antero-posterior radiograph. b The major landmarks by the various lines as follows: the iliopectineal line (anterior column) - - -; the ilioischial line (posterior column) – – –; the anterior lip of the acetabulum ——; the posterior lip of the acetabulum ⋯. c Anteroposterior radiograph of the left hemipelvis with the major landmarks outlined. (From Tile 1984)

Iliac Oblique View. The iliac oblique view is taken by externally rotating the affected hemipelvis. A foam wedge is inserted under the opposite hip of the patient allowing external rotation of 45° (Fig. 11.7a, inset). This view clearly shows the entire iliac crest and best depicts the extent of the posterior column and the anterior lip of the acetabulum (Fig. 11.7).

Obturator Oblique View. The obturator oblique view is obtained by internally rotating the affected hip 45° with the appropriate foam wedge under

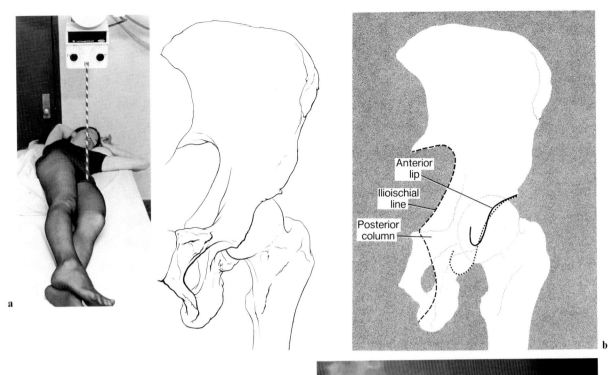

Fig. 11.7a–c. Iliac oblique radiographic view. This view is taken by rotating the patient into 45° of external rotation by elevating the uninjured side on a wedge (*inset*). **a** The anatomical landmarks of the left hemipelvis on the iliac oblique view. **b** The various acetabular lines (for key, see Fig. 11.6 legend). **c** Iliac oblique radiographic view of the left hemipelvis with the superimposed lines. This view best demonstrates the posterior column of the acetabulum outlined by the ilioischial line as well as the iliac crest and the anterior lip of the acetabulum. (**a, b** Adapted from Tile 1984)

the affected hip (Fig. 11.8a, inset). In this view, the iliac crest is seen perpendicular to its normal plane, so displacement of the iliac wing in the coronal plane is best noticed here. This view also best shows the anterior column and the posterior lip of the acetabulum (Fig. 11.8 b, c).

11.2.2.3 Tomography

Prior to computed tomography, plain tomography gave much helpful information especially on the state of the acetabular dome (Fig. 11.9). It may still be helpful in select cases or where CT is not available.

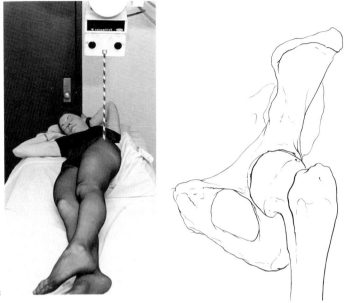

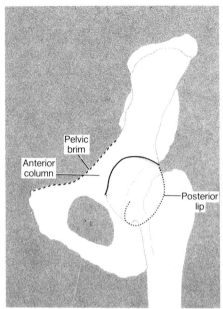

Fig. 11.8a–c. Obturator oblique radiographic view. This
view is taken by elevating the affected hip 45° to the horizontal by means of a wedge and directing the beam through
the hip joint with a 15° upward tilt (*inset*). a The anatomy
of the pelvis on the obturator oblique view. b The important
anatomical landmarks as indicated by various lines (for key,
see Fig. 11.6 legend). c Obturator oblique radiograph of the
left hemipelvis with the superimposed lines. In this view
note particularly the pelvic brim, indicating the border of
the anterior column and the posterior lip of the acetabulum
(a, b Adapted from Tile 1984)

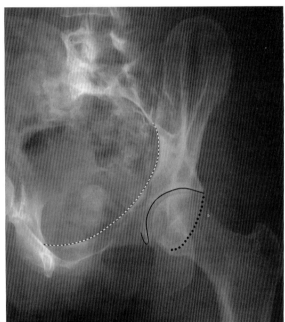

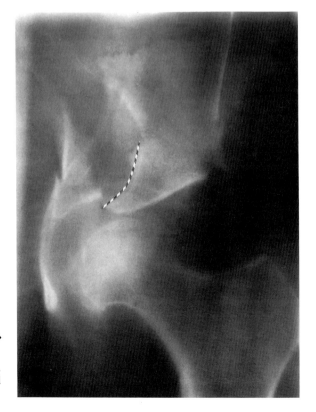

Fig. 11.9. Tomogram showing a dome fragment rotated 90°.
This fragment remained unreduced in spite of an attempted
closed reduction and traction. (From Tile 1984)

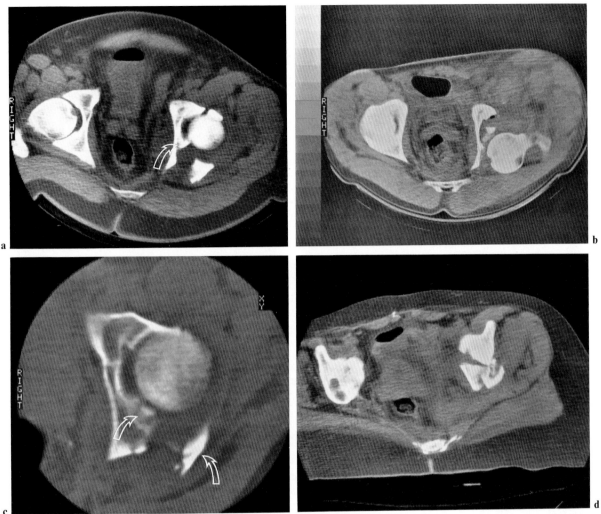

Fig. 11.10. a CT scan demonstrating a transverse fracture of the acetabulum; both the anterior column fracture and the large posterior wall fracture are clearly seen. The *arrow* points to a comminuted rotated bony fragment. **b** CT scan through the central portion of the acetabulum, showing a posterior dislocation of the hip with two large posterior wall fragments trapped within the joint, preventing reduction. The CT scan is most helpful in determining the presence and size of retained bony fragments in the joint. **c** CT scan through the central portion of the acetabulum. Note the large displaced posterior wall fracture on the *lower right*. The *arrow left* points to an impacted fracture of the articular surface. These depressed articular fractures are best seen on CT scanning. **d** CT scan through the acetabular dome of a patient with a severely comminuted acetabular fracture. Note the comminuted fragments and the degree of displacement of the posterior column. (From Tile 1984)

11.2.2.4 Computed Tomography

Computed Tomography (CT) has revolutionized our diagnostic abilities in the pelvis and acetabulum. Although the general acetabular pattern can be determined from the plane radiographs, the computed tomogram gives much additional information regarding for instance, impacted fractures of the acetabular wall, retained bone fragments in the joint, the degree of comminution, unrecognized dislocation, and sacroiliac pathology (Fig. 11.10). Major advances in CT include the ability to reconstruct the pelvis into its ring form, allowing the overall pattern to be visualized (Fig. 11.11).

The newest development in CT is the three-dimensional visual reconstruction of a fracture. This is truly an exciting advance which will greatly aid in decision making (Fig. 11.12a–c). The femoral head may be subtracted by this technique and the articular surface of the acetabulum seen (Fig. 11.12d).

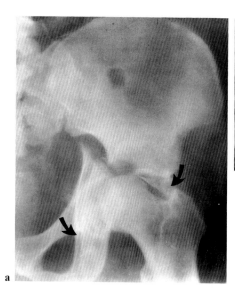

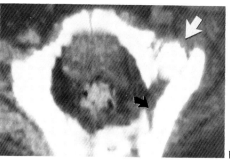

Fig. 11.11. a Anteroposterior radiograph of a comminuted transverse fracture of the acetabulum with a subluxated sacroiliac joint. Note the large fragment within the joint (*upper arrow*) and the split in the medial wall of the acetabulum (*lower arrow*). b CT scan of the same patient with reconstruction of the pelvic ring. Note the marked displacement of the transverse fracture by the interposition of the femoral head (*upper arrow*). Note also how clearly the sacroiliac opening is seen on the scan (*lower arrow*)

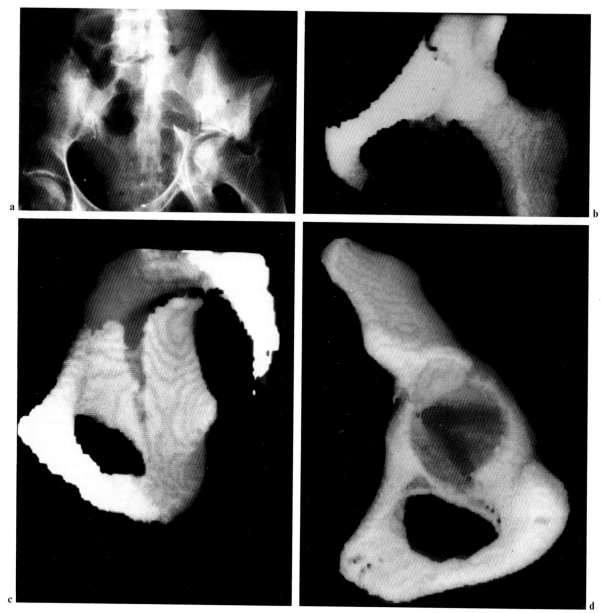

Fig. 11.13a, b. Classification of acetabular fractures. All fractures of the acetabulum are a combination of the major anatomical areas which may be fractured, such as the anterior or posterior lip (**a**) or the anterior or posterior column (**b**)

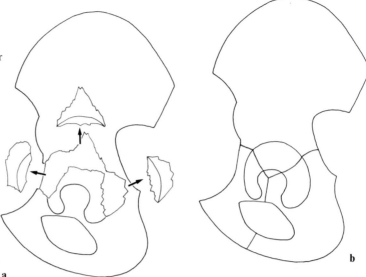

11.3 Classification

Classifications are useful for two purposes: (a) in assisting the decision-making process for the individual case, and (b) for documentation of case material for academic purposes.

For decision making, many factors must be built into any classification and no perfect classification exists. For this purpose, the degree of displacement, the amount of comminution, the presence or absence of a dislocation and the state of the bone, whether osteopenic or normal, must be considered. For documentation, an anatomical classification is best, but incorporating the parameters mentioned above.

Although several classifications exist in the literature, some simple facts should be examined first in order to remove the confusion that surrounds this subject. Basically, the acetabulum consists of four anatomical areas: an anterior and posterior column and an anterior and posterior wall of lip (Fig. 11.13). *All fracture types involve one or a combination of more than one of these.* Therefore, the

following types are possible: an isolated anterior column fracture or an isolated posterior column fracture, a combined anterior column fracture with an anterior lip fracture or a combined posterior column fracture with a posterior lip fracture.

If both columns are broken, we arbitrarily call that injury a *transverse fracture*, and if both columns are broken and separated from each other, that is a *T fracture*. Either of those two main types, the transverse or T, may be associated with an anterior or posterior lip fracture as well.

Finally, there is an unusual fracture of the acetabulum called the double-column (both-column) fracture which gives rise to a true floating acetabulum, that is, no portion of the weight-bearing surface of the acetabulum remains attached to the axial skeleton. The fracture through the iliac wing separating off the dome is usually in the coronal plane.

Therefore, in decision making, the surgeon must examine the plain radiographs and the CT scans available, either plain or three-dimensional, and draw the fracture lines on a dry skeleton. All cases have individual features and many defy classification. Hence, no attempt should be made to pigeonhole any particular case into a published classification for individual decision making. However, the pigeonholing of cases is important for academic purposes, namely clinical reviews. In these, more than just an anatomical classification is necessary.

The Letournel and Judet classification (1981) is given in Table 11.1. It is devided into simple and complex types. Our previously published clas-

Fig. 11.12a–d. Three-dimensional CT. **a** Anteroposterior view of the pelvis showing a transverse fracture of the left acetabulum. **b** Three-dimensional reconstruction showing the transverse fracture. **c** Three-dimensional reconstruction showing the quadrilateral plate. **d** Subtraction of the femoral head showing the interior of the acetabulum. (Courtesy of Dr. Dana Mears)

Table 11.1. Classification of acetabular fractures. (Letournel and Judet 1981)

Elementary fractures
  Posterior wall
  Posterior column
  Anterior wall
  Anterior column
  Transverse

Combination fractures
  T fracture
  Posterior column and posterior wall
  Transverse and posterior wall
  Anterior column (or wall) with posterior hemitransverse
  Double-column

Table 11.2. Classification of acetabular fractures. (From Tile 1984)

Undisplaced fractures

Displaced fractures

Type I
Posterior types ± posterior dislocation
A. Posterior column
B. Posterior wall
  – associated with posterior column
  – associated with transverse fracture

Type II
Anterior types ± anterior dislocation
A. Anterior column
B. Anterior wall
C. Associated anterior and transverse fracture

Type III
Anterior types ± central dislocation
A. Pure transverse
B. T fractures
C. Associated transverse and acetabular wall fractures
D. Double column fractures

Table 11.3. Classification of acetabular fractures. (According to AO Documentation Center)

I. Fractures involving one column or wall

II. Fractures involving both columns with a portion of the dome attached to the axial skeleton

III. Fractures involving both columns with *no* portion of the dome attached to the axial skeleton

of the superior dome is connected to the axial skeleton (Table 11.3).

11.4 Management

Management must begin with a careful clinical and radiographic assessment to define the personality of the injury. As mentioned previously, this includes a careful assessment of the patient profile including age, general medical state, and the severity of other injuries. Assessment of the limb to include ipsilateral femoral fractures, knee injuries, or neurovascular injury is essential.

Specific radiographic examination of the fracture includes the degree of displacement, the amount of comminution, the presence or absence of a dislocation and, most importantly, the state of the bone: whether it be osteopenic or not. The precise anatomical features according to the classifications given above are also essential.

11.4.1 Decision Making

The decision-making process then proceeds according to the algorithm shown in Fig. 11.14.

11.4.1.1 General Resuscitation

Since these patients are often severely injured or polytraumatized, aggressive early resuscitation is essential as previously outlined in Chap. 10 following the guidelines of the American College of Surgeons (Aprahamian et al. 1981).

11.4.1.2 Assessment of the Fracture Personality

Careful assessment of the anatomical features of the particular fracture may allow one to classify it as one with *minimal displacement* or one with *significant displacement*. A fracture with minimal displacement may be treated nonoperatively with the expectation of a good result. Nonoperative

sification by the direction of displacement was an attempt to incorporate surgical decision making into the classification (Table 11.2). Thus, fracture types may be anterior, posterior, medial, or transverse fractures associated with anterior, posterior, or medial displacement.

A new classification recently originated by the AO Documentation Center divides the fractures into those involving one column, those involving both columns in which a portion of the superior dome is attached to the axial skeleton, and, thirdly, those involving both columns in which no portion

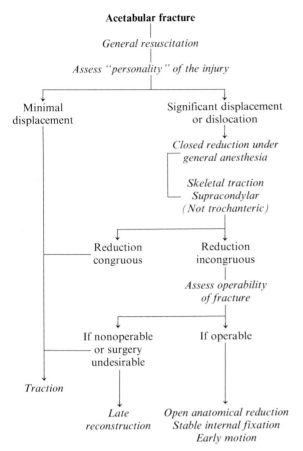

Acetabular fracture

General resuscitation

Assess "personality" of the injury

Minimal displacement

Significant displacement or dislocation

Closed reduction under general anesthesia

Skeletal traction
Supracondylar
(Not trochanteric)

Reduction congruous

Reduction incongruous

Assess operability of fracture

If nonoperable or surgery undesirable

If operable

Traction

Late reconstruction

Open anatomical reduction
Stable internal fixation
Early motion

Fig. 11.14. Algorithm for decision making in acetabular fractures

Table 11.4. Management of acetabular fractures

A. Nonoperative
Displacement less than 2 mm
Distal anterior column fractures
Distal transverse fractures
Double-column (both-column) fracture without major displacement of the posterior column

B. Operative management
Posterior fracture types with hip instability

Displaced dome fractures:
– displaced fragments
– high transverse or T types

Double-column (both-column) with displaced posterior column
Retained bone fragments
Fractures of the femoral head

Other indications:
– nerve injury
– vascular injury
– ipsilateral femoral fracture

management, therefore, may be appropriate for the fracture types described below (Table 11.4).

Minimal Displacement

Displacement Less Than 2 mm. If a fracture is displaced less than 2 mm, no matter what the anatomical type, nonoperative treatment should yield good results. With minimal displacement, skeletal traction is not essential. If the surgeon is concerned about hidden instability, examination under image intensification will help in the decision whether traction is necessary.

Distal Anterior Column Fractures. Prior to the advent of CT, the anterior column fracture was considered a rare acetabular injury. From examination by CT in our pelvic fracture population, we noted that fractures of the superior pubic ramus often entered the inferior portion of the acetabulum, violating the joint. Since these fractures are distal and do not involve the major weight-bearing

portion, surgery is virtually never indicated and good results are obtained (Fig. 11.15).

Low Transverse Fractures. A transverse fracture occurring low on the acetabulum, that is, through the acetabular fossa area, may often be treated nonoperatively with skeletal traction with the expectation of good results. In the five cases so treated in our recent series, four achieved excellent results, the one poor result being from an unrelated problem in the patient. In these particular fracture types, the intact medial aspect of the acetabular wall acts as a buttress, preventing further displacement (Fig. 11.16).

Double-Column (Both-Column) Fracture without Major Posterior Column Displacement. In this injury a two-column fracture with no portion of the weight-bearing dome attached to the axial skeleton, both columns are separated from each other and from the axial skeleton, resulting in a true floating acetabulum. This fracture occurs in the coronal plane. The transverse portion may be superior to or cephalic to the acetabulum and be truly extra-articular. If the posterior column is minimally displaced, skeletal traction may suffice as definitive treatment. Displacement of the posterior column is best seen on the iliac oblique radiograph and especially on the CT scan. CT often shows a major split in the superior surface of the acetabulum, making nonoperative treatment inappropriate (Fig. 11.19).

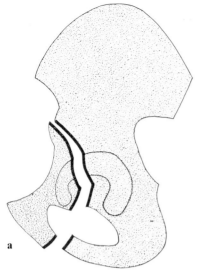

Fig. 11.15a–c. Fracture of the anterior column. **a** Diagram of a typical anterior column fracture dividing the anterior column just distal to the anterior inferior iliac spine. **b** The anteroposterior radiograph of the pelvis clearly demonstrates the fracture of the superior and inferior pubic rami (*arrows*). **c** The CT scan shows the comminution of the anterior column (*curved arrow*) and the intact posterior column (*straight arrow*). (From Tile 1984)

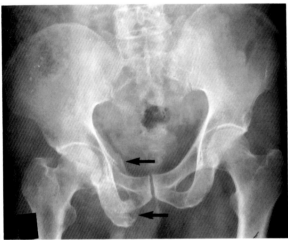

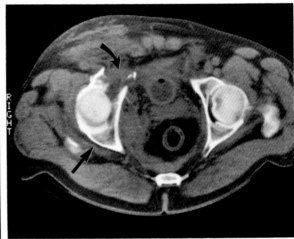

Significant Displacement

If significant displacement has occurred, operative management is indicated, especially in the fracture types described below.

Posterior Fracture Types with Hip Instability. If the posterior lip of the acetabulum is significantly displaced, allowing instability of the hip joint, open reduction and internal fixation are always indicated (Fig. 11.18). Posterior wall fractures may be isolated or they may be associated with posterior column, transverse, T, or double-column fractures. Since the posterior wall injury is usually caused by a blow on the flexed knee, the surgeon must look for knee injuries, including fractures of the patella, or posterior subluxation of the knee with posterior cruciate ligament tears. Also, with posterior dislocation of the hip, a high number

of transient or permanent sciatic nerve palsies may be expected.

Displaced Dome Fractures. Displacement of the acetabular dome may occur in several varieties of injury:

1. Displaced triangular dome fragment. A typical large triangular fragment involving the dome portion of articular cartilage may be displaced and even rotated 90°, as shown in Fig. 11.9. Open reduction and internal fixation are essential to restore the anatomical relationship of that fragment to the remainder of the hip joint.

2. High transverse or T fractures. These shearing type injuries involving the superior portion of the dome are extremely difficult to reduce by closed means. Often fragments of bone are interposed, making reduction impossible. In my opin-

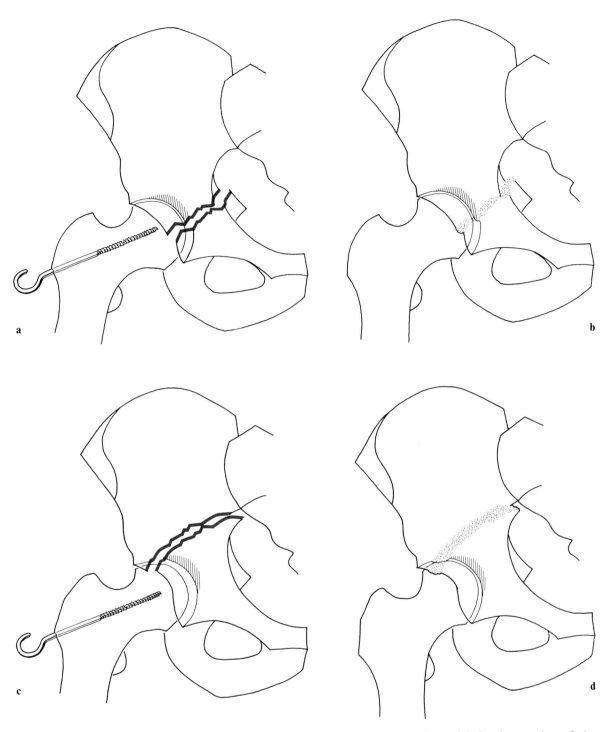

Fig. 11.16a–g. Transverse fracture of the acetabulum. **a** Diagram indicating a low transverse fracture at the level of the acetabular fossa. Closed reduction in this particular injury usually results in a congruous joint. Because the main portion of the weight-bearing dome is intact, as indicated by the striped lines, the medial portion of the dome acts as a buttress to the femoral head preventing redisplacement. **b** With healing, the femoral head retains its congruous rela- tionship with the major weight-bearing portion of the acetabulum. **c** In this diagram a high transverse fracture divides the mid portion of the superior weight-bearing dome. This shearing injury is difficult to manage with trac- tion and usually results in incongruity because the medial fragment remains displaced and the femoral head is congruous with that portion rather than the dome portion **(d)**

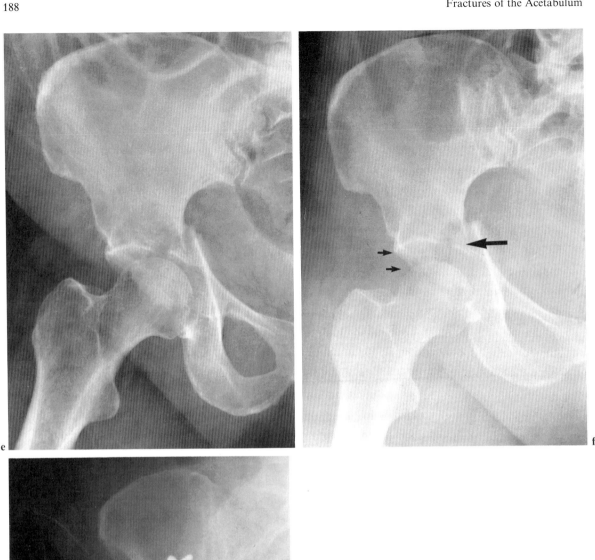

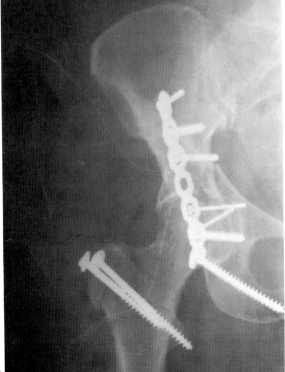

Fig. 11.16 (continued). **e** Anteroposterior radiograph of a patient with a transverse fracture of the acetabulum. Note that the femoral head is congruous to the medial fragment rather than to the dome. **f** Nine kilograms of traction were applied through a supracondylar pin (*small arrows*), but the medial portion of the acetabulum did not reduce (*large arrow*). Restoration of the joint anatomy was possible only with internal fixation (**g**). (From Tile 1984)

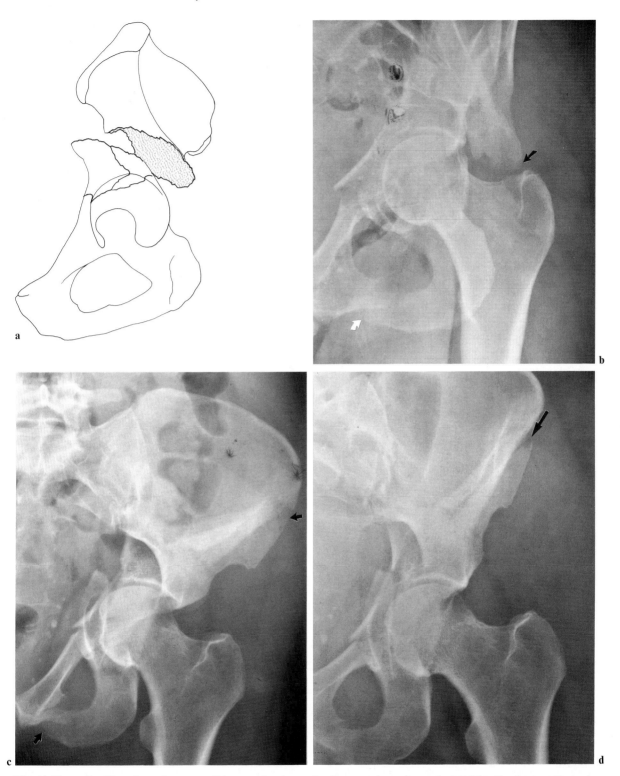

Fig. 11.17a–g. Double-column fracture. **a** Diagram showing the typical appearance of a double-column fracture (both-column fracture). The obturator oblique radiograph (**b**) shows the classic spur sign (*black arrow*). Note the split in the posterior column depicted by the fracture through the obturator foramen (*white arrow*). The iliac oblique (**c**) and anteroposterior (**d**) views show the fracture through the iliac crest (*arrows*).

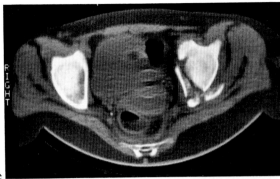

e

Fig. 11.17 (continued). The CT scan through the dome (**e**) shows the complex nature of the fracture, with a coronal split through the dome and a fracture in the posterior column. However, in this particular case, note that the femoral head is largely enclosed by the dome fragment. In this patient, a 49-year-old woman, traction was used as definitive treatment. At 2 years, the final result shows a congruous hip joint. The patient rated 90 on the Harris hip scale with only minimal discomfort from the partially united posterior column (**f, g**). (From Tile 1984)

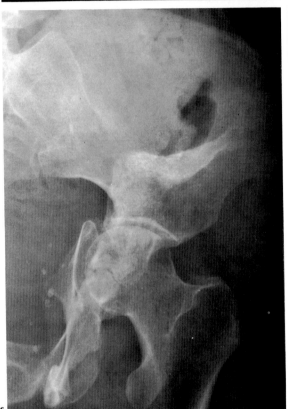

f

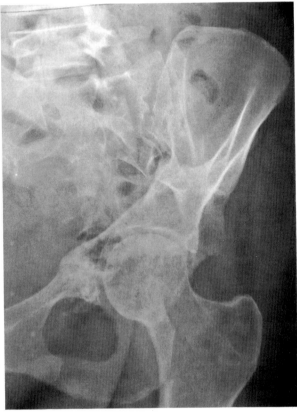

g

ion, these high-energy shearing injuries are extremely difficult to manage nonoperatively because anatomical reduction cannot be maintained and poor results will ensue (Fig. 11.16c–g).

Displaced Double-Column Fracture. In the double-column (both-column) or floating acetabulum fracture, the coronal split of the ilium may extend directly into the joint with gross displacement visible in the coronal plane, best seen on the CT scan. Note the coronal split in the dome in Fig. 11.19a–c, as compared to the split in the dome parallel to the quadrilateral plate, indicating a transverse type fracture, in Fig. 11.19d, e. This type of dou-

ble-column fracture is best managed by open reduction and internal fixation.

Retained Bone Fragments. Large retained bone fragments within the acetabulum may act as a block to anatomical reduction or may prevent normal biomechanical function of the joint. These fragments are best seen on the CT scan (Fig. 11.22 b). They should be removed surgically as soon as possible following injury.

Occasionally, a small fragment of bone will be seen within the fovea on a CT scan (Fig. 11.20). This fragment often represents an avulsion of the pelvic attachment of the teres femoris ligament.

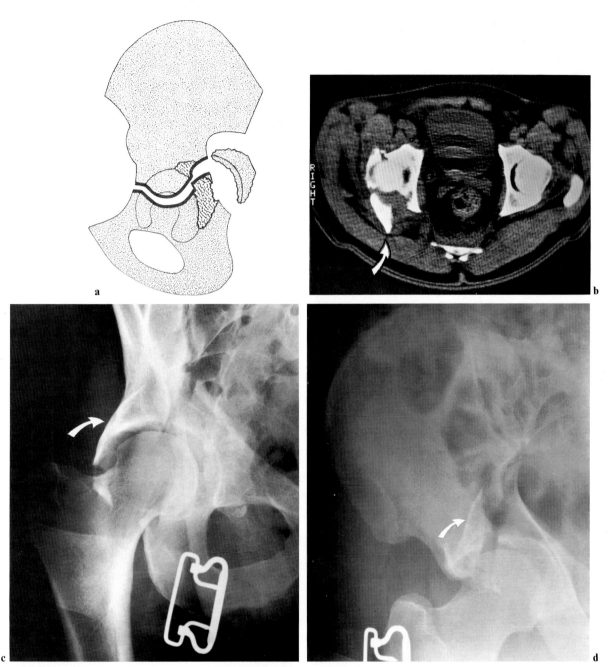

Fig. 11.18a–d. Posterior fracture with instability. **a** Diagram of a transverse fracture associated with a posterior wall fracture. The CT scan (**b**) shows gross displacement of the large posterior wall fragment through which the posterior dislocation of the hip had occurred. The hip was grossly unstable and the fracture dislocation required operative fixation. The obturator oblique view (**c**) and iliac oblique view (**d**) show the large posterior wall fragment (*white arrows*) and the transverse nature of the fracture. (From Tile 1984)

Avulsion of a small fragment of bone from the femoral head may also be seen. Neither of these requires removal, since they do not interfere with joint function or joint congruity.

Fracture of the Femoral Head. With dislocation of the femoral head, large bone fragments may be avulsed, usually with an intact teres ligament. This type of injury may occur with a pure dislocation or with a concomitant acetabular fracture. If the head fragment is large enough to cause instability of the hip joint or is displaced enough to cause incongruity, it should be restored anatomically and fixed with screws (Fig. 11.21).

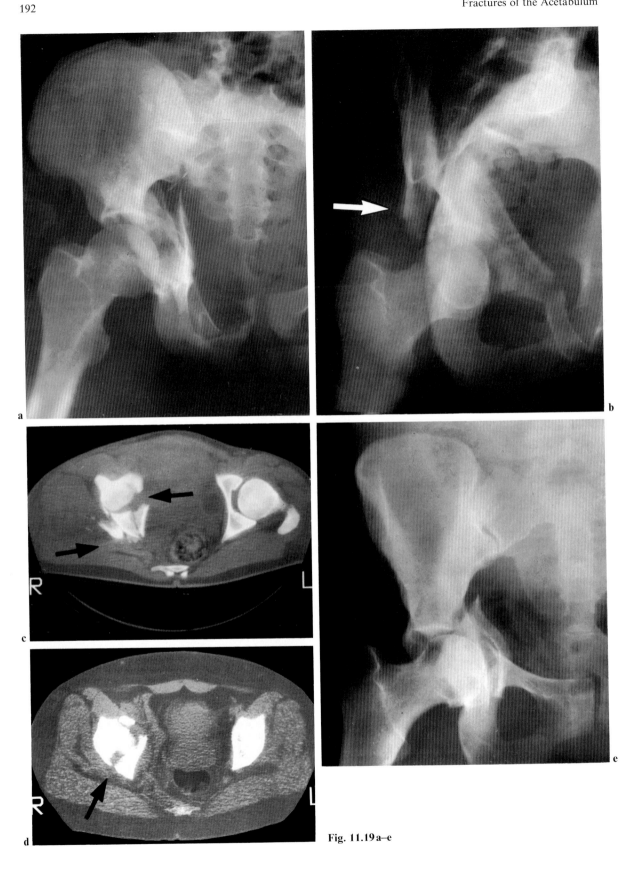

Fig. 11.19 a–e

Fig. 11.19a–e. Double-column fracture requiring open reduction and internal fixation. **a** Anteroposterior and **b** obturator oblique radiographs of the right hip of a 19-year-old student with a severe double-column fracture of the acetabulum. Note the classic spur sign in **b** (*arrow*). **c** The CT scan through the dome shows the coronal split with marked displacement of the quadrilateral plate (*upper arrow*). Note also the CT appearance of the spur sign (*lower arrow*) at this level. **d** CT appearance of a transverse fracture. Note the split in the direction parallel to the quadrilateral plate rather than through it, indicating a transverse fracture (*arrow*). **e** Radiological appearance of this case

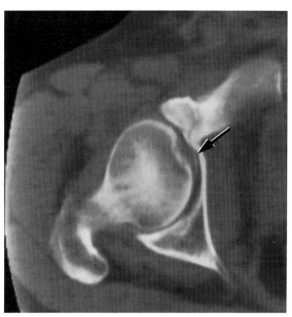

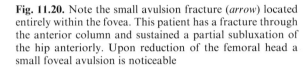

Fig. 11.20. Note the small avulsion fracture (*arrow*) located entirely within the fovea. This patient has a fracture through the anterior column and sustained a partial subluxation of the hip anteriorly. Upon reduction of the femoral head a small foveal avulsion is noticeable

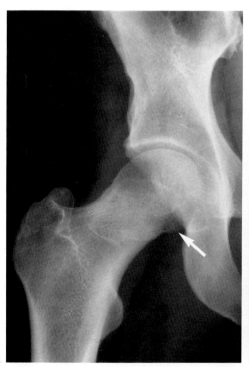

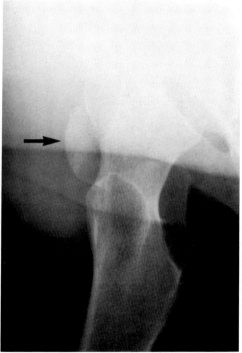

a   b

Fig. 11.21 a–i. Fracture of the femoral head. **a** Anteroposterior view of a 39-year-old man with a fracture of the femoral head secondary to a posterior dislocation. Note the large defect on the inferior aspect of the head (*arrow*). **b** On the lateral radiograph a large fragment is noted anterior to the femoral neck; this is clearly seen on the CT scan (**c**; *arrow*).

Note the posterior wall fracture on the CT scan cut through the dome (**d**, *arrow*). **e** The operative appearance of this fragment is indicated by the *arrow* and its size is readily appreciated following reduction (**f, g**). The fragment was fixed with two 4-mm cancellous screws (**h, i**). The final result at 4 years is excellent

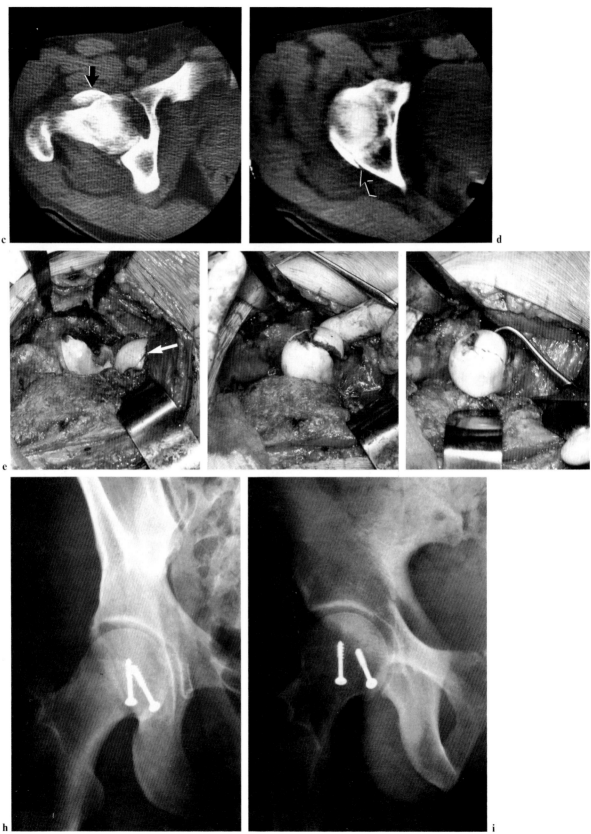

Fig. 11.21 c–i. (Legend see p. 193)

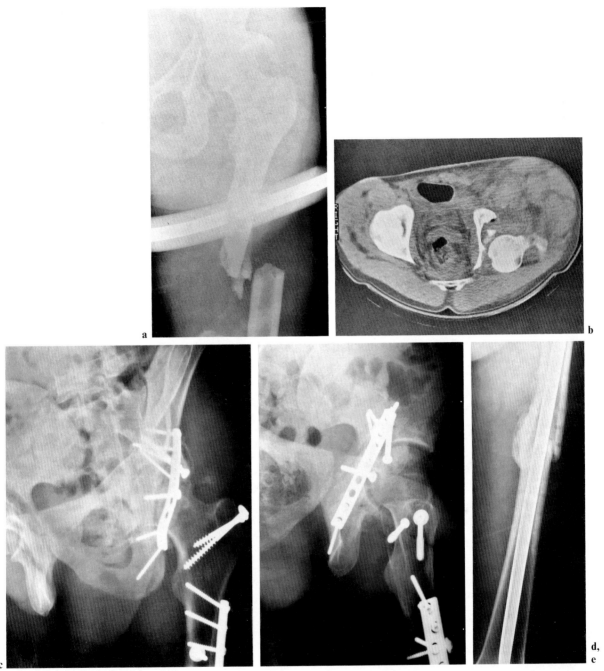

Fig. 11.22. a Anteroposterior radiograph showing a transverse fracture of the left acetabulum with a posterior wall fragment, associated with a comminuted fracture of the shaft of the femur. This patient also had severe involvement of his left sciatic nerve. The severe nature of this injury is best seen on the CT scan showing the posterior dislocation and the retained bony fragment (**b**). Because of his sciatic nerve lesion, his femoral and acetabular fractures were internally stabilized on the night of admission, the femur with a plate and interfragmental screws and the acetabulum through a transtrochanteric approach, using interfragmental screws for the posterior fragment and a neutralization 3.5-mm dynamic compression plate, as shown on the obturator oblique (**c**) and iliac oblique (**d**) radiographic views. Also, since we had planned to use the transtrochanteric approach to the hip, an intramedullary nail would have been technically difficult and undesirable. This patient had excellent restoration of congruity of his hip with an excellent clinical result. However, his femur failed to unite. Following a fracture through the plate at the site of the nonunion, an intramedullary nail was inserted (**e**), eventually resulting in sound union. The peroneal division of the sciatic nerve never recovered. In this situation, primary stable plating of the femur allowed full control of the femoral head without concern that the femoral fracture would redisplace. (From Tile 1984)

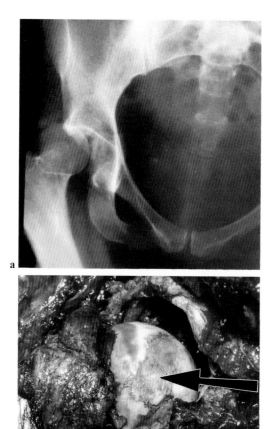

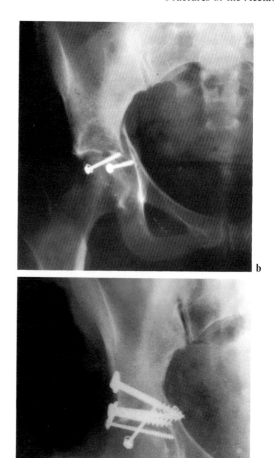

Fig. 11.23a–d. Pressure necrosis of articular cartilage. a Anteroposterior radiograph of the right hip of a 48-year-old woman with a posterior fracture dislocation. b The postoperative radiograph at 6 weeks shows the fixation of the posterior wall fracture. The previously undisplaced transverse fracture of the acetabulum displaced in the 6-week period. c Intraoperative photograph showing the large zone of pressure necrosis of the articular cartilage on the femoral head (*arrow*). d Postoperative radiograph showing the transverse fracture of the acetabulum fixed with four interfragmental screws. The reduction is anatomical. In spite of the large zone of pressure necrosis the patient has an excellent result at 2 years

Other Operative Indications. These include:

1. The development of a sciatic or femoral nerve palsy after reduction of the acetabular fracture, indicating the possible entrapment of the nerve at reduction.

2. The presence of a femoral arterial injury associated with an anterior column fracture of the acetabulum. In this circumstance, the fracture should be fixed at the time of primary vascular repair.

3. Fracture of the ipsilateral femur, which makes closed treatment of the acetabulum virtually impossible; open reduction is therefore indicated for both the fractured femur and the acetabular fracture (Fig. 11.22). The same is true for an ipsilateral knee disruption.

11.4.1.3 Early Management

If the patient has a *dislocation of the hip joint*, a general anesthetic should be administered to reduce the dislocation. During the same anesthetic, the stability of the fracture should be assessed under image intensification.

If the patient has *significant displacement* and traction fails to reduce it, this should also be reduced under general anesthesia. This is especially true for marked medial displacement of the femoral head, since failure to reduce the femoral head from the pelvis may cause early pressure necrosis of articular cartilage (Fig. 11.23), which may occur within 14 days of injury. Therefore, the femoral head should not be allowed to ride on the sharp lateral fragment of bone in these high transverse injuries. If the head can be easily reduced without an anesthetic, as will be indicated on image intensification or the plain radiograph, then a general anesthetic is not required.

Following reduction of the dislocation or the fracture under anesthesia or by traction without anesthesia, a skeletal traction pin is placed in the supracondylar area of the femur. *Do not insert a trochanteric pin at this stage, since the final method of treatment has not been determined.* If surgery is required and is delayed because of other factors, sepsis around that pin may jeopardize a surgical approach. Therefore, we feel that *there is no place for trochanteric traction in the immediate phase of fracture management.*

11.4.1.4 Assessment of Congruity

When traction has been applied, usually using 30 lb (13.5 kg) two possibilities arise:

1. Reduction Congruous. If the reduction of the acetabulum is congruous on the plain radiographs and CT scan, traction may be continued as the primary form of treatment. With anatomical restoration, a good result may be expected. We have already indicated those types of fracture which are most likely to result in a congruous reduction and those which are not.

2. Reduction Incongruous. If the reduction is clearly incongruous, then further decision making is required. In most instances, incongruity may be suspected immediately and would be rarely altered by the appearance in traction.

Fig. 11.24. a Anteroposterior radiograph of a 19-year-old male who jumped from a height sustaining multiple injuries as well as a fracture dislocation of the right acetabulum. This fracture was severely comminuted. Fixation was attempted by a surgeon not versed in acetabular surgery. **b** The postoperative radiograph at 3 days. The fracture is not anatomically reduced, is inadequately fixed, and the femoral head is dislocated. (From Tile 1984)

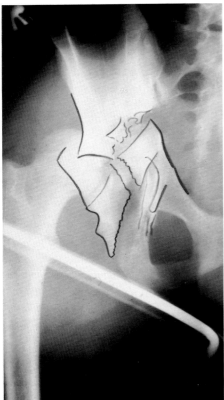

a

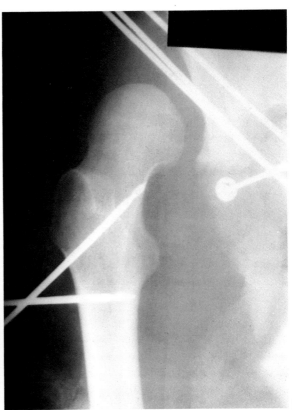

b

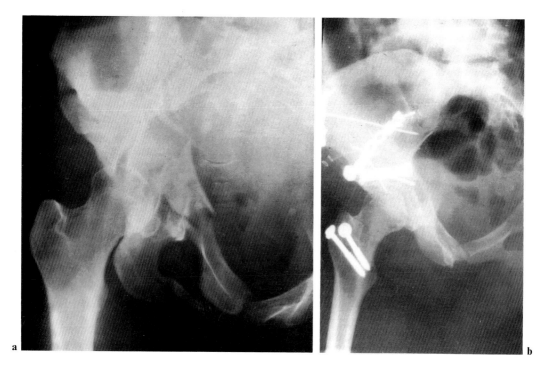

Fig. 11.25. a Severely comminuted double-column fracture of the right acetabulum. This fracture at first glance appears inoperable, but, with careful planning, surgical reconstruction was performed, resulting in an anatomical reduction and excellent internal fixation of this fracture (**b**). The result at 3 years is excellent

11.4.1.5 Assessment of Operability

If the reduction is incongruous, the next step is to assess the *operability* of the fracture and any potential contraindications to surgery. The important determinants concerning the operability of a fracture are the experience of the surgeon making the decision and the age and general state of the patient. As one's experience grows, the number of one's seemingly inoperable cases become greatly reduced. In the case shown in Fig. 11.24, that of a 19 year old male who jumped from a bridge, the surgeon recognized the difficulty involved but did not have the technical expertise to perform an adequate open reduction and internal fixation, with disastrous results. The patient would have been far better managed in traction than by the method used. These types of injuries are best sent to centers where the volume of cases is sufficient to afford adequate experience with these difficult problems (Fig. 11.25). Therefore, if the patient's general state or age preclude surgery or the fracture cannot be technically fixed – and this latter contraindication is rare indeed – then traction

should be continued and a late reconstructive procedure, namely, a total hip arthroplasty or arthrodesis anticipated.

Where the fracture is incongruously reduced but deemed technically operable, open reduction is indicated and the results will be improved if congruity is restored. The results will not be improved if surgery fails to achieve congruity (Fig. 11.3); therefore, if surgery is performed at all, the surgeon must strive for anatomical reduction and stable fixation of all major components of the fracture (Fig. 11.26). Early motion is then possible, allowing early rehabilitation of the hip joint.

11.4.2 Surgical Considerations

11.4.2.1 General

Timing

We prefer to operate electively as early as is feasible following the traumatic incident, usually on the 4th–7th day after trauma. The surgical procedures may be lengthy, often requiring 6 or more hours. Also, the best possible operating room team must be available. This is rarely possible at night.

There are indications for immediate open reduction including entrapment of the sciatic nerve following closed reduction, and rupture of the femoral artery, necessitating immediate vascular repair. In the latter instance, the incision should be

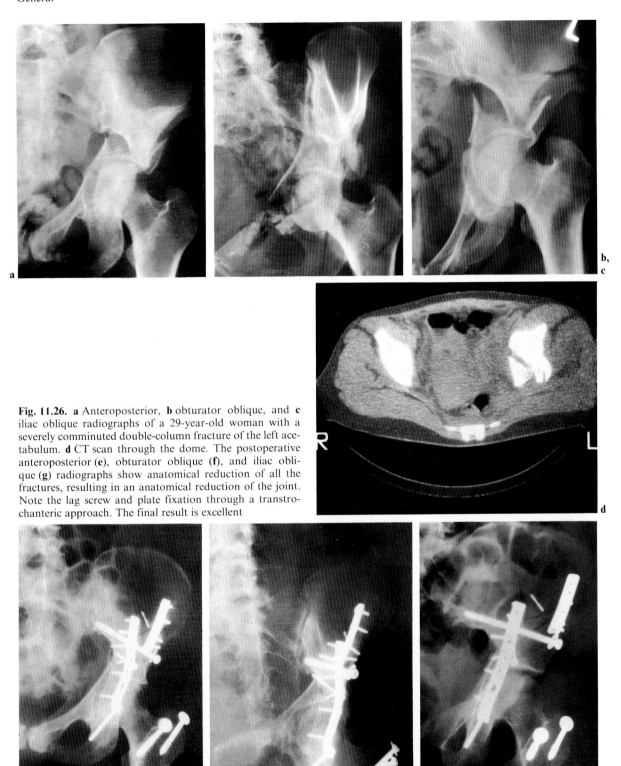

Fig. 11.26. a Anteroposterior, **b** obturator oblique, and **c** iliac oblique radiographs of a 29-year-old woman with a severely comminuted double-column fracture of the left acetabulum. **d** CT scan through the dome. The postoperative anteroposterior (**e**), obturator oblique (**f**), and iliac oblique (**g**) radiographs show anatomical reduction of all the fractures, resulting in an anatomical reduction of the joint. Note the lag screw and plate fixation through a transtrochanteric approach. The final result is excellent

carefully planned with the vascular surgeon to allow open reduction of the anterior column of the
acetabulum, the usual offending bone, which penetrates the femoral artery and occasionally the femoral nerve. An irreducible dislocation is another
indication for emergency surgery.

Antibiotics

Prophylactic intravenous antibiotics are given just
prior to surgery and for 48 h following surgery.

Blood

Six to eight units of blood are usually required
during the operative procedure. In rare instances,
a previously ruptured and clotted superior gluteal
artery may be manipulated, dislodging the clot.
If the patient has had major blood transfusions
preoperatively, bleeding may be profuse because
of ineffective coagulation. In such cases, the area
must be packed in the hope that clotting will ensue.
If the artery cannot be visualized and bleeding
continues, a safe procedure would be to close the
wound, take the patient to the angiography department and use an arterial clot of Gelfoam (Upjohn Pharmaceutic Co.) or other substance to stop
the bleeding. If the patient is in extremis, a direct
surgical approach in the pelvis is essential.

11.4.2.2 Approaches

The choice of surgical approach is determined by
the type of fracture. Several approaches are available to the surgeon and may be summarized as
follows:

1. Anterior
   (a) Iliofemoral
   (b) Ilioinguinal

Table 11.5. Guidelines for choice of approach in acetabular
fractures

Type of fracture	Approach
Anterior types	
– cephalad to iliopectineal eminence	Iliofemoral
– complex patterns requiring exposure to the symphysis and quadrilateral plate	Ilioinguinal
Posterior wall or posterior column	Posterior Kocher-Langen-beck
Transverse or T types ± posterior lip	Posterior transtrochanteric
Double-column (both-column)	Triradiate transtrochanteric Extended iliofemoral Ilioinguinal

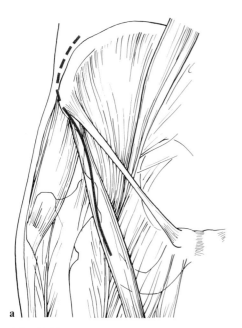

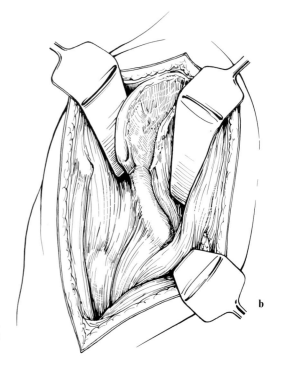

Fig. 11.27a, b. Iliofemoral approach. **a** Skin incision.
b Deep dissection by removal of muscles of inner and often
outer surface of the pelvis

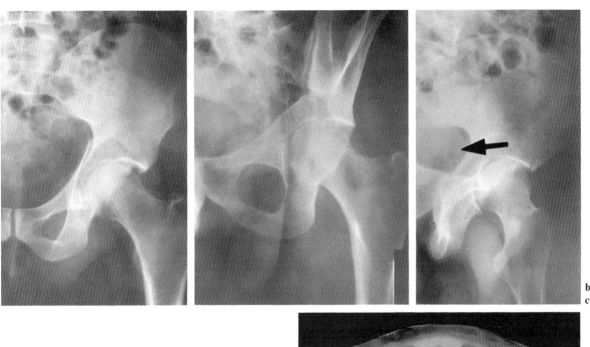

a   b,
                                                        c

Fig. 11.28 a–f. Fixation of a high anterior column fracture. The anteroposterior radiograph (**a**) shows a high anterior column fracture of the left acetabulum. Note the medial displacement of the femoral head causing incongruity of the hip joint. This is more clearly seen on the obturator oblique view (**b**). The iliac oblique view (**c**) shows the posterior column to be intact (*arrow*) as does the CT scan (**d**). The fracture was fixed through an anterior iliofemoral approach. Note the fixation by two interfragmental lag screws and a neutralization plate. The postoperative anteroposterior (**e**) and obturator oblique (**f**) radiographs, show congruity restored to the hip joint. The result at 2 years is excellent

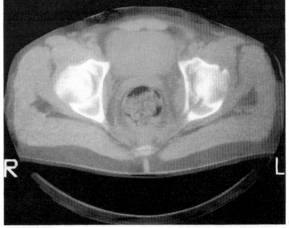

d

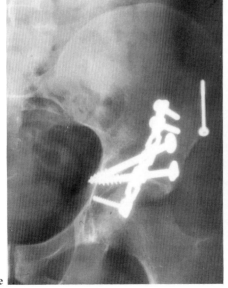

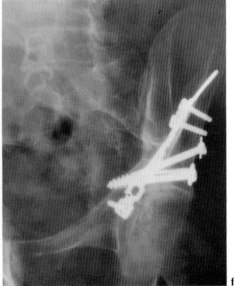

e   f

2. Posterior
   (a) Posterior Kocher-Langenbeck
   (b) Posterior transtrochanteric

3. Extensile
   (a) Triradiate transtrochanteric
   (b) Extended iliofemoral
   (c) Combined approaches

We have found the guidelines given below helpful in determining the type of surgical approach we use (Table 11.5).

Anterior

Iliofemoral. For fractures of the *anterior column*, where the main displacement is superior to the hip joint, the iliofemoral approach will suffice (Fig. 11.27). With this incision, the surgeon cannot gain access to the anterior column distal to the iliopectoral eminence, but in many cases this is unnecessary. Increased exposure may be obtained by adduction and internal rotation of the hips. Through this approach, lag screw compression of the anterior joint fracture is possible, but a plate cannot be fixed to the anterior column distal to the joint. Proximal plates may be fixed to the ilium with ease. This approach has the advantage of relative simplicity and safety but its restricted exposure limits its use. Therefore, this approach is used for anterior column fractures (Fig. 11.28), anterior wall fractures, and anterior column with posterior hemitransverse fractures, since the posterior hemitransverse segment is often undisplaced.

Ilioinguinal. For difficult fractures with anterior displacement where access to the whole anterior column is essential, the ilioinguinal approach is ideal (Fig. 11.29). This approach allows access to the entire anterior column as far as the symphysis pubis, as well as to the quadrilateral plate. Some double-column (both-column) fractures are also amenable to this approach, mainly those fractures with a large single fragment of posterior column. With these fractures, the posterior column may be approached anteriorly by exposing the quadrilateral plate. The posterior column forms the posterior portion of the quadrilateral plate and may be reduced and fixed by lag screws through this approach.

Because the original description of the ilioinguinal approach makes intra-articular visualization of the hip impossible, we usually make a *T* extension of the incision just medial to the anterior superior spine to allow exposure of the hip joint anteriorly (Fig. 11.30). This approach to the hip joint is really the iliofemoral, exposing the articular surface of the joint, so necessary in these intra-articular fractures.

The *T* extension extends between the tensor fasciae latae and the sartorius muscles, exposing the rectus femoris muscle. The lateral portion of the rectus femoris muscle is incised, exposing the anterior capsule of the hip joint which is incised medially approximately 2 mm beyond the acetabular labrum.

The anterior surface of the joint is now clearly visible. This approach allows the surgeon to see

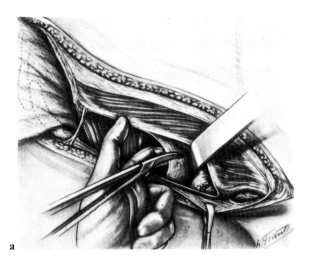

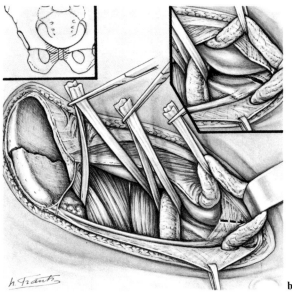

Fig. 11.29 a, b. Ilioinguinal approach. Note the importance of complete division of the iliopsoas fascia. (From Letournel and Judet 1981)

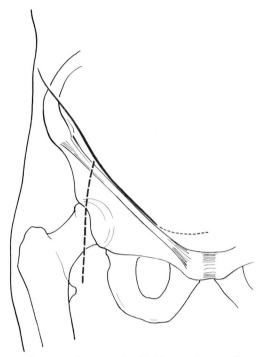

Fig. 11.30. Ilioinguinal approach with T extension to allow intra-articular visualization of hip joint

the anterior column, and the quadrilateral space, as well as the interior of the joint. It is extensile and allows fixation of the symphysis pubis if required. However, the approach requires considerable surgical expertise. It is recommended that it be done in the anatomy department or on a cadaver prior to its use in a patient. The approach is relatively safe, but care must be taken to protect the femoral nerve within the psoas sheath and the femoral vessels.

Posterior

We have adopted the following philosophy where posterior approaches are indicated.

Kocher-Langenbeck. In *isolated posterior lip* injuries as well as *posterior column injuries*, either isolated or associated with a posterior lip, a posterior Kocher-Langenbeck approach is made (Fig. 11.31 a–c). The incision extends from a point distal to the posterior superior spine of the ilium obliquely to the greater trochanter and then distally down the shaft. The gluteus maximus muscle is split and the tensor fasciae latae muscle incised along the femoral shaft, exposing the greater trochanter and the short external rotators of the hip. The insertion of the piriformis tendon into the pos-

terior aspect of the greater trochanter and the obturator internus tendon more distally into the greater trochanter are identified and tagged. In most cases, the sciatic nerve exits the sciatic notch anterior to the piriformis muscle and posterior to the obturator internus muscle. The piriformis, the obturator internus, and the gemelli muscles are divided. The obturator internus protects the sciatic nerve and the underlying obturator bursa is the guide to the posterior column. In this manner, the greater and lesser sciatic notch and the ischial tuberosity can be identified. Interfragmental compression with screws and posterior plates can be applied in this area through this approach.

Posterior Transtrochanteric. For difficult injuries involving the dome of the acetabulum, such as the *transverse T types* with or without a *posterior lip* component, we use the same posterolateral Kocher-Langenbeck skin incision but remove the greater trochanter for increased visualization (Fig. 11.31 d, e). The approach through the gluteus maximus and tensor fasciae latae muscles is the same, and the piriformis muscle and external rotators are divided to expose the posterior column as previously described. However, we feel that removal of the greater trochanter greatly simplifies the operative procedure.

Prior to removal, the greater trochanter is predrilled with the 3.2-mm drill anteriorly and posteriorly to accept the 6.5-mm cancellous screws at the end of the operative procedure. Stable fixation of the trochanter is obtained by this method.

The trochanter is removed transversely and retracted superiorly. The plane between the hip joint capsule and the gluteus minimus muscle is developed, leading the surgeon to the superior aspect of the acetabulum as shown in Fig. 11.31 e. Excellent exposure of the dome and posterior column is obtained with this approach. Further exposure of the anterior aspect of the joint is made possible by dissection anteriorly to expose the anterior inferior spine and the rectus femoris muscle. Removal of the rectus femoris will allow the surgeon to examine the anterior column of the acetabulum. If necessary, fixation of the anterior column will require retrograde lag screws.

The hip joint capsule is often torn. Exposure of the femoral head should be made by dividing the capsule 2 mm beyond the acetabular labrum. Insertion of a corkscrew device into the femoral neck will allow adequate distraction of the femoral head and excellent visualization of the articular surface (Fig. 11.31 e).

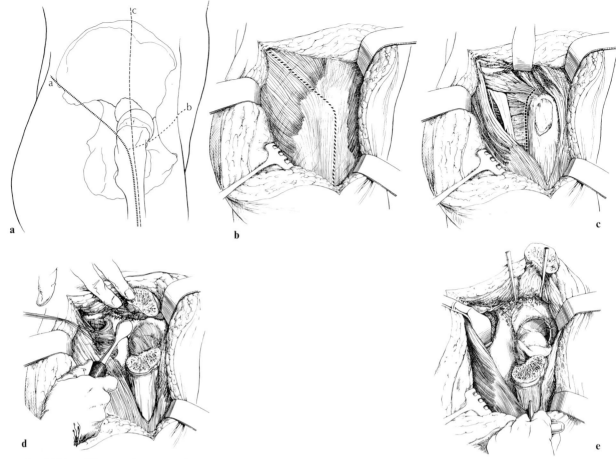

Fig. 11.31. a Diagram demonstrating the incisions for the posterior Kocher-Langenbeck approach (*a*), a modified Ollier approach (*a+b*) or a straight lateral approach (*c*). For posterior wall fractures the standard posterior approach (*a*) is adequate but for complex fractures the transtrochanteric approach combining *a+b* is much preferred. Both columns can be exposed, anatomically reduced, and fixed through that approach. **b** Following division of the skin and subcutaneous tissue the tensor fasciae latae and the gluteus maximus muscle are identified. These structures are divided by splitting the muscle fibers of the gluteus maximus and dividing the tensor fasciae latae longitudinally, as shown by the *striped line.* **c** Following division of the gluteus maximus and tensor fasciae latae, the posterior structures of the hip joint are identified. These include the piriformis, the short external rotators, the quadratus femoris, and the sciatic nerve. The tendons of the short external rotators and the piriformis are divided along the *checkered line.* **d** Elevation of the short external rotators will identify the obturator internus bursa and lead the surgeon to the greater and lesser sciatic notch. The entire posterior column of the acetabulum is exposed. In order to expose the superior dome and allow access to the anterior column, the greater tuberosity is osteotomized, as shown. **e** Visualization of the posterior column, the superior dome, and the anterior column is excellent with proper exposure through the transtrochanteric approach. Note that the capsule has been opened just along the rim of the acetabular labrum, leaving enough capsular tissue to resuture following open reduction. By using a femoral head extractor inserted distal to the trochanteric osteotomy the femoral head can be pulled from the joint, visualizing the entire articular surface. This is essential if anatomical reduction is to be achieved. It is helpful to insert two Steinman pins under the abductor muscle mass for retraction. All fractures are stabilized provisionally with Kirschner wires, and definitely with interfragmental screws, wherever possible. Finally, the fractures are stabilized with neutralization plates. (From Tile 1984)

Extensile

Triradiate Transtrochanteric. Double-column fractures with major posterior displacement may be approached as previously indicated, that is, a posterolateral incision is made, the same deep dissection carried out, and the trochanter removed. With this fracture, access to the iliac crest is essential, so the incision is carried anteriorly in a triradiate fashion to the anterior superior spine or just distal to it (Fig. 11.32). The tensor fasciae latae muscle is divided, exposing the gluteus medius and minimus muscles which are dissected subperiosteally from the outer table of the ilium. The incision may

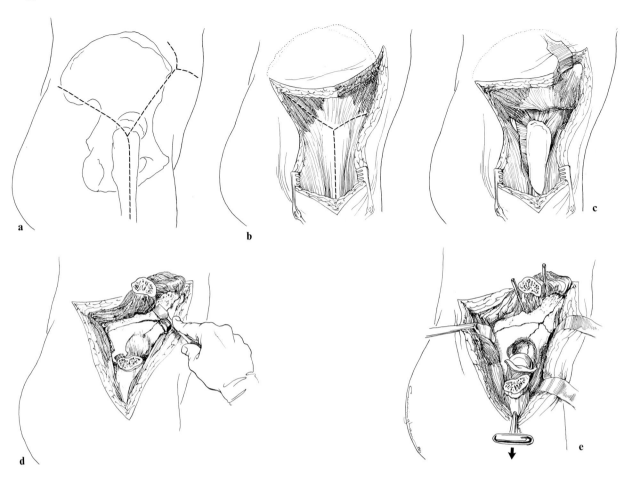

be carried posteriorly along the iliac crest. The addition of the triradiate skin incision and the subperiosteal dissection posteriorly allows excellent visualization of the outer table of the ilium, so essential in the double-column fracture.

The triradiate approach may also expose the inner aspect of the pelvis by extending the anterior limb of the incision to the symphysis, converting it into an ilioinguinal approach. Therefore, this approach is truly extensile, since it allows exposure of both the outer and inner table of the ilium including both columns.

A word of caution about the posterior approach. The *sciatic nerve* is in jeopardy in this approach and must be protected at all times by flexion of the knee and careful retraction using the muscle belly of the short external rotators for protection, otherwise intraoperative damage to the nerve will be unacceptably frequent.

Injury to the *superior gluteal artery and nerve* must also be avoided. These can be visualized exiting the greater sciatic notch; in this location, they can be easily injured when one is stripping the periosteum from the notch area. If injured, the

Fig. 11.32 a–e. Triradiate transtrochanteric approach. **a** Skin incision. No skin flaps must be raised: all dissection must be through fascial planes. **b** Exposure of the tensor fasciae latae muscle. **c** Division of the tensor fasciae latae and gluteus maximus muscles. **d** Removal of the greater trochanter and exposure of the lateral and posterior aspect of the pelvis. **e** Capsulorraphy of the hip capsule 2 mm from the pelvic attachment and insertion of a traction device into the femoral head facilitate access to the joint

artery may bleed massively and retract into the pelvis. Packing, embolization, or a direct surgical approach may then be necessary as described above. Of equal importance is the superior gluteal nerve. This nerve supplies the major hip abductors, the gluteus medius and minimus muscles. Injury may be caused either by a periosteal elevator or by retraction of the abductor muscles superiorly in order to gain visualization of the superior aspect of the acetabulum. Removal of the greater trochanter diminishes this risk, but throughout the operative procedure one must be aware of the possibility of a traction injury to this nerve.

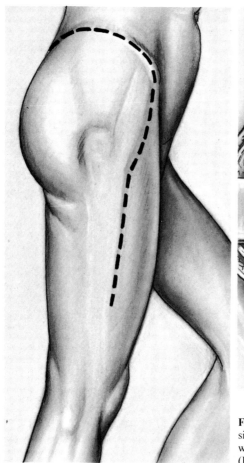

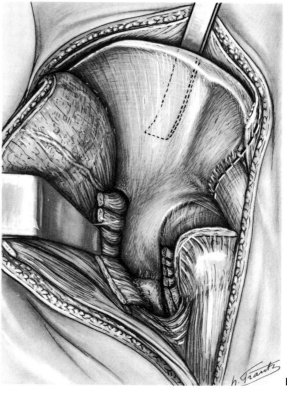

Fig. 11.33a, b. Extended iliofemoral approach. **a** Skin incision. **b** Deep dissection showing the exposure of the lateral wall of the ilium and posterior column of the acetabulum. (From Letournel and Judet 1981)

Extended Iliofemoral. The extended iliofemoral approach gives excellent visualization of the outer table of the ilium, the superior dome, and the posterior column and may be further extended to include the inner wall of the ilium as well (Fig. 11.33). We have removed the trochanter in the usual fashion rather than divide the abductor muscles.

Heterotopic ossification is a major complication of this approach, as in all approaches which require removal of the abductor muscle mass from the outer table of the ilium. Although visualization is excellent, we have some concern about the vascularization of the very large abductor muscle flap. This abductor flap is based primarily on the superior gluteal artery and vein as they exit from the greater sciatic notch. Venous engorgement may occur, resulting in some vascular insufficiency to the outer end of the muscle, causing necrosis. For this reason, we tend to use the triradiate approach, which keeps a layer of skin intact over the iliac crest to ensure adequate skin healing.

Combined. A simultaneous combined anterior and posterior approach is possible; however, we feel that adequate visualization of the entire acetabulum is preferable to two separate approaches, which we therefore rarely use.

11.4.2.3 Reduction

Resources

Reduction may be the most difficult aspect of acetabular surgery even with a good exposure. In order to achieve an excellent reduction, the surgeon must have available the following human and material resources:

1. Assistants. At least two and occasionally three assistants are necessary for these operative procedures. Of even greater help than the number is the quality of the assistants, since the surgeon cannot continuously keep an eye on the vital structures, such as the sciatic nerve.

2. Special instruments. Essential instruments include pointed fracture forceps, fracture reduction

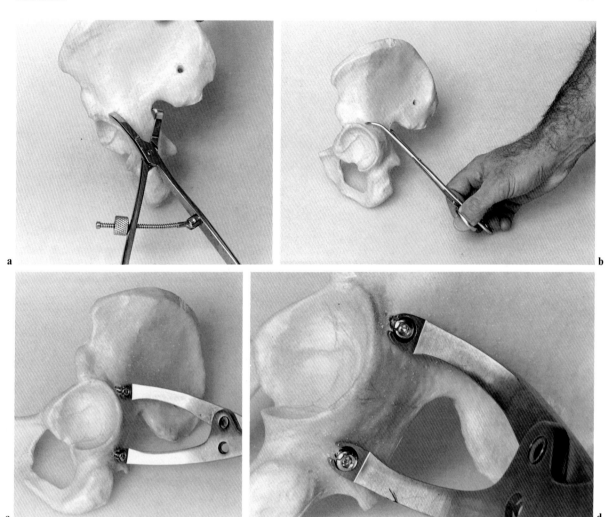

clamps, fracture pushers, and other standard fracture clamps (Fig. 11.34). Special pelvic reduction clamps are also available and others are being developed. The pelvic reduction clamp is screwed directly to the bone using two 4.5-mm cortical screws or 6.5-mm cancellous screws. This clamp can be extremely helpful by applying direct forces to the fracture.

Helpful Hints for Reduction

The following tricks may be helpful during this stressful aspect of the surgery:

1. The articular surface of the joint *must* be adequately visualized by a wide capsulorrhaphy. Only by direct visualization of the fracture lines within the joint can the adequacy of the reduction be confirmed (Figs. 11.31, 11.32).

2. A corkscrew in the femoral neck will allow better retraction of the femoral head and visualization of the articular surface (Fig. 11.35a).

Fig. 11.34. a Photograph demonstrating the use of the AO fracture reduction clamp. One limb of the clamp is placed through the greater sciatic notch, the other in a hole drilled to accept it, as shown. Reduction of the posterior column is accomplished by closing and locking the clamp. Much greater forces can be achieved with this type of clamp than with traction applied to the leg. Another invaluable instrument is the sharp-tip, self-locking fracture clamp (**b**). Again, one point is inserted through the greater sciatic notch, the other on the superior dome and the clamp closed. These sharp points will penetrate the bone, thereby giving stability. No predrilling is usually necessary. **c** Photograph of the pelvic reduction clamps, fixed to the pelvis by 4.5-mm cortical bone screws, shown in close-up in **d**. Again, tremendous forces may be applied through this clamp, enabling the surgeon to reduce the posterior column. (From Tile 1984)

3. A 5- or 6-mm Schantz pin with a T handle should be inserted into the ischial tuberosity in high transverse or T type fractures to allow rotation of the posterior column, which in some instances cannot be reduced by any other method (Fig. 11.35b).

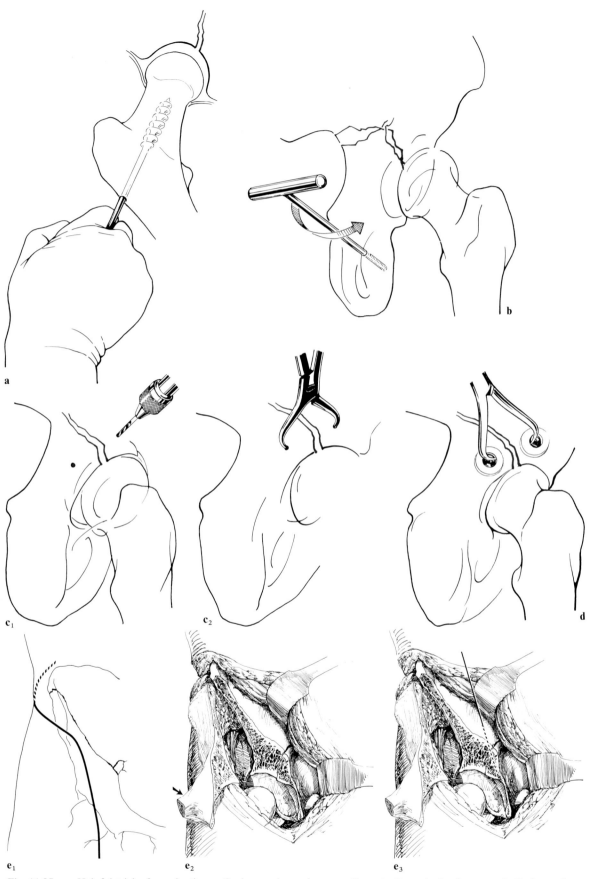

Fig. 11.35a–e. Helpful tricks for reduction. **a** Corkscrew in femoral head. **b** Schantz screw with T handle in ischial tuberosity. **c₁**, **c₂** 2-mm holes drilled to accept pointed fracture reduction clamp. **d** Washers to hold pointed reduction clamps. **e** Operate through the fracture: 1: iliofemoral approach; 2: anterior fragment (*arrow*) rotated to expose deep intra-articular fragment; 3: reduction of the intra-articular fragment and provisional fixation with Kirschner wire

4. Holes should be drilled to accept the pointed forceps (Fig. 11.35c).

5. Washers with extensions have been developed for use with the pointed fracture forceps (Fig. 11.35d).

6. Work within the fracture (Fig. 11.35e). In visualizing impacted fragments from either an anterior or posterior approach, it is important to move the major fracture out of the way so that the impacted fragment can be visualized. This is akin to the tibial plateau fracture where the lateral fragment is retracted like a book to allow reduction of the impacted fragment. Therefore, work within the fracture where possible.

11.4.2.4 Internal Fixation

Implants

Screws

- 6.5-mm cancellous lag screws
- 4.0-mm cancellous lag screws (lengths up to 120 mm)
- 6.5-mm fully threaded cancellous screws
- 3.5-mm cancellous screws

For lag screw interfragmental compression of the major fractures, we prefer the 6.5-mm cancellous screw. However, in some instances the 4.0-mm cancellous screws are essential, especially when fixing smaller fragments. These screws are available in lengths to 120 mm.

For fixation of the plate to the bone, fully threaded cancellous screws are desirable, the 6.5-mm screw for the large reconstruction plate (4.5-mm) and the 3.5-screw for the 3.5-mm reconstruction plate.

Plates. A 3.5-mm reconstruction plate is the implant of choice for acetabular reconstruction. These plates can be molded in two planes and around the difficult areas such as the ischial tuberosity. Also, precurved 3.5-mm plates are available for anterior column fixation. These plates are fixed with the 3.5-mm cancellous screws. In large individuals, and in pelvic fixation, the 4.5-mm reconstruction plates are also useful, with fixation by the 6.5-mm fully threaded cancellous screws (Fig. 11.36).

Sites of Application

The plates may be applied to the anterior column from the inner table of the ilium to the symphysis pubis (Fig. 11.37a). Plates may also be applied to

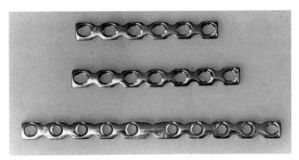

Fig. 11.36. 3.5-mm and 4.5 mm reconstruction plates for pelvic fixation

the posterior column and the superior aspect of the acetabulum (Fig. 11.37b). On the posterior column, the distal screw should be anchored in the ischial tuberosity. *Great care should be taken to ensure that screws in the central portion of the plate do not penetrate the articular cartilage of the acetabulum.* In most instances, no screws should be put into that danger area, but if screws are necessary for stable fixation, they should be directed away from the joint (Fig. 11.38). Screws within the joint are a not uncommon cause of chondrolysis (Fig. 11.39).

Plates may be nested to buttress small fragments (Fig. 11.40).

Methods of Stable Fixation

Internal Fixation. Stable fixation in the acetabulum, as in all areas, is best achieved by *interfragmental compression using lag screws.* Therefore, after provisional fixation of all fractures with Kirschner wires, screw fixation of the fractures is essential. The joint must be visualized at all times to ensure that anatomical reduction has been achieved and that no screw penetrates the articular cartilage. After fixation by interfragmental lag screws, plates may be used to neutralize the fracture. Plates may be placed either on the anterior or posterior column, depending on the approach.

Adequate contouring of the plates is essential. Otherwise, displacement of the opposite column may occur (Fig. 11.41).

11.4.3 Postoperative Care

The postoperative care is dependent upon the ability of the surgeon to achieve stable internal fixation which, in turn, will be dependent on the quality of the bone and the adequacy of the reduction. In general, we have maintained skeletal traction

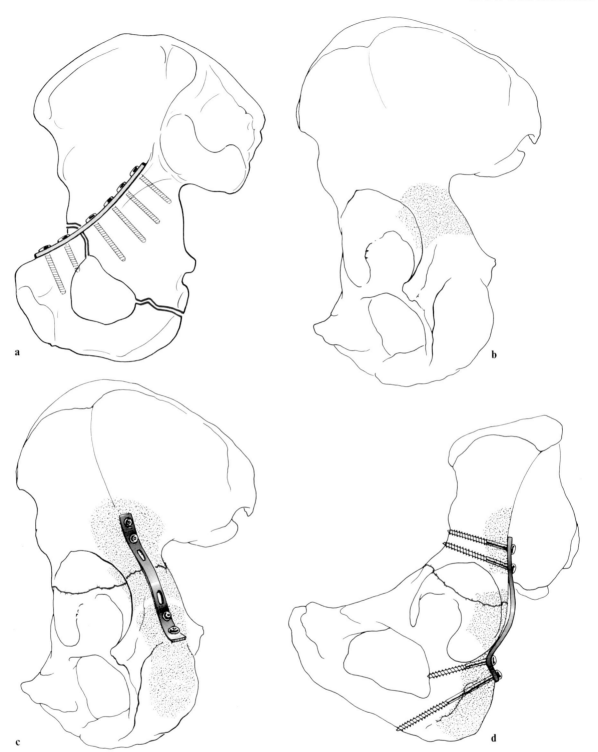

Fig. 11.37 a–d. Sites of application of plates. **a** Fixation of an anterior column fracture with an anteriorly placed plate. **b** Diagram indicating the danger zone for screw fixation in the midportion of the posterior column superior to the ischial spine, demonstrated by the red shading. The posterior column in this area is extremely thin and misdirected screws will commonly penetrate the hip joint. No screws should be placed in this area unless absolutely essential, and then only if directed away from the articular surface. **c** Diagram demonstrating the correct position of a plate placed on the posterior column of the acetabulum. Note that no screws are used in the central posterior portion of the acetabulum to avoid penetration of the articular surface. The most distally placed screw fixes the plate to the ischial tuberosity, best seen in **d**. (**b–d** From Tile 1984)

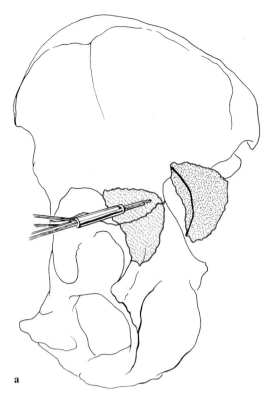
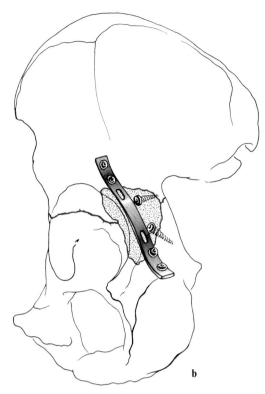

Fig. 11.38 a, b. Diagrams demonstrating the correct fixation of a posterior wall fracture. **a** The drill bit is positioned in a direction away from the joint so that the articular cartilage cannot be penetrated. After reduction of the fracture Kirschner wires are used for provisional fixation. This will allow the surgeon to carefully plan the position of the interfragmental screws and the neutralization plate along the posterior column (**b**). (From Tile 1984)

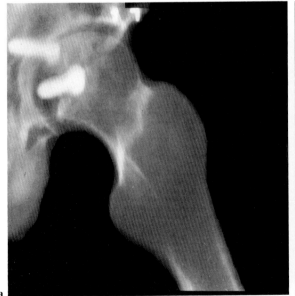
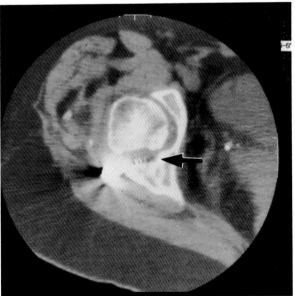

Fig. 11.39 a, b. Screw in the hip joint. **a** Fixation of a posterior wall fracture with two screws. The inferior screw has entered the hip joint and has eroded the femoral head. **b** CT scan showing the threads within the joint (*arrow*) and the posterior erosion of the femoral head

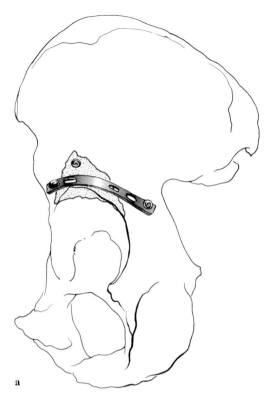

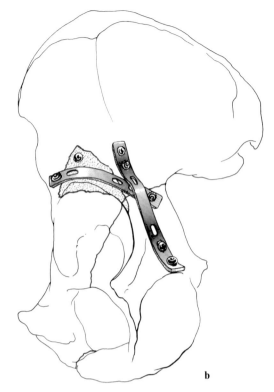

a

b

Fig. 11.40 a, b. Diagrams depicting the internal fixation of a superior dome fragment. In **a** the dome fragment is fixed with one interfragmental screw and a neutralization plate. Occasionally in complex fractures, the plates may be over-

lapped as seen in **b**. This will allow fixation of the superior dome fragment as well as the posterior column. (From Tile 1984)

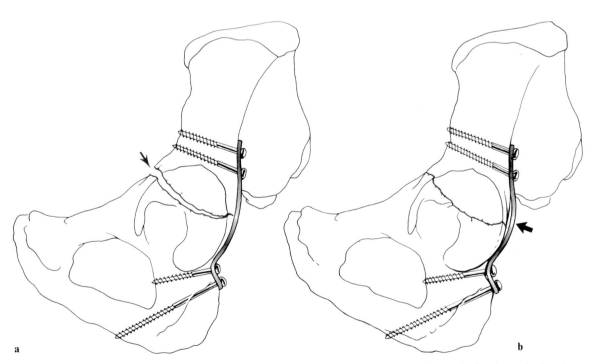

a

b

Fig. 11.41 a, b. Proper contouring of the plate is essential. If the plate is not contoured properly, a fracture which ap-

pears reduced posteriorly may in fact be malreduced anteriorly (**a**). Note the proper contour of the plate (**b**) with the patient in continuous passive motion in the immediate postoperative period for 7 days, and then gradually weaned the patient from the machine. If stability is deemed to be excellent, the traction may be removed and the patient ambulated. Weight bearing is not started until some signs of union are present, usually by the 6th postoperative week; however, the patients may be ambulatory with crutches during this period.

If one is concerned about the quality of the bone, about gross comminution, especially of the medial wall of the acetabulum, or about inadequate stability, traction should be continued for 6 weeks until some healing of the fragments has occurred. Ambulation may then begin with crutches, followed by progressive weight bearing at approximately 12 weeks.

11.5 Complications

Complications associated with acetabular fractures are common. As in all hip surgery, general complications include thromboembolic disease, wound necrosis, and sepsis. More specific complications include:

Nerve Injury

1. Sciatic Nerve. This nerve may be injured at the time of trauma or during the surgery. Most injuries to it occur with posterior type lesions or with posterior approaches to the hip. In our first 102 cases, there were 22 sciatic nerve lesions, 16 post-traumatic and six postoperative. All of the postoperative cases recovered, but in the 16 post-traumatic types, only four showed full recovery, while eight showed partial and four no recovery.

2. Femoral Nerve. This nerve may be injured by the spike of the anterior column or during surgery using an ilioinguinal approach. We have seen one post-traumatic case associated with a femoral artery injury. A nerve cable graft was performed with poor results, that is, no quadriceps function was restored.

3. Superior Gluteal Nerve. This nerve is situated in a vulnerable position in the greater sciatic notch, where it may be injured during trauma or during surgery, resulting in paralysis of the gluteus medius and minimus muscles.

Heterotopic Ossification

This remains our major postoperative complication. In our series, there were 18 cases of significant heterotopic ossification, all associated with posterior approaches to the hip. At the moment there is no known method of preventing this complication; the diphosphonates have been shown to be ineffective and radiotherapy may cause long-term problems in young patients.

Avascular Necrosis

Avascular necrosis of the femoral head is a devastating complication, developing in 6.6% of Letournel's 302 fractures (Letournel 1980). It was only seen in the posterior types in our series, and was 18% in that group.

Avascular necrosis of the acetabular segments may also occur, causing collapse of the joint.

References

Aprahamian C, Carrico CJ, Collicott PE et al. (1981) Advanced trauma life support course. Committee on Trauma, American College of Surgeons

Judet R, Judet J, Letournel E (1964) Fractures of the acetabulum: classification and surgical approaches for open reduction. J Bone Joint Surg 46A(8):1615–1647

Letournel E (1980) Acetabular fractures: classification and management. Clin Orthop 151:81–106

Letournel E, Judet R (1981) Fractures of the acetabulum. Springer, Berlin Heidelberg New York

Pennal GF, Davidson J, Garside H, Plewes J et al. (1980) Results of treatment of acetabular fractures. Clin Orthop 151:115–123

Rowe CR, Lowell JD (1961) Prognosis of fractures of the acetabulum. J Bone Joint Surg 43A(1):30–59

Tile M (1984) Fractures of the pelvis and acetabulum. Williams and Wilkins, Baltimore

Tile M, Joyce M, Kellam J (1984) Fractures of the acetabulum: classification, management protocol and early results of treatment. Orthopaedic Transaction of the J Bone Joint Surg. 8(3)

**Part IV
Fractures of the Lower Extremity**

12 Subtrochanteric Fractures of the Femur

J. SCHATZKER

12.1 Biomechanical Considerations

12.1.1 Mechanical Forces

The subtrochanteric segment of the femur extends from the lesser trochanter to the junction of the proximal and middle thirds of the diaphysis. This segment of the femur is subjected not only to axial loads of weight bearing, but also to tremendous bending forces because of the eccentric load application to the femoral head (Fig. 12.1). Recent strain-gauge studies in vivo (Schatzker et al. 1980)

have confirmed Pauwel's and the AO/ASIF contention that the bending forces cause the medial cortex to be loaded in compression and the lateral in tension. Furthermore, they have shown that the compressive stresses in the medial cortex are significantly higher than tensile stresses in the lateral cortex. An appreciation of this asymmetrical loading pattern is important in determining the suitability of internal fixation devices for fixation of these fractures, in understanding the causes and the prevention of failure of these devices, and in appreciating the causes of nonunion or malunion. Factors important for the stability of a reduction and fixation are, in order of importance:

1. Degree of comminution
2. Level of the fracture
3. Pattern of the fracture

12.1.2 Degree of Comminution

As we have emphasized elsewhere (see p. 248), the stability of a reduction depends on structural continuity. A simple fracture which is reduced anatomically and fixed with the aid of compression is stable and shows little tendency to redisplacement. Under load the forces are conducted directly from one fragment to the other, with relatively little stress being borne by the internal fixation. In a comminuted fracture, on the other hand, where the cortex opposite the plate ("the medial buttress") is deficient or where a segment of bone is so shattered that structural stability cannot be restored, the forces of loading are borne almost entirely by the internal fixation. The reduction is unstable and the only factor preventing redisplacement is the internal fixation. Hence, failure is common. The internal fixation either pulls out of bone, breaks because of overload, or undergoes fatigue failure because of cyclic loading. Thus, irreconstructible medial cortical comminution (shattered medial buttress) and irreconstructible segmental

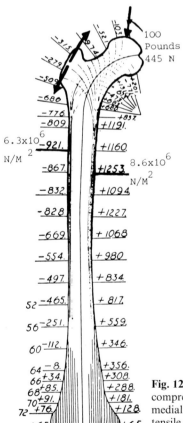

Fig. 12.1. Note the very high compressive stresses in the medial cortex and smaller tensile stresses in the lateral cortex. (From Cochran et al. 1980)

comminution stand out as the most important causes of failure.

12.1.3 Level of the Fracture

Next in the order of importance in determining the prognosis of a subtrochanteric fracture is the level of the fracture. The significance of this factor will be appreciated if we consider the difference between the two extreme situations, namely, a high fracture almost at the level of the lesser trochanter and a low fracture at the junction of the proximal and mid thirds of the femur. The closer the fracture to the lesser trochanter, the shorter the lever arm and the lower the bending moment.

12.1.4 Pattern of the Fracture

The pattern of the fracture is more important in determining the mode of internal fixation and only indirectly influences the outcome of treatment. In a transverse or short oblique fracture we rely on axial compression for stability. To achieve such compression we use a tension band plate. In a long oblique or spiral fracture primary stability is obtained by interfragmental lag screw fixation, which is then protected by a neutralization plate. If we are dealing with a transverse or short oblique fracture with a long proximal fragment, we can also consider intramedullary fixation with a conventional or, preferably, with a locking nail.

12.1.5 Deformity

The proximal femur is surrounded by very large and powerful muscles. In case of a fracture, their spatial arrangement, combined with their origin and insertion, results in a very characteristic deformity. The proximal fragment, as a result of contraction of the abductors, the external rotators, and the iliopsoas muscle, is flexed, abducted, and externally rotated. The adductors cause the shaft to be adducted and the force of gravity causes the distal fragment to fall into some external rotation. All the muscles which span the fracture combine to cause shortening. Thus, the resultant deformity is one of an anterior and lateral bowing of the proximal shaft, combined with considerable shortening and variable degrees of external rotation (Fig. 12.2).

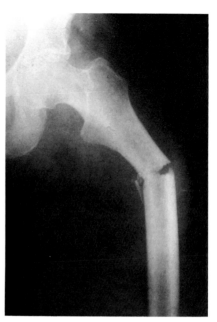

Fig. 12.2. Characteristic deformity following a subtrochanteric fracture. There is anterior and lateral bowing of the proximal shaft combined with external rotation and shortening

12.2 Natural History

Nonoperative treatment of a subtrochanteric fracture is difficult and frequently unsatisfactory (Schatzker and Waddell 1980). All nonoperative forms of treatment involve the use of traction, exerted by either a supracondylar pin or a pin in the tibial tubercle. Longitudinal traction can correct the shortening but it will not correct the deformity. The proximal fragment remains flexed, abducted, and externally rotated, and a large gap frequently remains between the fragments. In order to correct the deformity and close the gap, the distal fragment must be realigned with the proximal one. This involves traction in the so-called 90/90 position, with the hip and knee flexed to 90°. This position is not only very difficult to maintain in the adult, but also frequently fails to give a satisfactory reduction, and a significant degree of deformity often persists.

A malunion is not compatible with normal function. Patients with malunited subtrochanteric fractures walk with a Trendelenburg lurch and frequently complain of pain in the front of their thigh. A lift in the shoe to compensate for the leg length discrepancy neither stops the lurch nor abolishes the pain. The lurch and the pain are the

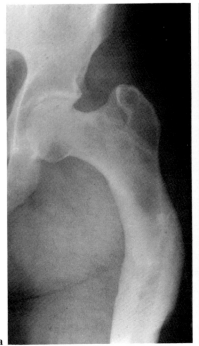
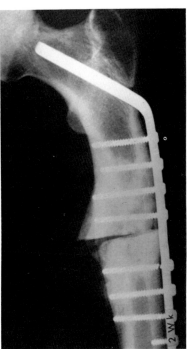

Fig. 12.3. a The varus bow of the shaft causes the tip of the greater trochanter to rise above the center of rotation of the femoral head. This causes a functional varus deformity of the hip and abductor insufficiency. **b** The deformity has been corrected by means of an osteotomy. A wedge with a lateral and anterior base had to be resected to achieve correction in two planes **a** **b**

result of the disturbed biomechanics about the proximal femur. The varus or lateral bow of the proximal femur causes the tip of the greater trochanter to rise above the center of rotation of the femoral head (Fig. 12.3a). This brings about a functional varus deformity of the hip and laxity of the abductors. The laxity and inefficiency of the abductors is responsible for the Trendelenburg lurch. The anterior bowing is probably the cause of the anterior distal thigh pain. Both the pain and the lurch persist until the deformity is corrected surgically and the biomechanical relationships are restored to normal (Fig. 12.3b).

12.3 Indications for Open Reduction and Internal Fixation

It is our opinion that subtrochanteric fractures should be treated by open reduction and stable internal fixation, as this is the only form of treatment which ensures a high percentage of satisfactory results (Schatzker and Waddell 1980; AO Fracture Documentation, Bern). Nonoperative methods are not only fraught with all the serious complications of prolonged bed rest; in the adult, as already indicated, they also frequently fail to reestablish acceptable alignment of the fragments.

Undoubtedly, the surgical zeal of many surgeons is tempered by the unhappy memory of a frustrating surgical experience of trying to put together a badly comminuted subtrochanteric fracture. The inherent difficulties of a surgical procedure cannot, however, be used as an argument to justify nonoperative treatment, which, apart from the dangers of enforced and prolonged bed rest, frequently fails to yield satisfactory results because of malunion.

12.4 Surgical Techniques

12.4.1 Diagnosis

The precise diagnosis of a subtrochanteric fracture can only be made radiologically. The history, however, should not be neglected, because it yields valuable information on the manner of injury, on associated injuries, and on the patient's state of health and expectations of treatment.

In addition to anteroposterior and lateral radiographs of the involved femur, which must include the joints above and below, one should order corresponding anteroposterior and lateral radiographs of the normal femur which will serve as a template for the reconstructive plan.

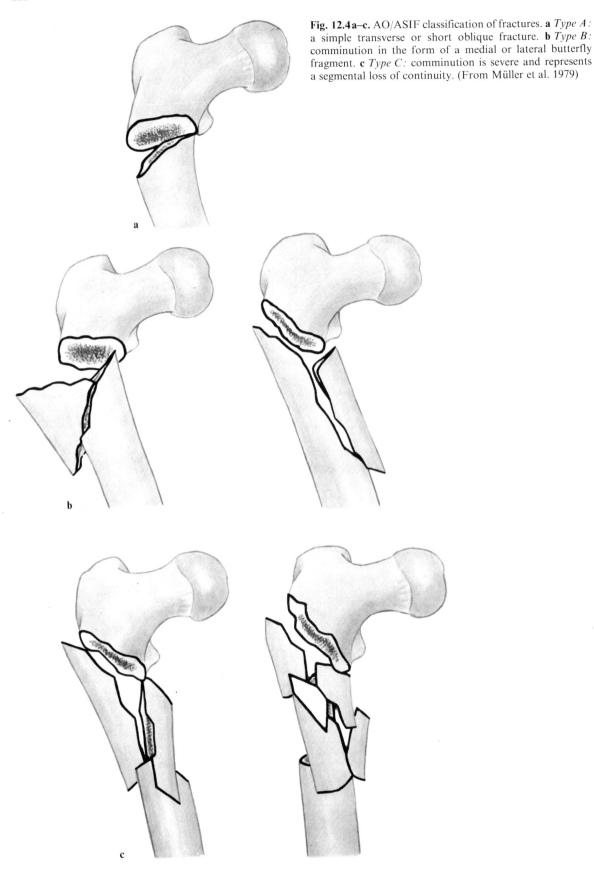

Fig. 12.4a–c. AO/ASIF classification of fractures. **a** *Type A:* a simple transverse or short oblique fracture. **b** *Type B:* comminution in the form of a medial or lateral butterfly fragment. **c** *Type C:* comminution is severe and represents a segmental loss of continuity. (From Müller et al. 1979)

12.4.2 Classification

For a classification to be useful it must not only identify the fracture pattern, but also serve as a guide to treatment, and therefore indicate prognosis.

As we have seen in the discussion of biomechanical factors, the most important factor determining the outcome of treatment in subtrochanteric fractures is the degree of comminution. We therefore favor the AO/ASIF classification of subtrochanteric fractures, because it identifies – in addition to the fracture pattern – the most important feature: namely, the type of comminution. Thus, there are the simple "type A" fractures, which may be transverse, oblique, or spiral, the "type B" fractures, which have either a medial or a lateral butterfly but which can still be reconstructed to yield a stable structural unit, and the "type C" fractures, which have as their hallmark comminution to such a degree that a stable unit cannot be achieved. This group includes fractures with an irreconstructible medial buttress or such segmental comminution that it represents a segmental loss (Fig. 12.4).

12.4.3 Planning the Surgical Procedure

12.4.3.1 Implants

Once the diagnosis has been established and open reduction and internal fixation decided upon, it becomes necessary to formulate a careful plan of all the steps of the operative procedure. Let us begin with a discussion of the different methods of internal fixation available.

a) Intramedullary Nailing

Intramedullary nailing has played a role in the stabilization of subtrochanteric fractures. As with fractures of the mid-diaphysis, only transverse and short oblique fractures could be considered ideally suited for this technique. Unfortunately, the majority of subtrochanteric fractures are spiral and comminuted, and therefore only a relatively small number can be considered suitable for conventional intramedullary nailing.

The stability of the fixation provided by an intramedullary nail (see p. 242) depends on the length of contact and the degree of fit between the nail and bone on both sides of the fracture. The medullary canal of the subtrochanteric segment is very wide just below the lesser trochanter and narrows down like a cone toward the isthmus. The isthmus, or the narrowest portion of the medullary canal, is usually at the upper or mid portion of the middle third of the diaphysis. Thus, a nail which snugly fits the isthmus obtains little fixation in the proximal fragment. Conventional intramedullary nailing of subtrochanteric fractures has been successful in teenagers and young adults, because in such patients the proximal femur is still filled with very dense cancellous bone which gives the nail excellent purchase. In older individuals this cancellous bone becomes sparse. The nail fails to obtain purchase and the proximal fragment frequently drifts into varus. To overcome this complication Küntscher devised a "Y-nail" (Küntscher 1967), which in more recent years has been modified by Zickel (Zickel 1976). Our experience with the Zickel nail has not been favorable. We were able to use it as the sole means of fixation only in transverse and short oblique fractures. Spiral and comminuted fractures required supplemental fixation, as described by Zickel (1976), which obviates the advantages of this technique. In addition, in some of the short oblique or transverse fractures the distal fragment demonstrated rotational instability, and rotational deformities were common. The difficulties of the technique and its complications have led us to the conclusion that, in comparison with other techniques, the Zickel nail has little to offer, and we have abandoned it in the treatment of subtrochanteric fractures.

Ender rekindled interest in the intramedullary mode of stabilization of these fractures with the introduction of his elastic nails (Ender 1970; Pankovich and Tarabishy 1980). Once again, we have found that this technique has considerable shortcomings. Stable subtrochanteric fractures, i.e., simple transverse or oblique fractures with little comminution, could be treated successfully with Ender's nailing. The "problem" subtrochanteric fractures, however, the ones with extensive comminution and segmental loss of continuity, fared badly. We were unable to maintain length or sufficient stability to keep the patients ambulant; patients with these unstable fractures treated with Ender's nailing had to be placed in skeletal traction for 3–6 weeks. In our opinion, an operative procedure which has to be combined with complete bed rest and traction is not justified. Long spiral fractures could be reduced and stabilized with cerclage wiring prior to the introduction of Ender's nailing. Such a combined mode of fixation is sufficiently strong to allow early ambulation, but the need for open exposure of the fracture defeats the biological advantages of the closed nailing, and we have abandoned the technique in preference to locked nailing.

The recent introduction of the locking intramedullary nailing system has greatly enlarged the scope of intramedullary nailing of subtrochanteric fractures (Kempf et al. 1985). We have found it an excellent technique for the severely comminuted, segmental defect fracture which has a long proximal fragment. Locking the proximal fragment to the nail, which this system makes possible, has overcome the tendency of the proximal fragment to drift into varus, and locking the distal fragment to the nail has prevented shortening. The locking of the fragments has made supplemental internal fixation of the fragments, such as cerclage or lag screw fixation, superfluous. This allows one to take full biological advantage of intramedullary

nailing. Also, the development of "intramedullary bone grafting" (M. Chapman, personal communication) has permitted grafting of major defects while keeping the procedure closed. The fact that we do not have to interfere with the soft tissue envelope and the remaining blood supply of the bony fragments and soft tissues has resulted, in our hands, in a more rapid consolidation than with any other technique. The locking of the fragments provides exceptional rotational stability, which has also permitted us to deal with oblique or spiral fractures. Thus, we feel that of all the intramedullary devices, the locking intramedullary nail is the only device suitable for subtrochanteric fractures, as long as the proximal fragment is sufficiently long to permit stable locking (Fig. 12.5). Fractures with a short proximal fragment or with intertrochanteric extensions require blade-plate or compression screw fixation.

b) Nail Plate

In a stable, strong internal fixation an equal number of screws must traverse the plate and the bone on each side of the fracture. If one attempts

Fig. 12.5a–d. A severely comminuted subtrochanteric fracture stabilized with a statically locked Grosse–Kempf intramedullary nail. **a** Anteroposterior and **b** lateral radiographs. Note the abundant callus. **c, d** Radiographs taken after nail removal 2 years after fracture. Note the advanced degree of remodeling of the cortex

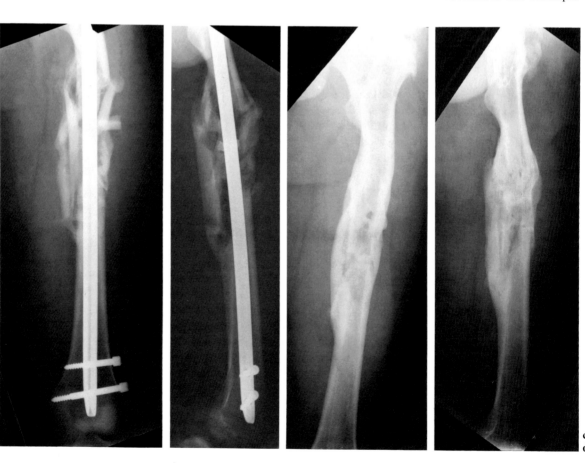

a,
b

c,
d

to fix a subtrochanteric fracture with a straight plate, the fixation in the proximal fragment is frequently deficient. This is particularly true if the fracture line extends close to the lesser trochanter, because the femoral neck makes fixation in the proximal fragment with simple screws virtually impossible. This problem has been solved with a nail-plate type of device; the introduction of the nail up the neck into the head greatly increases the fixation of the device in the proximal fragment.

Modern "nail-plate devices" all have a fixed angle between the "nail" and the plate. They fall into two categories: those with sliding "nail" or screw assemblies and those with a fixed segment which is inserted into the proximal femur.

The best example of the "sliding" nail-plate is the compression hip screw (Richards Surgical Ltd.) or the dynamic hip screw (Synthes Ltd.). The design of this device is such that a large-diameter screw is screwed into the femoral head. The screw fits into a collar of the plate, which in turn is fixed to the femoral shaft. The two are so designed that the smooth shaft of the screw can slide within the collar of the plate and yet retain rotational stability. Thus, with these devices one can impact those fractures which are crossed by the sliding mechanisms.

The sliding nail principle was developed for the impaction of subcapital and intertrochanteric fractures. It has a wide appeal to surgeons who, in surgery on the proximal femur, desire guidewire insertion with two-plane radiographic control as well as the use of the fracture table and traction (Fig. 12.6). What, then, about its use for the fixation of subtrochanteric fractures?

Its advocates have made claims that the device allows impaction of the subtrochanteric fracture and medialization of the shaft. The medialization in turn reduces the bending moment and reduces the resultant of forces, which leads to a large varus moment, and by these mechanisms increases the stability of the fixation. This reasoning is unfortunately wrong. In order for the device to have secure fixation in the proximal fragment, it is essential to prevent secondary displacement in the frontal plane (varus) or in the sagittal plane due to rotation. Instability due to rotation of the proximal fragment about the screw can result in flexion or extension with consequent deformity and malunion (see Fig. 12.7). To prevent such rotation the compression screw fixation must be supplemented with at least one screw inserted through the plate into the proximal fragment. This is impossible to achieve in most high subtrochanteric

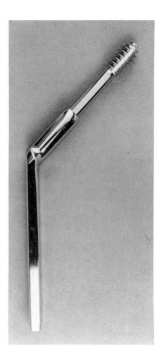

Fig. 12.6. A dynamic hip screw

fractures when a 130° angled device is used for fixation. Furthermore, once a screw is inserted through the plate into the proximal fragment, the sliding mechanism is blocked, the fracture cannot be impacted, and the shaft cannot be medialized. Thus, the device is not ideal for use in high subtrochanteric fractures (Fig. 12.7). The only advantages to its use in lower subtrochanteric fractures are its strength and the fact that it can be inserted into the proximal fragment with the aid of guidewires and radiographic control. The only time the shaft can be medialized is when the fracture is at the level of the lesser trochanter, but even in such cases rotational instability of the proximal fragment and possible shortening of the extremity must still be considered.

The 130° intertrochanteric and the 95° condylar angled plates of the AO (Fig. 12.8) are two useful devices for the treatment of subtrochanteric fractures. The 130° angled plate, like the compression screw or the dynamic hip screw, is useful only in low subtrochanteric fractures, where fixation of the device in the proximal fragment can be supplemented by the insertion of one or two cortical screws. Thus, its use is limited, and when a 130° angled device is to be used we prefer the dynamic hip screw because of its greater ease of insertion. The 95° condylar plate is the one we prefer and commonly use, because its proximal extension makes it usually possible to insert two or more cortical screws through the plate into the calcar.

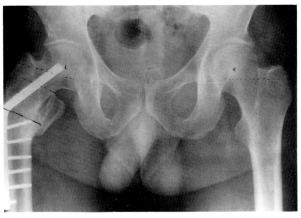
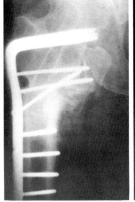
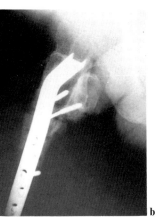

Fig. 12.7. a Malunion resulting from an improper choice of implant. A high subtrochanteric fracture cannot be stabilized with a 130° angled device, as the fixation of the device in the proximal fragment must be supplemented with at least one screw, which in this case is impossible. The result is instability with varus deformity in the frontal plane and rotation about the axis of the blade in the sagittal plane. **b** A corrective osteotomy was fixed with the 95° condylar blade plate. This would also have been the better device for the initial fixation of the fracture

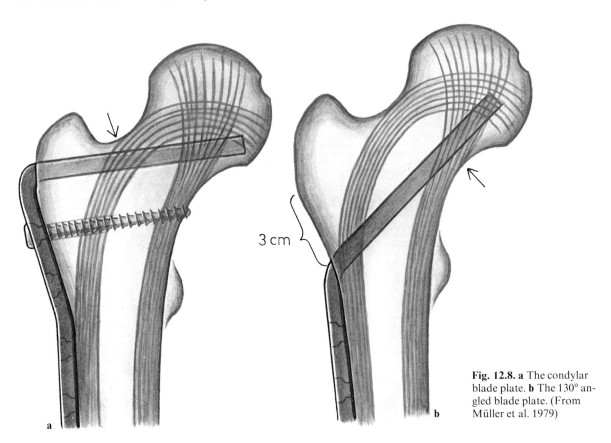

3 cm

Fig. 12.8. a The condylar blade plate. **b** The 130° angled blade plate. (From Müller et al. 1979)

This greatly strengthens its hold in the proximal fragment and prevents varus or rotational deformities. Thus, this plate can be used for the fixation of not only high subtrochanteric fractures but even those combined with intertrochanteric fractures. It can also be employed for lower subtrochanteric fractures, providing a sufficiently long plate is used. The greatest benefit of the 95° condylar plate is that it can be introduced into a short proximal fragment prior to the reduction of the subtrochanteric fracture (Fig. 12.9). This is a decided advantage when one is faced with a highly comminuted

Fig. 12.9. Note that the condylar plate has been inserted into the proximal fragment prior to the reduction of the fracture. (From Müller et al. 1979)

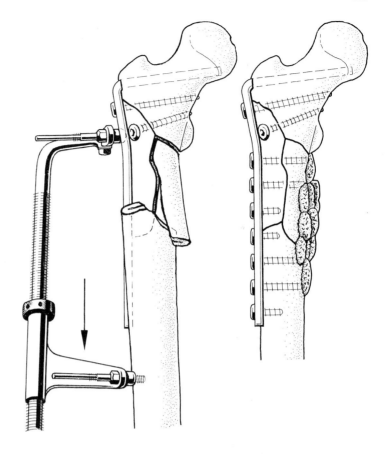

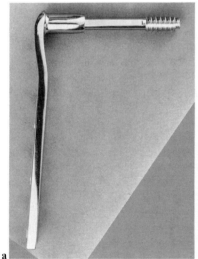

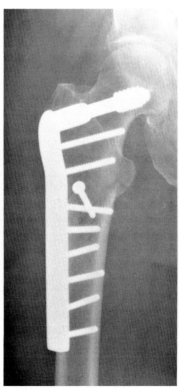

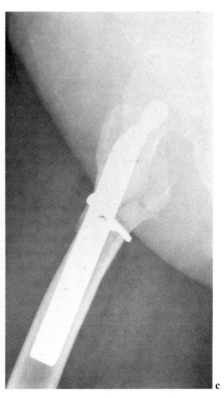

Fig. 12.10. a The dynamic condylar screw. **b** Anteroposterior and **c** lateral radiographs showing its use for the fixation of a subtrochanteric fracture

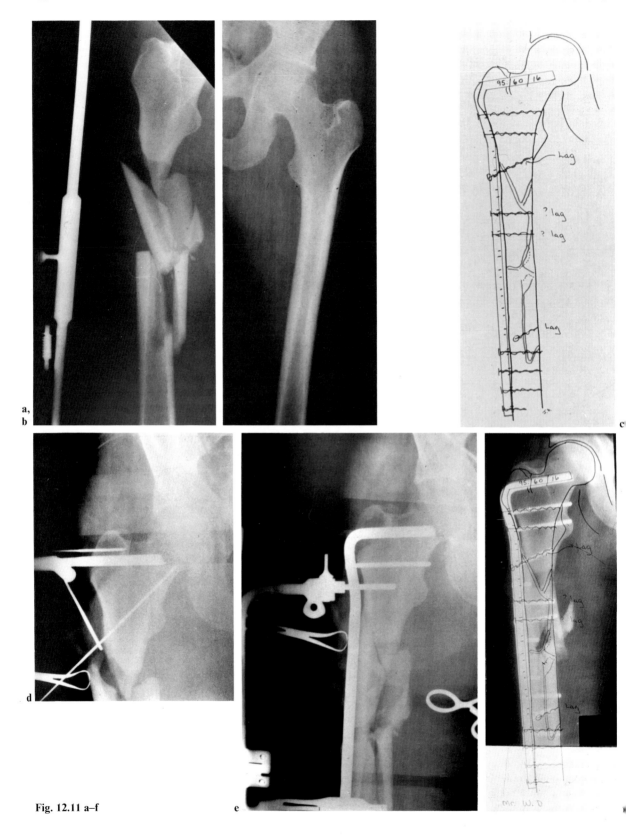

Fig. 12.11 a–f

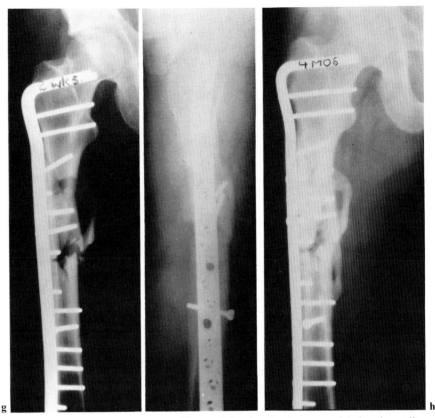

g   h

Fig. 12.11a–h. Preoperative planning for open reduction and internal fixation of a subtrochanteric fracture. **a** A comminuted subtrochanteric fracture. **b** Radiograph of the opposite extremity. Reversed, it serves as a template. **c** Preoperative drawing of the planned internal fixation. **d** Intraoperative radiograph to check position of the seating chisel. **e** Intraoperative radiograph. Note the use of the distractor to achieve length and reduction of the comminuted frag-ments. **f** Internal fixation has been completed and a radiograph obtained in the recovery room. **g** Radiograph at 2 weeks after surgery. **h** At 4 months the fracture is solidly united. Note the formation of abundant callus in this "biological" internal fixation, where great care was exercised not to damage the blood supply to the comminuted fragments

fracture in which reconstruction of the comminuted segment is impossible and in which locked nailing cannot be performed because of the shortness of the proximal fragment. When the 95° condylar plate is inserted into the femur the anatomical landmarks of the proximal femur are used as a guide. If desired, the position of the guidewires can be checked radiologically prior to insertion of the blade. As will be clear from the discussion of the insertion technique (see 12.4.4.4), if a careful preoperative plan is executed, and if the guidewires are carefully inserted under direct visual control using the anatomical bony landmarks and templates as guides, accurate insertion of the blade becomes relatively easy and accurate. The radiograph is used not as a guide to insertion but rather as a check of its accuracy. Recently, a dynamic condylar screw has become available (Fig. 12.10). It has a 95° angle like the condylar blade plate.

However, it is cannulated and uses a guidewire whose position can be checked radiologically. It is also easier to insert into bone because, like the dynamic hip screw, once proper positioning of the guidewire has been achieved the screw can be inserted with great ease. It can also be used in every situation in which a condylar blade plate would be indicated. This is a new device, still undergoing clinical trials. If it lives up to expectations, however, it will probably supplant the condylar plate.

12.4.3.2 Preoperative Planning

Once the diagnostic radiographs and those of the opposite, uninvolved extremity are available, a careful preoperative plan can be prepared (see Fig. 12.11c). The radiograph of the normal proximal femur is reversed and the outline of the bone traced onto a sheet of tracing paper. If the fracture

extends distally into the mid-diaphysis and is comminuted, so that identification and reduction of
the fragments is difficult, the outline of the whole
normal femur may have to be traced. The position
of the proximal and distal fragments must be then
marked on the tracing of the uninvolved femur
and the gap between the main fragments measured. A further guide to length is to select the
plate of correct length for the uninvolved femur
and note at what point the distal fragment makes
contact with the plate, i.e., how many screw holes
of the plate are opposite the distal fragment. In
this way correct length can be established intraoperatively. Where comminution is not so great,
the most proximal and the most distal fracture
lines are then carefully marked on the tracing of
the proximal femur. It should be carefully noted
where the fractures cross the medial and lateral
cortices both proximally and distally. If the comminuted fragments are major and large they are
carefully drawn in. If the comminution is such that
the outline and arrangement of the fragments is
not identifiable, this is also noted. Any places
where lag screws can be inserted between the fragments are marked. One should decide at this point
and mark on the drawing which holes will be
drilled first and their order, and which will be gliding and which will be thread holes. The principle
of converting a fracture with many fragments into

one consisting of two major fragments which are
then reduced at the end like a simple fracture applies to large major fragments only. One should
not attempt to fix a fragment if it means that in
doing so it will be stripped of its soft tissue and
thus rendered avascular. It is better to leave it unreduced with its blood supply preserved. In this
way it can act as a living bone graft and lead to
much more rapid consolidation than would a dead
piece of cortex in its normal anatomical position.

Once the fragments are marked, a template is
placed under the drawing, and the position of the
plate and its length are carefully noted. In addition
to the blade length and the length of the plate,
one must carefully note the exact position of the
entry of the blade into the lateral cortex of the
greater trochanter, since a window must be cut
prior to the insertion of the seating chisel. The
distance of the blade from the superior cortex of
the neck is also noted, as is the position of the
tip of the blade in relation to the center of the
femoral head, where the tension and compression
trabeculae intersect. These are all important landmarks. They can be identified at surgery and will
give the surgeon the correct insertion of the blade
into the proximal fragment, even when this is so
small that the condylar guide cannot be employed
intraoperatively as a check of the position of the
seating chisel or the guidewire for the dynamic
condylar screw. The position of the cortical window is best related to the rough line (easily identified intraoperatively) where the gluteus medius
and vastus lateralis muscles meet. If comminution
is present, one should also note the placement of
the bone grafts to be used (Fig. 12.11).

Fig. 12.12. The magnification factor: *a* the actual length of
the femur; *b* the projected length. The thicker the thigh,
the greater the distance between the femur and the X-ray
cassette; thus, the greater the magnification

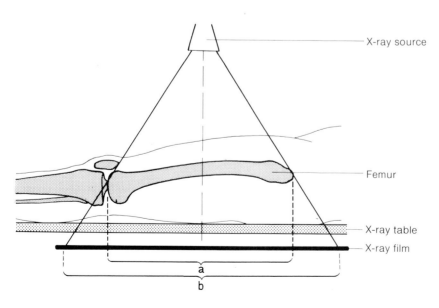

Locked intramedullary nailing is a closed procedure, and the reduction is achieved by closed manipulation and traction. Length cannot be judged intraoperatively; it must be carefully measured preoperatively. The most accurate method is to measure the sound extremity from the tip of the trochanter to the joint line and then subtract 2 cm. Next, a nail judged to be of the correct length or a ruler of suitable length is taped to the lateral side of the thigh in its midposition, and then an anteroposterior radiograph of the femur is made. A more accurate assessment of length is obtained if the nail or ruler is taped to the lateral side of the thigh rather than placed on the table beside the leg. If the patient's thigh is large and the nail is taped to the X-ray cassette, there is a real danger of choosing a nail which is too long, because of X-ray magnification of the femur (the thicker the thigh, the longer the nail; Fig. 12.12). Once the correct length is confirmed radiologically, it gives the length of the nail to be used. All that is then necessary at surgery is to make certain that the tip of the nail is driven as far into the distal fragment as planned. When the femur is distracted and the nail is locked in its proper position, both proximally and distally, correct length will have been achieved.

Rotational malalignment is a problem with closed intramedullary nailing. This cannot be avoided by any preoperative planning. One must be aware of this complication and remember to take the usual intraoperative measures to avoid it.

12.4.4 Surgery

12.4.4.1 The Operating Table

Because the techniques which we employ, with the exception of locked intramedullary nailing, do not require intraoperative radiographic control or traction, the surgery can be carried out on an ordinary operating table with the extremity draped free. We do advise, however, that the operating table have an attachment for holding X-ray cassettes which allow for intraoperative radiographs. Although radiographs are not used as a guide for the insertion of the implant, we feel that once the implant is inserted, anteroposterior and lateral radiographs should be obtained to make certain that the blade has not penetrated into the hip joint (see Fig. 12.11 d, e). Intraoperative traction is unnecessary – it may actually increase the difficulty of the surgery rather than ease the reduction. An

AO distractor allows a more direct and accurate application of traction without tying down the extremity. For details on its use, please see Sect. 12.4.4.4 below.

For locked intramedullary nailing, a special table designed for closed intramedullary nailing is employed.

12.4.4.2 Positioning the Patient

For plating the patient should be positioned supine. We prefer to keep the pelvis level, and we do not use a roll to elevate the involved hip since this may lead to a rotational malreduction. The iliac crest and the anterior and lateral aspects of the hip and the leg are draped free. This allows for full lateral access to the hip, it leaves the anterior iliac crest exposed as a donor site for bone graft, and it leaves the leg free to be manipulated as necessary during the reduction. In a badly comminuted fracture the only guide to correct rotational alignment is the range of hip motion. If the leg is in traction, or if it is draped in such a way that rotation of the hip is not possible, malreduction can easily occur. Furthermore, if the hip cannot be flexed to 90° it will become impossible to obtain a lateral radiograph of the hip during the procedure.

For *locked intramedullary nailing* we position the patient supine.

12.4.4.3 Surgical Approach for Plating

The surgical approach is through a straight lateral incision made in the skin along an imaginary line joining the greater trochanter with the lateral femoral condyle. It should extend from a point above the greater trochanter to approximately a hand's breadth below the fracture. The fascia lata is incised in line with the skin. As the next step, the surgeon should identify the interval between the tensor fasciae latae muscle anteriorly, the anterior edge of the gluteus medius and gluteus minimus muscles cephalad, and the vastus lateralis muscle caudad. Once this interval is defined, the anterior and superior aspects of the hip joint capsule should be cleared and a Hohmann retractor inserted over the anterior pillar of the acetabulum (see Fig. 12.13).

In order to be able to insert an angled blade plate into the femur without radiological control one must make an arthrotomy to define the bony landmarks, such as the anteversion of the femur, the center of the femoral head, and the superior aspect of the neck. In order to carry out this ar-

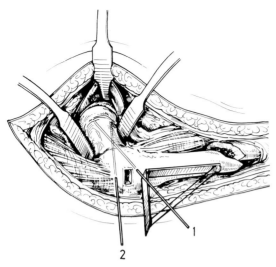

Fig. 12.13. Exposure of a subtrochanteric fracture. The vastus lateralis muscle is held retracted together with the inferior half of the joint capsule. The tip of the most anterior Hohmann retractor is passed through the capsule and then over the anterior pillar of the acetabulum. This ensures anterior exposure of the hip. Note the tip of a narrow Hohmann retractor driven into the cephalad superior aspects of the neck; this prevents the retractor from slipping and damaging the retinacular vessels posteriorly on the neck. Kirschner wire *1* indicates antiversion; Kirschner wire *2* indicates direction of seating chisel. It is parallel to *1*

In the region of the fracture the vastus lateralis muscle should not be detached from any loose comminuted fragments since this completely devitalizes them. Proximally, in the region of the hip, the vastus lateralis is reflected medially and distally, together with the inferior half of the hip joint capsule. In this way, full exposure is gained of the shaft, of the fracture, and of the hip joint (see Fig 12.13). The necessary Kirschner guidewires can then be inserted and the open reduction and internal fixation executed. To maintain the exposure we have found it useful to keep the muscle reflected with broad Hohmann retractors. The anterior exposure of the hip is maintained with the Hohmann retractor which is passed over the anterior pillar of the acetabulum. The superior aspect of the neck is exposed by reflecting the cephalad flap of the hip capsule and driving the tip of a narrow Hohmann retractor into the middle of the superior cortex of the femoral neck. This prevents the tip of the retractor from slipping posterosuperiorly and possibly damaging the retinacular vessels in their course to the femoral head. The inferior aspect of the neck and of the calcar is kept exposed by passing the tip of a retractor below the neck (Fig. 12.13).

12.4.4.4 Technique of Open Reduction and Internal Fixation

Once the fracture is exposed, the surgeon must go back to the preoperative drawings and plan. If one is dealing with a type A or a type B fracture, reduction of the fracture should precede the introduction of the angled blade plate. If the fracture is spiral or oblique, the gliding and thread holes should also be drilled prior to reduction of the fragments. If one is dealing with a type C fracture, i.e., one with severe comminution and segmental loss, we have found it far easier – even if the proximal fragment consists only of the portion of the femur above the lesser trochanter – to insert the condylar plate into the proximal fragment prior to reduction of the fracture.

The first Kirschner guidewire ("1" in Fig. 12.13) is placed inferiorly to mark the anteversion. The second guidewire ("2" in Fig. 12.13) will mark the direction of the seating chisel. Ideally, it should be inserted at 95° to the anatomical axis of the femur. In a comminuted femur which cannot be reduced, the anatomical axis cannot be determined from the bone at the time of surgery, and one has to go to the preoperative drawing in order to find the direction of this guidewire

throtomy, the exposed capsule is incised in line with the axis of the femoral neck and then a "T" is made at the base of the neck.

The fracture and the femoral shaft are exposed by reflecting the vastus lateralis muscle anteriorly. The femur should not be exposed through the substance of the vastus lateralis, because such an exposure is often associated with unnecessary bleeding from the perforating branches of the profunda femoris artery and, after surgery, with considerable muscle scarring. The anterior arthrotomy incision is extended laterally just distal to the rough line on the lateral aspect of the greater trochanter. The rough line separates the fibers of the vastus lateralis muscle and those of the gluteus medius muscle. The incision is then carried distally through the fascia of the vastus lateralis, just anterior to its posterior attachment, and the vastus lateralis is freed with a periostial elevator from its attachment to the lateral intermuscular septum. The perforating branches of the profunda femoris artery should be cross-clamped and ligated. If cauterized and cut they may cause troublesome bleeding, since the posterior part may retract through the posterior intermuscular septum. Once retracted, a bleeding vessel is very difficult to find.

in relation to such identifiable bony landmarks as the superior cortex of the neck, the center of the femoral head, and the rough line of the greater trochanter. The preoperative drawing was made using the uninvolved side as the template for the femur. The plate was then fitted to the proximal femur using the template as a guide. The exact placement in bone and the exact direction of the seating chisel and the plate were therefore predetermined with accuracy. Kirschner wire "2" is now driven into the tip of the trochanter to be out of the way of the seating chisel (see Fig. 12.13). It is driven in parallel to Kirschner wire "1", which indicates the anteversion of the femoral neck, and in the same relationship to the superior cortex of the neck and the center of rotation of the femoral head as that marked on the preoperative drawing.

Before the seating chisel can be inserted, a window in the lateral cortex of the greater trochanter must be cut. The correct placement of this window is very important. It bears different relationships to the midpoint of the lateral surface of the femur in the region of the greater trochanter and in the region of the shaft. If the femur is viewed end-on from above (see Fig. 12.14), it can be clearly seen that the neck is more anterior and not in line with the midpoint of the greater trochanter. Thus, for a blade to enter the middle of the neck when it is inserted through the greater trochanter, it must straddle the junction between the anterior and middle thirds of the greater trochanter (Fig. 12.14a). If the window for the seating chisel is cut, in error, too far posteriorly, it is deflected anteriorly as it enters the neck, and one runs the danger of entering the hip joint anteriorly with the tip of the implant. Similarly, if the window is cut too far posteriorly in the region of the shaft (Fig. 12.14b) – which is easily done, particularly if the leg is in traction and the shaft internally rotated – the blade of a 130° angled plate or the compression screw will be deflected anteriorly. The window in the trochanter for the condylar plate or the dynamic condylar screw should also be so situated that the seating chisel enters the neck 1 cm from the superior cortex of the neck. If the seating chisel is driven in too close to the superior cortex, it will be deflected downward, because the superior curve of the neck will not accommodate the width of the chisel. If the window is made too far distally, the seating chisel will strike the calcar. This is not such a disaster in itself, but it may bring about two complications: if the proximal fragment is short, then the lower the blade lies within the prox-

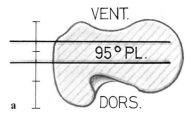

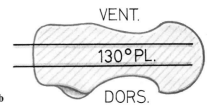

Fig. 12.14. a When viewed from above, the neck is more anterior and not in line with the midpoint of the greater trochanter. Thus, in order to enter the middle of the neck, a plate must be inserted through the junction between the anterior and the middle thirds of the trochanter. **b** In the region of the shaft (e.g., for a dynamic hip screw), the window must be cut in the middle of the lateral cortex. (From Müller et al. 1979)

imal fragment, the less room one has to supplement the fixation with a screw through the plate into the calcar. Furthermore, if one is guided by the calculated length of the blade as determined in the preoperative drawing, one may not recognize the arrest of the seating chisel by the calcar, particularly if the latter is osteoporotic or the individual very young and the cancellous bone within the proximal femur very hard. Further blows of the mallet will drive the seating chisel into the calcar, which may shatter. In driving the seating chisel into bone, one further plane must be carefully observed. The flap of the seating chisel guide must be in line with the long axis of the greater trochanter to ensure that the proximal fragment will be neither flexed nor extended. Once the seat for the blade is cut, the seating chisel is withdrawn and the angled plate inserted. Once the plate is impacted into bone and is sitting flush against the cortex of the proximal fragment, it is secured in the proximal fragment by the insertion of a 4.5-mm cortical screw through the plate into the calcar. A 6.5-mm cancellous screw is too wide and may splinter the calcar; hence, its use in this position has been abandoned.

The reduction of the fracture can now proceed with relatively little effort. The shaft of the femur is lined up with the plate. Its rotation is adjusted and it is then held to the plate with a Verbrugge bone clamp (see Fig. 12.11 e). No attempt is made to identify or reduce any of the comminuted fragments. The distractor is now inserted with one bolt through the second hole of the plate, and its second bolt is inserted into a predrilled 4.5-mm hole distal to the plate (see Fig. 12.9). One must note on the preoperative drawing the relationship of the most distal fracture line to the holes of the plate. This helps one to judge when the correct length of the femur is restored. The rotation should be restored as close to normal as possible prior to insertion of the distal bolt of the distractor, since only limited rotational correction can be achieved with the distractor in place.

The distractor is now used to distract the femur and gradually regain the correct length. The Verbrugge clamp may have to be loosened but it should not be removed completely, since it guides the femoral shaft in the correct axial alignment as length is being regained. Once the correct length is restored the comminuted fragments should be inspected. Occasionally, the fracture may have to be overdistracted in order to ease the reduction of the comminuted fragments. The majority realign as length is regained and the soft tissues are placed under tension.

Occasionally, some fragments have to be turned to achieve a reduction. Once reduction is achieved the distractor is turned back until the correct length is regained. At this point we like to secure the position of the plate to the shaft with one screw distally and check the rotational alignment of the leg by flexing the hip and checking the degree of internal and external rotation. This is also a convenient moment to get anteroposterior and lateral radiographs of the hip (see Fig. 12.11 e). Since we have chosen an operating table with facility for an anteroposterior radiograph, the anteroposterior radiograph is simple. In order to get a perfect lateral view of the femoral neck, the hip should be flexed to 90° and, while held flexed, abducted 20° in neutral rotation. A second anteroposterior exposure with the hip held in this position gives a perfect lateral projection of the femoral neck and head.

If the placement of the plate is correct, the internal fixation can now be completed. If there are major butterfly fragments, these should have been noted on the preoperative drawing, as well as the possibility of securing these together with lag screws (see Fig. 12.11 c). The lag screws are now inserted, together with the remaining screws which secure the plate to the shaft.

12.4.4.5 Bone Grafting

If one is dealing with a comminuted fracture, the fracture must be bone grafted in order to ensure union and prevent fatigue fracture of the implant. We feel that the bone grafting should be performed at the same time as the internal fixation. Because the femur is eccentrically loaded, there are major compressive stresses on the medial side. If there is a defect on the medial side, i.e., the side opposite the plate, the plate will be bent with loading of the femur, which may be no greater than that of simple muscular contraction. With unloading, because of its elasticity, the plate will spring back to its original shape. If allowed to continue unchecked, such cyclic loading will result in a fatigue fracture of the implant. In addition to the bending forces, there are shearing forces which contribute to the failure of the implant. The cyclic loading may be prevented by bridging the comminuted segments with a second plate applied to the medial side, but, apart from the technical difficulties of applying such a plate medially, one would incur a very heavy biological price, the risk of rendering a segment of the femur next to the fracture avascular. This would delay healing and would heighten the chance of nonunion.

The autogenous cancellous bone is applied opposite the plate to bridge the defect. If it is successful, usually by the end of 6–8 weeks, it results in a radiologically visible bony bridge opposite the plate. Such a bridge is then ideally situated. The compressive stresses lead to its hypertrophy (Fig. 12.11 h). Because it is opposite the plate it arrests all bending movements, brings all motion to a standstill and protects the implant from failure. At this point, i.e., once a radiologically visible bridge appears, loading can be rapidly increased to full without fear of implant failure. Actually, with increased stress the medial bridge is usually seen to hypertrophy and gain further strength.

12.4.5 Postoperative Care

The patient recovering from surgery on the proximal femur does not require any special positioning or splinting. We believe that early ambulation is far more effective and safer than any anticoagulants in preventing thrombophlebitis. All patients, if able, are up with crutches on the day after surgery. We discourage sitting, since in a patient with a swollen thigh and groin the sitting posture leads to compression of vessels in the groin and contributes to venous thrombosis. The amount of weight bearing is determined by the stability of the reduction and of the internal fixation. Generally, in the type C fractures, weight bearing is avoided until there is some evidence of osseous bridging medially, which usually takes up to 8 or 10 weeks to make its appearance. In stable fracture configurations, such as type A and type B, partial weight bearing of 10–15 kg is begun almost immediately. The above regimen applies to patients with plating or locked intramedullary nailing. In patients with locked intramedullary nailing, once there is evidence of bridging callus, the bolts are removed to allow the bone to resume its function of weight bearing.

12.4.5.1 Signs of Instability

The absence of callus in the presence of stable fixation makes it difficult to judge the progress of healing. We must rely more on indirect evidence of union, such as the gradual disappearance of the fracture line, the absence of irritation callus, the absence of resorption around the screws and under the plate, the maintenance of the reduction without recurrence of deformity, and, clinically, on the absence of pain. The patient who either continues to have pain after an open reduction and stable fixation or develops pain after a period of painless mobilization must be considered to have either instability of the fixation or a deep-seated infection. In each instance the patient will have pain, local tenderness, and even redness with swelling. The latter applies more to the subcutaneous bones, such as the tibia, than to the femur. Usually, redness with swelling in the thigh signifies sepsis. Other confirmatory evidence, such as a temperature, the white blood cell count, and the sedimentation rate, will aid in the diagnosis.

12.4.5.2 Infection

If the diagnosis of a deep-seated infection is made, then, in addition to the intravenous antibiotics, the patient must have the wound reopened and thoroughly débrided, and a suction irrigation system must be set up or the wound packed open. Most infections are deep-seated and go right to the fracture. Superficial wound infections are rare and occur only in the immediate postoperative period. If redness, tenderness, and swelling appear a month or so after surgery, particularly in a case where prophylactic antibiotics were used during the surgery, one can be almost certain that the patient has a deep-seated infection. A new course

of antibiotic therapy may bring all the manifestations of the disaster under control, but only the inexperienced surgeon will take solace from this seeming cure. Usually the flare-up of sepsis makes its inevitable appearance a few weeks later. At this point the situation is usually more complex, because the smoldering infection has led to bone resorption and to some loss of stability. One can usually recognize radiologically, in addition to some periosteal bone formation at the ends of the plate, resorption of bone deep to the plate and a widening of the fracture line. At this stage it is not enough to treat the infection aggressively with débridement and suction irrigation. One must determine whether the internal fixation is stable. If stability has been lost because of loosening of the fixation it must be revised. If stability exists or if it has been restored, the fracture must be bone grafted with autogenous cancellous bone to accelerate union and prevent failure of the implant.

If the diagnosis is instability and failure of the fixation, then the situation must be treated aggressively, or fatigue fracture of the implant is certain. The only ways to lessen the load on the proximal femur are to immobilize the patient in traction with complete bed rest or to immobilize the patient in a hip spica. Unloading of the extremity as described, although in itself unwise because of the complications of such treatment, can lead to union only in the presence of a well-marked irritation callus which can convert to a fixation callus. If the diagnosis of delayed union is made on the basis of a widening fracture line and an ill-defined irritation callus, or if the diagnosis is one of failed internal fixation because of loosening, then the only sensible course to follow is to revise the internal fixation and to bone graft the fracture to promote union. Procrastination in the face of instability and failing fixation only protracts the patient's disability.

References

Cochran GVB, Zickel RE, Fielding JW (1980) Stress analysis of subtrochanteric fractures: effect of muscle forces and internal fixation devices. In: Uhthoff HK (ed) Current concepts of internal fixation of fractures. Springer, Berlin Heidelberg New York

Ender SW (1970) Die Fixierung der Trochanterbrüche mit runden elastischen Kondylennägeln. Acta Chir Austriaca 1:40–42

Kempf I, Grosse A, Beck G (1985) Closed locked intramedullary nailing. J Bone Joint Surg 67A:709–720

Küntscher G (1967) Practice of intramedullary nailing. Thomas, Springfield, p 178

Müller ME, Allgöwer M, Schneider R, Willenegger H (1979) Manual of internal fixation, 2nd edn. Springer, Berlin Heidelberg New York

Pankovich AM, Tarabishy IE (1980) Ender nailing of inter-trochanteric and subtrochanteric fractures. J Bone Joint Surg 62A:635–645

Schatzker J, Waddell JP (1980) Subtrochanteric frac-tures of the femur. Orthop Clin North Am 11(3):539–554

Schatzker J, Manley PA, Sumner-Smith G (1980) In vivo strain-gauge study of bone response to loading with and without internal fixation of fractures. Springer, Berlin Heidelberg New York, pp 306–314

Zickel RE (1976) An intramedullary fixation device for the proximal part of the femur. J Bone Joint Surg 58A:866–872

13 Fractures of the Femur

J. Schatzker

13.1 Introduction

The femur, the largest tubular bone in the body, is surrounded by the largest mass of muscles and is designed to withstand greater forces than any other bone. Fractures of the femur are almost always the result of great violence and are sometimes a threat to the patient's life, not only because of the immediate complications such as bleeding or associated injuries, but also because of subsequent complications related either to the treatment of the fracture, or to the complications of the associated injuries.

13.2 Factors Important in Evaluating the Mode of Treatment

Any fracture of the femoral shaft, if it goes beyond an undisplaced crack, is unstable and displaces further under the influence of physiological forces. The fragments always shorten, rotate, and angulate. Early systems for the immobilization of the femur frequently involved the immobilization of the whole patient as well as immobilization of the leg, including the hip and knee joint. Immobilization of the fracture was recognized as essential for union. The development of splints, such as the Thomas splint, and the subsequent combinations of the splints with traction methods, either fixed or balanced, allowed for better control of the fracture.

Patients nevertheless had to remain in traction for 3 months or longer before the fracture was sufficiently stable to allow ambulation. Even at this point, a number had to be protected in ischial-bearing long leg calipers to prevent refracture. A hip plaster spica could not be used as a successful method to treat fresh fractures because it did not allow control of angulation or shortening. It was recognized that an initial period of traction of 6–8 weeks was necessary before a fracture became sufficiently stable for the patient to be transferred into a hip spica. This freed the acute treatment bed, but did not influence the rate of union, nor did it improve the result of treatment.

Certain complications of prolonged traction, such as decubitus ulcers, can be overcome by better nursing, but the complications of prolonged bed rest such as bladder and bowel derangements, deep vein thrombosis, osteoporosis, and muscle wasting, to mention only a few, cannot be prevented. Furthermore despite the most expert care, a disturbing number of patients end up with significant shortening of 2 cm or more, angulation of sufficient degree to effect the biomechanical function of their extremity, and, above all, knee joint stiffness. A return of 90° of knee joint flexion was often considered as a most successful result of treatment, which could be achieved only at the end of a prolonged period of rehabilitation requiring many hours of hard work, not only from the patient, but also from the attending rehabilitative staff.

The resurgence of cast bracing (Sarmiento 1972; Sarmiento and Latta 1981) spurred many enthusiasts to apply this method to fractures of the femur. It was found, however, that it is not a method which can be used to treat fresh fractures. Initial reduction still has to be obtained and the limb has to be treated on a splint in traction until such time as callus renders the fracture sufficiently stable for the limb to be transferred into a cast brace. The average stay in hospital with this method is still between 6 and 8 weeks. Cast bracing, although suitable for fractures of the distal third of the femur, has been abandoned even by the enthusiasts of this technique for fractures of the mid and proximal third, because of complications of shortening and angulation.

Initial attempts at internal fixation of the femur were disastrous. The stability obtained with plates and screws was inadequate to nurse the extremity without the protection of splints, traction, or both. Despite the supplemental protection, failure of the internal fixation and resulting nonunion was common. Furthermore, the stiffness which resulted from surgery followed by immobilization was far greater than the stiffness from nonoperative methods alone. Thus, until the advent of the intramedullary nail, open reduction and internal fixation played a negligible role in the treatment of fractures of the femoral shaft. In 1940, Gerhard Küntscher introduced intramedullary nailing of the femur and revolutionized the treatment of femoral shaft fractures (Küntscher 1967). The stability obtained with his method of internal fixation was sufficient to render the patients pain-free, allow them early mobilization, and in certain cases, even allow early weight bearing. Later on, Küntscher recognized that stability could be further increased by increasing the diameter of the medullary nail. In 1950, he introduced intramedullary reaming and further improved the results of his technique (Küntscher 1967). There remained, however, all the fractures not suitable for the intramedullary nailing technique, such as fractures of the proximal or distal third, long oblique and spiral fractures, and comminuted fractures with loss of segmental continuity.

The introduction of stable internal fixation with the aid of compression by the Swiss AO group in the early 1960s further revolutionized the surgical treatment of femoral shaft fractures (Müller et al. 1965). It now became possible, after a careful atraumatic anatomical reduction of the fracture, to achieve an absolute degree of stability by means of lag screws and tension band or neutralization plates. This rendered the extremity completely pain-free. The stability achieved was such that supplemental protection of splints or traction was no longer necessary. The patient could begin early active mobilization of the extremity, often with partial weight bearing. This led to a rapid recovery of the soft tissue envelope and to a rapid return of motion of the adjacent joints. Because of the absolute degree of stability achieved, union occurred in a very high percentage of the cases without loss of position and malunion or nonunion. Thus, the scope of internal fixation was greatly expanded and the indications for nonoperative treatment of the femur correspondingly reduced to a very small number.

The most recent advance in the treatment of femoral shaft fractures has been the development of the locking intramedullary nail (Kempf et al. 1985), which we describe in some detail later on in this chapter. This technique has made it possible to deal surgically with the most extreme degrees of comminution of the shaft which are completely beyond the scope of conventional intramedullary nailing or plating.

The techniques which we have described, conventional intramedullary nailing, the AO/ASIF methods of open reduction and internal fixation by means of screws and plates, and the most recent development of locking intramedullary nailing, are by no means devoid of complications, nor are they simple to execute. They comprise, however, together with external skeletal fixation, the best methods of treatment for femoral shaft fractures. Nonoperative means have a very small role to play as definitive methods of care for fractures of the femoral shaft. We must emphasize again and again that the decision to pursue a particular course of treatment must be based on the analysis of the personality of the fracture, that is, the nature of the fracture and of the patient: age, functional demands, etc. It must also be based on the environment where the care is being administered, and lastly on the skill of the surgeon with a particular technique. If a surgeon does not have the necessary skills to execute complex internal fixation, then it is clearly best to pursue nonoperative means. However, a surgeon who is going to treat fractures should acquire the skills to execute the forms of treatment generally accepted as the best, and recognize that nonoperative treatment for fractures of the femoral shaft should be viewed as nondefinitive and temporizing, and that the patient should be referred, if at all possible, to a center where appropriate treatment can be carried out safely and expertly.

13.3 Surgical Treatment

13.3.1 Timing of Surgery

Once the decision is made to pursue surgical treatment, the next important decision to be made is the timing of surgery. The decision as to when to operate must be based on a number of factors, the most important being the associated injuries.

13.3.1.1 Multiple System Injuries

Recent experience from trauma centers (Riska et al. 1976; Winquist et al. 1984; Sibel et al. 1985) indicates that immediate fixation of long bone fractures, particularly of the femur, has been instrumental in preventing or reversing progressive respiratory failure by allowing the chest to be nursed in a vertical position. Furthermore, these studies have demonstrated that there has been no increase in fat embolism as a result of immediate intramedullary nailing of femoral shaft fractures (Riska et al. 1976; Riska and Myllenen 1982; Winquist et al. 1984). By immediate, we mean as soon as possible after the general priorities such as airway, bleeding, and volume replacement, and cranial, abdominal, and thoracic priorities of patients with multiple injuries have been satisfied. Frequently, stabilization of long bone fractures can be begun while a general surgeon is dealing with injuries to chest or abdomen. If the position of the patient on the table renders internal fixation logistically not feasible, it should be executed under the same anesthetic as soon as the position can be changed. A previously healthy patient with multiple injuries will never be as fit for surgery as after the initial resuscitation and stabilization, while well oxygenated under endotracheal anesthesia, with fluid and electrolyte status under full control. This is true as long as there is no rise in the intracranial pressure or as long as no complications develop, such as ventilatory problems or coagulopathies.

13.3.1.2 Head Injury

A head injury with unconsciousness was formerly considered a contraindication to any internal fixation. The nursing of unconscious patients with femoral shaft fractures was extremely difficult. They could not be nursed supine with limbs in traction. They demanded frequent turning to prevent respiratory complications, and their limbs could only be immobilized by propping them up and splinting them with pillows, with the traction adjusted as well as possible. The cardiorespiratory complications that ensued from the moving about of fractured femora, and from the enforced supine position, cannot be overemphasized. In addition, we have all witnessed the unnecessary lifelong crippling of accident victims whose skeletal injuries, such as dislocated hips, fractured hips, or fractured femora, were neglected because of their head injury and initial unconsciousness. Many such patients awoke 3–4 weeks after their injury with a clear sensorium and undamaged intellect, only to find their extremities permanently shortened and deformed. Neglect of skeletal injuries because of an associated head injury must be avoided.

An unconscious patient whose cerebral status is stable and who does not have an enlarging intracranial mass with rising intracranial pressure

(these would be clear priorities in treatment) should have most of the significant musculoskeletal lesions treated definitively on an emergency basis, either operatively or nonoperatively. In the case of a fractured femur, the definitive treatment must be operative. This will not only prevent permanent deformities and disability, but will greatly enhance the ease and quality of the nursing care of such patients and greatly diminish morbidity. The advent of computed tomography and intracranial pressure monitoring has greatly eased the initial evaluation of intracranial injuries and has helped immeasurably in defining the fitness of patients for definitive care of their skeletal injuries.

13.3.1.3 Open Fractures

The débridement of an open wound should be carried out on an emergency basis. Whether internal fixation of an open fracture should be carried out is still a matter of some controversy. We believe that stable fixation of an open fracture is not only the single most important maneuver after débridement in preventing sepsis, but also that it is the only maneuver which will safeguard the optimal return of soft tissue function (Matter and Rittman 1978). How stability is achieved will depend upon the type of fracture. This will be discussed at length later in this chapter. However, at this point, it must be said that we believe that an open fracture must be stabilized at the time of surgical débridement, either by means of screws and plates or by means of an external fixator. As a rule, we prefer not to use intramedullary nailing in the more severe open fractures.

13.3.1.4 Vascular Injury

Vascular injury clearly demands immediate intervention to safeguard the survival of the extremity. Although experience from the war in Vietnam war suggested that vascular reconstruction would not be jeopardized if the extremity were subsequently treated in traction, we feel that in the event of a vascular injury, immediate fixation of the femur should be carried out, either by means of internal or external skeletal fixation, but preferably by the former. To minimise the complications of ischemia, a temporary vascular shunt should be inserted before the internal fixation is undertaken.

13.3.1.5 Ipsilateral Neck Fracture or Dislocation of the Hip

Both injuries, but particularly the latter, create an emergency situation. The incidence of avascular necrosis is directly related to the time that the head remains out of the joint, to the degree of intra-articular hypertension, and to the displacement. If a closed reduction of the dislocation or of the fracture is to be attempted, then the shaft fracture must be first reduced and fixed. It is also best to stabilize the shaft fracture before the neck lest any manipulation of the shaft should dislodge an internal fixation of the neck or trochanteric region. Also, it may be necessary for a number of reasons to do an open reduction of the dislocation. If so, the shaft fracture should be fixed at the same time and not treated in traction.

13.3.1.6 Ipsilateral Fracture of the Femoral Shaft and Ligamentous Disruption of the Knee

One cannot apply traction across a disrupted knee. Therefore, if, for some reason, surgery has to be delayed, skeletal traction should be applied through a supracondylar pin. Otherwise, it is best to proceed to an internal fixation of the fracture and to an immediate reconstruction of the disrupted ligaments.

13.3.1.7 Floating Knee Syndrome

Patients who sustain fractures of the ipsilateral femur and tibia have the so-called floating knee syndrome. This syndrome has recently received considerable attention. All who have concerned themselves with the care of these injuries agree that a proper evaluation of the knee is only possible once the knee and tibia have been stabilized by means of internal fixation, and that the best results of treatment of these and their associated ligamentous or intra-articular injuries are obtained if they are treated as soon as the general condition of the patient allows.

13.3.1.8 Isolated Fractures of the Femoral Shaft

After resuscitation of the patient with an isolated fracture of the femoral shaft, the surgeon has the option of either proceeding with definitive surgical treatment or delaying the treatment for a few days. Those who favor delay have frequently cited the difficulties encountered in attempting an immediate open reduction of a femoral shaft, particularly in athletic and muscular individuals. This can no longer be accepted as an indication for the delay of treatment. The distractor (Fig. 13.1) will facilitate the early reduction out to length of even the most muscular thigh. Furthermore, immediate intramedullary nailing is not associated with an increased incidence of fat embolism syndrome (Riska et al. 1976; Riska and Myllenen 1982; Winquist et al. 1984; Schatzker to be published). Some authors (Charnley and Guindy 1961; Lam 1964; Smith 1964) have reported an increased incidence of union of fractures of long bones if open treatment was delayed for 1 week or longer. This initial lag period allowed the initiation of all events which lead to the formation of callus. Although of no particular value in a fracture with a simple fracture pattern (for these can be easily stabilized by means of screws and plates or by means of intramedullary nails, with a high rate of uncomplicated union), the delay is of some value in a badly comminuted shaft fracture if plate fixation is chosen. In these, because of comminution, stability is difficult to achieve. Furthermore, many of the comminuted fragments lose their blood supply, further increasing the risk of nonunion and failure of the fixation. In these, therefore, if plating is to be carried out, it is better to wait for 7–10 days before carrying out an open reduction and internal fixation. During this interval, the blood supply to many of the

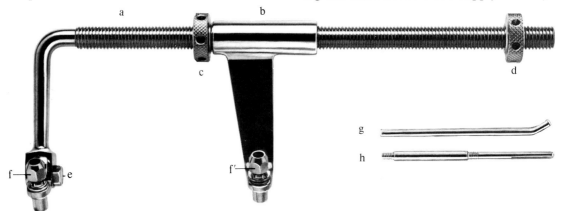

Fig. 13.1. The femoral distractor. The screw spindle (*a*), its movable wing (*b*), the distraction screw (*c*), the compression screw (*d*), the hinged joint for rotational correction (*e*), the fixation screw (*f*), the lever (*g*) and connecting bolt (*h*) (From Müller et al. 1979)

small fragments will have improved and by the time one operates, many of the events which lead to union will already have been set in motion and one has the benefit of a second injury which frequently leads to a rapid formation of callus.

If surgery is to be delayed, the fracture must be properly splinted and the extremity placed in skeletal traction with the fragments in the best possible alignment. One should attempt to overdistract the fracture. This will ease subsequent reduction. Where circumstances dictate immediate intervention, an immediate internal fixation should be executed. The advent of locked intramedullary nailing has made it technically possible to stabilize even highly comminuted shaft fractures immediately, without running a higher risk of failure (see Fig. 13.12).

13.3.2 Surgical Technique

13.3.2.1 Positioning the Patient, Skin Preparation, and Draping

Open reduction and internal fixation of the femoral shaft fracture by means of screws and plates or open intramedullary nailing should not be attempted on the fracture table with the extremity in traction. The traction results in such tension of the soft tissue envelope that exposure and manipulation of the fragments is extremely difficult, if not impossible. Visualization is difficult, retraction of necessity is forceful, and unnecessary devitalization of the fragments is inevitable. An accurate anatomical reduction is almost impossible to obtain, and as a result, fixation is often not as stable as it should be.

We prefer to position the patient lying on the uninjured side on an ordinary table, and support the trunk with chest rests to stop the pelvis from flopping back and forth. An open reduction and internal fixation can be performed with equal ease if the patient is supine. If the patient is positioned supine, then the table top must be radiolucent to permit intraoperative radiography.

During surgical scrubbing, the extremity must be elevated and kept in traction to prevent telescoping of the fragments which could lead to further soft tissue damage and further comminution of the fracture. Ipsilateral posterior and anterior iliac crests should be included in the surgical scrub and should be subsequently draped free to serve as donor sites for bone grafting, should it prove necessary. The leg should be scrubbed almost to the ankle and, in draping, the knee should be left

free so that it can be flexed as necessary during the procedure. If a Steinmann pin has been used for preoperative traction, it should be draped out of the field and left in until the internal fixation is complete. Sometimes, despite the best of intentions, the limb may have to be placed in traction again. It is best not to use pillows for padding between the legs, but to rely on sterile folded sheets which are placed under the scrubbed leg. These can then be rearranged as necessary during the reduction to support the bone and prevent redisplacement.

A tourniquet is not used. Even if a sterile tourniquet were used, it would get in the way of the incision. If vascular reconstruction has to be carried out at the same time as the internal fixation, then it is best to place the patient supine on the table to provide free access to the groin and medial aspect of the popliteal fossa.

13.3.2.2 Surgical Approach

The standard approach to the whole femoral shaft is through a straight lateral incision which is made along an imaginary line joining the greater trochanter with the lateral femoral condyle (Fig. 13.2). The fascia lata is incised in line with the skin. One should not approach the bone through the substance of the vastus lateralis mus-

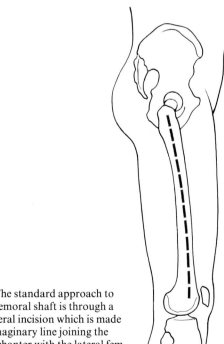

Fig. 13.2. The standard approach to the whole femoral shaft is through a straight lateral incision which is made along an imaginary line joining the greater trochanter with the lateral femoral condyle

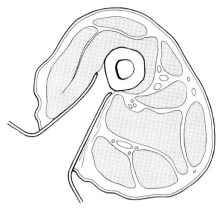

Fig. 13.3. The vastus lateralis muscle is dissected from its attachment to the intermuscular septum and is lifted forward and medially to expose the shaft

cle, even if the latter has been pierced by bone. The vastus lateralis should be carefully dissected with a sharp periostial elevator from its attachment to the intermuscular septum and should be lifted forward and medially to expose the shaft (Fig. 13.3). The perforating vessels which are found within the substance of the vastus lateralis 4–8 mm from the bone should be cross-clamped and ligated. If they are cauterized and cut, the posterior portion of the vessel may retract through the intermuscular septum and begin to bleed. Bleeding from it during surgery is a nuisance because it is difficult to find the vessel and to stop the bleeding. It may also begin to bleed after closure and result in a large, troublesome hematoma.

13.3.2.3 Technique of Open Reduction

The key to the execution of an open reduction is to be "atraumatic". The muscle should be stripped as little as possible from the bone fragments to preserve the blood supply. Small comminuted fragments are best left unexposed. Large fragments must be exposed because they must be

reduced in order to achieve structural stability; however, every effort must be made not to strip them from their muscle attachment. The periosteum is reflected only at the edges of the fracture which are also cleared of all clot and soft tissues so that any undisplaced fracture fissures can be detected and an accurate reduction executed. The periosteum is not stripped from under the plate. In order to ease the manipulation of the main fragments, they should be gripped with a reduction clamp. It is best to use the special reduction clamps with narrow jaws (Fig. 13.4). This keeps the devitalization to a minimum. In manipulating the fragments, care must be taken not to squeeze the handles of the reduction clamps as this could result in crushing of the bone and in extensive comminution.

The trick in reducing a comminuted fracture with one or two large butterflies is to reduce the butterflies and fix them with lag screws to one or both fragments. In this way, the comminuted fracture is converted to a simple fracture. This greatly eases the final reduction (Fig. 13.5). It is very difficult to regain length by longitudinal traction. If possible, the main fragments should be grasped and angulated through the fracture until the cortices can be hooked on. Length is then reestablished by simple realignment of the bones while the cortices are maintained engaged. If this is impossible to achieve because of the obliquity of the fracture or because of comminution, then the simplest and safest way to achieve length and reduction is to use the distractor (see Fig. 13.1). If reduction is going to be difficult because the fracture was allowed to foreshorten, then preliminary overdistraction with the distractor should be executed before any reduction is attempted. The distraction must be carried out very slowly to allow the soft tissues to stretch without tearing.

We have come to rely on the distractor more and more, even for simple fractures, as it ensures reduction with the least amount of soft tissue

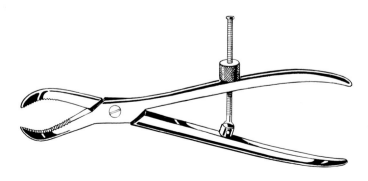

Fig. 13.4. Special reduction clamps with narrow jaws. They keep devitalization of fragments to a minimum

Fig. 13.5. In a comminuted fracture, the fragments are fixed with lag screws to each other and to the main fragments where possible. This converts a comminuted fracture into a simple fracture. (From Müller et al. 1979.) Do not strip the muscle from the fragments. This devitalizes them and greatly prolongs the time to union. It is more important to preserve the blood supply than to secure fixation of small fragments

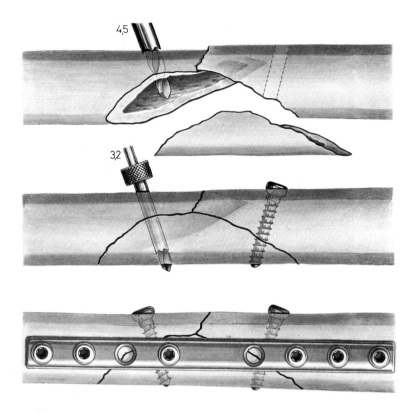

trauma. It is invaluable in dealing with comminuted fractures. In these, length can be easily restored by slight overdistraction. As the soft tissue envelope is stretched, the comminuted fragments frequently reduce spontaneously or require only minimal manipulation to be fitted in place. The larger fragments can then be lagged together with the least damage to their blood supply.

13.3.2.4 Technique of Fracture Fixation

There are three methods available for achieving stable fixation of the femur. These are intramedullary nailing, internal fixation by means of screws and plates, and external skeletal fixation.

a) External Skeletal Fixation

External skeletal fixation of the femur is used chiefly to stabilize severe open fractures and infected pseudoarthroses. The large muscle mass, the proximity of the other leg near the groin, and the medial course of the femoral artery and the posterior course of the sciatic nerve present specific problems to be dealt with when erecting an external skeletal fixation frame. For stability to be achieved in the femur, one would ideally require three-plane fixation. In the proximal femur, however, the pins cannot exit medially because of the proximity of the other leg and the perineum. Thus, in the proximal third, only a half-frame can be erected laterally.

If one wishes to insert transfixing pins through the shaft, this must be done under direct vision from the medial side with identification of the femoral artery in order to prevent its damage with the pins. Transfixing pins can be inserted safely only through the condyles and through the immediate supracondylar area. Transfixing pins cannot be inserted in the anteroposterior plane because of the sciatic nerve which is directly behind the femur. Hence, only an anterior half-frame can be erected, with the pins stopping just at the point of exit through the posterior cortex. The difficulty with all the pins except those in the frontal plane in the condylar area is that they penetrate large muscle bellies; this frequently gives rise to pin track sepsis. The anterior half-frame transfixes the quadriceps muscle mechanism and blocks any knee movement. Therefore, it can be used only if knee motion must be sacrificed or if it is already absent, as in an infected pseudoarthrosis. Half-frame systems, such as the Wagner leg lengthening device, the Judet external fixator, or a unilateral AO tubular frame, do not provide a high degree of stability if used on fresh fractures. The Wagner device provides a greater degree of stability if used

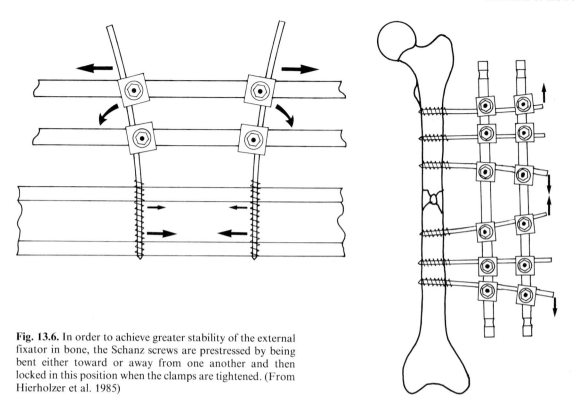

Fig. 13.6. In order to achieve greater stability of the external fixator in bone, the Schanz screws are prestressed by being bent either toward or away from one another and then locked in this position when the clamps are tightened. (From Hierholzer et al. 1985)

for leg lengthening because it is pulling against the resistance of tight soft tissues. Such soft tissue tension is absent in fresh fractures. Stability is further influenced by the question of comminution and whether axial compression can be exerted or not. In order to achieve greater stability, the fragments should be compressed, or, if this is impossible because of comminution, then the pins should be prestressed against one another (Fig. 13.6). This is possible to achieve with such devices as the AO tubular external fixator system, but not with the Wagner leg-lengthening device. The stability of the system can be further increased by erecting the system in such a way that the pins transfix the bone close to the fracture.

b) Intramedullary Nailing

Gerhard Küntscher is credited with the development of modern intramedullary nailing (Küntscher 1967). He reasoned that, if one were to introduce into the rigid bone of the medullary canal an elastic, deformable nail somewhat larger than the medullary canal, the nail would be squeezed and its elastic recoil would result in the nail gripping the bone along its endosteal surface (Fig. 13.7). The initial nail was V-shaped in profile. It was subse-

quently changed to the familiar cloverleaf configuration. It was elastic and slit along its full length to make it compressible. It was bowed anteriorly to correspond to the physiological curvature of the femur with its slit coming posteriorly.

Recent studies have shown that the holding power of the nail depends on a combination of a number of factors. If we think of the nail as a tube within a tube of bone, several of the biomechanical properties of this type of fixation become obvious. A nail has to overcome the forces of bending, rotation, and shortening. The resistance to bending depends on the length of intimate contact between the two tubes. Thus, a nail introduced without reaming would have contact only over a short area at the isthmus and, theoretically, bending could occur, with the fulcrum at the isthmus and the amplitude of displacement corresponding to the distance between the nail and the endosteum at each end (Fig. 13.8). In the young, the metaphyseal areas are filled with dense cancellous bone which resists this angular displacement, but in the elderly the metaphyses are filled with sparse, weak trabeculae which offer virtually no resistance to it. Intramedullary reaming enlarges longitudinally the area of contact between the nail and the bone (Fig. 13.8). In clinical practice, we aim for at least

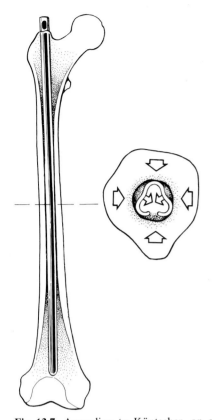

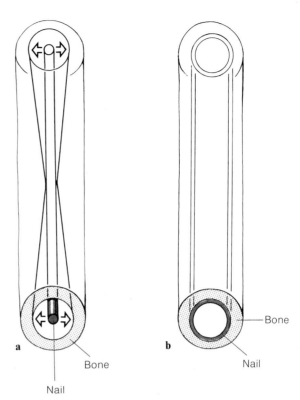

Fig. 13.7. According to Küntscher, an elastic deformable nail, when inserted into a slightly smaller medullary canal, will be deformed. Its elastic recoil results in the nail gripping the bone which provides fixation for the fragments. (Adapted from Küntscher 1967)

Fig. 13.8. a A nail introduced without reaming has contact only along the narrowest segment of the medullary canal. Bending can occur at either end. **b** After reaming, the length of contact of the "tube within a tube" is significantly increased, as is stability

5 cm contact on each side of the fracture. Therefore, the exact diameter of the nail can best be determined only at the time of surgery, although one can arrive at an approximation from preoperative measurement of the endosteal diameter.

Resistance to rotation of the bone about the nail depends on the degree of friction between the two surfaces. The greater the surface area of contact, the greater the friction. The concept of the bone squeezing the elastic, deformable nail which in its elastic recoil grips the bone is not entirely correct. Viewed under high magnification, the channel cut by the reamers is seen to be a series of peaks and valleys. The fixation is in reality an interference fit between the nail and the bone. As the contours of the nail and bone do not correspond exactly, there are areas of greater pressure where the bone is forcing the nail to follow its contour. Where the reduction is such that the fracture fragments are in contact, rotational control is achieved by the interdigitation of the fragments, and not by friction. Axial muscle force keeps the fragments in opposition. This applies to short oblique and transverse fractures. Longer oblique and spiral fractures lack rotational stability for two reasons. The first is that a long split decreases the available areas of bone for contact and thus decreases rotational control, and the second is that the long spiral fracture can open. This not only interferes with rotational stability, but also with longitudinal stability.

Intramedullary reaming not only enhances the resistance to bending and rotation, but also allows one to use a thicker nail which will be able to withstand the physiological forces of bending. A nail, because of its special orientation in relationship to the mass of the femur, is in a much more advantageous position than a plate to withstand deformation. Because of this, it can be used as a load-sharing device and permit much earlier weight bearing.

The nail has to substitute for the bone while the bone is uniting; therefore, it must be just as strong. The bending strength of a nail is related to its cross-sectional configuration and to the orientation of this configuration. Thus, for example, in a diamond-shaped nail, the longer diameter affords a greater resistance to bending than the short diameter. The spatial distribution of the material is also important: a tube has greater bending resistance than a solid rod.

The bending strength is also related to the diameter of the nail. Thus, the average adult female and male will usually require a 14- and 15-mm nail, respectively. The nail should extend from the tip of the greater trochanter almost to the subchondral bone of the distal metaphysis. It should not be allowed to jut out into the abductors because it often causes pain, lurching, or both, and may result in heterotopic calcification and/or ossification, which may result in permanent malfunction of the abductors. The slit in the nail weakens its torsional resistance. The nail, however, never fails in torsion because the bone will spin about the nail long before nail failure threatens.

Fig. 13.9 a, b. Severely comminuted fracture of the femoral shaft. Longitudinal stability was restored by reduction and cerclage wiring of the fragments prior to nailing. Note that all the fragments are large. Today this case would be an ideal indication for a "locked" intramedullary nailing

Longitudinal stability depends on the ability of the bone to withstand axial compression. Thus, it is dependent on the fracture pattern, as already mentioned, and on the degree of contact between the main fragments. The ideal fracture pattern for axial stability is the transverse fracture, but even here the degree of stability is a function of the degree of contact. If there is comminution, the less the circumferential contact between the main fragments, the less the stability. If the contact falls below 50%, then the likelihood of collapse increases significantly unless the comminuted fragments can be reduced and kept in place by supplemental fixation such as cerclage wiring. This applies, of course, only to open nailing. In closed nailing where supplemental fixation cannot be carried out, one must carefully assess the degree of contact between the main fragments in order to assess accurately the degree of stability and the applicability of the technique.

Loss of reduction of long or spiral fractures can be prevented either by cerclage wires or by the insertion of lag screws between the main fragments (Fig. 13.9). Longitudinal splits can be prevented by cerclage if the comminution is not too extensive and the fragments not too small. If the segmental loss of contact cannot be restored by

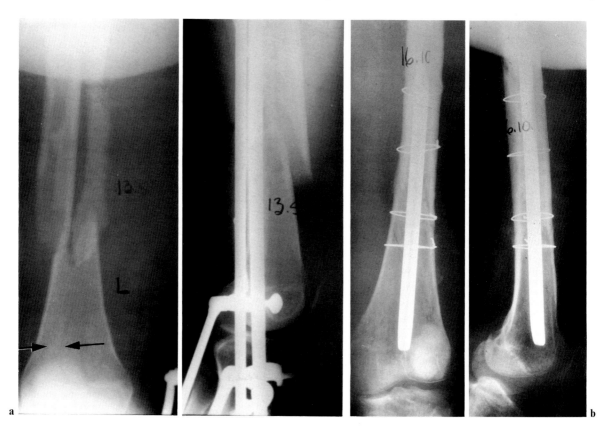

a   b

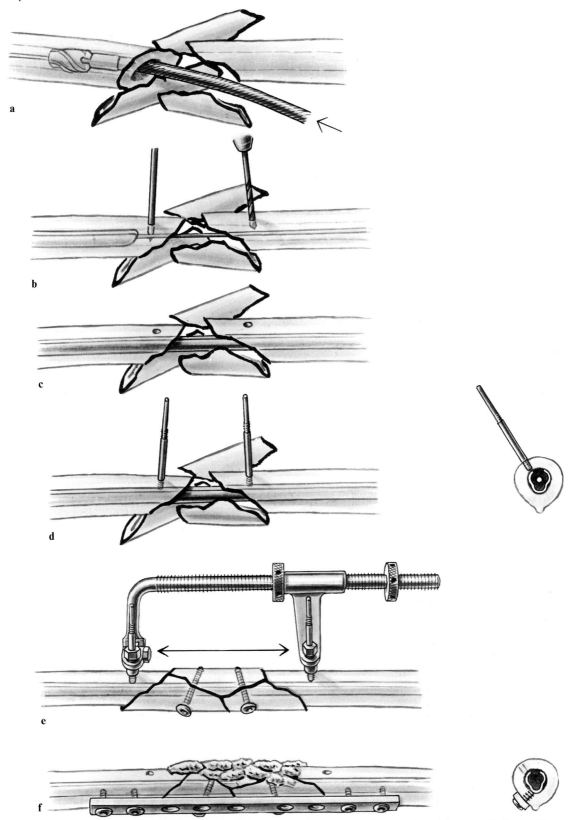

Fig. 13.10a–f. Schematic representation of **a**, reaming, **b–d**, nailing, **e**, reducing with the aid of a distractor, and **f** finally, with the aid of screws and a narrow plate, securing fixation of a severely comminuted fracture of a femur. (From Müller et al. 1979.) Note the bone graft. In this type of "locked" open intramedullary nailing a bone graft is a must

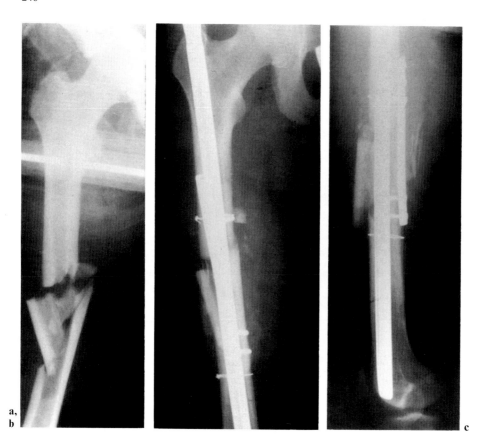

a,
b
c

Fig. 13.11. a A severely comminuted fracture of the middle third of the femoral shaft. Some of the fragments are too small for cerclage wiring. b The fixation has been achieved with a combination of an intramedullary nail, cerclage wiring, and a plate. The main function of the plate is to maintain length and rotational stability. c Note the extreme posterior position of the plate, just in front of the linea aspera. Note also the bone graft in (b)

an open reduction and internal fixation, then, once the femur is nailed with the main fragments out to length, shortening can be prevented by bridging the zone of comminution with a narrow plate. The medullary canal is anterior to a thick ridge of bone which represents the linea aspera. Thus, a plate can be screwed to the posterolateral aspect of the femur with the screws passing posterior to the nail. If a zone of comminution is bridged by a plate, then only the main fragments are reamed prior to the reduction, in order to keep the devitalization of the comminuted segment to a minimum (Figs. 13.10, 13.11). The fixation of oblique spiral fractures, the fixation of comminuted segments, and the bridging of defects implies open intramedullary nailing with exposure of the fracture. If closed intramedullary nailing is chosen, then re-

duction of the unstable fracture must be maintained either by traction or in a hip spica.

From the foregoing, it should be evident why conventional intramedullary nailing is suitable as a method of internal fixation only for fractures of the middle third of the femur and ideally only for transverse and short oblique fractures. Its use for other fracture patterns is an extension of the technique beyond the ideal indications and, if employed, often requires combination with cerclage, lag screws, or plates.

The recent development of the locking intramedullary nail (Kempf et al. 1985) has greatly increased the indications for closed intramedullary nailing of femoral fractures not only of the middle third, but also of the proximal and distal thirds (Fig. 13.12). The advantage and biological prerequisite of this technique is that the nailing must be done closed. This preserves any remaining soft tissue attachment and viability of the comminuted fragments, which, coupled with the bone grafting effect of the reaming debris, greatly accelerates the formation of callus and stability.

The locking feature of the nail is achieved by the insertion of bolts through the bone and nail which lock the two together. Thus, if a bolt is

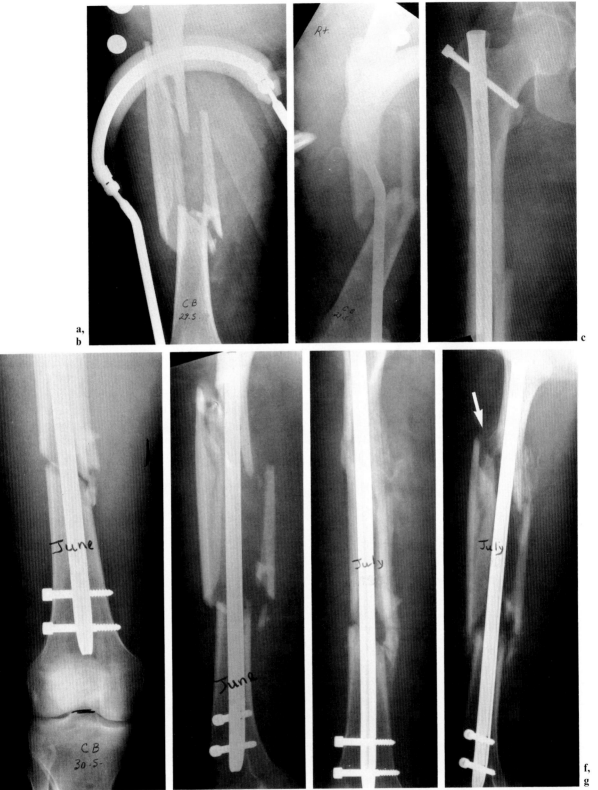

Fig. 13.12a–i. A comminuted fracture of the femoral shaft treated with a locking intramedullary nail. **a, b** Note the severe comminution and displacement of the diaphyseal fragments. Such displacement and comminution usually denote a high-velocity injury. **c, d** Anteroposterior and **e** lateral view of the proximal and distal fragments. Note the proximal and distal locking screws which traverse the bone and the nail. **f** Anteroposterior and **g** lateral views of the same femur 6 weeks after surgery. Note the rapid formation of callus, which is a biological advantage of closed intramedullary nailing. **h** Anteroposterior and **i** lateral views at 2 years after surgery. The proximal screw was removed at 3 months to dynamize the nail. Usually the distal screws are removed at the same time. Note at this time just prior to nail removal the advanced remodeling of the cortex and the full incorporation of severely displaced fragments

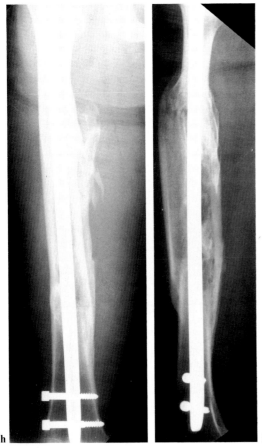

h   i

Fig. 13.12 h, i

inserted proximally and distally, a femur, even with extreme comminution of the diaphysis, can be kept out to length and rotationally stable. Similarly, fractures of the proximal and distal femur can be stabilized by the insertion of the corresponding bolts proximally or distally. While the bolts are in place, the nail acts as a distracting device; thus, instead of being a weight-sharing device, it becomes a weight-bearing device. Once callus begins to form and the fracture becomes progressively more stable, the bolts can be removed and weight bearing gradually begun.

c) Plate Fixation

The principles of stable internal fixation do not vary. However, the forces acting on the femur are much greater than those acting on any other bone; therefore, the biomechanical considerations must be observed much more closely.

The femur is an eccentrically loaded bone. Recent in vivo strain gauge work has demonstrated that in vivo the lateral cortex is loaded in tension and the medial in compression (Schatzker et al. 1980; Fig. 13.13). Therefore, the femur is suitable for tension band fixation with plates (compression plates). In this bone, the integrity of the medial buttress for stable tension band fixation is more important than in any other bone because of the enormous bending forces. In order to achieve sta-

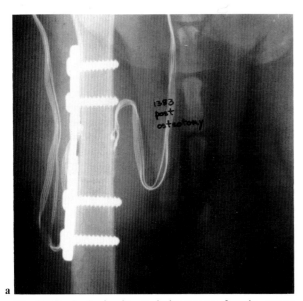

a

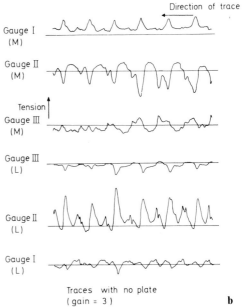

b

Fig. 13.13a, b. An in vivo study by means of strain gauges of the bone response to loading in the dog. **a** One rosette of strain gauges was placed on the medial cortex and one on the lateral cortex just under the milled-out portion of the plate. **b** A tracing of the deflections produced as the dog walked about; note gauge II (M (medial) and L (lateral)). The principal medial strain is compression and the principal lateral strain is tension

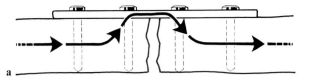

a

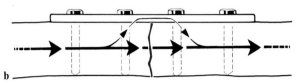

b

Fig. 13.14. a A fracture has been fixed with a plate, but the reduction is incomplete: a gap has been left between the fragments and there is no structural continuity. Under load, the whole force must be transmitted by the plate from one fragment to the other. **b** The fracture has been reduced anatomically. There is structural continuity and no gap between the fragments. Under load, the force is transmitted from bone fragment to bone fragment and only partially through the plate

ble fixation, the reduction must be anatomical to regain structural continuity (Fig. 13.14). Stability of fixation is secured as elsewhere by means of compression. All oblique and spiral fractures are stabilized first by means of lag screw fixation which assures interfragmental compression. The primary fixation with lag screws, as elsewhere, is then protected by means of plates which are fixed to the main fragments (Fig. 13.15). These plates are referred to as neutralization plates. When used to bridge zones of comminution where longitudinal continuity of the cortex is lost, these plates cannot be prestressed under tension to secure axial compression and in this way increase the stability of the fixation, as placing the plates under tension would result in shortening of the bone. If axial continuity of bone exists under the plate, then, even when primary lag screw fixation of the fragments has been obtained where possible, the neutralization plate should be placed under tension. In this way, it acts as a neutralization and as a tension band plate.

Short oblique and transverse fractures of the middle third of the femur are ideally stabilized by means of intramedullary nailing. Fractures of the proximal and distal third of the femur are not suitable for intramedullary nailing except by the specialized technique of locked nailing. Hence, if internal fixation is indicated, plate and screw fixation must be used. In addition to lag screw fixation and correct application of the plate, an attempt should be made, if at all possible, to insert at least

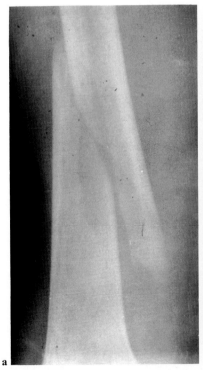

a

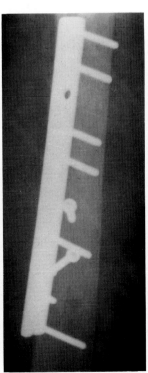

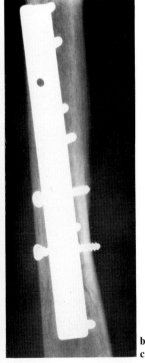

b, c

Fig. 13.15. a A spiral fracture of the femur. **b, c** Lag screws used to secure interfragmental compression between the fragments. Plate is used to neutralize the forces of bending, shear, and torque, and to protect the lag screw fixation

one lag screw through the plate and across the fracture. This greatly enhances the rotational and bending stability of the fixation.

The femur must be fixed with broad plates. The length chosen should be such that the cortex is traversed by screws in at least seven places on each side of the fracture. This rule applies to young individuals with strong cortical bone. In osteoporotic bone, the plate should be correspondingly longer to permit the use of a greater number of screws to compensate for the decreased holding power of screws in osteoporotic bone. Two plates should not be used for the fixation of a normal diaphysis. The stress protection of two plates is so great that a segment of bone so plated undergoes intense osteoporosis and is greatly weakened. At one time, it was thought that two-plate fixation would be the answer to all difficult problems of internal fixation of the femur. Experience has shown, however, that double-plating is associated with a much higher failure rate. It should be recognized that this applies to the diaphysis only. In metaphyseal areas where the cortex is thin and filled with a network of trabecular bone instead of a medullary canal, two plates may be used and, indeed, at times comprise the only possible means to stable internal fixation. Under exceptional circumstances where the cortex of a diaphysis is very much thickened, such as in a hypertrophic pseudarthrosis (Fig. 13.16), two plates may be employed as necessary. One should be shorter than the other to allow for a more gradual transition between the rigid double-plated segment and the remainder of the bone. The posterolateral side of

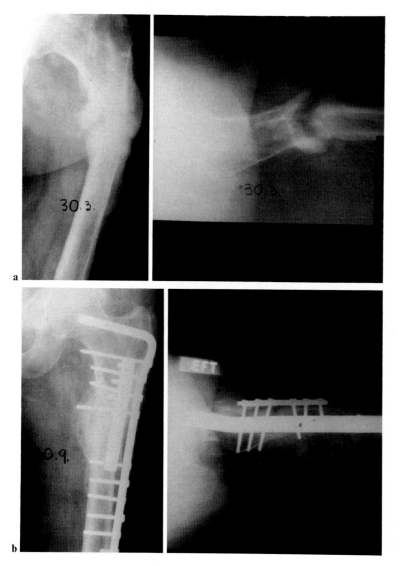

Fig. 13.16. a A hypertrophic pseudarthrosis of the femur. **b** Two plates have been used for fixation. The cortex is flared and hypertrophied and stress shielding will not result in any significant weakening of the bone

the femur just in front of the linea aspera is the ideal site for plate application. If two plates are used, they should be inserted at 90° to one another.

13.3.2.5 Bone Grafting

Whenever a femur is plated, no matter how perfect the internal fixation, it should be bone grafted to diminish the incidence of failure. In open intramedullary nailing, bone grafting should be carried out whenever a delayed union is foreseen, such as would occur with extensive stripping and devascularization of the fragments, in segmental fractures, and whenever there is comminution with loss of bone which would leave a portion of the nail exposed.

13.3.2.6 Wound Closure

In elective incisions for closed fractures, wound closure is rarely a problem. If tension should exist and threaten the survival of the wound edges, then the wound should be left open. Because the plate is under the cover of the vastus lateralis muscle, it is not exposed if the wound is left open. The muscle is usually rapidly covered by granulation tissue. If a secondary closure cannot be achieved within the 1st week, then the wound can either be left open to re-epithelialize slowly or be skin grafted.

13.3.3 Postoperative Care

Because the object of the open reduction and internal fixation is the rapid return to function of the soft tissue envelope and adjacent joint, the details of postoperative care are as important as those of the operative procedure. Compressive dressings should not be used in an effort to prevent wound hematomas: suction drainage is much more efficient. The drains should be withdrawn 24–36 h after surgery.

Following any surgery on the shaft of the femur, the knee should be immobilized for the first 4–5 days, in 90° of flexion. This will prevent postoperative knee stiffness and greatly reduce the time spent on postoperative rehabilitation. With flexion of the knee, the vastus lateralis muscle descends 3–4 cm. If the reflected vastus lateralis is allowed to fall back into place at the end of a procedure and the knee is then kept extended for 5 days or more, the muscle fibers reattach rapidly in the pre-shortened position. Any effort at flexion pulls on these muscle fibers and stretches the joint capsule.

Both give rise to pain which results in protective splinting. This sets up a vicious circle which takes many weeks or months to be reversed. If, however, the knee is kept flexed, the capsule is kept stretched, and the muscle fibers attach more distally. Once the splint is removed on the 4th or 5th day, the patient is usually able within 30–60 min to regain full extension. Extensor lag or a flexion deformity has never been seen; patients can usually maintain the 90° of flexion and continue to regain further flexion in the ensuing days. If one considers that, in patients treated in traction on a Thomas splint and Pearson knee piece, a 90° range of flexion achieved at the end of a rehabilitative period was considered an excellent result, then a method which at the start of the rehabilitative period guarantees 90° of flexion must be considered superior.

It is best to support the knee in 90° of flexion in a very well padded, light cast which leaves the foot free. To facilitate drainage, the extremity can be supported on a special splint or pillows, but the patient must be cautioned not to roll the leg into external rotation, lest this lead to compression of the peroneal nerve. We like to leave the foot free so that the patient can exercise the ankle and in this way activate the venous pump. We prefer the padded cast to a padded splint because the patient is not immobilized and can stand up with crutches or be sat up. This is very important if the chest is to be kept upright and respiratory insufficiency prevented. The time of mobilization cannot be governed by the calendar alone. If wound healing is not progressing satisfactorily, then knee mobilization may have to be postponed for a day or two. Since continuous passive motion machines have become available we have used them in preference to splinting because mobilization of the knee is more rapid, as is the dissipation of edema and decrease of pain.

13.4 Special Considerations: Open Fractures of the Femur

We cannot emphasize enough that the most important goal in the treatment of an open fracture is the prevention of infection. Stability of the bone fragments is, next to the débridement of the wound, the most important prophylactic maneuver in preventing infection. In addition to preventing infection, stability of the bone fragments allows early mobilization of the damaged soft tissue envelope which promotes the optimal recovery of soft tissue function.

The grade I open fracture of the femur rarely presents a serious problem in management (for classification of open fractures, see pp. 21). If the fracture is received early for treatment and its contamination is relatively minor, then the open wound is débrided and is left open. The fracture is then treated as if it were a closed injury. Initially, we felt that one should not carry out intramedullary nailing of open fractures because of the increased risk of sepsis. Thus, isolated fractures of the femur with minimal soft tissue damage, if considered best suited for intramedullary nailing, were first thoroughly débrided and then kept in skeletal traction for 7–10 days; they were nailed only if one could be certain that infection had been prevented. The other fracture patterns were either stabilized immediately by means of plates and screws or, if too comminuted and definitely beyond the scope of internal fixation, initially stabilized in an external fixator. Recent experience of Winquist et al. (1984) with immediate intramedullary nailing of grade II and at times, even of grade III open fractures in patients with multiple injuries would indicate that fears of an increased occurrence of sepsis with immediate intramedullary nailing of the femur were exaggerated. We feel, however, that caution must be exercised because an infected intramedullary nailing is the most difficult type of infection to eradicate. Thus, we would execute an immediate intramedullary nailing only under the most ideal conditions, and prefer to rely on internal fixation by means of plates and screws for the remainder.

While delay of definitive bone stabilization may be argued for the isolated grade I open fracture because the care of the wound is never a problem since the tissue necrosis is minimal and the likelihood of sepsis small, such an argument cannot be advanced for the treatment of a patient with multiple injuries or one with grade II or grade III injuries. The care of these wounds, if they involve any part of the thigh except its anterior surface, becomes agony for the patient. If the limb is in traction or a splint, the wounds are inaccessible. Attempts at dressing changes result in movement of the fragments which is extremely painful. Thus, wound care is significantly interfered with. The more severe the wound, the more severe is the associated tissue necrosis, which is a very significant contributing factor in the development of sepsis. If we add to this the effect of movement of the bone fragments, which results in an increase in local tissue damage and in repeated breakdown of tissue barriers to infection, then we see that in many cases an infection must be the inevitable outcome. Thus, the principle of treatment of such an open wound is to achieve initial stability of the bone which will prevent further tissue damage, promote humoral and cellular defense mechanisms, and greatly facilitate wound care.

We feel that the safest approach to the severe grade III open fracture is to provide skeletal stability by means of one of the modern external fixators. If the fracture pattern is such that one can achieve stability by means of lag screw fixation, this may be carried out, as long as fixation does not significantly increase the exposure or the devitalization of the fragments. The primary fixation is then provided by the lag screws and the external fixator takes the place of a neutralization plate.

Difficulties invariably arise when surgeons seek to complete the care of an open fracture in one operation. We consider the surgical care of an open fracture as a series of surgical procedures timed and executed as directed by preceding events and by the progress of the fracture and the wound. Thus, after the débridement and stabilization of the bone, the wound is left open. Within the 1st 48–72 h the patient returns to the operating room, the dressing is removed, and the wound is inspected. If further débridement is necessary, this is carried out. Once the wound is clean and beginning to granulate, a cancellous bone graft is added and a secondary closure is executed as far as possible. The remaining open wound is left to granulate in or a split-thickness skin graft is applied. Once closure is achieved and infection prevented, the next most important decision is made, usually 4–6 weeks after fracture. This is the decision whether the external fixator will be used as the definitive method of skeletal stabilization or whether the fixation will be revised to one involving plates and screws. (We must emphasize that this applies only when sepsis has been prevented.) Occasionally, one might even consider intramedullary nailing, but one must not forget that in a previously open fracture or one where external skeletal fixation was used, this carries an increased risk of sepsis. If nailing is decided upon, the external fixator is removed and the leg is placed in traction. If all pin tracts heal rapidly without any sign of sepsis, a closed nailing is carried out 7–10 days later.

If the external fixator has been used in combination with internal fixation and functions as a neutralization plate, it is frequently safe to continue unless complications arise such as pin tract sepsis or stiffness of the knee because of the irritation around the pins and inhibition of quadriceps muscle function. In our experience, an external fixator alone, if not bone grafted, frequently fails to induce union. If the fracture is bone grafted, and no complications arise, the external fixation can be continued until union occurs. Usually, if union has not occurred by the end of the 3rd month and evidence exists that a delayed union or nonunion is developing, it is best to intervene and convert the fixation to one with a plate and screws. If a large gap still exists which has to be bridged, it may be of advantage to use the modified broad AO plates which Wagner has developed for use in leg lengthening. Because these plates have no holes in their mid zone, they are stronger and fail less readily when subjected to bending.

If complications arise early in the course of treatment with an external fixator, then, as soon as one can be certain that infection has been prevented, one should convert the external fixation to internal fixation as outlined already. If the knee has stiffened, it may be manipulated at the time of the conversion to internal fixation in order to regain a useful range of flexion.

References

Charnley J, Guindy A (1961) Delayed operation in the open reduction of the fractures of long bones. J Bone Joint Surg 43B:664–671

Hierholzer G, Allgöwer M, Rüedi T (1985) Fixateur-externe-Osteosynthese. Springer, Berlin Heidelberg New York Tokyo

Kempf I, Grosse A, Beck G (1985) Closed locked intramedullary nailing. J Bone Joint Surg 67A:709–720

Küntscher G (1967) Practice of intramedullary nailing. Thomas, Springfield, p 34

Lam SJ (1964) The place of delayed internal fixation in the treatment of fractures of the long bones. J Bone Joint Surg 46B:393–397

Matter P, Rittman WW (1978) The open fracture. Huber, Bern

Müller ME, Allgöwer M, Willenegger H (1965) Technique of internal fixation of fractures. Springer, Berlin Heidelberg New York

Müller ME, Allgöwer M, Schneider R, Willenegger H (1979) Manual of internal fixation, 2nd edn. Springer, Berlin Heidelberg New York

Riska EB, Myllenen P (1982) Fat embolism in patients with multiple injuries. J Trauma 22:891–894

Riska EB, von Bonsdorff H, Hakkinen S, Jaroma H, Kiviluoto O, Paavilainen T (1976) Prevention of fat embolism by early internal fixation of fractures in patients with multiple injuries. Injury 8:110–116

Sarmiento A (1972) Functional bracing of tibial and femoral shaft fractures. Clin Orthop 82:2–13

Sarmiento A, Latta LL (1981) Closed functional treatment of fractures. Springer, Berlin Heidelberg New York

Schatzker J (to be published) The Toronto experience with fractures of the femur

Schatzker J, Manley PA, Sumner-Smith G (1980) In vivo strain-gauge study of bone response to loading with and without internal fixation. In: Uhthoff HK (ed) Current concepts of internal fixation of fractures. Springer, Berlin Heidelberg New York, pp 306–314

Sibel R, Laduca J, Hassett J, Babikian G, Mills B, Border D, Border J (1985) Blunt multiple trauma (ISS36) femur traction and the pulmonary failure-septic state. Ann Surg 202:283–295

Smith JEM (1964) The results of early and delayed internal fixation of fractures of the shaft of the femur. J Bone Joint Surg 46B:28–31

Winquist RA, Hansen ST, Clawson DK (1984) Closed intramedullary nailing of femoral fractures. J Bone Joint Surg 66A:529–539

14 Supracondylar Fractures of the Femur

J. SCHATZKER

14.1 Introduction

A supracondylar fracture of the femur (Fig. 14.1) is a grave injury which for years represented an unsolved problem in trauma, and was considered to result almost always in varying degrees of permanent disability. It was felt that the fate of the joint was determined by the injury rather than by its treatment. Treatment was almost always closed and consisted principally of splinting and traction. The traction was applied either through a two-pin system, one through the supracondylar fragment and one through the tibial tuberosity, or through a single pin through the tibial tuberosity. The reduction was accomplished by traction or, if necessary, under general anesthesia. The extremity was then immobilized on a splint. Padding, flexion of the knee, and skeletal traction were used to maintain reduction. The difficulties with these methods were, first and foremost, an inability to control displaced intra-articular fragments which did not reduce with manipulation or traction, and secondly, that occasionally the supracondylar fragments displaced posteriorly. Further major drawbacks consisted of knee stiffness and the necessity for prolonged hospitalization and bed rest in the supine position which often exceeded 6–8 weeks.

Open reduction and internal fixation was attempted from time to time, but the results were largely unsatisfactory, because the techniques of internal fixation and the devices available did not allow stable fixation which would allow early motion without deformity and nonunion. Stewart et al. and Neer et al. gave good summaries of the state of the art as it was in the mid 1960s. In 1966, Marcus Stewart et al. published a review of 442 patients who were treated over a period of 20 years. The purpose of his review was a comparison of methods of treatment. Some 213 patients were closely analyzed and followed. Of the 114 patients treated by closed methods, 67% had an excellent or good result, whereas of the 69 patients treated by open reduction with internal metallic fixation or some type of bone graft, only 54% had an excellent or good result. Patients treated with skeletal traction stayed an average of 62 days in hospital, whereas patients who had surgery had an average stay of 33 days. The ten nonunions and ten delayed unions were all in the operated group. The authors concluded that "the additional trauma of surgery and the proximity of metallic implants to the joint predispose to excessive reaction and subsequent adhesions. Even though one obtains an excellent roentgenographic result with solid union, final function may be quite poor. No doubt, a few surgeons have mastered the technique of operative correction and internal fixation..., but they are in the minority.... Conservatism should be taught and practiced more universally."

In 1967, Charles Neer et al. reviewed a series of 110 unselected supracondylar fractures in order to analyze the results of internal fixations compared with those of closed methods of treatment. Only 52% of those treated by open means obtained a satisfactory result, whereas closed treatment yielded satisfactory results in 90% of patients. It must be noted, however, that in this review, patients were satisfied if they could flex the knee 70°! Thus, a patient whose knee flexed only 80° lost only 40% in the numerical rating used to assess function. This considerably boosted the seeming excellence of nonoperative treatment.

It must be noted that the patients who were included in the reviews of Stewart and Neer et al. were treated at a time when the techniques of internal fixation and the implants used were very limited. If accurate reduction was achieved, it was very difficult to maintain. Stability achieved was never sufficient to render the extremity painless. Thus, active motion was inhibited by pain and complicated further by frequent loss of position of the fragments, which led to malunion or nonunion with further loss of function.

In conclusion, Neer et al. felt that "no category of fracture at this level seemed well suited for inter-

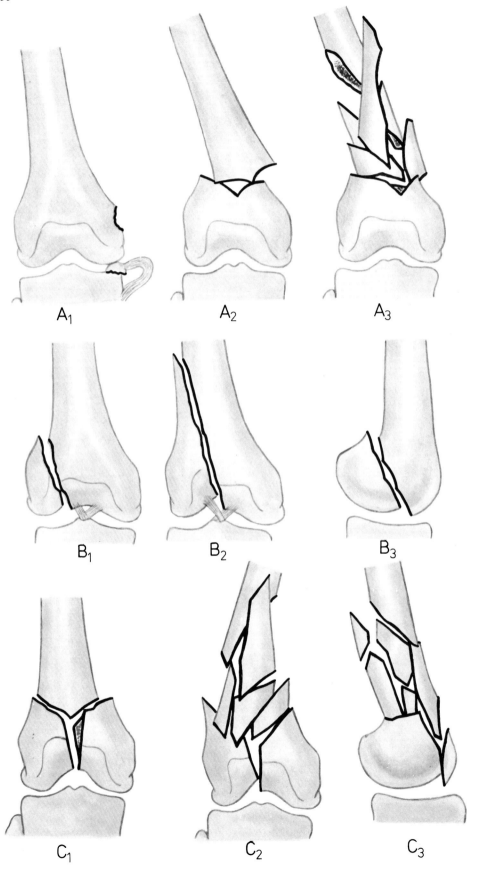

A_1 A_2 A_3

B_1 B_2 B_3

C_1 C_2 C_3

nal fixation, and sufficient fixation to eliminate the need for external support or to shorten convalescence was rarely attained." They felt that surgery should be limited only to the instances of an open fracture or to the internal fixation of a fracture associated with an arterial injury or some other unusual problem.

In 1970, the AO group published its first review of 112 patients with supracondylar fractures who were treated according to the principles of accurate anatomical reduction, stable internal fixation, and early motion (Wenzl et al. 1970). Of these patients, 73.5% achieved a good to excellent result. This result was certainly better than any previously published results of open treatment. Surgeons steeped in the older methods advanced arguments against this new surgical method. They felt that these AO results were obtained by master surgeons who were the innovators of their technique and that the results in the hands of other surgeons would be no better than those previously published.

In 1974, Schatzker et al. published a review of the Toronto experience with supracondylar fractures from 1966 to 1972. Patients whose fractures were treated in accordance with the AO principles obtained 75% good to excellent results which contrasted sharply with the 32% of good to excellent results of patients who were treated nonoperatively. The study clearly demonstrated the superiority of the AO method not only as a surgical technique, but as a method of treatment, because the Toronto surgeons were not members of the Swiss AO group and were considered very skilled in the nonoperative methods of treatment of the supracondylar fracture.

In 1979, Schatzker and Lambert published the results of the surgical treatment of a further 35 patients. Of the 17 patients who were treated in accordance with the AO principles, 71% achieved good to excellent results. In 18 patients, the surgeons employed the AO implants, but failed to achieve anatomical reduction and stable internal fixation. The results in this group of patients were very poor, with only 21% having good to excellent results. When this second group of patients was further analyzed, it became evident that elderly patients with severe osteoporosis were in the ma-

jority. The failure on the part of the surgeon to treat these patients in accordance with AO principles was not always due to neglect of the principles. The comminution frequently associated with osteoporosis and the poor holding power of osteoporotic bone presented a challenge which could not be met with any consistency. The study also clearly outlined the dictum that stable internal fixation is not achieved automatically by carrying out an open reduction and by the insertion of the AO implants. In those patients in whom the goals of surgery were realized (that is, in whom an accurate anatomical reduction was achieved, the internal fixation was absolutely stable, and early unencumbered mobilization could be carried out), the results continued to be excellent. This study further illustrated that, despite the excellence of the treatment, the results were tempered by the severity of the trauma, the type of fracture, and by osteoporosis. An analysis of the age incidence as related to the type of trauma revealed two groupings of patients. The younger patients in their 20s and 30s had sustained high-velocity trauma, which often results in a more severe fracture with greater intra-articular disruption or segmental comminution. Severe comminution, particularly of the joint, had an adverse effect on the final result. Other factors which tended to temper the excellence of the final outcome were the presence of other fractures, such as fractures of the ipsilateral tibial plateau or tibia or of the contralateral femur, and the presence of major ligamentous disruptions.

The older patients often sustained their fractures in a low-velocity injury, such as might result from a simple fall. Because of severe osteoporosis, despite the low-velocity nature of their injury, the comminution of the fracture was occasionally quite marked. The advent of cast bracing has improved the results of nonoperative treatment because patients can be mobilized earlier. Cast bracing, however, has had no beneficial effect on residual joint disorganization or on fractures which could not be controlled in traction.

14.2 Guides to Treatment and Indications for Surgery

In evaluating the criteria for surgery in the supracondylar fracture, the surgeon must carefully weigh the results achieved by nonoperative and operative treatment and the factors which adversely affect the results in each group. The experience

Fig. 14.1. Supracondylar fractures of the femur. Type A: extra-articular fractures; type B: fractures which involve one condyle; type C: intra-articular and supracondylar fractures. Note: the complexity of the fractures increases from *left* to *right*. (From Müller et al. 1979)

in Toronto between 1966 and 1972 with nonoperative treatment, where only 32% of patients
achieved a good to excellent result, serves to emphasize that if the same strict criteria are applied
in evaluating the final result, it becomes evident
that conservatism as advocated by Stewart et al.
(1966) and Neer et al. (1967) is not a panacea for
the supracondylar fracture and can be undertaken
only with great reservations. If surgery is to be
undertaken, however, the surgeon must be certain
that the objectives of treatment, namely accurate
anatomical reduction, stable fixation, and early
motion will be achieved, for failure to achieve
these might lead to results worse than those
achieved by closed means. Therefore, the surgeon
must carefully assess the personality of the fracture, which includes the patient's age, level of ac-
tivity, and functional demands, the severity of the
trauma, whether it was caused by high- or low-
velocity impact, the individual fracture pattern,
and the type and severity of associated injuries.
The surgeon must also evaluate honestly his or
her own skill and environment. The evidence from
clinical studies as well as from the experimental
investigations of Mitchell and Shepard (1980), on
the effects of anatomical reduction and stable fixation on cartilage regeneration, and of Salter and
Harris (1979), on the effects of rest and continuous
passive motion on cartilage regeneration, indicates
irrefutably that the goals in the treatment of all
intra-articular fractures should be:

1. Accurate anatomical reduction of the joint surface
2. Accurate anatomical reduction of the metaphyseal component of the fracture with restoration of normal axial alignment
3. Stable internal fixation
4. Early motion

In the majority of fractures, these goals are attainable only by surgical means. Indications for
surgical treatment are either absolute or relative.
The absolute indications relate to fractures which
have to be treated surgically because nonsurgical
methods are certain to lead to poor results.

14.2.1 Absolute Indications

14.2.1.1 Intra-articular Fractures in which Adequate Joint Congruity Cannot be Restored by Manipulation

Under this heading, we would like to single out
particular fractures as given below.

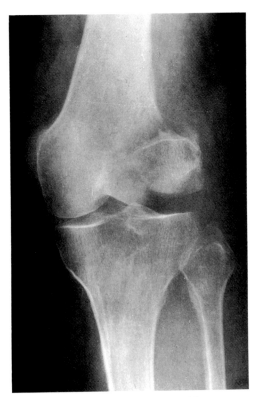

Fig. 14.2. Unicondylar fracture of the femur

a) Unicondylar Fracture

In our experience, this fracture, if treated in a cast
brace, traction, or plaster, frequently displaces
with joint incongruity and axial nonalignment
(Fig. 14.2).

b) Bicondylar Fracture in the Coronal Plane

This intra-articular fracture (the Hoffa fracture)
cannot be reduced by closed means because the
only soft tissue attachment (if any) is the synovial
reflection and posterior capsule of the joint. Thus,
traction has little effect on the position of the fragment (Fig. 14.3).

c) The T or Y Bicondylar Fracture with Rotational Displacement of the Condyles

The classic displacement of the supracondylar
fragments is posterior angulation (rotation about
the knee joint axis) due to the pull of the gastrocnemius muscle and anterior displacement of the
shaft due to shortening (Fig. 14.4). If the displacement cannot be corrected by flexion of the knee
and traction, then only an open operation can effect a reduction. This is particularly true if treatment is delayed for 1 week or longer.

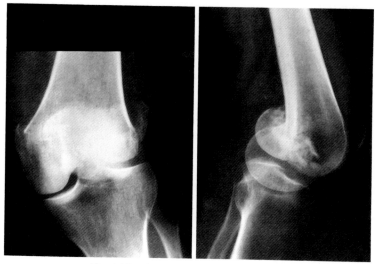

Fig. 14.3. Bicondylar fracture of the femur in the coronal plane (Hoffa fracture)

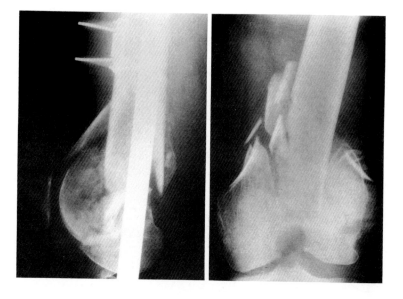

A more important displacement is the rotation of one condyle with respect to the other. Manipulation and traction cannot effect a reduction and, if left, this displacement results in permanent joint incongruity.

14.2.1.2 Open Intra-articular Fractures

In any open fracture, the main cause of permanent disability is sepsis, because it leads to scarring of the soft tissue envelope and to joint stiffness. In the treatment of an open fracture, therefore, all efforts must be directed to the prevention of sepsis.

Fig. 14.4. Supracondylar and intracondylar fracture C_2. Note the rotation of the condylar fragments. Their fracture surface faces posteriorly

Mounting clinical evidence, as well as experimental work (Rittman and Perren 1974), indicates that after thorough surgical débridement, the next most important factor in the prevention of sepsis is absolute stability of the bony fragments. Therefore, after débridement, one should carry out an internal fixation of the fracture in order to achieve stability to prevent infection. Recent evidence disputes the conclusion of Stewart et al. that the proximity of metal to joints increases the likelihood of sepsis and of stiffness (Olerud 1972).

14.2.1.3 Associated Neurovascular Injuries

Stability of the skeleton is most useful in the protection of any neurovascular repair.

14.2.1.4 Ipsilateral Fracture of the Tibial Plateau

The presence of two separate fractures on opposite sides of the joint makes an open operation mandatory in order to reduce displaced fragments.

14.2.1.5 Ipsilateral Fracture of the Tibia

In the presence of these two fractures, control of the knee by closed means is impossible and, in order to preserve function, an open reduction and internal fixation is necessary.

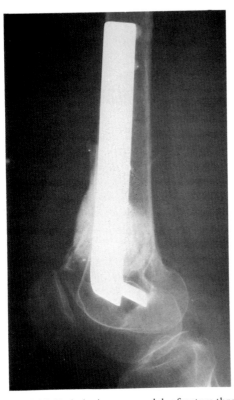

Fig. 14.5. Pathologic supracondylar fracture through a large metastatic deposit from a breast carcinoma. Methyl methacrylate was used to fill the eroded portion of the bone. Note that at 18 months the posterior cortex has united

14.2.1.6 Multiple Injuries

In a patient with multiple injuries, the stabilization of the fracture may be desirable for reasons other than the fracture itself.

14.2.1.7 Pathologic Fractures

These fractures cannot be treated successfully by immobilization in plaster, because of the bone destruction caused by the presence of tumor. An open reduction with the evacuation of the tumor and a composite type of internal fixation which employs methyl methacrylate and metal is necessary (Fig. 14.5).

14.2.2 Relative Indications

As we have already indicated, we believe that a major intra-articular or periarticular fracture is best treated by open reduction and stable internal fixation because it is the most certain way of preserving the best possible function of the joint. We must caution, however, that these are technically very difficult fractures and that the first one tried should not be a badly comminuted intra-articular fracture, as these are far too demanding.

14.3 Surgical Treatment

14.3.1 Timing of Surgery

A major intra-articular or periarticular fracture is a difficult surgical undertaking which should not be executed in the middle of the night without a very careful evaluation of the fracture and without the necessary help. Clearly, the condition of the patient with multiple injuries may dictate that surgery be carried out at a less than optimal time. It may even have to be carried out as an emergency if the fracture is open or if there is an associated vascular injury. If circumstances permit, however, a short delay, during which proper preparations are done, is time well spent and will often be an important factor in effecting a favorable outcome of surgery. The delay should not be protracted. We have reconstructed supracondylar fractures at 3–4 weeks from the time of the injury, but the longer the delay, the more difficult the reconstruction. The limb shortens, the fragments become embedded and covered by soft tissue and new granulations. An even greater difficulty is the healing of the compacted cancellous bone, which obliterates the fracture lines and makes their definition as well as the reduction very difficult.

The limb should be splinted while the patient awaits surgery. If surgery is to be delayed for more than a few hours, then we prefer to splint the extremity on the Thomas splint in skin traction to maintain some length and immobilization. If surgery has to be delayed for a few days, then we feel the extremity should be splinted on a Thomas splint with a Pearson knee piece with the knee in 20°–30° of flexion. Instead of skin traction, we use skeletal traction through the tibial tubercle which should be sufficiently strong to pull the limb out to length and even overdistract the fracture. This greatly eases the subsequent open reduction. Care must be taken to insert the Steinmann pin a hand breadth or so below the projected lowermost point of the skin incision so as to avoid the risk of contamination and sepsis from the pin tract.

14.3.2 History and Physical Examination

A careful history is of importance in determining whether the injury is high- or low-velocity. Physical examination is the most readily available and the simplest method to determine whether there is an associated nerve or vascular injury. A radiological examination, however, is necessary to obtain a detailed view of the fracture.

14.3.3 Radiological Examination

We begin this examination by obtaining an anteroposterior, a lateral, and two oblique roentgenograms of the injured side as well as an anteroposterior and lateral view of the uninjured side which serve as a template for the surgical reconstruction of the fracture. If necessary, anteroposterior and lateral tomograms of the fracture are obtained. These are invaluable in evaluating the intra-articular components and in evaluating the extent of the supracondylar comminution. In complex fractures we also use CT scanning. This portrays the distal femur in cross section, which is particularly helpful in identifying fracture lines in the frontal plane.

14.3.4 Classification

We rely on the AO classification of supracondylar fractures because this classification defines the fracture, indicates its prognosis, and helps one decide which is the best type of internal fixation to use. Thus, the fractures are divided into type A, which are extra-articular, type B, which are intra-articular but do not have a supracondylar component, and type C, which have both an intra-articular and a supracondylar component (see Fig. 14.1). These major types are further subdivided into subtypes in ascending order of complexity. Thus, the C_3 supracondylar fracture is one with extensive intra-articular and extra-articular comminution and, as such, is the most difficult to stabilize and has the worst prognosis.

14.3.5 Planning the Surgical Procedure

Once a detailed radiographic assessment is available, it is possible to make an accurate diagnosis of the fracture and plan its treatment. The surgical treatment begins with a careful preoperative plan of the procedure. Tracing paper is used together with the radiograph of the patient's normal extremity. The anteroposterior radiograph is turned over to give the outline of the opposite side (Fig. 14.6).

An outline of the distal femur is now drawn on the tracing paper. The radiographs and tomograms of the fracture are now used to draw in carefully all the fracture lines as well as any bony defect present. A similar drawing is made of the lateral projection. One is now ready to plan the internal fixation. In the properly executed plan of the surgical procedure, one must draw in and number every step.

Thus, drawings a_1 and a_2 show the outline of the bone in the anteroposterior and lateral projection with all the fracture lines drawn in. Drawings b_1 and b_2 are copies of a_1 and a_2, respectively, on which the position of the window for the condylar plate has been marked in as step I. Step II shows the position of the lag screws used to secure fixation of the condyles. Step III shows the position of any gliding holes or thread holes which should be drilled prior to the reduction of the fracture.

Drawings c_1 and c_2 are copies of b_1 and b_2, respectively. They are the definitive drawings on which one marks in the internal fixation. The plate is drawn in with the aid of a transparent template (obtainable from Synthes on request: Synthes USA, Wayne, Pennsylvania, or Synthes AG, Chur, Switzerland). This helps one to judge the length of the blade required as well as the length of the plate and the number of screws. If lag screws are to be used, they are now drawn in and numbered in the order in which they will be inserted. To

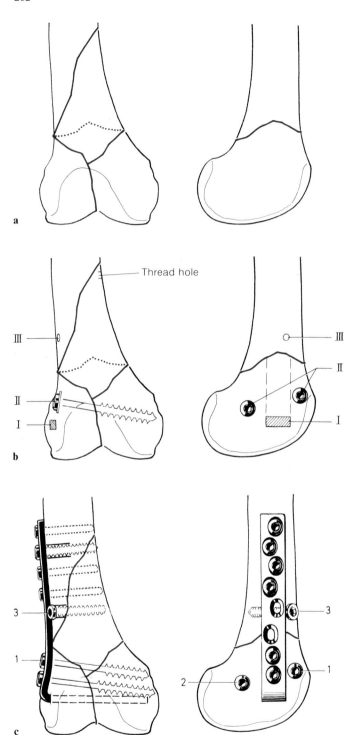

Fig. 14.6. a₁, a₂ Anteroposterior and lateral outlines of the distal femur drawn with the aid of an anteroposterior and lateral radiograph of the opposite femur. Note the fracture lines have been drawn in. **b₁, b₂** Copies of **a₁** and **a₂**, respectively. Step I: the position of the window for seating chisel is marked; step II: lag screws used to secure fixation of the condyles; step III: note the position of any gliding holes or thread holes which should be predrilled prior to reduction of fragments. **c₁, c₂** Copies of **b₁** and **b₂** on which the plate has been drawn in with the aid of a template and the screws numbered in order of insertion

complete the drawing, the remainder of the screws are sketched in and also numbered in the order in which they will be inserted.

Such careful preoperative planning helps the surgeon with every step of the operative procedure. We are critical of the surgeon who thinks that the fixation can be planned properly only after the fracture has been exposed. Often, one sees much less at surgery than on the preoperative radiographs. If the type and size of the implant has not already been determined, it may not be available when required. Furthermore, at the time of surgery, one is rushed to keep the wound open for as short a time as possible in order to keep down the infection rate. Thus, one cannot afford the time required to plan the surgical procedure in detail.

14.3.6 Surgical Anatomy of the Distal Femur

The anatomical axis of the knee joint does not coincide with the weight-bearing axis. The latter crosses the center of the femoral head and the center of the knee. The anatomical axis is in valgus and subtends an angle of 81° with the knee joint axis (Fig. 14.7).

If one views the femur from one side (Fig. 14.8) and projects the posterior cortex distally on a line, one will note that the posterior positions of the condyles appear as if they were tacked on to the posterior cortex of the shaft with the anterior position of the condyles appearing as a continuation of the shaft. The application of this anatomical fact is illustrated in Fig. 14.8: the blade of the condylar plate must be inserted into the anterior part of the condyles which is the distal projection of the shaft, or the plate will not fit the femur.

The distal femur, when viewed in cross section, is seen to be a trapezoid (Fig. 14.9). The anterior articular surface is not parallel to a line joining the posterior cortices of the condyles. Furthermore, the distance anteriorly between the medial and lateral wall is less than the distance posteriorly because the medial and lateral walls are inclined toward one another. The medial wall has the greater slope of the two and is inclined at 25° to the vertical. These facts are important to remember when one is selecting the length of the blade of the condylar plate. The projected width of the femur on a radiograph is the maximum width and represents the most posterior distance between the medial and lateral wall and not the distance in the anterior half where the blade must come to lie. Therefore, a blade which would corre-

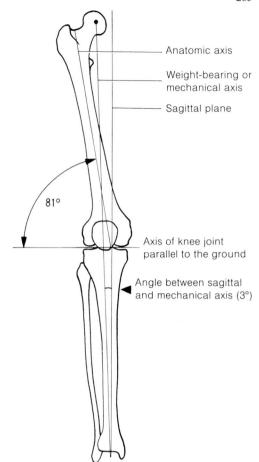

Fig. 14.7. The mechanical axis is a line projected through the center of the femoral head, knee joint, and ankle joint. It subtends an angle of 3° with the sagittal plane and an angle of 6° with the anatomical axis of the femur. The knee joint is parallel to the ground. The anatomical axis subtends an angle of 81° (79°–82°) with the knee joint axis

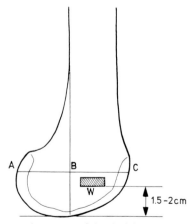

Fig. 14.8. When the posterior cortex of the shaft is projected distally as a line, it divides the epiphysis into an anterior and posterior half. The condyles appear as if they were tacked on posteriorly to the shaft. Note that the longest diameter *AC* is at 90° to the axis of the shaft. The window *W* for the condylar plate is in the middle of the anterior half *BC* and 1.5–2 cm from the distal end of the femur

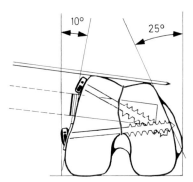

Fig. 14.9. The distal femur in cross section is a trapezoid. Note that the anterior and posterior surfaces are not parallel and that both the medial and lateral walls are inclined. This results in the anterior diameter being smaller than the posterior diameter. (Adapted from Müller et al. 1979)

spond in length to the posterior cortex would be too long and would jut out through the bone intra-articularly just deep to the anterior fibers of the medial collateral ligament.

14.3.7 Positioning and Draping the Patient

We prefer to carry out the surgery with the patient supine on an ordinary operating table. The leg should not be put in traction on a fracture table, as traction only tightens the soft tissue envelope and makes the visualization and manipulation of fragments almost impossible: thus, instead of making the reduction easier, it makes it more difficult. We like to cleanse the skin to the umbilicus above and to the ankle below. This permits us to drape the limb in such a fashion that the anterior iliac crest is left exposed should it be necessary to obtain a bone graft during the procedure. We expose at least half of the leg and drape the leg free. In this way, if we wish, we can extend the incision. The leg has to be free so that the knee can be flexed over one or two rolled-up, sterile sheets. This greatly facilitates the exposure and the reduction. We do not use a tourniquet, even if a sterile one is available, because bleeding can be readily controlled if the perforating vessels, when encountered, are clamped and ligated and all other vessels cauterized.

14.3.8 Surgical Exposure

The skin is incised along an imaginary line joining the greater trochanter with the midpoint of the lateral condyle. The incision is then curved for-

ward, aiming for a point just distal to the tibial tuberosity. The length of the skin incision will depend on the type of fracture. With a type A fracture the incision often stops at the joint line, whereas in type C fractures it is often curved to a point distal to the tibial tuberosity. The fascia lata is incised in line with the skin just anterior to the iliotibial tract (Fig. 14.10 a). Distally, the incision is extended through the lateral quadriceps retinaculum capsule and synovium. Even in type A fractures it is necessary to expose the joint so that the guide wires for the insertion of the blade plate can be positioned. Proximally, the femur is exposed by reflecting the vastus lateralis muscle from the lateral intermuscular septum. The perforating vessels are usually encountered close to the femur, but not directly over the bone. They should be cross-clamped, divided, and ligated (Fig. 14.10 b). When one is dealing with type A_3 fractures, and even more with type C_3 fractures, which have severe and complex intra-articular and supracondylar comminution, it becomes necessary to increase the intra-articular exposure so that the distal femur can be viewed from directly in front (Müller et al. 1979). To achieve this we extend the skin incision distally and medially, expose the tibial tubercle, and osteotomize it in such a way that the infrapatellar tendon can be lifted with a piece of bone approximately 1.5 cm × 3 cm × 0.5 cm. Once the fat pad is detached from the tibia and the synovium divided in the supracondylar region, the whole quadriceps muscle can be folded over upwards and medially, which exposes not only the whole joint but also the medial side of the shaft (Mize et al. 1982). One can then work unobstructedly on the whole joint surface, and also, if necessary, fix a second plate to the medial side of the femur without having to make a second incision.

14.3.9 Techniques of Reduction and Internal Fixation

The techniques of reduction and subsequent stable internal fixation of supracondylar fractures of the femur pose many problems. At times, the reduction and subsequent internal fixation may be so difficult that it will tax the surgical judgment and technical expertise of the most skilled surgeon to the limit. We feel, therefore, that it would be most worthwhile to discuss each fracture type in considerable detail.

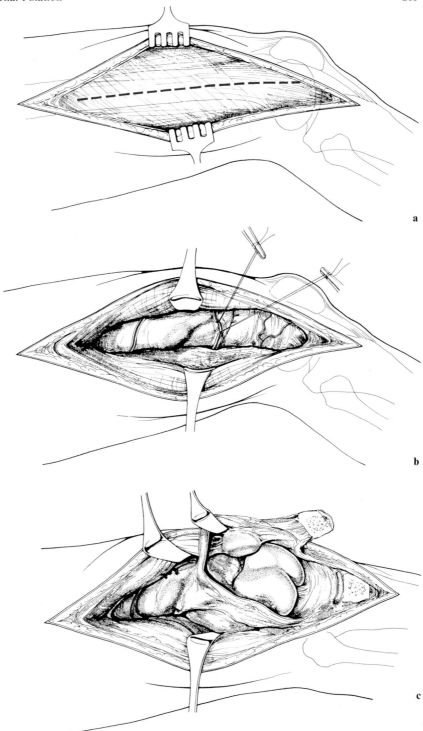

Fig. 14.10. a The skin incision is along an imaginary line joining the greater trochanter with the lateral condyle. The incision is aimed distally for a point just past the tibial tubercle. The fascia lata is incised in line with the skin incision. **b** The vastus lateralis muscle is reflected from the intermuscular septum. The perforating vessels should be clamped, divided, and ligated. **c** An extensile exposure of the distal femur. The insertion of the infrapatellar tendon is osteotomized and the quadriceps muscle insertion is reflected upward. The release of the vastus lateralis muscle from the septum allows full exposure of the distal femur and of the medial side of the shaft which is sufficient to permit the fixation of a plate to the medial side. A medial counterincision is unnecessary

14.3.9.1 Type A Fractures

a) Type A_1

This fracture represents the avulsion of the medial collateral ligament from its proximal insertion, together with a piece of the surrounding bone. The exposure for the disruption of the medial collateral ligament is usually through a medial parapatellar incision. The type of internal fixation employed will depend on the size of the piece of bone avulsed. If the fragment is large enough, it should be put back and screwed in place with a lag screw. One can also make use of a special washer with small protrusions which bite into the surrounding soft tissue as the lag screw is tightened. This helps considerably in the fixation of the ligament. If the surrounding bone is small, as is frequently the case, the fixation of the ligament can still be carried out with the lag screw and a special washer, or with a stable or sutures. In each instance, the internal fixation has to be protected until healing of the soft tissues has been achieved.

b) Types A_2 and A_3

A_2 and A_3 are supracondylar fractures without an intra-articular extension. The difference between these two is the degree of comminution (see Fig. 14.1). The surgical exposure is (as already described for a supracondylar fracture) through a lateral incision with an opening into the joint to permit the visualization of the articular surface and the insertion of two guide wires (Fig. 14.11a, b). The first guide wire to be inserted (a) guides the inclination of the anterior articular surface of the femur, that is, of the patellofemoral joint (Figs. 14.9, 14.11). The second guide wire to be inserted (b) will denote the axis of the knee joint and be parallel to the distal articular surface of the femoral condyles (Fig. 14.11).

If the fracture is type A_2, the reduction is simple, and once accomplished, it can be provisionally held with two crossed Kirschner wires inserted between the proximal and distal fragment. One can then insert guide wires a and b and guide wire c, which must be parallel to a in the coronal plane and to b in the frontal plane (Fig. 14.11). Guide wire c is the definitive guide wire for the insertion of the seating chisel. The design of the 95° condylar plate is such that, as long as its blade is inserted parallel to the knee joint axis (that is, to guide wire c), the normal anatomical axis of the femur will automatically be restored when the shaft is screwed to the plate.

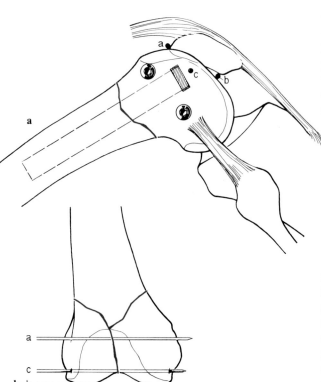

Fig. 14.11a, b. On **a** the lateral and **b** the anteroposterior drawing of the distal femur note the position of the three Kirschner wires a, b, and c. Guide wire a indicates the plane of the patellofemoral joint. Guide wire b indicates the plane of the knee joint axis. Guide wire c is the final guide wire, denoting the direction of the seating chisel and of the blade of the condylar plate. It is parallel to a and b

Inexperienced surgeons and those who have some difficulty with conceptualization and visualization in three dimensions may find it hard to grasp how one wire (c) can be parallel to two other wires (a and b) which are not parallel to one another. They forget that guide wires a and b are in different planes, the one horizontal (cross section) and the other coronal (frontal or anteroposterior).

In simple fractures, such as A_2 without comminution, where the main fragments can be held together provisionally with crossed Kirschner wires, the direction of guide wire c in the coronal or frontal plane can be further checked with the condylar guide (Fig. 14.12). Once the fracture is reduced

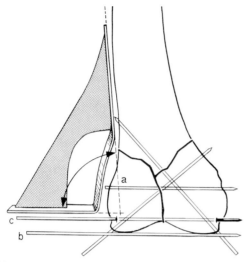

Fig. 14.12. In simple fractures such as A_2 or C_1 the reduction can be provisionally held with crossed Kirschner wires. The position of guide wire c can be checked with the condylar guide

and the guide wires inserted, all that remains is to insert the seating chisel and then the condylar plate. The condylar blade plate has to be inserted into the anterior half of the femoral condyles which are the distal continuation of the femoral shaft (see Fig. 14.8).

The simplest and most reliable way of determining the anterior half of the lateral femoral condyle is to palpate the most posterior margin of the lateral femoral condyle, then determine the direction of the longest diameter of the condyle, and divide that distance in two. The anterior half of this line denotes the anterior half of the lateral condyle. The condylar plate or the condylar screw was designed to be inserted 1.5–2 cm proximally to the distal articular surface of the femoral condyle. If we now take the midpoint of the anterior half of the lateral femoral condyle at a point 1.5–2 cm from the distal articular margin, we will have determined accurately the center of the window to be cut for the insertion of the seating chisel and subsequently of the condylar blade plate (see Fig. 14.8).

The insertion of the seating chisel in very young people can be difficult because their distal femoral epiphysis is filled with very dense, hard cancellous bone. The difficulty is not only the resistance the bone offers to the insertion of the seating chisel, but also the fact that dense cancellous bone does not yield as the seating chisel is hammered in and it can explode. In order to ease the insertion of the seating chisel and prevent this serious complication of splitting the supracondylar fragment, one should predrill the slot for the seating chisel with the 3.2-mm drill bit. It is enough to make three or four holes parallel to the guide wire c, and drill the central one of these all the way through the opposite medial cortex. With a depth gauge, one can then determine the depth of this hole and in this way check exactly the width of the femur at this point against the preoperative drawing; any necessary adjustment in the selection of the implant should now be made.

Because of the difficulties encountered with the insertion of the condylar plate, the AO/ASIF has recently developed a "dynamic condylar screw" (DCS). In its design and conception it is identical to the dynamic hip screw (Synthes). The difference is that instead of "hammering in" a seating chisel, if one is using a DCS, all that one has to do is insert the reaming guide wire in the center of the area where the window for the seating chisel would have been cut and parallel to guide wire c (its position can be verified radiologically at this point if desired). The seat for the DCS screw-plate combination is then precut with a special triple reamer and a tap. The insertion of the implant into bone has thus been greatly simplified. The DCS has one further advantage: the sagittal plane is not as critical as it is for the condylar plate. Any malalignment of the DCS in the sagittal plane is simply corrected by sliding off the plate and turning the screw the desired amount to achieve correction of the malalignment. Apart from the differences mentioned, the DCS is identical to the condylar plate in indications and use.

The holding power of the condylar plate in the distal fragment is not interfered with by predrilling the slot because the plate does not rely for its holding power on a tight fit. The strength of the fixation of the plate in the distal fragment is determined, first, by the pressure between the broad surface of its blade and the bone as compression is generated, and secondly, by one or preferably two cancellous screws which must be inserted through the plate into the distal fragment. These screws are essential to give the implant rotational stability, and in those fractures where, because of comminution, no axial compression is used, they are the only fixation of the implant in the distal fragment. These two screws are also needed when the DCS is used.

Once the window is precut and the slot for the seating chisel predrilled, the seating chisel is hammered in. The flap of the seating chisel guide is

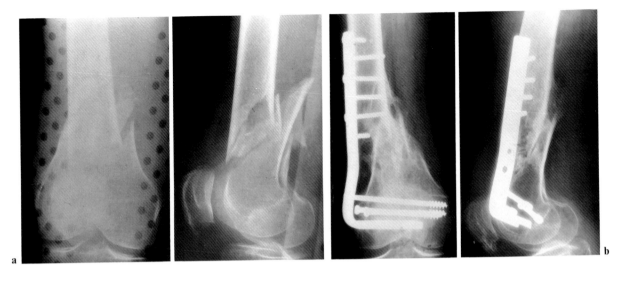

Fig. 14.13. a A$_3$ fracture before reduction. b Same fracture after reduction and insertion of the condylar plate. The plate was not inserted into the anterior half of the condyles, but more posteriorly. Note the resultant malreduction and medial translocation of the distal fragment

used to determine the sagittal plane. As long as it is parallel to the long axis of the femur as viewed from the side, the condylar plate will fit the femur when hammered in, and its plate will not point either forward or backward.

If the slot is not cut in the anterior half, but in error is cut at the midpoint of the lateral condyle or further back, then it becomes impossible to insert the angled plate sufficiently into bone for the plate to come to be flush with the lateral cortex. When the blade is fully inserted in this position, a gap of 1 cm or so between the plate and the reduced shaft always arises (Fig. 14.13). One must not destroy the cortex above the blade in order to drive the blade deeper. This will gravely weaken the supracondylar fragment, decrease the holding power of the device in the distal fragment, and drive the tip of the blade out through the medial cortex. Similarly, the shaft must not be lateralized to fit the plate because this destroys the stability of the reduction and functionally medializes the distal fragments which may have subsequent adverse biomechanical consequences on the function of the knee joint.

Once the condylar plate is inserted and the fracture reduced, the fracture should be placed under axial compression, either with the aid of a tension device or, if the reduction is anatomical and there are no gaps in the fracture, by means of the self-

compressing principle of the DC plate. This also applies for the DCS. One should strive, if at all possible, to cross the supracondylar fracture line with a lag screw which should be inserted through the plate. This greatly increases the stability of the fixation.

If the supracondylar fracture is very low and the supracondylar fragment small, then it may be impossible to use the condylar plate because it may be impossible to fix the distal fragment to the plate with at least one cancellous screw. If that should be the case, then fixation should be carried out with the condylar buttress plate (Fig. 14.14). Once its distal portion is fixed to the supracondylar fragment with screws, the fixation proceeds in exactly the same manner as with a condylar plate. This buttress plate can be placed under tension with the tension device, and thus axial compression can be achieved.

The reduction and fixation of an A$_3$ fracture or a C$_3$ fracture is very much more difficult because the supracondylar fracture cannot be reduced before the condylar plate is inserted into the distal fragment. Thus, the problems which face the surgeon are: (a) correct insertion of the condylar plate into the distal fragment prior to reduction of the supracondylar fracture; (b) subsequent reduction of the femur out to length and in proper rotational alignment. The exposure of an A$_3$ fracture is similar to an A$_2$ fracture, although the incision may have to be extended distally and proximally.

The first difficulty which the surgeon will encounter is the proper orientation of the distal fragment. This fragment frequently rotates about its axis because of the pull of the gastrocnemius mus-

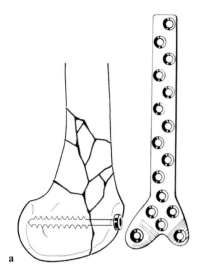

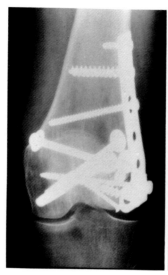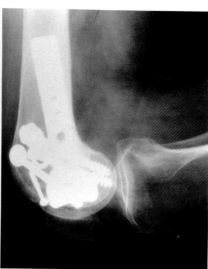

a

b

cles so that, when exposed, the distal articular surface is actually pointing anteriorly (see Fig. 14.4).

The best guide to the orientation of this fragment is the long diameter of the lateral condyle. One must carefully palpate the outline of the lateral femoral condyle and expose parts of it as necessary to determine the orientation of its long diameter. Once the orientation of the long diameter is determined, one should mark its direction and its midpoint on the bone with methylene blue. Through the midpoint, one should drop a line which is at 90° to the long diameter. This blue line indicates the direction of the long axis of the femur (see Fig. 14.8). Next, with methylene blue, one should mark in the position of the window in the anterior half of the lateral condyle. The Kirschner guide wires a, b, and c should now be inserted. One must be extremely careful with this step because the alignment in the frontal plane of the guide wire c cannot be double-checked with the condylar guide. Any error will result in either a valgus or varus misalignment of the distal fragment.

The window in the lateral cortex of the condyle is now cut, and the slot in the supracondylar fragment is predrilled with the 3.2-mm drill bit as already described. The next crucial step is the insertion of the seating chisel into the supracondylar fragment. It must be very carefully inserted parallel to the guide wire c with the flap of its guide parallel to the line drawn at 90° to the long diameter of the lateral femoral condyle. Once inserted, it is carefully withdrawn, and the condylar plate is inserted and fixed with one cancellous screw to the distal fragment.

Fig. 14.14. a The condylar buttress plate is used either when the distal fragment is too small for the insertion of the condylar plate or when the fracture lines are in the frontal plane, as in a C_3 fracture, in which the blade of the condylar plate would interfere with the lag screws which must be inserted from front to back. **b** A Hoffa fracture fixed with a T plate. A condylar buttress plate could also have been used

The length of the condylar plate will have been previously determined from the preoperative drawing and checked with the depth gauge. The length chosen should be such that, depending on the quality of the bone, there are at least four holes above the zone of comminution through which screws will be inserted to fix the plate to the proximal main fragment.

The plate in the distal fragment is now aligned with the shaft, the rotational alignment is checked, and the plate is fixed to the femur with a Verbrugge clamp before any attempt is made to reduce any of the comminuted fragments or apply traction. The supracondylar fracture with a segmental bone loss because of comminution is a very difficult problem, particularly if the comminution is such that one cannot reduce some of the fragments and fix them with lag screws to decrease the complexity of the fracture. Simple traction on the leg is rarely sufficient to regain length. One can increase one's mechanical advantage and apply traction by flexing the knee over a rest which is raised up from the table. This is more efficient than simple traction, but is awkward and also rarely adequate. The best, least traumatic, and most efficient way to restore length to the femur is to correct rotational alignment and then use the AO

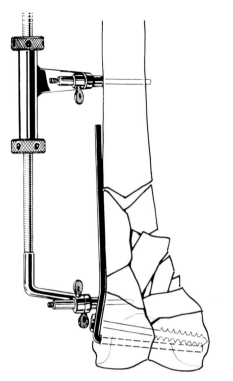

Fig. 14.15. The distractor makes the reduction of comminuted fractures relatively easy

distractor (Fig. 14.15). One of the bolts of the distractor is inserted into the proximal shaft above the plate, and the second is inserted through the first hole or, if a screw has already been inserted, through the second hole of the condylar plate into the distal fragment. With the distractor, one can gradually pull the femur out to length. It is often advantageous to overdistract slightly. This permits one to rearrange some of the comminuted fragments and improve on the reduction which occurred spontaneously as traction was applied. The plate can now be fixed to the shaft with one screw and the rotational alignment checked clinically by checking the internal and external rotation of the hip and comparing it with the normal range of the uninjured extremity, which has to be determined preoperatively. At this point, one should also obtain a radiograph to check the alignment of the extremity and check the reduction. If all is well, the internal fixation is completed by first easing off the overdistraction. The comminuted fragments are then fixed to one another with lag screws as well as to the plate, and the plate is fixed to the proximal and distal fragments by inserting the remainder of the screws.

14.3.9.2 Type C Fractures

The reduction and internal fixation of type C fractures is further complicated by one or more fractures of the epiphysis splitting the femoral condyles. The first step in the open reduction of any intra-articular fracture is the careful reconstruction of the joint. Thus, in C_1 and C_2 fractures, the vertical component of the supracondylar fracture must be reduced and fixed. C_1 and C_2 correspond in their supracondylar components to A_2 and A_3, respectively, so the steps in the open reduction and internal fixation will be identical once the supracondylar fragment is reduced and stabilized.

In simple intra-articular fractures, e.g., C_1 and C_2, it is not necessary to free and reflect the insertion of the quadriceps muscle. If the supracondylar fracture is left unreduced, the shortening of the leg slackens the quadriceps which usually allows all the retraction necessary to expose the articular surface and permit an accurate reconstruction.

As the first step in the reconstruction, one should assess the lateral condyle and mark in with methylene blue the position of the window for the seating chisel as well as the position of the plate. This step is important because one must know exactly where the condylar plate is going to be before any of the cancellous lag screws are inserted; otherwise, the one may be in the way of the other (see Fig. 14.11).

Once the condyles are anatomically reduced, they are fixed with two cancellous lag screws, which should be inserted over washers to prevent their heads from sinking through the cortex as the screws are tightened.

The window is then prepared by first drilling three 4.5-mm holes in the lateral cortex. These are then enlarged and joined with a router. A bevel is cut with an osteotome proximally in the lateral cortex to make room for the bend in the plate. The three guide wires a, b, and c are now inserted as described on p. 266.

The condyles which have been reduced and fixed with the cancellous screws can be easily driven apart by the seating chisel, particularly if the patient is young and the cancellous bone dense, offering resistance to the advancement of the seating chisel. How to avoid this complication has been described on p. 267. An assistant should also apply counterpressure as the seating chisel is being driven in. The seating chisel must be parallel in both planes to the definitive guide wire c, and the flap of the seating chisel guide must be parallel to the line drawn at 90° to the long diameter of the femoral condyle which represents the long axis of the femur. Once the seating chisel is introduced to the predetermined depth for the blade, it is removed, and the condylar plate is inserted. One is now ready for the reduction and fixation of the supracondylar fracture.

If the fracture is simple, as in C_1, the reduction usually follows without difficulty. The more severe the supracondylar comminution, the more difficult is the reduction. The steps one should follow are those described in the reduction and fixation of A_2 and A_3 fractures and use the AO distractor to regain length.

The most difficult fracture type is C_3. In order to be able to reduce the joint and subsequently fix the shaft with two plates, which is often the case, one is frequently forced to free and reflect the quadriceps mechanism by detaching the patellar tendon from its insertion together with a surrounding block of bone as described in Sect. 4.3.8 (see Fig. 14.10 c).

The joint reconstruction begins by careful reduction of all articular fragments and their provisional fixation with Kirschner wires. The definitive fixation of these articular fragments is secured with lag screws which are inserted wherever possible through nonarticular portions of the joint. Occasionally, it may be necessary to insert a screw through articular cartilage. Such a screw must be countersunk below the articular level and must not be inserted through weight-bearing surfaces. Wherever possible, one should endeavor to use a condylar plate or a DCS for the fixation of C_3 fractures. Because of the fixed angle, once properly inserted the plate ensures, the normal axial alignment of the femur. At times, the fracture pattern of the condyles and the path of screws necessary for the fixation of the fracture are such that a condylar plate cannot be used. In these instances, we use the condylar buttress plate which, instead of a blade portion, relies on screws for its fixation to the distal femur (see Fig. 14.14). With this plate, it is more difficult to achieve the correct axial alignment of the femur because one lacks the constant relationship of a fixed angle device to the joint axis. Therefore, before such a plate is securely fixed to the supracondylar fragment, one should check its position radiographically. This applies to the anteroposterior or frontal plane because the axial alignment in the sagittal plane is the same as for a condylar plate, namely, at 90° to the long diameter of the lateral condyle. The buttress plate, like the condylar plate, must be fixed to the anteri-

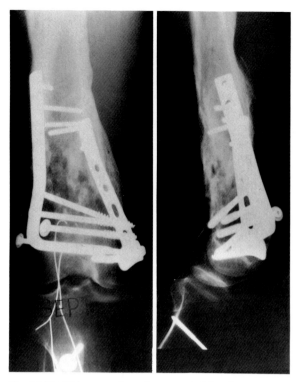

Fig. 14.16. This comminuted supracondylar fracture was fixed with a condylar plate laterally and with a T plate medially. The two plates were necessary to secure fixation of a severely comminuted segment which had resulted in loss of continuity between the shaft and the distal fragment

or half of the lateral condyle. If it is fixed more posteriorly, not only will it fail to fit the shaft, but there is also the great danger that the posterior screw will damage the lateral collateral ligament of the knee.

If the supracondylar comminution is very severe, or if there is actual loss of bone, two plates may have to be used to achieve the desired stability. We have found the T plate to be most useful as the medial plate, although any plate, if properly positioned, can serve this purpose (Fig. 14.16). One must take great care, of course, not to damage the femoral artery and accompanying veins as they pass through the adductor canal. The lateral plate is applied first and the medial plate second, with the comminuted fragment of bone or bone graft between them.

14.3.10 Bone Grafting

The intra-articular epiphyseal portion of a supracondylar fracture is through well-vascularized cancellous bone and usually goes on the heal, even if inaccurately reduced and not well fixed. This is not true, however, of fracture lines which are subjected to a major shear stress, such as the B type fractures of the condyles.

The supracondylar extra-articular portion of the fracture involves the expanded portion of the diaphysis where, particularly in the older patient, the cancellous bone filling the medullary canal is very sparse and the cortex thin and brittle. Internal fixation in this area is difficult and if comminution exists, stability may be difficult to obtain. We feel, therefore, that any supracondylar segment with bone loss or severe comminution should be bone grafted with autogenous corticocancellous and cancellous bone. This will accelerate union and will protect the internal fixation from failure.

14.3.11 Methyl Methacrylate

Occasionally, it may be necessary to carry out an open reduction and internal fixation for a patient whose bone is extremely osteoporotic. Such bone offers very poor holding power for the screws and, as a result, stability may not be obtained despite an accurate reduction and proper position and insertion of the implant. Under these circumstances, we have made use of methyl methacrylate to increase the holding power of the screws. In order to retard the setting time of the cement, both the powder and the liquid should be cooled in the deep freeze. The internal fixation is then carried out. The crucial screws, the holding power of which has to be supplemented, are withdrawn, and the hole in the near cortex is overdrilled with a 4.5-mm drill bit. The tip of a 20-ml disposable plastic syringe is drilled out with a 3.5-mm drill bit. This enlarges the hole and eases the injection of the cement. The precooled cement is now mixed, and as soon as it reaches a uniform liquid phase, it is poured into the syringe and injected into the screw holes under pressure. This creates a cement plug which spreads out in the medulla and extends through both cortices. The screws are then inserted into their corresponding holes, and once the cement polymerizes, they are retightened. An amazing degree of purchase for the screws is usually obtained with this technique.

14.4 Postoperative Care

At the end of the surgical procedure, it is necessary to splint the joint to prevent a contracture which would result in a loss of movement and function.

The knee joint has been traditionally splinted in full extension in the so-called position of function to ensure that if stiffness were to ensue, at least the extremity would be in a position in which it could function to some degree. The AO group recommended immobilization of the knee in 90° flexion for 3–4 days following surgery (Müller et al. 1979). We adopted this unorthodox position at first with some reservations, but we have since become very strong advocates of it. We have not had one instance which could be attributed to positioning where a patient failed to regain full, active extension after a period of immobilization in flexion. The decided advantage of this position is the rapid return of flexion. This is the arc of motion which has been repeatedly noted by previous authors to be the range frequently lost and the range responsible for permanent disability (Stewart et al. 1966; Neer et al. 1967). When the flexion splint is removed, patients are instructed to begin active flexion and extension exercises. Usually within the first hours, the patients regain full extension, but more important is the fact that all patients maintain the 90° flexion, and most go on to increase their range of flexion from that position. In recent years, we have employed continuous passive motion machines in the immediate postoperative period and for the first 4–7 days and have found them extremely helpful in the rehabilitation of intra-articular fractures.

Not all patients can begin unprotected active exercises. A ruptured lateral collateral ligament must be repaired at the time of the open reduction and internal fixation, such repairs are never sufficiently strong to withstand unprotected active movement. After the initial period of splinting and rest or continuous passive motion, we have transferred patients with this injury into a cast brace with polycentric hinges without blocks. This has allowed early, active mobilization of the knee with full protection from the undesirable valgus/varus forces.

Ruptured cruciate ligaments should be repaired only if they have been avulsed with a piece of bone which can be securely fixed either with a tension band wire or a lag screw. Such fixation is usually sufficiently secure to permit early motion. An insubstance tear or an avulsion without bone is best ignored and treated later if cruciate insufficiency becomes a problem. We have adopted this attitude because experience has taught us that in dealing with intra-articular fractures following an open reduction and internal fixation, the immediate goal must be motion. Early motion will not only ensure a useful range of movement, but also aids articular cartilage regeneration.

This applies also to unstable internal fixation. At the end of an open reduction and internal fixation, the surgeon must judge the stability of the internal fixation. Only the surgeon knows how many screws stripped at the time of insertion, how strong the bone really was, and how good its holding power. If, at the end of an internal fixation, the surgeon judges that the internal fixation is not stable, then once again early motion must be begun to ensure return of joint motion, but external protection must be employed to prevent overload which could result in loss of fixation and malunion or nonunion. It is very important to judge the degree of instability correctly. Very unstable fixation is best protected in skeletal traction. Other fractures which are more stable can be protected in a cast brace.

14.5 Complications

An analysis of the patients whose results of surgery were less than satisfactory revealed that the most common errors responsible for failure were technical, and therefore preventable (Schatzker and Lambert 1979). The most common error of all was incomplete reduction. The stability of an internal fixation depends on the inherent stability of bone. Inaccurate reduction fails to restore structural continuity and thus fails to reestablish the inherent stability of the fragments, so that the bone cannot take part in force transmission. The internal fixation therefore takes the full brunt of all the bending, shearing, and twisting stresses, and thus frequently fails. Furthermore, inaccurate reduction of joints results in incongruency of joint surfaces and rapid development of post-traumatic osteoarthritis. This is often accelerated by concomitant axial deformity with overload. Axial varus or valgus deformities are often the result of malreduction, but at times are also the result of error in insertion of the implant.

The second most common error found was failure to achieve interfragmental compression with lag screws or to apply axial compression where possible. The failure to achieve compression resulted in the fragments of bone being aligned and held coapted by means of the plate. The resultant gaps led to early instability, loss of fixation, delayed union, nonunion, and failure of the implant.

The third most common error found was improper selection and insertion of the condylar plate. Blades which are too long penetrate the medial cortex, irritate the joint, cause synovitis, and come to lie deep in the medial collateral ligament where they cause pain and lead to joint stiffness. Furthermore, the blade plates were sometimes inserted without observance of the three planes of reference, which resulted in deformity with subsequent failure.

14.6 Conclusions

The supracondylar fracture is a difficult problem. The modern techniques of open reduction and stable internal fixation, however, if properly executed, can ensure the majority of patients an excellent result (Olerud 1972; Schatzker et al. 1974; Schatzker and Lambert 1979; Mize et al. 1982). The only patients in whom a poor result can be accepted are those with C_3 fractures in which the articular portion of the fracture is irreconstructible.

References

Mitchell N, Shepard N (1980) Healing of articular cartilage in intra-articular fractures in rabbits. J Bone Joint Surg 62A:628–634

Mize RD, Bucholz RW, Grogan DP (1982) Surgical treatment of displaced comminuted fractures of the distal end of the femur. J Bone Joint Surg 64A:871–879

Müller ME, Allgöwer M, Schneider R, Willenegger H (1979) Manual of internal fixation, 2nd edn. Springer, Berlin Heidelberg New York

Neer CS, Grantham S, Shelton L (1967) Supracondylar fracture of the adult femur. J Bone Joint Surg 49A:591–613

Olerud S (1972) Operative treatment of supracondylar-condylar fractures of the femur. Technique and results in fifteen cases. J Bone Joint Surg 54A:1015–1032

Rittmann WW, Perren SM (1974) Cortical bone healing after internal fixation and infection. Springer, Berlin Heidelberg New York

Salter RB, Harris DJ (1979) The healing of intra-articular fractures with continuous passive motion. American Academy of Orthopaedic Surgery Lecture Series 28:102–117

Schatzker J, Lambert DC (1979) Supracondylar fractures of the femur. Clin Orthop 138:77–83

Schatzker J, Horne G, Waddell J (1974) The Toronto experience with the supracondylar fracture of the femur 1966–1972. Injury 6:113–128

Stewart MJ, Sisk TD, Wallace SH Jr (1966) Fractures of the distal third of the femur. A comparison of methods of treatment. J Bone Joint Surg 48A:784–807

Wenzl H, Casey PA, Hébert P, Belin J (1970) Die operative Behandlung der distalen Femurfraktur. AO Bulletin, December

15 Fractures of the Patella

J. Schatzker

15.1 Introduction

The patella is a sesamoid bone which develops within the tendon of the quadriceps muscle. Any fracture which results in displacement of the fragments in the longitudinal axis represents a disruption of the quadriceps mechanism.

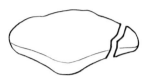

Fig. 15.1. Osteochondral fracture of the medial facet sustained in a lateral dislocation of the patella. This fracture is usually not visible on an anteroposterior or lateral radiograph of the knee and must be looked for on a "skyline" view of the patella

15.2 Methods of Evaluation and Guides to Treatment

Just as one cannot expect a return of function without repair of a ruptured flexor tendon in the hand, one cannot expect a return of function of the quadriceps mechanism if the displaced fracture of the patella is left unreduced. Loss of quadriceps function means loss of active extension of the knee and loss of the ability to lock the knee in extension. Individuals with such lesions can neither walk on the level without the knee being unstable and buckling, nor can they walk upstairs or downstairs or on inclined planes. The disability is profound. Thus, the indication for open reduction and internal fixation of the patella is any fracture which leaves the quadriceps mechanism disrupted. The patella is intimately bound to the quadriceps tendon proximally, to the infrapatellar tendon distally, and on either side to the retinacular expansions which are adherent to the capsule. We have come to differentiate three groups of fractures of the patella, each requiring different treatment.

15.3 Classification

15.3.1 Osteochondral Fractures

Osteochondral fractures of the patella (Fig. 15.1), which usually involve varying portions of the medial facet and subjacent bone, are the result of patellar dislocation. Surgery is required to remove the intra-articular loose body and repair the quadriceps mechanism to prevent recurrences of the dislocation. In this injury, the extensor mechanism as such is not interfered with. This fracture may only be visualized in the "skyline" radiographic projection of the knee and therefore is frequently missed in routine radiographs of the knee.

15.3.2 Stellate Fractures

A stellate, undisplaced fracture of the patella (Fig. 15.2), or a vertical fracture, is usually the

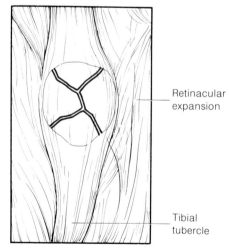

Fig. 15.2. In a vertical or stellate fracture of the patella, the retinacular expansions remain intact. The patient is able to execute straight leg raising against gravity

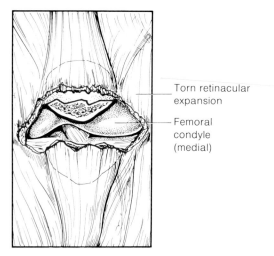

Torn retinacular
expansion

Femoral
condyle
(medial)

Fig. 15.3. In a displaced transverse simple or comminuted fracture of the patella, the retinacular expansions are torn and the patient loses the ability to extend the knee against gravity

result of a direct blow to the patella. The continuity of the quadriceps mechanism is undisturbed and the retinacula are not torn. The fracture is stable and will not displace under the normal physiologic stresses of active motion. Surgery is unnecessary.

15.3.3 Transverse Fractures

A sudden, violent contraction of the quadriceps muscle, such as might occur when an individual stumbles and tries to stop the fall, may disrupt the quadriceps mechanism. Thus, there may be an avulsion of the quadriceps tendon, or of the infrapatellar tendon, or there may be a transverse fracture of the patella, together with a tear into the retinacular expansion (Fig. 15.3).

15.4 Surgical Treatment

We shall concern ourselves here only with disruptions of the extensor mechanism.

15.4.1 Undisplaced Fractures

A transverse, undisplaced fracture of the patella is an avulsion fracture. The function of the quadriceps mechanism is not disrupted and the patient is able to maintain the knee extended because the retinacula on either side of the patella are not torn.

The fracture is, however, potentially hazardous because, with further sudden strong contractions of the quadriceps, the retinacular expansions might tear. The fracture will displace and the quadriceps function will be disrupted. The knee requires simple protection. Excellent results have been achieved either by allowing motion, but keeping the patient on crutches, or by immobilizing the knee in a cylinder cast and allowing weight bearing.

15.4.2 Displaced Fractures

A transverse fracture, either simple or comminuted, has, as an integral part, an associated disruption of the quadriceps retinacula (see Fig. 15.3). Thus, the quadriceps function is lost and surgical repair is necessary.

15.4.2.1 Surgical Approaches

We prefer to expose the patella through a transverse incision made directly over the defect. The transverse incision does not pull apart when the knee is flexed and it heals with the least noticeable scar. It can also be readily extended if greater exposure is needed to visualize the retinacular tears. These must be exposed so that the articular surface is visible as the patella is being reduced and fixed.

15.4.2.2 Biomechanical Considerations

Fractures of the patella and fractures of the olecranon are the two ideal indications for tension band fixation with wire (Müller et al. 1979). If the patella is reduced and held together with a cerclage wire passed circumferentially, reduction is maintained as long as the knee is not flexed or the quadriceps muscle is not contracted. The moment the knee is flexed, the fracture gapes anteriorly, the contour of the patella is changed, and congruency is lost (Fig. 15.4). This will also happen as the result of a strong quadriceps contraction, even if the knee is immobilized in extension in a plaster cylinder. With tension band fixation, flexion of the knee results in an increase of compression across the fracture (Fig. 15.5), and contraction of the quadriceps if the knee is extended will not cause the fragments to gape.

15.4.2.3 Techniques of Internal Fixation

The tension band wire is passed through the quadriceps and patellar tendons before it is tied over the anterior surface of the patella. We like to use

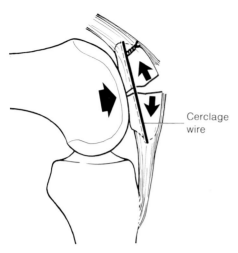

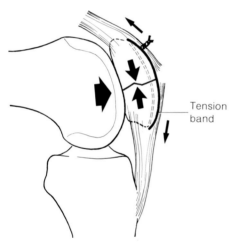

Fig. 15.4. Circumferential cerclage wiring of the patella is unable to neutralize the pull of the quadriceps and infrapatellar tendons. Under load, such as flexion of the knee, the fracture gapes anteriorly and stability of the fracture and congruity of the patella are lost

Fig. 15.5. A tension band wire applied to the anterior surface of the patella absorbs the distracting forces. In flexion, the patella is pulled against the intercondylar groove and the fracture closes with the fragments under axial compression. This is an example of dynamic compression

a large-bore needle (gauge 12–14) to guide the wire through the tendons. This ensures its accurate placement and allows its passage through the substance of the tendon. The fracture must be reduced and the knee extended before the wire is tied under tension. We like to observe the fracture as the wire is tightened and we tighten the wire till a slight overcorrection occurs and the articular fissure begins to gape. The knee is then flexed to beyond 90°. This maneuver places the whole fracture surface under compression, impacts the frag-

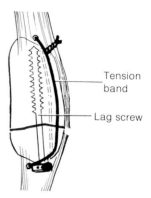

Fig. 15.6. Small fragments of the patella, such as an avulsed inferior pole or a lateral fragment, are best fixed to the remainder of the patella with a lag screw. This fixation must be further protected with a tension band wire

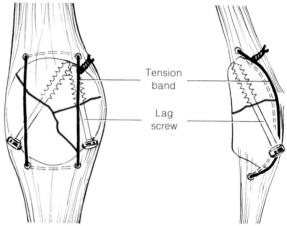

Fig. 15.7. Major comminuted fragments of the patella can be lagged together. This is best for vertical or oblique fracture lines because a tension band applied about the quadriceps and infrapatellar tendons will not compress a vertical fracture line. The remaining fracture lines are fixed with a tension band

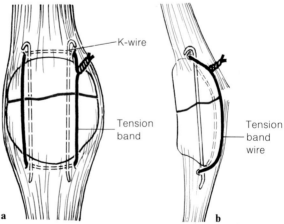

Fig. 15.8a, b. Kirschner wires provide rotational and lateral stability. If used, they must be inserted parallel or they will block interfragmental compression of the tension band

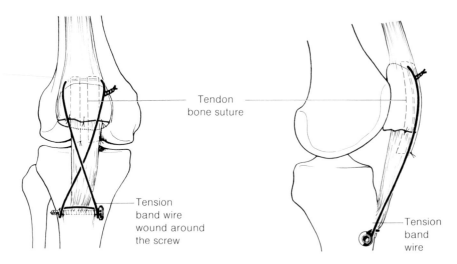

Fig. 15.9. If the inferior half of the patella is sacrificed because of severe comminution, the infrapatellar tendon is sutured to the remaining bony fragment. The suture line is protected with a tension band wire which allows early mobilization of the knee

ments, and closes the articular fissure without an anterior gap or distortion of the patella. Compression can also be achieved with lag screws, a technique which is particularly necessary with fractures of the distal pole because if only tension band wiring is used, the small distal fragment displaces and tilts into the joint (Fig. 15.6). The tension band wire is applied once the lag screw is tightened. It serves to protect the lag screw fixation. Similarly, if there are major comminuted fragments, we like to reduce and fix them in place with lag screws (Fig. 15.7). If Kirschner wires are used to secure fixation of the fragments, they must not be crossed or impaction and compression of the fragments will not occur. If the tension band is placed around the Kirschner wires rather than through the tendon, there is great danger of pulling the Kirschner wires forward, deforming them, and having the tension band wire slip off (Fig. 15.8). This can be prevented proximally by bending the wire over on itself 180° and by turning the free end toward the joint. The other end of the wire must not be turned over but must be left straight. If both ends are turned over, it becomes extremely difficult to remove the wire at the time the metal is removed. We use Kirschner wires only if the patella is grossly comminuted and the wires are necessary for stability. We feel that the patella should be preserved at all cost and we feel that a primary patellectomy should be performed only if the fracture is such that it is impossible to save

even a portion of the patella. If a portion of the patella is retained, the suture of the tendon to bone is protected with a tension band wire (Fig. 15.9).

15.5 Postoperative Care

The joint is immobilized in 40°–60° flexion for 2–3 days and the extremity is kept elevated on a Böhler–Braun splint. On the 4th or 5th day, if we judge that the wound is healing satisfactorily, we instruct the patient to begin active flexion and extension exercises, but we allow only partial weight bearing for the first 6 weeks. It is wrong to immobilize the knee after open reduction and internal fixation of an articular fracture. Not only is motion required to enhance the healing of the articular cartilage, but also knee flexion is necessary to enhance the stabilizing effect of dynamic compression on the fracture interface, and this is exerted only when the knee is flexed. Thus, we do not use cylinder casts to protect the internal fixation. Usually, in 6 weeks or so the fracture will have consolidated and the patient will have regained a good range of movement. At this point, the patient can begin full weight bearing. Some protection is advisable until full quadriceps strength has been regained. We have also used continuous passive motion machines to advantage in the postoperative management of patellar fractures, as in other intra-articular fractures (see Chap. 7).

Reference

Müller ME, Allgöwer M, Schneider R, Willenegger H (1979) Manual of internal fixation, 2nd edn. Springer, Berlin Heidelberg New York, pp 42–47

16 Fractures of the Tibial Plateau

J. SCHATZKER

16.1 Introduction

A survey of the recent literature indicates that many authors continue to report only slightly better than 50% satisfactory results with either closed or operative methods of treatment of this fracture. The failures of treatment are usually due to residual pain, stiffness, instability, deformity, recurrent effusions, and give-way episodes. Our own review of over 140 of these fractures treated by both closed and operative methods has shed considerable light on the reason for the failures (Schatzker et al. 1979).

Fractures of the tibial plateau are intra-articular fractures of a major weight-bearing joint. They occur as a result of a combination of vertical thrust and bending (Kennedy and Bailey 1968). This mechanism of fracture usually leads to varying degrees of articular surface depression and axial malalignment. When part of the articular surface be-

comes depressed, the articular surface becomes incongruous and a smaller portion of the joint comes to bear all the weight which increases the stress borne by the articular cartilage. If, in addition, there is an axial malalignment, the weight-bearing axis is shifted to the side of the depression (Fig. 16.1). These two mechanisms of overload alone can give rise to post-traumatic osteoarthritis. If this destructive mechanism is combined with traumatic damage to the articular cartilage, the destruction of the joint will progress more rapidly.

Fig. 16.1. a In a normal knee, the articular surfaces are congruous and, when weight bearing, the medial and lateral compartments share the load almost equally, the medial taking slightly more than the lateral. b When fractured and partially depressed, the articular surface becomes incongruous and a smaller portion of the joint carries the full load. The load can be further increased by axial malalignment

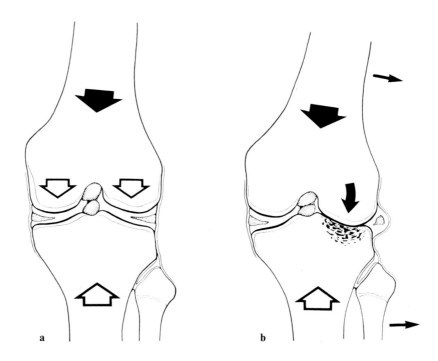

a   b

Occasionally, at the time of fracture, the deforming force may be such that, in addition to the fracture, the corresponding collateral ligament and even the cruciate ligament may rupture (Roberts 1968; Rasmussen 1973; Hohl and Hopp 1976; Schatzker et al. 1979; Hohl and Moore 1983). This results in joint instability. Instability may also be present as a result of joint depression and incongruity without ligamentous disruption (Hohl and Moore 1983). From whatever cause, the instability interferes with normal joint function because of insecurity and the concomitant axial malalignment and overload. Thus, joint incongruity, axial malalignment, and instability will act in concert or alone to produce post-traumatic osteoarthritis. Thus, to be successful, treatment of a tibial plateau fracture must ensure that the joint remains stable, that the articular surfaces remain congruous, that the joint is painless, and that it retains a satisfactory range of motion.

Our experience with the tibial plateau fractures has led us to the conclusion that it is wrong to speak of these fractures collectively because they differ, not only in their pattern of fracture and required therapeutic approach, but also in their prognosis. Thus, we have developed a classification which groups the fractures into six types (Schatzker et al. 1979). Each type represents a group of fractures which are similar in pathogenesis and pattern, pose similar problems in their treatment, and have a similar prognosis.

16.2 Classification and Guides to Treatment

16.2.1 Type I

This is the wedge fracture of a lateral tibial plateau (Fig. 16.2). It occurs mostly in young people since the dense cancellous bone of the lateral plateau resists depression. If undisplaced, these fractures require early motion and protection from weight bearing because, under stress, displacement may occur. There are three basic patterns of displacement. The lateral wedge fragment is either spread apart from the metaphysis, which results in a broadening of the joint surface, or it is depressed, or it may be both spread and depressed. In our experience, all of these fractures, if significantly displaced, have had the lateral meniscus trapped in the fracture. Thus, we believe that, when displaced, these fractures should be operated upon, because if the lateral meniscus is trapped in the fracture line, it prevents any manipulative reduction. Furthermore, if trapped and displaced, the meniscus will give rise to a major intra-articular derangement which will grossly interfere with future joint function. Clearly, the effect of the widening of the lateral plateau depends on the degree to which it occurs. If minimal, the split is partially covered by the lateral meniscus and is of no consequence. If major, not only may the meniscus be trapped in the fracture line, but the spread may also result in joint incongruity and in varying degrees of instability. Both the incongruity and instability are incompatible with normal function. As this fracture type occurs most commonly in young people under 30 years, we must strive for the best possible result of treatment. Thus, for displaced

Fig. 16.2. a Wedge fracture of the tibial plateau. **b** In young people, the proximal tibia is filled with strong cancellous bone. Lag screws alone suffice for fixation

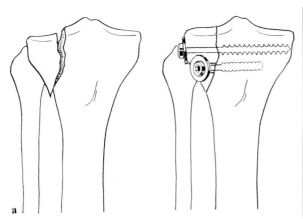
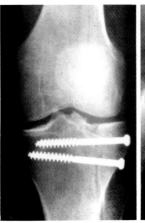
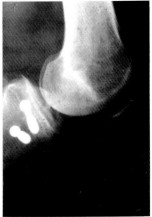

fractures, we feel that open reduction and internal fixation are justified because of the potential internal derangement, joint incongruity, instability, and axial overload. If the displacement is minor and the indications for surgery not clear-cut, then one should at least examine the joint with an arthroscope to make certain that the meniscus is not trapped in the fracture. All patients who had this joint carefully reconstructed ended with excellent function.

16.2.2 Type II

In this type, the lateral wedge is combined with varying degrees of depression of the adjacent remaining weight-bearing portion of the lateral tibial plateau (Fig. 16.3). The depressed segment may be anterior, central, posterior, or a combination of all three. Similarly, the wedge may vary from being simply a rim fracture to one involving almost one-third of the articular surface. The displacement of this fracture consists of a widening of the joint with spreading apart of the wedge, in combination with a central depression of the lateral plateau. We have graded the depression by measuring the vertical distance between the lowest recognizable point on the medial plateau and the lowest depressed fragment of the lateral plateau. We have found that a depression greater than 4 mm was significant and, if left unreduced, it resulted in joint incongruity, valgus deformity, and a sense of instability. The degree of these was proportional

to the degree of joint widening and the central depression. The patients' average age was around 50 years and about half of them had evidence of osteoporosis.

All poor results of open or closed treatment could be related to residual joint depression, incongruity, and joint instability, either because it was accepted in the first place, or because the reduction was not perfect, or because redisplacement occurred in the postoperative period.

Closed manipulative reduction combined with traction, or traction alone, was associated with varying degrees of success. The displaced lateral wedge sometimes reduced surprisingly well; however, the anterior or posterior wedge fragments remained relatively unaffected. Furthermore, depressed articular fragments which were impacted into the metaphysis could never be dislodged by closed means (Fig. 16.4). If the depression of the fragments was significant and was responsible for joint instability, this instability remained and was present at the end of conservative treatment. The joint depression did not fill in with fibrocartilage, but remained as a permanent negative articular defect. Plaster immobilization of these intra-articular fractures, even of short duration, resulted in marked irreversible stiffness. The advantage of traction, even if it failed to yield an acceptable reduction, was in the relief of pain and in the ability of the patient to start early motion while in traction. If a disruption of a collateral ligament was coexistent with a fracture, it was repaired. After surgery, immobilization of the joint in plas-

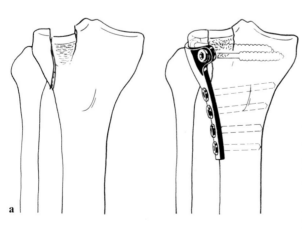
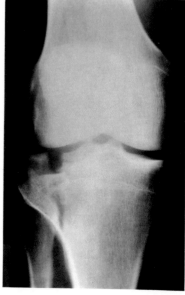

Fig. 16.3. a Type II wedge fracture combined with depression of the adjacent weight-bearing surface. **b** Because of frequent comminution of the articular surface and osteoporosis of the condyles, it is best to combine the fixation with a buttress plate

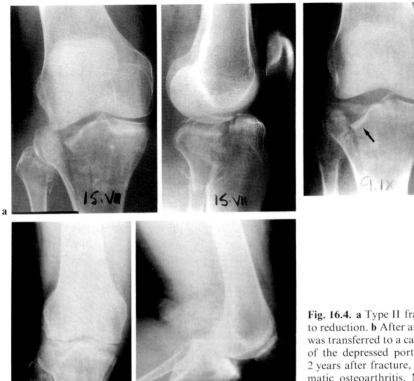

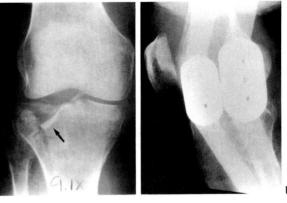

Fig. 16.4. a Type II fracture in a 56-year-old woman prior to reduction. b After an initial period of traction, the patient was transferred to a cast brace. Note the failure of reduction of the depressed portion of the articular surface. c Some 2 years after fracture, the patient shows signs of post-traumatic osteoarthritis. Note, in flexion, the subluxation of the femoral condyle into the depressed posterior portion of the articular surface, which was left unreduced

ter for a few days resulted frequently in a serious permanent loss of motion. Therefore, we have made immediate use of the cast brace to protect the ligamentous repair. We have also found the cast brace to be an ideal method of external splintage of unstable internal fixation, and a very satisfactory method of protection of undisplaced fractures in unreliable and noncompliant patients. Certain displaced fractures which were not operated upon but which were treated in traction were transferred into the cast brace once they became "sticky." The cast brace maintained axial alignment of these unstable fractures with joint depression, but the malalignment frequently recurred once the brace was removed. The cast brace could not be used as a method of reduction, but it served as an excellent method of functional treatment once reduction was obtained, allowing motion while unloading the damaged portion of the articulation.

We feel, therefore, that significant displaced lateral wedge fragments associated with central depression greater than 4 mm should be treated by open reduction, elevation of the depressed fragments, stable fixation, and early motion. If the patient is elderly, or if there are contraindications to surgery, then the patient should be treated by closed manipulative reduction, skeletal traction, and early motion, and should be transferred into a cast brace as soon as the fracture is no longer displaceable, even though it may be still deformable. At no time should the fracture be immobilized in plaster, as such treatment frequently results in significant degrees of joint stiffness.

16.2.3 Type III

This fracture type represents a central depression of the articular surface of the lateral plateau without an associated lateral wedge fracture (Fig. 16.5). It is usually the result of a smaller force exerting its effect on weaker bone. Indeed, it commonly affects a somewhat older age group (55–60 years) than type II fractures, and one in whom osteoporosis is more marked. This fracture pattern is the most innocent of all the tibial plateau fractures. The stability of the joint is rarely affected and excellent function without joint incongruity is the usual outcome. The degree of joint involve-

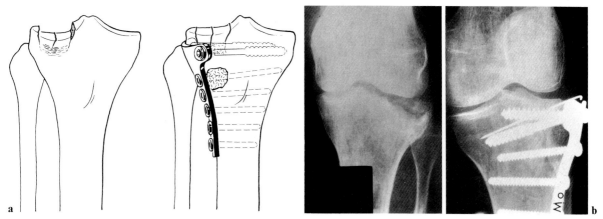

Fig. 16.5. a Type III fracture. There is depression of the articular surface, but no associated wedge fracture. **b** In this patient, the whole plateau was depressed, the joint was unstable, and an open reduction was necessary

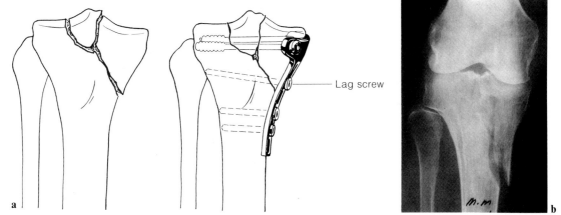

Lag screw

Fig. 16.6a, b. Type IV fracture of the medial tibial plateau. Note the associated fracture of the intercondylar eminence

ment may vary, however, from a small central plateau depression to one involving the whole plateau (Fig. 16.5b). Thus, it is important when evaluating this fracture to examine the knee under anesthesia in full extension and in different degrees of flexion. If no valgus instability is found, it is safe to treat such a fracture with early motion without weight bearing. If valgus instability is demonstrated, then, depending on the degree of instability and other factors (patient's age, expectations, etc.), open reduction and internal fixation should be performed.

In our experience, this fracture pattern was the most common. The few patients who required an open reduction and internal fixation did well as long as their reduction and joint congruity was maintained. Patients whose joints were stable when examined under anesthesia and who were treated by early motion did well.

16.2.4 Type IV

This is a fracture of the medial tibial plateau (Fig. 16.6). It occurs either as a result of a high-velocity injury or as a result of a rather trivial varus force and carries the worst prognosis of all the tibial plateau fractures, for the following reasons. If the fracture occurs as a result of a rather trivial low-velocity injury, it usually occurs in an elderly person with grossly osteoporotic bone in whom the medial tibial plateau simply crumbles into an irreconstructible mass of fragments. The poor prognosis is that of a fracture which is technically beyond reconstruction. Traction rarely results in a reasonable alignment of the medial condyle and of the articular surface, and the poor result is due to joint incongruity and instability. The medial plateau is more difficult to overload

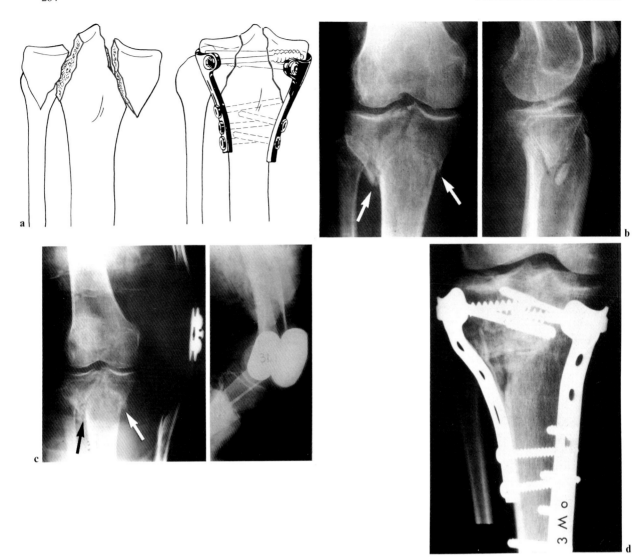

and fracture than the lateral; therefore, the force which gives rise to a fracture of the medial plateau is of higher magnitude. If this fracture is the result of a high-velocity injury, it usually involves a younger individual. The medial plateau splits as a relatively simple wedge, similar to the wedge fracture of the lateral plateau, but there is often an associated fracture of the intercondylar eminence and adjacent bone with the attached cruciate ligaments. Furthermore, there is frequently a concomitant disruption of the lateral collateral ligamentous complex (which may be through the substance of the ligament or be an avulsion of bone such as the proximal fibula) and a rupture of the peroneal nerve as a result of traction. In some cases there may also be damage to the popliteal vessels. A disruption of this magnitude represents a subluxation or a dislocation of the knee which has been realigned. Thus, in the younger patient

Fig. 16.7. a Type V fracture. Note that the fracture lines begin close to the intercondylar eminence. There is frequently no depression of the articular cartilage. **b** A bicondylar fracture in traction. Note the slight overriding of the cortices, indicating shortening. **c** The position of the fragments and alignment is maintained in a cast brace. **d** Two buttress plates are necessary in addition to lag screws to maintain a stable fixation

the poor prognosis of this injury is not the result of the fracture, but the result of the associated injuries and other complications such as compartment syndrome, Volkmann's ischemia necrosis, or foot drop.

If undisplaced and not associated with significant soft tissue lesions, type IV fractures can be treated successfully by closed means as long as motion is begun early and axial malalignment is prevented. If displaced and/or associated with ligamentous or neurovascular lesions, these fractures must be treated open with repair of the soft tissue components of the injury and stable internal fixation of the fracture.

16.2.5 Type V

This is a bicondylar fracture which consists of a wedge fracture of the medial and lateral plateaux (Fig. 16.7). It results from an equal axial thrust on both plateaux. There is usually no associated depression of the articular surface, although this may occur. Because of the soft tissue attachment to the split wedge fragments, traction frequently results in an acceptable reduction and, once the fracture has become "sticky," it is easily managed in a cast brace. Although the cast brace can maintain alignment, it cannot prevent minor degrees of shortening. As a result, once transferred to a cast brace, many of these fractures tend to telescope, with some spreading of the tibial condyles (Fig. 16.7b, c). This leads to a relative lengthening of the collateral soft tissue hinges which results in minor varus/valgus instability. In an individual without athletic aspiration, this minor varus/valgus instability is of no consequence. In younger, athletically inclined individuals, however, the varus/valgus rocking can constitute a significant disability. Thus, in younger individuals, if the fracture is displaced, we prefer to carry out open reduction and internal fixation. The same would apply, of course, to an older individuals in whom traction had failed to yield an acceptable reduction (Fig. 16.7d).

16.2.6 Type VI

These are the most complex tibial plateau fractures. Their hallmark is a fracture which separates the metaphysis from the diaphysis (Fig. 16.8). The significance of this is that traction tends to separate the diaphysis from the metaphysis without any reduction of the metaphysis or of the articular components. This makes this fracture less amenable to nonoperative treatment. The fracture pattern of the articular component is variable and can involve one or both tibial condyles and articular surfaces. The fracture is almost always the result of a high-velocity injury and therefore is often associated with marked displacement and depression of the articular fragments. Such articular disorganization can be corrected only through direct surgical intervention.

A word of caution is in order. These fractures may be so comminuted as to defy even the most skilled surgeon, and must therefore be very carefully evaluated. If there is doubt whether an open reduction can be successfully performed, it is best to treat such a fracture by nonoperative means, despite its limitations. *The result of a failed open reduction and internal fixation is always worse than the result of a failed closed treatment.* Despite the severity of this injury, 80% of the patients who came to surgery ended up with a most satisfactory result (Schatzker et al. 1979).

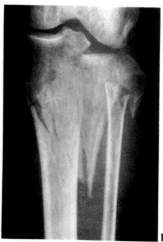

Fig. 16.8a, b. Type VI fracture. The hallmark of this fracture is the separation of the metaphysis and diaphysis. Comminution and displacement are frequently marked

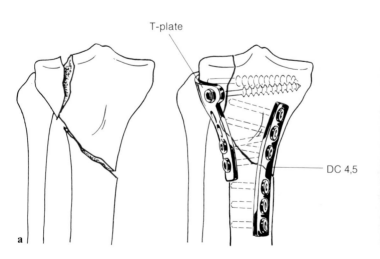

16.2.7 Absolute Indications for Surgery

In considering the therapeutic approach required to ensure the best possible result, certain situations must be isolated and added to what has just been said above. These, because of their nature or potential effects, demand operative rather than closed treatment and can be considered to comprise absolute indications for operative intervention.

16.2.7.1 Open Fractures

As stability is the mainstay of prophylaxis against sepsis, in addition to débridement, stable internal fixation of an open intra-articular fracture is a necessity.

16.2.7.2 Acute Compartment Syndrome

Occasionally, while one is contemplating whether a fracture should be treated open or closed, one's hand is forced by the development of an acute compartment syndrome. Once a compartment is decompressed and a previously closed fracture converted to an open one, we feel that stable internal fixation of the fracture is the most advisable course, because the same considerations now apply as in an open fracture.

16.2.7.3 Associated Vascular or Neurologic Injury

Vascular injury is most often associated with type IV tibial plateau fractures. They usually represent fracture dislocations (Hohl and Moore 1983).

The popliteal vessels must be repaired. The fracture should then be stabilized and the associated ligamentous tears repaired.

16.3 Methods of Assessment

Before one is able to classify a tibial plateau fracture and thus arrive at a plan of treatment, one must carefully assess the patient and the fracture. We cannot overemphasize the importance of an accurate diagnosis: it identifies all the components of the injury, facilitates the therapeutic approach, and effects a better recovery from the injuries in the patient.

16.3.1 History

A case history is important because it allows one to determine whether the injury was caused by low- or high-velocity force. Although the patient is rarely able to relate the exact mechanism of the injury, it is usually possible to determine the direction of the force as well as the deformity produced. These are important clues. A history also allows one to evaluate the patient's expectations and level of function.

16.3.2 Physical Examination

Physical examination is the only accurate method of evaluating the state of the soft tissue cover. Tenderness elicited on physical examination is often the only clue available to indicate a concomitant disruption of a collateral ligament. Examination for any neurological or vascular deficits as well as for the presence of a compartment syndrome is also very important.

Fig. 16.9. Internal and external oblique X-rays are necessary for a complete visualization of the tibial plateau

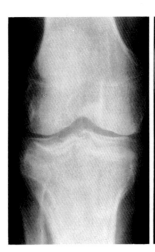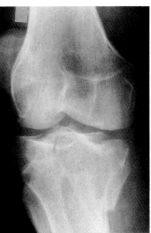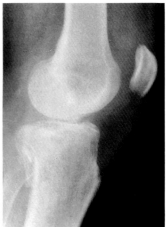

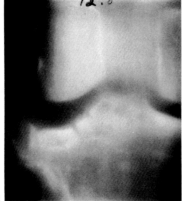
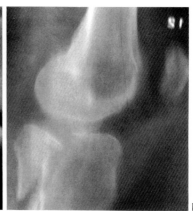

a   b

Fig. 16.10a, b. Note the information obtained from the **a** anteroposterior **b** and lateral tomogram of a knee injury. Frequently, plain radiographs fail to reveal important fracture lines, the number of fragments, and their depression. Note the posterior subluxation of the femoral condyles

16.3.3 Radiological Examination

A radiological assessment of the injury is indispensable because this is the only means available which leads to an accurate evaluation of the fracture pattern and its severity. Anteroposterior and lateral radiographs alone are inadequate: they must be supplemented with at least an internal and an external oblique view. The degree and location of the articular surface depression are best seen on the oblique projection (Fig. 16.9). Frequently, the four standard exposures are inadequate and it is necessary to resort to tomography in order to be able to evaluate accurately all fracture lines in their extent and position, determine the degree of comminution of the fracture and thus judge its operability, and determine the presence and extent of articular depression. In ordering the tomography, it is important to order both anteroposterior and lateral tomographic cuts. These complement one another and permit the surgeon to get a much more accurate three-dimensional concept of the fracture (Fig. 16.10).

Computed tomography is useful in evaluating the degree and extent of the comminution as well as in demonstrating the cortex circumferentially in cross section. If available, this greatly eases the three-dimensional reconstruction of the injury – it is very useful, but it is not essential.

16.4. Surgical Treatment

16.4.1 Planning the Surgical Procedure

Having carefully evaluated the patient and the radiographs, the surgeon is now able to decide on the best plan for treatment. If an open surgical approach is chosen, the surgical procedure must be carefully planned. This involves a reasoned choice of the approach, a detailed drawing of the fracture pattern, a careful plan of all the steps necessary in the open reduction, and a plan of the internal fixation. The latter must include a detailed position of all the screws and their function, together with the appropriate implant and its position.

16.4.2 Approaches

The essence of a good surgical approach is maximum visualization combined with minimum devitalization and the preservation of all vital structures. Initially, we employed the exposures as recommended in the second edition of the *AO Manual* (Müller et al. 1979). We changed the shape of the skin incisions, and their placement, as we became aware of certain difficulties which an improper skin incision may pose if the surgical procedure fails and some years later a total joint arthroplasty becomes necessary. Thus, we have abandoned the triradiate "Mercedes" incision recommended by the AO group for complex tibial plateau fractures (Müller et al. 1979) and prefer all approaches to be as straight and as close to the midline as possible (Fig. 16.11). One should also remember that the skin incisions must be planned in such a way that they do not come directly over an implant. The flaps which are raised must be full thickness, consisting of the subcutaneous fat down to the fascia lata and the quadriceps retinacular expansions. This will ensure the survival of the flaps and prevent wound edge necrosis or partial loss of the flap due to ischemia.

We have also come to appreciate the importance of the meniscus in safeguarding subsequent

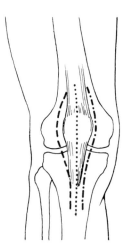

Fig. 16.11. The incisions should be straight. Increase in exposure is gained by extension of the incision proximally and distally

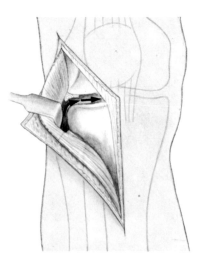

Fig. 16.12. The arthrotomy should be made by incising the capsule transversely below the meniscus. (From Müller et al. 1979)

joint function. The meniscus appears to share in weight transmission and distributes the weight over a broader surface area (Schrive 1974; Walter and Erkman 1975). This cushioning effect protects the elevated articular cartilage fragments and enhances cartilage healing. We therefore feel that the meniscus must be preserved in the execution of a surgical exposure; it should *never* be excised to facilitate exposure. We believe that the capsule should be incised horizontally below the meniscus. This allows the surgeon to pull up on the meniscus together with the capsule to which it remains peripherally attached, thus achieving an unobstructed view of the articular surface (Fig. 16.12). (If the arthrotomy is made above the meniscus, the meniscus will keep most of the articular surface hidden from view and will interfere with the attempts to execute an accurate open reduction.) If a peripheral detachment of the meniscus is encountered, or even a tear into the meniscal body, this should be meticulously repaired at the end of the procedure. Every effort should be made to preserve the meniscus (Wirth 1981; Hohl and Moore 1983).

In order to gain exposure of the depressed articular fragments, one should make use of the fracture. Thus, if there is a peripheral wedge fragment, regardless of its size, it should be hinged back on its soft tissue attachment, like the cover of a book. This allows perfect visualization of the joint depression (Fig. 16.13). The soft tissue attachment preserves the blood supply to the wedge fragment.

The collateral ligaments must be preserved, but on the lateral side it is best to cut horizontally across the iliotibial band at the level of the joint to facilitate exposure. At the end of the procedure, the iliotibial band should be resutured with a nonabsorbable suture. We have done this many times with complete impunity and have not encountered a single instance of varus instability as a result.

Occasionally, in the very severe fractures which involve both tibial plateaux, it may become necessary to reflect the quadriceps mechanism upward so that, as the knee is flexed, both sides of the joint are simultaneously exposed. The infrapatellar tendon should not be detached from the tibia together with its surrounding bone. In the severe fractures, the tibial tubercle and adjacent cortex may be the only intact anterior cortex. If destroyed, the reduction is made considerably more difficult and it may prove impossible to reattach the tubercle, particularly if the posterior cortex is also comminuted. If necessary for exposure, we have found it best to cut the infrapatellar tendon in a Z fashion (Fig. 16.13). At the end of the procedure, we have resutured the tendon together with the horizontally incised quadriceps retinacula and capsule. In order to secure the resuture, the repair can be protected with a tension band wire which is passed through the quadriceps tendon just above the patella, crossed over the front to form a figure eight, and then passed either through bone or tied around a transverse screw inserted through the anterior cortex, just below the tibial tubercle. We have had no complications with this approach and have had no secondary ruptures of the tendon or any extensor lags (Fig. 16.14). Occasionally, an additional major posterior fracture may demand a

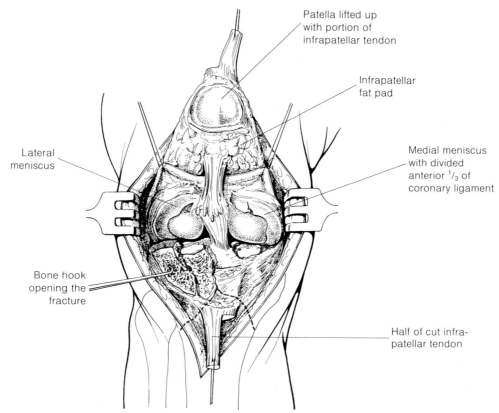

Fig. 16.13. The best exposure of the depressed fragments is gained by opening the fracture. The lateral wedge is pulled to the side like the cover of a book. In order to achieve exposure of bilateral tibial plateau fracture lines, it is best to divide the infrapatellar tendon in a Z fashion and divide across the medial and lateral capsule below the menisci. The capsule, the attached menisci, and patella are then lifted up to give unlimited exposure of the whole proximal tibia. Osteotomy of the tibial tubercle could enter the main fracture lines and make subsequent fixation very difficult

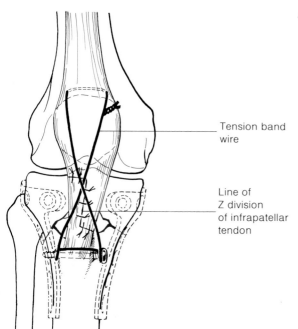

◀**Fig. 16.14.** The resuture of the Z division of the infrapatellar tendon is protected by means of a tension band wire. This allows immediate mobilization of the knee

posterior counterincision to facilitate the reduction and fixation of the fracture (Hohl and Moore 1983). We have found, however, that most often one can reach posteriorly by simply lengthening the anterior incision by undermining the full thickness flap more posteriorly and then by flexing the knee.

16.4.3 Positioning the Patient

The patient should be positioned supine on the operating table in such a way that the table can be broken during the procedure and the knee flexed. Flexion of the knee improves visualization of the joint. If the table is tilted to induce a slightly inclined Trendelenburg position, the patient will not slide forward. The dependent position of the leg applies traction, frees an assistant from holding the leg, and allows the surgeon to apply a varus or valgus force by simply pushing on the foot in the desired direction.

16.4.4 Timing the Surgical Procedure

There are only three situations in which a tibial plateau fracture has to be treated as an emergency. These are: an open fracture, an acute compartment syndrome, and a fracture associated with a vascular injury. The guide to the timing of the surgical procedure in all others is provided by the state of the patient, the state of any associated injuries, the state of the limb, and, finally, the state of the soft tissue envelope. In some cases the initial swelling or contusion of the soft tissue envelope may be so severe as to preclude an early surgical repair. If there are no contraindications, the simple plateau fracture may be dealt with immediately. In the more complex fracture patterns, particularly if the comminution is severe, we prefer to perform the repair on an elective basis after a careful evaluation of the fracture with all the necessary ancillary studies completed. If a delay of more than 1–2 days is necessary, then the leg should not be immobilized in a long leg plaster or other type of splint because this does not prevent shortening, which will result in further displacement and telescoping of fragments. It is best to place the leg in skeletal traction until such time as the surgical procedure can be executed (Apley 1979). The placement of the Steinmann pin for traction is very important. If placed too high, it will either be in the fracture or interfere with the safety of subsequent surgical repair. It should be inserted a handbreadth below the most distal discernible fracture line.

16.4.5 Methods of Open Reduction and Internal Fixation

Before discussing the open reduction and internal fixation of each type in detail, we would like to point out certain generalities which are important. The lateral plateau is convex from front to back and side to side, whereas the medial one is concave. The lateral plateau is higher than the medial one. Both the medial and lateral plateaux slope approximately 10° from front to back. Therefore, in a standard anteroposterior radiograph of the knee, the plateaux appear elliptical in shape, and the posterior joint edge is represented by the lower of the two lines (Moore and Harvey 1974).

The medial plateau is usually much less comminuted than the lateral, hence, if both plateaux are fractured, one can usually get better purchase with screws in the medial one. Because the lateral plateau is higher, one has to be careful with the insertion of the proximal screws medially from the lateral side so as not to enter the medial joint space and damage the medial plateau. In a bicondylar fracture the reconstruction should begin with the simple fracture, which is usually the medial of the two.

In elevating the depressed articular cartilage fragments, it is best to elevate them "en masse" from below. If one attempts to lift up the fragments through the joint, one is usually left with a number of totally devitalized loose articular fragments which cannot be successfully put back and fitted together. When the articular fragments are driven into supporting cancellous bone of the metaphysis, the cancellous bone compacts and holds the fragments together. When the fragments are elevated together with the compacted cancellous bone, they do not fall apart, but behave as if they were held together by a skin. Thus, to initiate the elevation, a periosteal elevator should be pushed deep into the compacted metaphysis. With upward pressure, the whole segment is gradually dislodged. A broad bone punch is then introduced from below and the fragments are gradually tapped back into place until they are slightly overreduced.

Once the fragments are elevated, one faces, of course, the problem of how to keep them from falling back. There are two maneuvers which are helpful. The first is to insert a massive bone graft below the fragments into the hole in the metaphysis which is created when the fragments are elevated. The second is to compress them circumferentially by means of the remaining intact portion of the plateau. This is accomplished with lag screws which, when tightened, tend to squeeze and narrow the proximal tibia. Some authors have suggested the use of cortical slabs to hold up the elevated fragments. Cancellous bone allograft stored appropriately has also been used successfully in these areas with good healing and incorporation of the grafted bone (A. Gross, 1983, personal communication). We prefer pure cancellous bone autograft such as one can obtain either from the iliac crest or the greater trochanter. The cancellous bone adapts better to the shape of the hole and, when compacted, provides excellent support for

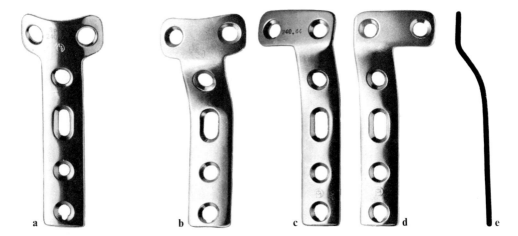

Fig. 16.15a–e. The different plates available for internal fixation of the proximal tibia: **a** Four-hole T plate; **b** T buttress plate; **c, d** L-buttress plates. **e** In profile the tibial plateau buttress plate shows its double bend. (From Müller et al. 1979)

the articular fragments, strong enough to permit early movement but not early weight bearing.

The plates which are used to support the cortex of a metaphysis from crumbling or displacing under axial thrust fulfill the function of buttressing and are called buttress plates (see Fig. 16.3b). Any plate, if it is carefully contoured to the shape of the metaphysis, can be made to function as a buttress plate. Because metaphyses in different areas of the body have specific contours, the AO/ASIF, to save time in contouring, have made available several precontoured plates for use. Thus, for the proximal tibia, we have the regular T plate which best fits the medial side. For the lateral side, we have the precontoured T buttress plate and the L buttress plate which comes in a right and a left version (Fig. 16.15).

A buttress plate must be accurately contoured to the cortex it is supposed to buttress. Even the precontoured plates must be adjusted to fit, for if a buttress plate were to be accidentally placed under tension, it could lead to the very displacement it is trying to prevent. Therefore, whenever a buttress plate is fixed to the bone, the first screws should be inserted through the distal end of the plate and the remainder inserted in orderly fashion one after another as one approaches the joint. If the two ends of the plate are fixed to bone first and there is a gap between the plate and bone, as the remaining screws are inserted, the plate is brought under tension, which in a buttress plate could result in displacement and deformity.

On the medial side, as already stated, the plate is applied to the anteromedial face of the proximal metaphysis deep to the pes anserina and the anterior fibers of the medial collateral ligament. On the lateral side, because of the proximal fibula, the plate has to be fixed slightly obliquely with its

distal end flush with the anterior tibial crest and its proximal end as far posterolaterally as is necessary. The L plate allows more lateral buttressing without getting in the way of the proximal fibula. We have usually found it best, as already stated, to fix the plate first distally and then advance proximally with the screws as the plate is fixed. The proximal lag screws are usually inserted through the most proximal holes at the very end, or above or beside the plate. Their position is governed by the configuration of the fracture and not the placement of the plate.

In type V and type VI fractures, one should always begin with the less comminuted tibial plateau so that one side can be reduced and provisionally buttressed while the other side is reconstructed. For provisional fixation, the proximal cancellous screws should be directed posteriorly to engage the posterior cortex, which may in some cases be the only cortex left intact. As in fractures of the distal tibia, it is necessary first to reestablish the normal length, and this is clearly best and easiest to accomplish on the side of least comminution. Occasionally, however, the comminution may be so severe that it is impossible to reconstruct either side. Under these circumstances, we have found it best to fix a T plate distally on the medial side and a T buttress plate or a longer plate similarly contoured on the lateral side. These two plates are then used as a lateral scaffolding between which the fragments of the tibia are erected. A bar bolt can then be inserted through the plates proximally to tie them together.

We prefer to carry out the articular reconstruction with the limb exsanguinated and a pneumatic tourniquet inflated. This controls bleeding and improves visualization, which leads to a more accurate articular reconstruction. In order to shorten the tourniquet time as well as the time the tibial wound is left open, we prefer to obtain our cancellous bone from the donor site and close that incision before the tibial reconstruction is begun.

16.4.6 Internal Fixation of Different Fracture Types

16.4.6.1 Type I

This wedge fracture of the lateral plateau (see Fig. 16.2) can usually be fixed with only cancellous lag screws and washers. In young people with a strong cortex, buttressing is not required, but this fracture type in an older individual requires a buttress plate to prevent redisplacement which could occur on axial loading, the result of muscular contraction alone without actual weight bearing.

16.4.6.2 Type II

This fracture has, in addition to the lateral wedge, a central articular depression (see Fig. 16.3). Because it occurs in older, more osteoporotic bone, one cannot rely on lag screws alone to prevent redisplacement of the fragments. A buttress plate is almost always a must.

16.4.6.3 Type III

In this central depression fracture, the lateral cortex is intact circumferentially (see Fig. 16.5). Thus, theoretically, there is no need for a buttress plate and no need for any lag screws because, first, there is nothing to lag together and, secondly, the lag screws cannot support the articular fragments nor can they hold up the bone graft. The hole which one has to make in the lateral cortex weakens the bone. The cortex is also very thin and fragile. Although these factors have to be judged at the time of surgery, we have nevertheless frequently buttressed the lateral cortex to prevent its possible subsequent fracture and displacement. Also, the lag screw, if passed under the elevated portion of the plateau, will be of some help in keeping it elevated.

16.4.6.4 Type IV

This fracture of the medial plateau (see Fig. 16.6) can, in the young individual, be satisfactorily fixed with lag screws; otherwise, it should be buttressed. The frequently avulsed intercondylar eminence with the attached cruciate ligaments should be either fixed back in place with a lag screw or held reduced with a loop of wire tied under tension over the intact anterior cortex.

16.4.6.5 Type V

This bicondylar fracture, if it comes to surgery, requires buttressing on both sides (see Fig. 16.7). Lag screws alone are never enough to prevent displacement.

16.4.6.6 Type VI

In this fracture, the metaphysis is dissociated from the diaphysis; therefore, at least one of the two buttress plates must be strong and long enough to bridge to the diaphysis and act either as a compression or a neutralization plate (see Fig. 16.8). It should be a narrow 4,5 DC-plate rather than a long T plate. The T plate is too flexible for this purpose.

16.4.7 Ligament and Meniscal Repair

Every effort should be made to preserve the menisci. Torn menisci should be repaired if at all technically possible (Wirth 1981; Hohl and Moore 1983; see also Sect. 16.4.2). We have practiced open meniscal repair for years, with the view that even a failed repair which would subsequently lead to a meniscectomy would be better than immediate meniscectomy, because of the protective effect of the meniscus on the underlying articular cartilage. To date we have not had to carry out a secondary meniscectomy. We believe that disrupted collateral ligaments and capsules should also be meticulously repaired. Similarly, if a cruciate ligament is avulsed with a piece of bone, the bone should be reduced and fixed in place. If the cruciate ligament is disrupted in its substance, then we believe that such a disruption should be ignored and repaired at some point in the future if instability makes it necessary. Such a rupture requires a primary ligamentous substitution, which necessitates a period of immobilization to ensure healing. In the presence of a fracture the joint must not be immobilized because it becomes permanently stiff.

16.4.8 Postoperative Care

The postoperative care of fractures of the tibial plateau is governed by the findings at surgery and the degree of stability achieved by the internal fixation. If, at the time of the open reduction and internal fixation, a satisfactory reduction has been achieved of both the joint and metaphysis, and if the internal fixation is stable, then we apply a padded dressing to the knee and elevate the extremity with the knee in 45°–60° flexion on a Böhler–Braun splint. We do not believe in padded compression dressings as an effective means of controlling postoperative swelling: this is far better achieved with the suction drainage which we use routinely for the first 24–48 h. After the first 2–3 days, once we are satisfied that the wound is healing without any complications, we encourage the patient to begin active motion of the knee. Usually by the end of the 1st week, the patient has regained full extension and at least 90% flexion, and by the end of the 2nd or 3rd week, full flexion. The advent of continuous passive motion machines has greatly facilitated the postoperative care of these patients and improved their prognosis. At the end of the surgical procedure, a light, unobstructive dressing is applied to the extremity and the extremity is positioned on a machine while the patient is still asleep. The machine is set to permit full extension and flexion to 40°–60°, which is increased to 90° as quickly as the patient will allow. Initially, the patients do not tolerate rapid cycling. We have found that one full flexion and extension every 2 min is a comfortable pace. With the passage of time, it is possible to increase the rate as well as the degree of flexion. Usually at the end of 1 week, it is possible to cease continuous passive motion, and the patients are able to carry on with their rehabilitation without reliance on passive aids. We have noted that with the machines, the patients very rapidly lose power in their quadriceps muscle and often have to stay in hospital just as long as before, concentrating on regaining strength instead of motion. We have instituted faradic stimulation of the quadriceps muscle in conjunction with the continuous passive motion machines during the extension phase, and this has helped considerably in speeding up the recovery.

We feel that major intraarticular fractures should be treated immediately after surgery with CPM because of its influence on articular cartilage healing. Splinting as described should be used only if a CPM is not available.

Regardless of how stable the reduction, we do not allow weight bearing for 10–12 weeks. We believe in early active motion since it not only ensures a return of motion to the knee and good function of the soft tissue envelope, but also has a beneficial effect on the healing of the articular cartilage (Mitchell and Shepard 1980; Salter et al. 1980, 1986). Early weight bearing can not only lead to loss of reduction, joint incongruity, and malalignment, but it can interfere with the healing of articular cartilage by loading the tissue when it is not sufficiently mature to accept the load.

If, at the time of surgery, the diagnosis of a disrupted collateral ligament is either confirmed or established, then the disruption is repaired. Because early motion is necessary to prevent stiffness and because the ligamentous repair must be protected from lateral bending forces which could disrupt the repair, we protect such a knee in a cast brace. This protects the ligamentous repair from lateral bending forces and permits full mobilization. In the presence of a fracture, we use polycentric joint hinges, but do not restrict the range of motion. The knee in the brace is then mobilized with CPM as described.

If, at the end of surgery, we judge the internal fixation to be unstable, then we protect it from overload. If only one plateau is involved, a cast brace with the knee stressed in the direction of the uninvolved plateau provides adequate protection. If both plateaux are involved, one must decide whether sufficient longitudinal stability has been achieved to prevent shortening. If doubt exists, then such a knee must be mobilized on a splint with skeletal traction for at least 3–4 weeks before it is transferred into a cast brace for the remainder of healing.

16.5 Summary and Conclusions

Fractures of the tibial plateau involve a major weight-bearing joint. Thus, to achieve good joint function one must strive to achieve joint congruity, axial alignment, stability, and a satisfactory range of motion. If the fracture is stable, the joint congruous, and the alignment acceptable, then closed treatment is the method of choice (Fig. 16.16). Early motion must be instituted, however, because if immobilized, even with closed treatment, the knee will stiffen permanently. Joint instability and significant incongruity are clear indications for surgical treatment. The majority of these fractures occur in the fifth and sixth decades, and at least

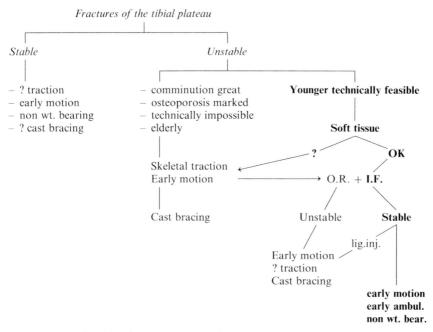

Fig. 16.16. An algorithm for the treatment of tibial plateau fractures. *O.R. + I.F.*, open reduction and internal fixation

50% of the patients who underwent surgical treatment had some degree of osteoporosis (Schatzker et al. 1979). Thus, age and osteoporosis cannot be employed as an argument against open treatment. The patients who underwent surgical treatment had, on average, at least three times the degree of depression of their articular surface, and yet the overall results of surgical treatment were better than those of closed treatment (Schatzker et al. 1979). Therefore, the degree of joint depression should not mitigate against surgery. We have stressed the following:

1. *Anatomical reduction.* This ensures the reconstruction of joint congruity and axial alignment which, in the presence of intact ligaments, will also ensure joint stability.

2. *Elevation of the plateau en masse.* Depressed comminuted impacted articular fragments must be handled as a continuum and elevated by pushing from below on the whole area of depression till it reexpands. This ensures the proper reduction of the fragments, enhances their stability, and where possible, preserves their blood supply.

3. *Bone grafting of the defect in the metaphysis.* The elevation of the depressed articulation leaves a defect in the metaphysis which must be bone grafted to prevent redisplacement.

4. *Stable internal fixation.* The vertical fracture lines in the articular surface and metaphysis must be stabilized with the aid of compression by means of lag screws. This greatly enhances articular cartilage healing and regeneration (Mitchell and Shepard 1980). The metaphysis must be buttressed to prevent redisplacement due to axial load. Stable fixation eliminates pain and makes early motion possible.

5. *Early motion.* Early motion is necessary for the preservation of joint motion and soft tissue function. Furthermore, it has a profoundly beneficial effect on cartilage regeneration (Salter et al. 1980, 1986).

Our results of treatment, based on these principles, have shown an 89% acceptable result, which is better than other methods of treatment (Schatzker et al. 1979).

References

Apley AG (1979) Fractures of the tibial plateau. Orthop Clin North Am 10:61–74

Hohl M, Hopp E (1976) Ligament injuries in tibial condylar fractures. J Bone Joint Surg 58A:279 (abstract)

Hohl M, Moore TM (1983) Articular fractures of the proximal tibia. In: McCollister Evarts C (ed) Surgery of the musculoskeletal system, vol 7. Churchill Livingstone, New York, pp 11–135

Kennedy JC, Bailey WH (1968) Experimental tibial plateau fractures. J Bone Joint Surg 50A:1522–1534

Mitchell N, Shepard N (1980) Healing of articular cartilage in intra-articular fractures in rabbits. J Bone Joint Surg 62A:628–634

Moore TM, Harvey JP Jr (1974) Roentgenographic measurement of tibial plateau depression due to fracture. J Bone Joint Surg 56A:155–160

Müller ME, Allgöwer M, Schneider R, Willenegger H (1979) Manual of internal fixation, 2nd edn. Springer, Berlin Heidelberg New York, p 257

Rasmussen PS (1973) Tibial condylar fractures. J Bone Joint Surg 55A:1331–1350

Roberts JM (1968) Fractures of the condyles of the tibia. J Bone Joint Surg 50A:1505–1521

Salter RB, Simmonds DF, Malcolm BW, Rumble EJ, MacMichael D (1980) The biological effects of continuous passive motion on the healing of full-thickness defects in articular cartilage: an experimental investigation in the rabbit. J Bone Joint Surg 62A:1232–1251

Salter RB, Hamilton HW, Wedge JH, Tile M, Torode IP, O'Driscoll SW, Murnaghan J, Saringer JH (1986) Clinical application of basic research on continuous passive motion for disorders and injuries of synovial joints: preliminary report of a feasibility study. Techniques Orthop 1(1):74–91

Schatzker J, McBroom R, Bruce D (1979) The tibial plateau fracture. The Toronto experience. Clin Orthop 138:94–104

Shrive N (1974) The weight-bearing role of the menisci of the knee. J Bone Joint Surg 56B:381 (abstract)

Walker S, Erkman MJ (1975) The role of the menisci in force transmission across the knee. Clin Orthop 109:184–192

Wirth CR (1981) Meniscus repair. Clin Orthop 157:153–160

17 Fractures of the Tibia

M. Tile

17.1 Introduction

The management of the tibial fracture remains controversial despite advances in both nonoperative and operative care. Orthopedic opinion is often cyclic, and in no area of orthopedic endeavor is this better seen than in the management of the fractured tibia. Orthopedic surgeons with an interest in orthopedic history would be well advised to study this particular fracture which reflects the cyclic changes in opinion so clearly.

During our orthopedic residency and careers as clinicians, we have been subjected to this full cycle. During our residency, we were taught that most tibial fractures were best treated by open reduction and internal fixation; unfortunately, the surgery was often inadequately performed and indifferent results were achieved, with many serious complications. This, in turn, led to an extreme nonoperative approach, championed on the North American continent by Dehne (Dehne et al. 1961) and Sarmiento (1967). In the preceding era, this nonoperative approach had been popularized by Böhler (1936) of the Viennese School.

The introduction of the AO/ASIF method of fracture care led to a renewed interest in internal fixation based on sound biomechanical and biological principles. In the hands of the AO/ASIF surgeons, marked improvement was reported in the results of operative fracture care (Allgöwer 1967). However, many problems remained.

It is obvious that there is no perfect method of treating all tibial fractures. Different circumstances demand differing approaches to the same problem. At the present time, improved methods of both nonoperative care of the fractured tibia, using functional casts, cast braces, or splints and operative care, using the principles and implants of the AO group (Müller et al. 1979), where indicated, should allow decision making to be based on logical principles, which in turn should resolve the so-called controversy of the fractured tibia. We

should reject the theories of dogmatists which state that "all tibia fractures must be treated nonoperatively" or, conversely, that "all tibia fractures should be treated operatively." It is time to remove this type of dogma from our thinking and to individualize the treatment for each patient.

Logical management of any tibial fracture can only flow from a precise knowledge of its natural history. For the individual case, the natural history is dependent upon the personality of the particular fracture to be treated. Once the personality has been determined by a careful clinical and radiographic assessment, and compared to the natural history of similar fracture types, a treatment protocol for that particular patient will become relatively clear. This knowledge will also allow the surgeon to carefully weigh and balance the alternative methods of management and clearly outline them to the patient. Where clear-cut alternative treatment methods exist, the surgeon should not play God, but should allow the patient to share in the decision-making process.

17.2 Natural History

Most fractures of the tibia will heal if treated by nonoperative means – this fact is undeniable. Watson-Jones (1943) has stated that "if immobilized long enough, all fractures will eventually heal."

Charnley (1961) stressed the importance of the soft tissue hinge on the healing process of the tibial fracture. He recognized that fractures with an intact periosteal hinge did well, whereas those with gross displacement, indicating complete periosteal rupture, did less well. He recommended primary surgery for the tibial fracture with an intact fibula and for any tibia with a gap at the fracture following reduction. Astutely, he recommended early bone grafting procedures for fractures with predictably poor results.

Nicoll (1964), in a definitive study of 705 tibial fractures treated prior to the widespread use of the early weight-bearing method, was able to clearly describe the natural history of the tibial shaft fracture treated nonoperatively. It was he who coined the term *"personality of the fracture"*, by which the eventual outcome of each case could be predicted. The major factors affecting the outcome were:

1. The amount of initial displacement
2. The degree of comminution
3. The amount of soft tissue damage in the open fracture
4. The presence or absence of sepsis

The incidence of favorable outcome for fractures managed by nonoperative means ranged from 91% in the "good personality" types to 61% in the "poor personality" types, and to only 40% if sepsis was involved. These figures indicate a significant complication rate with many poor functional results in all categories. In order to improve upon these results, two major schools of thought evolved, one stressing the importance of early weight bearing to the ultimate function of the limb, the other, the importance of stable internal fixation.

17.2.1 Nonoperative School

Böhler (1936) had recommended that all major tibial fractures be treated with skeletal traction for 3 weeks followed by a weight-bearing plaster cast until healing was complete. However, Watson-Jones and Coltart (1943) clearly showed that traction for tibial shaft fractures had a deleterious effect on the rate of union.

Dehne eliminated the preliminary period of skeletal traction, and instituted immediate weight bearing for the patient in a long leg cast with the knee extended. In 1961, he and his colleagues reported good functional results with no nonunions.

Fig. 17.1a–d. Nonoperative management of a spiral tibial fracture. **a, b** Anteroposterior and lateral radiographs of a 59-year-old woman showing a markedly displaced fracture of the tibia and fibula. Note also the undisplaced butterfly fragment. Closed manipulation under general anesthesia and plaster immobilization for 12 weeks resulted in firm bony union and an excellent functional result with shortening of only 1.1 cm (**c, d**)

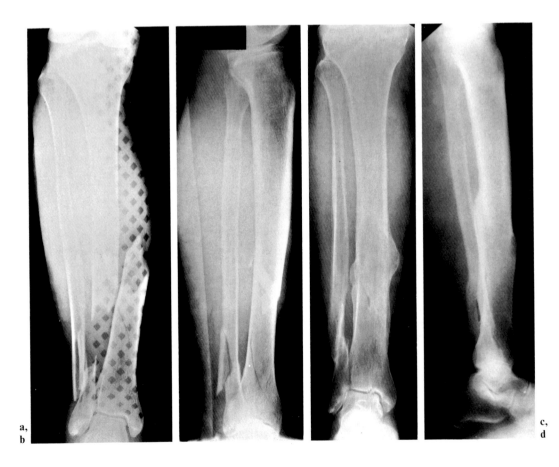

a,
b

c,
d

In 1967, Sarmiento, using the combination of early weight-bearing casts and functional braces, reported no nonunions in 100 consecutive fractures of the tibial shaft. His biomechanical and clinical studies indicated few complications with early weight bearing, and many benefits. Excessive shortening was not the problem it was expected to be – the fracture rarely shortened beyond its initial displacement, the average being 1.9 cm (Fig. 17.1). Weight bearing on the injured extremity allowed early functional rehabilitation, thus preventing joint stiffness, swelling, and other complications, while also having a beneficial effect on fracture healing. Other reports by the same author with Latta (1981) corroborated the above results.

Brown (1974) soon confirmed these improved results. Thus, the simple addition of early weight bearing positively altered the natural history of the tibial fracture without affecting the safety factor inherent in closed treatment.

Thus, all of these studies indicate that the vast majority of tibial fractures will heal with nonoperative treatment, and will result in good functional limbs, if the patients follow with the prescribed programs.

17.2.2 Operative School

In 1957 the AO group, studying the poor functional results then being obtained by nonoperative treatment, placed open reduction and stable internal fixation on a firm scientific basis. They believed that the failure of surgical treatment, leading to its widespread condemnation at the time, was mainly the result of poor surgery. Stable internal fixation would, they believed, eliminate the complications resulting from plaster immobilization, that is, "plaster disease". Careful documentation by devotees of that method have indicated excellent functional results with no sacrifice of fracture healing, as a study of the excellent papers of Rüedi, Webb and Allgöwer (1976), Allgöwer and Perren (1980), Karlstrom and Olerud (1974), and others will indicate. Complications in their hands were minimal (Tables 17.1, 17.2a–c).

Thus, it would appear that both schools have achieved the same end by markedly different means, that is, excellent functional results with few complications.

From the above reports, it is self-evident that nonoperative management will achieve satisfactory results in the majority of tibial fractures, without the need for surgery. Are the arguments of the proponents of the operative school cogent en-

Table 17.1. Results of 617 cases of fractured tibias, treated by stable internal fixation (total of 4 fully controlled series: 1958/59, 1959/60, 1961/62, 1962/63). No case received insurance compensation for permanent partial damage of more than 20% (total invalidity being taken as 100%). (From Allgöwer and Perren 1980)

Fracture			Late disability ($<20\%$)	
Site	Type	Number of cases	n	%
Shaft of the tibia	closed	535	6 =	1.1%
	compound	45	8 =	17.7%
Distal tibia	intra-articular	37	3 =	8.1%
Total		617	17 =	2.7%

Table 17.2a. Follow-up of 435 consecutive tibial shaft fractures with DCP fixation. (From Allgöwer and Perren 1980)

	Fracture		Total	
	Closed	Open		
DCP fixation	334	101	435	
Follow-up:	323	95	418	
– personal	300	88		388
– X-ray and questionnaire	23	7		30
– no follow-up	2	–	2	
– died	9	6	15	

Table 17.2b. Functional results 1–2 years after DCP fixation of 332 closed fractures of the tibial shaft (see comment Table 17.2c). (From Allgöwer and Perren 1980)

	Cases	in %
Good	317	98%
Acceptable	6	2%
Poor	–	
Total	323	

Table 17.2c. Functional results 1–2 years after DCP fixation of 95 open fractures of the tibial shaft; *good:* functional recovery compatible with normal professional and extraprofessional activities; *acceptable:* occasional complaints (pain, fatigue), normal professional, reduced extraprofessional (sport!) activities; *poor:* any of the following: significant pain in tibio-tarsal or knee joints, reduced professional activities, non-union, amputation. (From Allgöwer and Perren 1980)

	Cases	in %
Good	84	88.3%
Acceptable	8	8 %
Poor	3	3.5%
Total	95	

ough to sway us into adopting their approach –
that is, almost universal operative management of
displaced tibial fractures? We doubt it; therefore,
we recommend that most tibial fractures be managed nonoperatively, with the exceptions to be
noted later in this chapter. Even the argument
about plaster disease needs careful scrutiny.

17.2.3 Plaster Disease

As previously indicated, if patients comply with
their exercise program of early weight bearing,
plaster disease in nonoperative care is rarely significant. Is it, then, alone enough of a reason to recommend universal open reduction for the fractured tibia? Is it, in fact, a real entity and can
it be eliminated by an aggressive operative approach?

Plaster disease is, in our opinion, not a disease
but a syndrome. This syndrome, characterized by
swelling under the cast followed by permanent
stiffness in the immobilized joints, has many
causes, including:
1. An unrecognized compartment syndrome
2. Reflex sympathetic dystrophy
3. Thromboembolic disease
4. Severe soft tissue injury

While it may be true that eliminating the plaster
of Paris will improve early function in many cases,
it is not true that any of the above will necessarily
be eliminated by surgery. Failure to recognize that
fact may obscure an impending compartment syndrome and lead to a delay in its diagnosis.

What of the other causes of this syndrome?
To answer this question, each of them will now
be discussed in turn.

1. Compartment Syndromes. Plaster disease is often mistakenly diagnosed in patients suffering
from an unrecognized deep compartment syndrome, which is far more common in fractures
of the tibia than we have been led to believe. A
perusal of the recent literature will indicate the
growing importance of the compartment syndrome in determining the end result of a tibial
fracture. The advent of modern monitoring techniques, either intermittent or continuous, as advocated by Rorabeck (1977), Mubarek et al. (1978),
and others, makes it possible to prevent this disastrous complication by early diagnosis and aggressive management.

Patients with a tibial fracture who are placed
in a well-padded, above-knee plaster rarely have
undue or excruciating pain. If they do, a compart-

ment syndrome must be suspected. For example,
the patient shown in Fig. 17.2 a 17-year-old girl,
sustained a high-energy tibial fracture after being
thrown from a horse. She complained of severe
pain in the extremity, but never developed any
other symptoms or signs of vascular insufficiency.
The first 2 months of her treatment were agonizing
for her when she attempted to bear weight. As
treatment progressed, it became obvious that she
had developed an equinovarus foot deformity with
clawing of the toes (Fig. 17.2c, d). Union of the
fracture was also delayed for 7 months. This patient represents a typical case of a posterior compartment syndrome leading to Volkmann's
ischemic contracture of the deep posterior muscle
groups. This syndrome is often misread as plaster
disease. The residual equinovarus foot with a
cock-up deformity of the great toe is pathognomonic of this condition. Unfortunately, these patients may also have painful hyperesthesia of the
foot, a condition most difficult to eradicate.

2. Reflex Sympathetic Dystrophy. This complication, which may occur in any fracture, is occasionally seen in patients with a tibial fracture. The
patients often develop massive swelling under the
cast and will not bear weight, and a painful, stiff,
hyperesthetic foot is often the result. Since this
complication is not specific to the form of treatment, operative or nonoperative, it should not be
taken to be plaster disease.

3. Thromboembolic Disease. The functional result
is also affected by the presence of deep vein thrombosis in the injured extremity. This, in turn, may
lead to chronic edema in the extremity with all
the sequelae of that condition. We believe the incidence is higher in patients who have been kept
in plaster for long periods and that this is a true
indication of plaster disease. However, precise
data on this matter is unavailable at present, and
one must remember that deep thromboembolism
may also occur following surgery.

4. Severe Soft Tissue Injury. The functional result
is often compromised by significant soft tissue
damage. In some instances, when the soft tissue
damage is so major that it includes loss of muscle,
the damage will be permanent no matter which
mode of treatment is chosen. However, stabilization of the fracture in patients with major soft
tissue damage will allow early motion of the soft
tissues, ensuring more rapid rehabilitation and a
better final result. Recent studies by Salter (1980)
have stressed the importance of the postoperative
use of continuous passive motion. We believe that

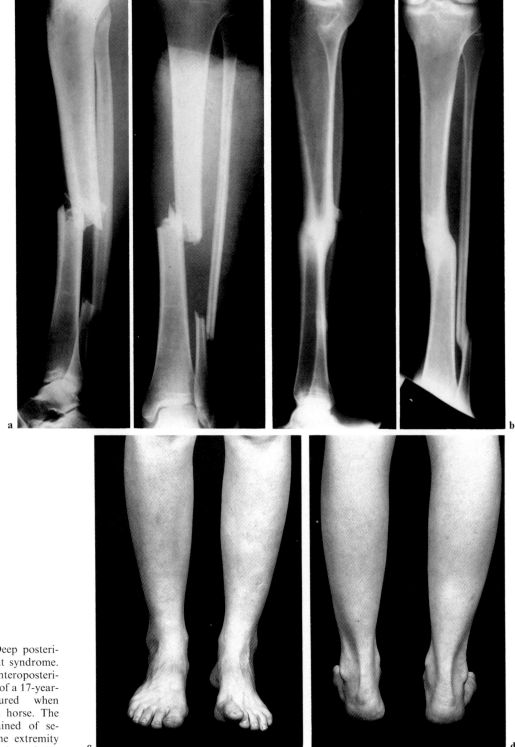

Fig. 17.2a–d. Deep posterior compartment syndrome. **a** Lateral and anteroposterior radiographs of a 17-year-old girl injured when thrown from a horse. The patient complained of severe pain in the extremity following reduction of this fracture but never developed any other signs or symptoms of vascular insufficiency. The fracture eventually united after 7 months in plaster (**b**).

c, d The photographs show the classic appearance of a deep posterior compartment syndrome. Note the equinovarus foot and the cock-up deformity of the left great toe, as well as the varus position of the heel on the posterior view. The patient also complained of painful paresthesia. Secondary reconstructive surgery (a triple arthrodesis) was required but success was only partial. (From Tile 1980)

this technique, when combined with stable fracture fixation, will in the future allow much quicker and better rehabilitation of the patient with a major soft tissue injury associated with fracture.

Thus, if plaster disease is not truly a disease, and open operative treatment aids only cases with major soft tissue injury, and perhaps lowers the incidence of thromboembolic disease, without altering the problem of the compartment syndrome or reflex sympathetic dystrophy, what factors, if any, favor operative treatment of the tibial diaphyseal fracture? The answer will be made clearer by a study of the factors influencing the natural history of the tibial fracture.

17.2.4 Factors Influencing the Natural History

In order to justify any open operation on the tibia, we must clearly define those characteristics of the fracture which adversely affect its ability to heal satisfactorily with normal function, that is, affect the natural history of the fracture. Such factors do exist, and may be present in the fracture itself, the limb, or the patient, and they are modified by the experience and expertise of the health care team (Fig. 17.3). By carefully weighing and balancing all of these factors for your particular patient, that is, by assessing the personality of the injury, the most logical method of treatment should become apparent.

17.2.4.1 Pathoanatomy of the Fracture

The tibia, like the ulna, is an unique anatomical structure. Its anteromedial surface is entirely subcutaneous and its location in the body makes it prone to injury, often associated with high energy. The pathoanatomy of the fracture (that is, the location, morphology, and degree of displacement) has a marked influence on the outcome of the fracture. As important as the pathoanatomy of the fracture itself is the state of the soft tissues. A careful analysis of the pathoanatomy of the fracture and the state of the soft tissues will allow the surgeon to identify the personality type to which it most closely relates, and thereby predict the expected outcome.

a) Anatomical Site

The natural history of the tibia fracture is influenced by the location of the fracture, whether it is in the diaphysis, the transition zone extending into the metaphysis, or the epiphysis, with or without joint involvement. The response of diaphyseal cortical bone is quite different from that of metaphyseal cancellous bone.

Articular (Epiphysis). If the fracture extends into either the knee (Fig. 17.8) or ankle joint (Fig. 17.9) and is displaced, then dealing with that aspect of the fracture assumes overriding importance, since the end result will depend upon obtaining a stable anatomic reduction and early motion of the joint.

Metaphysis and Transition Zone. Fractures in the metaphysis or in the transition zone between the metaphysis and the diaphysis may be caused by compressive or tensile forces. If caused by *compressive forces*, the fractures are often crushed and axially malaligned. Healing of this cancellous bone may be rapid, but in an unacceptable position. Closed reduction of this type of fracture may often leave a gap at the site of crush, with a tendency for the fracture to redisplace into it. Also, disimpaction of the fracture changes it from a stable to an unstable one.

Transition zone fractures caused by *shear forces* may be due to direct or indirect trauma. Those caused by direct trauma, especially in young people, are usually markedly unstable. The same may be true of those caused by indirect trauma, with torsional forces. The force required to fracture the

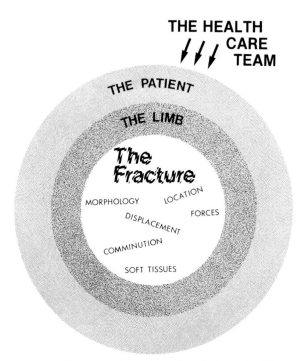

Fig. 17.3. The personality of an injury is determined by a careful appraisal of the patient, the limb, the fracture, and the expertise of the health care team. (From Tile 1984)

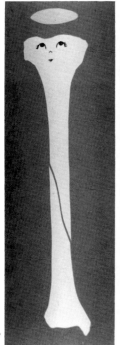
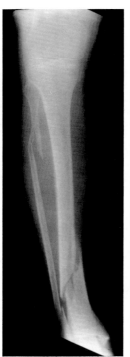
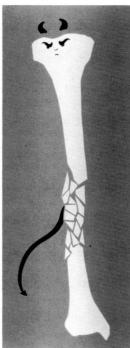
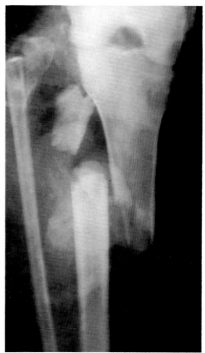

a,
b

c,
d

metaphysis of a young patient with normal bone is extreme. A shearing injury through the metaphysis or the transition zone between the metaphysis and diaphysis is therefore a high-energy one, and may be associated with considerable instability and displacement. If this displacement results in poor bone apposition, despite adequate nonoperative management, difficulties may arise. Since cancellous metaphyseal bone heals quickly if compressed and slowly if displaced, open reduction and compression of some fractures in the metaphysis or the transition zone may be desirable.

Diaphysis. Unstable, displaced diaphyseal fractures of the tibia may be slow to heal. In these cases, the soft tissue envelope, which includes both muscle and periosteum, may be grossly disrupted. As a result, maintenance of an acceptable reduction may be difficult and union may be delayed.

b) Morphology

The morphology of the fracture will suggest the type of violence that caused it, whether transverse, short oblique, or spiral, displaced or undisplaced, comminuted or not.

Transverse and short oblique fractures, unless associated with a pathologic lesion in the bone, are indicative of a more violent force than are spiral fractures. Marked comminution and gross dis-

Fig. 17.4a–d. Personality traits of tibia fractures. A "happy" tibial fracture (**a, b**), a low-energy spiral fracture caused by rotation, is contrasted to an "unhappy" tibial fracture (**c, d**), transverse, severely comminuted, and usually open

placement, suggesting complete disruption of the soft tissue envelope, further emphasize the violent nature of the injury.

Therefore, it is possible for a pattern of injury to emerge from a study of these factors. A high-energy injury caused by shearing forces is usually transverse, comminuted, and markedly displaced, while spiral fractures with minimal displacement and minimal comminution represent examples of low-energy injury (Fig. 17.4). Definite personality traits of the injury will become more apparent if one considers the state of the soft tissues.

17.2.4.2 The Soft Tissue Injury

The state of the soft tissues is at least as important as the morphological appearance of the fracture. Open fractures of the tibia will be considered in more detail later in this chapter. Suffice it to say here that the more violent the trauma, the more likely the presence of major soft tissue damage.

This soft tissue damage may be overt, with an open wound, or presumed, with massive swelling, ecchymoses, and instability of the fracture. These closed fractures may be accompanied by complete disruption of the soft tissue envelope, leading to hematoma and massive edema and thereby causing increased compartment pressure and tension on the skin. Fracture blisters may appear early, and will greatly influence the management decisions. If the fracture is open, the site and size of the laceration and the degree of muscle damage and possible contamination are all important factors. Recently, Tscherne and Gotzen (1984) have classified soft tissue injury associated with closed fractures. This classification is discussed fully in Chap. 18 and later on in this chapter (Sect. 17.3.1.2).

17.2.4.3 Other Injuries to the Limb

The presence or absence of other injuries in the same limb will greatly affect the natural history of a tibial fracture. Fractures of the pelvis and acetabulum may require long-term bed rest, and the beneficial effect of early weight bearing is thus out of reach. Fractures of the femur associated with fractures of the tibia usually have a major injury to the knee associated with them. This injury, known as the "floating knee", has a poor prognosis with nonoperative treatment.

The presence or absence of an arterial or nerve injury or an early compartment syndrome will greatly influence the decision making in the management of a tibial fracture. An arterial injury in particular has a gravely deleterious effect on the prognosis of a tibial fracture.

17.2.4.4 Factors in the Patient

a) General Considerations

It is important to carefully assess the general state of the patient. His or her age is important at the two extremes. In the skeletally immature patient, open reduction of the tibia is almost never indicated. In the older individual, on the other hand, having decided that open reduction and internal fixation are strongly indicated and important, the surgeon may find him- or herself faced with extremely osteoporotic bone in which it is impossible to achieve stable internal fixation. Therefore, the physiological age of the patient, especially with reference to the presence of osteoporosis, is important.

The patient's occupation and recreational habits should be known so that there can be no major disparity between the expectation of the patient and the expectation of the surgeon with respect to the quality of the end result. This is especially true in the case of the professional athlete.

Finally, the pretrauma general medical state of the patient must be considered prior to the patient's subjection to a general anesthetic.

b) The Polytraumatized Patient

Patients with injuries to many body systems have a high risk of developing respiratory complications. If these patients are rapidly mobilized, especially in the upright position, many of these complications may be prevented or reversed (Border et al. 1975). Therefore, current surgical practice would indicate that early stabilization of fractures and rapid mobilization of the polytraumatized patient are beneficial to both the fracture and the patient (McMurtry et al. 1984).

In the tibia, however, this is not a prime indication for surgery, since patients can be mobilized with a plaster cast. However, when associated with other fractures in the same limb, some type of stabilization of the tibia, whether internal or external, is often desirable.

17.2.4.5 The Health Care Team

A realistic assessment of one's health care team is often difficult, but in deciding upon the management of a tibial fracture this assessment becomes vital. Where clear alternatives to treatment exist, one must choose a route that will not only give superior results, *but will also be safest for the patient*. Good nonoperative management is far preferable to poor operative management, the results of which can be disastrous. The patient may be left with the worst of both worlds – the trauma of inadequate surgery superimposed upon the trauma of the injury, which often compromises the results and exposes the patient to needless risk, especially of sepsis. Therefore, as a surgeon one must appraise one's own ability and that of one's team to achieve the type of stable fixation that we have been stressing before embarking on operative care of a tibial fracture. The surgeon must have available a complete armamentarium of modern internal and external fixation devices. For open reduction and internal fixation, the infection rate in any institution should not exceed 2% and should preferably be well below 1% for elective orthopedic surgery. If the team is not experienced in modern biomechanical principles and methods of fixation, the surgeon should decide whether the surgical indications in a particular patient are definite or relative. If definite, the patient should be referred to another center, and if relative, nonoperative means should be employed.

17.2.5 Summary

At the worst end of the personality scale is the grossly displaced, highly comminuted, open fracture with skin loss and vascular compromise; at the best end, the spiral, minimally displaced, closed fracture (Fig. 17.4). Fractures, however, do not come in neat packages with specific labels, nor with absolute – that is, good or bad – personalities. Each patient is unique, his or her injury falling somewhere in the spectrum. By determining the specific characteristics of the fracture and by predicting how those characteristics will affect its natural outcome, the surgeon will have taken the first and most logical step in the management of that fracture. That initial management decision will have far greater influence on the final outcome of the fracture than any amount of attempted late rehabilitation.

17.3 Assessment

A careful clinical and radiographic assessment, looking for those factors which will affect the natural history, is the first important step in management.

17.3.1 Clinical

17.3.1.1 History

Precise details of the injury are important, as obtained either from the patient or from reliable witnesses. From the history alone, the surgeon may be able to suspect the nature of the injury.

The *general patient profile* is of great importance and will affect the medical treatment. Of importance are the age, both chronological and physiological, the general medical state, and especially the expectations. The expectations of a professional athlete will be considerably different from those of a sedentary, physically inactive individual, and this will affect the treatment decision considerably.

17.3.1.2 Physical

A careful *general* physical examination is mandatory, as it is in any injured patient corresponding to the primary survey of the American College of Surgeons Advanced Trauma Life Support System (1981). The limb must also be inspected *locally* for the degree of soft tissue damage, the presence of an open wound, the degree of deformity and instability, the neurovascular state, and the presence of a compartment syndrome. If a compartment syndrome is suspected, pressure measurements using a monitoring device are mandatory. Continuous monitoring is being successfully used in some centers to ensure early detection of a deep compartment syndrome (Fig. 17.5).

a) Soft Tissue Assessment

The evaluation of the skin and the soft tissues is of prime importance, as it will lead the surgeon to an appreciation of the degree of violence of the injury. Attempts have been made to grade the degree of injury for both closed (Tscherne and Gotzen 1984) and open (Gustilo 1982) fractures.

Closed Fractures

The medial border of the tibia is subcutaneous, and the skin and subcutaneous tissues are therefore immediately adjacent to the periosteum. The ends of the tibial fracture frequently puncture this skin, creating an open fracture. If a puncture of the skin does not occur, the soft tissue envelope may be stretched by the hematoma and fracture displacement. However, this skin is unable to stretch very much, which causes excessive pressure on the soft tissues, leading to diminished vascularity and pressure necrosis, as exhibited by fracture blisters and dead skin. Furthermore, the muscles in the leg are encased in firm fibrous compartments which are very sensitive to increases in intracompartmental pressure. Compartment syndromes involving all compartments of the leg, the anterior, the lateral, and the posterior, are not infrequent. Therefore, the degree of soft tissue damage in closed fractures is as important as in open fractures and has major prognostic significance.

Any grading system will be handicapped by individual variations in the patients and observer bias. In managing the individual case, therefore, a careful description of the injury is more valuable than assignment of a number (Fig. 17.3). However, for the purpose of comparing results between centers and different treatment regimens, a numerical grading system is helpful, but none has been universally accepted. The following is a suggested grading system (Tscherne and Gotzen 1984; see also Fig. 18.4):

Grade 0 – Little or no soft tissue injury
Grade 1 – Superficial abrasion with moderate swelling and bruising of the skin and subcutaneous tissue

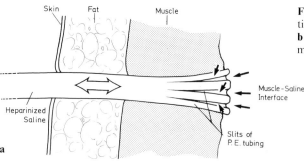

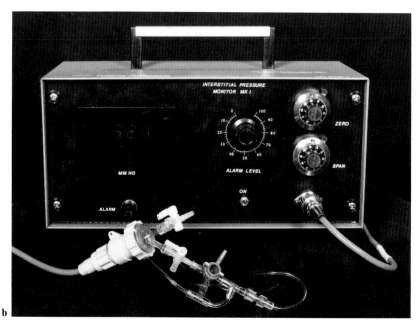

Fig. 17.5a, b. Continuous compartment monitoring. **a** Position of a slit catheter for measuring compartment pressure. **b** Measuring device for continuous compartment pressure monitoring. (Courtesy of Dr. Cecil Rorabeck)

Grade 2 – Deep contaminated abrasion with tense swelling, excessive bruising, and fracture blisters

Grade 3 – Extensive contusion, tense swelling, fracture blisters, with the addition of a compartment syndrome or injury to major vessels

Open Fractures

Many observers have attempted to grade open fractures but again, in the individual patient, a clear description of the injury is more important than a numerical grade. For example, a grade 1 injury is defined as a small puncture wound (less than 1 cm). However, the location of that small puncture wound is more important than its size. If the puncture wound is on the medial subcutaneous border of the tibia, it might have been caused by relatively low energy, since the skin lies immediately adjacent to the fractured bone. Muscle dam-

age in such a case may be relatively minor (Fig. 17.6a). However, if the puncture wound is located posteriorly, the bone ends must have penetrated a large mass of muscle to reach the skin. The puncture wound would have been the same size, but the amount of muscle damage is far greater than in the previous case (Fig. 17.6b). Failure to recognize this fact might have grave consequences for the patient, as inadequate management might lead to gas gangrene.

Therefore, any grading system of open fractures must consider the site of the lesion, the size of the lesion, the degree of muscle damage, the involvement of nerves, tendons, and blood vessels, and, finally, whether a traumatic amputation is present.

The following grading system is relatively widely accepted (Gustilo 1982):

Grade 1 – Small puncture wound (<1 cm) with little visible contusion or swelling

Fig. 17.6a, b. Open fracture of the tibia. **a** A high-energy open fracture of the tibia with an anterior subcutaneous puncture wound. Note that the skin may be easily punctured without great damage to muscle. However, in **b** the fracture has displaced posteriorly through a massive amount of muscle. Major muscle necrosis may be expected here under a seemingly small skin wound. In this particular situation inadequate management might lead to grave consequences including gas gangrene. (From Tile 1980)

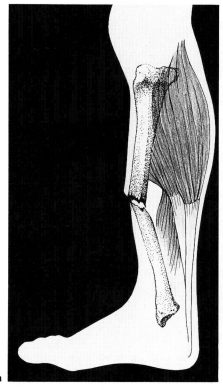
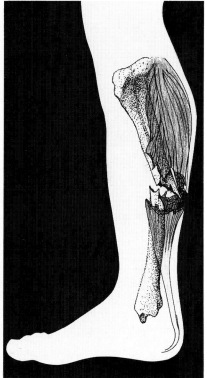

a   b

Grade 2 – Larger wound from without with visible contusion to skin

Grade 3 – Severe injury with skin contusion, skin loss, muscle crush or less severe periosteal stripping
   (a) With major muscle loss or nerve or tendon damage
   (b) With arterial injury
   (c) With traumatic amputation

b) Bony Assessment

The physical examination of the limb will allow the examiner to assess the stability of the fracture. A careful assessment of the bony injury is essential. All the factors noted in Sect. 17.2.4 must be considered, including the location (articular, metaphyseal, diaphyseal), the morphology (transverse, oblique, spiral), the degree of displacement (high- or low-energy force), and the amount of comminution. Recommendations of radiological techniques are given in the next section.

17.3.2 Radiological

In the standard examination an anteroposterior, a lateral, and an oblique radiograph will usually allow the surgeon to determine the morphology of the fracture. The radiographs must include views of both the knee and the ankle. If the fracture lines extend into a joint, tomograms are often helpful.

If vascular impairment is suspected, a special examination using arteriography may be indicated.

17.4 Management

17.4.1 Decision Making

The natural outcome of a tibial shaft injury should be a functionally excellent limb and a healed fracture. A decision favoring surgery cannot be taken lightly and must be justified by a careful assessment of the individual fracture. Only if the fracture possesses significant unfavorable personality traits and no major contraindications should surgery be contemplated, and then only by a surgeon and a team well versed in modern operative fracture care. In other words, logical decision making by the astute surgeon depends upon the natural history of the injury, altered by the specific personality traits of the individual case. *Therefore, if no clear*

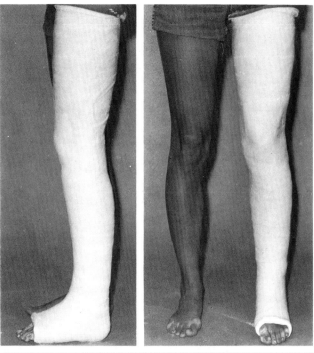

Fig. 17.7 a–c. Casts and splints in the treatment of ▶ tibial fractures. **a** Above-knee walking cast for early weight-bearing treatment in tibial fractures. **b** A functional patellar-bearing below-knee cast. **c** Functional brace allowing ankle and knee motion. (From Sarmiento and Latta 1981)

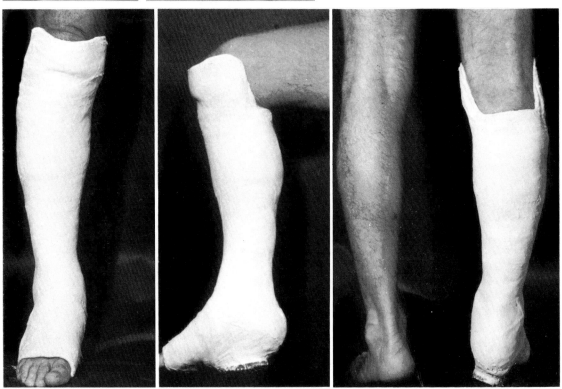

Fig. 17.7 c

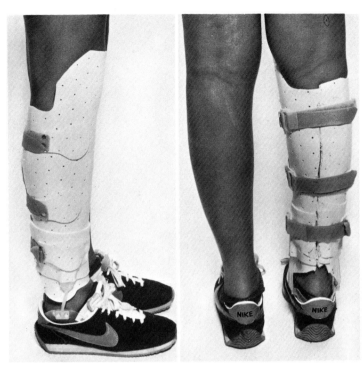

indication for surgery exists, the surgeon should proceed with nonoperative treatment.

17.4.1.1 Nonoperative Treatment

The fracture should be aligned and an above-knee *padded* plaster applied (Fig. 17.7a). A general anesthetic is rarely necessary if reduction is carried out shortly after the injury. Gravity reduction with the patient in the sitting position is often all that is required to align the fracture. If a padded plaster is not applied, the cast should be split immediately after drying to allow for soft tissue swelling. The patient should be admitted to hospital, the leg well elevated, and the patient closely monitored for any impending compartment syndrome. The use of a continuous monitoring device should rule out the potential catastrophe of a compartment syndrome, as changes in the monitored parameters occur more quickly than the clinical signs and symptoms of pain, pallor, paresthesia, paralysis, and pulselessness, and will allow the surgeon to react much quicker to a developing symptom complex.

Once the initial phase of the injury is over, usually in 2 or 3 days, the patient is encouraged to stand upright and begin weight bearing. Many patients have misconceptions about walking on their fractured limb, so a careful educational program should accompany this phase of the treatment. Patients may bear weight on the cast as much as they can tolerate. Usually between the 7th and 14th day, full weight bearing with the use of crutches may be achieved.

When fully weight bearing, the patient may switch to canes as tolerated. Depending on the type of fracture present, the above-knee cast may be converted to a below-knee patellar-bearing plaster (Fig. 17.7b) or to a functional cast brace between the 4th and 8th week (Fig. 17.7c). However, there are some fractures that are best left in an above-knee plaster, namely, those occurring close to the knee joint, and those associated with an intact fibula.

With progressive healing, a mobile foot and ankle device is added to the functional splint (see Fig. 17.7c).

The patient must be carefully monitored throughout the treatment phase: in the early phase to detect the presence of a compartment syndrome, and in the intermediate and later phases to prevent redisplacement of the fracture, leading to malunion, and to detect thromboembolic disease. Remember that many patients with slow fracture healing require protection for 4–6 months. Failure to recognize this may lead to permanent late displacement of the fracture.

Our motto should be "maximum function in minimum time." With this method, early function is restored to the limb, and most nonindustrial workers can return to their jobs quickly.

17.4.1.2 Indications for Surgery

If most tibial fractures can be managed successfully by nonoperative means, what, if any, are the indications for surgery?

We have already discussed those factors in the natural history of this injury which may compromise the final result, such as the degree of displacement or instability, the amount of comminution, the presence of an open wound with or without soft tissue or bone loss, and others. Careful assessment of the patient may lead the surgeon to choose an operative approach in order to fulfill the prime aim of fracture care, that is, a return of the injured limb to full function in the shortest possible time and with relative safety.

A tibial fracture should be fixed for the reasons given below and summarized in Table 17.3.

Primary Indications

a) Definite Indications

Early assessment of the patient may reveal that operative management of the fracture would be the preferable choice. Under ideal conditions, the situations described below form the more definite indications for surgical intervention as listed in Table 17.3. The word "definite," as used here, must be preceded by the word "more," indicating that considerable surgical judgment must be exercised in each case.

Associated Intra-articular and Shaft Fracture

Displaced intra-articular fractures in the lower extremity are prime indications for open reduction and internal fixation. If a tibial shaft fracture is associated with a displaced fracture into either the knee or ankle joint, the difficulties of nonoperative management are almost insurmountable. Optimal function can rarely be achieved in these joint injuries without adhering to the basic principles in the management of joint fractures; that is, anatomical reduction, stable internal fixation, and early motion. In a tibial plateau fracture, the only method by which the surgeon can achieve early motion without operative stabilization is with traction, but if a diaphyseal fracture is also present, this option becomes extraordinarily difficult, if not impossible. Therefore, stabilization of the fracture becomes not only desirable but almost imperative if an excellent functional result is to be obtained.

Table 17.3. Tibial fractures: operative indications

1. *Primary*
   Definite:
      Associated intra-articular and shaft fracture
      Open fracture
      Major bone loss
      Neurovascular injury
      Limb reimplantation
      The compartment syndrome
      Ipsilateral femoral and tibial fractures – the "floating knee"

   Relative:
      Unstable fractures – inability to maintain reduction
      Relative shortening
      Segmental fractures
      Tibial fractures with intact fibula
      Transition zone fractures
      The polytrauma patient
      Patient with enforced bed rest
      High expectation patient (professional athlete)

2. *Delayed* primary
   failure to maintain reduction

3. *Secondary*
      Unacceptable position
      Management of complications

Diaphyseal fractures of the tibia may be associated with either a tibial plateau fracture into the knee joint, or with a fracture into the ankle joint. These diaphyseal fractures with extensions into the joint must be anatomically reduced and stabilized using atraumatic techniques. Techniques describing fixation of displaced tibial condyle fractures are described in Chap. 16. Bone grafts are often required to maintain the depressed fragments in their reduced position. Following reduction of the intra-articular fracture, the diaphyseal portion of the injury should be dealt with by plating with a suitable implant. If the metaphysis is greatly comminuted, two buttress plates are often required to restore stability (Fig. 17.8), or occasionally an external fixation frame.

Fractures of the tibial diaphysis, especially those in the lower third, associated with a posterolateral butterfly fragment and a displaced lateral malleolar fracture are difficult to manage nonoperatively. Attempts at reducing the ankle often displace the tibial shaft component. Since the posterolateral butterfly is usually connected to the lateral malleolar fragment, only open reduction will allow accurate anatomical restoration and return good, early function to the ankle (Fig. 17.9). Discussion of the distal tibial metaphyseal injury will be found in Chap. 18.

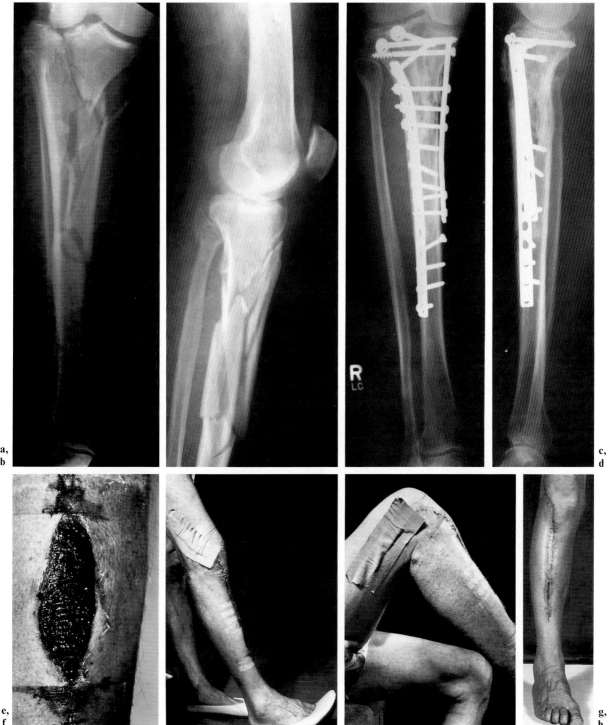

Fig. 17.8a–h. Associated intra-articular fracture of the knee with tibial shaft fracture. **a** Anteroposterior and **b** lateral radiographs of a 60-year-old man who fell 12 feet from a ladder. Note the severe depression of the lateral tibial plateau and severe comminution of both the metaphysis and diaphysis of this tibia. **c** Anteroposterior and **d** lateral postoperative radiographs showing reconstruction of the joint surface with cancellous lag screws and neutralization of the tibial fracture by a double plate. The medial buttress plate was necessary because of the extreme comminution area and porosity of the bone. A cancellous iliac bone graft was used to fill the gap. Immediate surgery was necessary because of a developing compartment syndrome which in this case was caused by an expanding hematoma rather than increasing edema in the muscle. Postoperatively the lower portion of the wound was left open to avoid tension (**e**). **f, g** The state of the limb 10 days postoperatively. Note the excellent knee movement, from full extension to 95° flexion. The lower portion of the incision was allowed to heal by secondary intention and fully epithelialized (**h**). The final functional result was excellent. (From Tile 1980)

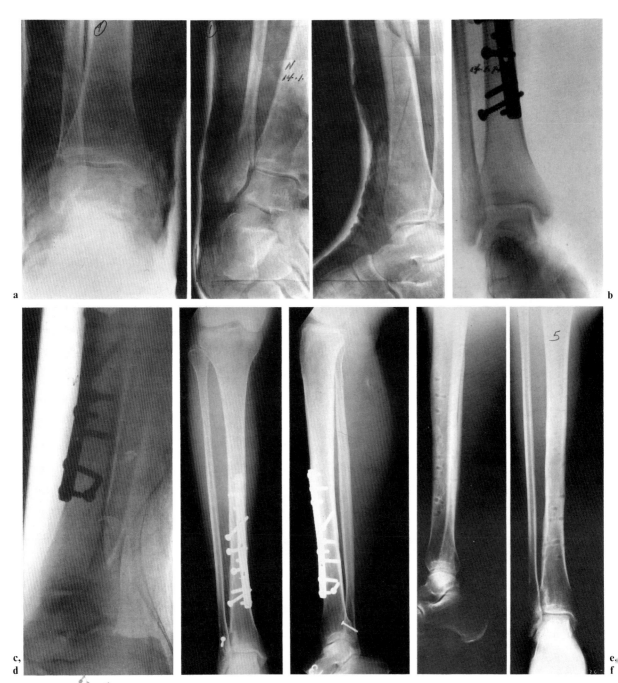

Fig. 17.9a–f. Fractured ankle associated with tibial diaphyseal fracture. This 29-year-old woman sustained a fracture of the tibia associated with an ankle fracture while skiing. **a** The tibial fracture has a posterolateral butterfly and the lateral malleolus is fractured at the level of the ankle mortise. All attempts to reduce the ankle fracture resulted in displacement at the tibial site, while all attempts to reduce the tibia fracture allowed the ankle to remain in valgus. **b** The anteroposterior intraoperative polaroid radiograph shows the stable internal fixation by means of three lag screws and a neutralization plate. Note that when the tibia was anatomically reduced the lateral malleolar fracture also reduced with no valgus deformity at the ankle. This is clearly seen on the lateral intraoperative polaroid radiograph (**c**). **d** Anteroposterior and **e** lateral radiographs 3 months after surgery show sound primary bone union. A single cancellous lag screw was used to immobilize the fibula. **f** The final appearance at 2 years. The anatomical appearance of the ankle is confirmed by an excellent functional result. (From Tile 1980)

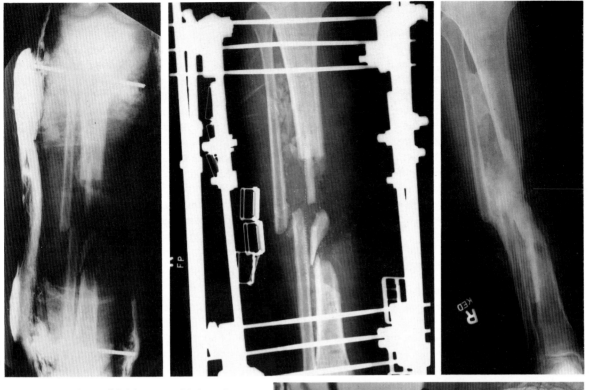

a,
b

d

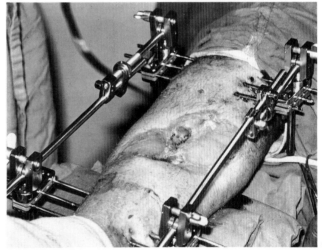

c

Fig. 17.10 a–d. Open tibial fracture with bone loss.
a Anteroposterior radiograph of a 22-year-old man
injured in a mine accident. This was an open fracture and much of the tibial shaft was débrided and
discarded. The patient was immobilized with a pin
above and below the fracture incorporated in plaster as seen in this radiograph. When seen at
5 weeks he had purulent drainage anteriorly. Treatment consisted of a bilateral external skeletal fixator and débridement of the anterior wound, followed 2 weeks later by a massive posterolateral
bone graft from the tibia to the fibula (**b**). **c** The
appearance of the extremity in the bilateral external
fixator. At 8 weeks, a second posterior bone graft
was carried out to span the proximal to distal tibia
after partial consolidation of the first bone graft
had taken place. **d** The final result at 1 year is of
good function in the foot and ankle and sound union of the fracture. (From Tile 1980)

The Open Fracture

Treatment of the open fracture of the tibia remains
controversial and will be discussed later. However,
a consensus of current surgical opinion favors primary stabilization of the open tibia fracture associated with major soft tissue damage. Movement
due to imperfect stabilization in plaster may compromise soft tissue healing and may impair the
functional result. In our opinion, an improved final result will be achieved by proper stabilization
of the fracture, whether by internal or external

means, and by sound surgical management of the
soft tissue injury.

Major Bone Loss

If a major degree of bone loss is present, the length
of the extremity can only be maintained by surgical stabilization of the fracture. Bone loss at the
time of injury is always associated with a major
open fracture, another definite indication for surgical intervention (Fig. 17.10).

Arterial or Nerve Injury

In the past, repair of arterial injuries at the tibial level has been infrequent, but with refinements in microvascular techniques, it is becoming more common. Although not essential, stabilization of the fracture enhances the possibility of successful microvascular repair, and we recommend it highly in such cases. Stabilization of the fracture is also desirable following primary repair of an injured lower extremity nerve. However, it must be understood that the combination of an open tibial fracture with a vascular injury gives a poor prognosis for the limb. In such cases, especially in a crushing injury, early amputation may be the best form of treatment in select cases.

Limb Reimplantation

The ultimate open arterial injury is the severed limb. The advent and advance of microvascular techniques have made the salvage of severed limbs both possible and desirable. The first step in such a procedure is to stabilize the fracture; therefore, limb reimplantation is an absolute indication. However, as stated above, in lesions through the tibia, especially with crushing, amputation is the treatment of choice.

The Compartment Syndrome

We have already stated that compartment syndromes are not uncommon following closed treatment of tibial fractures. The advent of continuous monitoring devices should prevent the disastrous complication of Volkmann's ischemic contracture from occurring. Early recognition, followed by immediate decompression of the involved compartment or compartments, will achieve this end. Following decompression, open reduction through the same incision and stable internal fixation of the unstable fracture are highly desirable, and will simplify the further management of the patient (Fig. 17.8). Stability of the fracture will prevent further damage to the soft tissues and will allow early motion of the extremity, which should reduce edema. Also, it will permit the limb to be handled during the many necessary dressing changes and secondary skin procedures without fear of losing the reduction. These advantages so outweigh any theoretical disadvantages that we regard the association of a tibial fracture with a compartment syndrome as a definite indication for stabilization.

Ipsilateral Fractured Femur and Tibia:
The "Floating Knee" Syndrome

The combination of a fracture of the tibia with a fracture of the ipsilateral femur has given rise to notoriously poor results when both fractures have been treated nonoperatively (Fraser et al. 1978). These fractures are often associated with a severe injury to the knee joint, frequently called the *floating knee*. Nonoperative care usually results in impaired knee function and difficulty with one or other fracture. Optimal management consists of stabilization of both fractures, followed by careful evaluation of the knee injury. This, in turn, may be managed by primary ligamentous repair, if necessary, and early active or continuous passive motion.

b) Relative Indications

If any or some of the factors listed below are present in the particular fracture to be treated, they should be taken as more relative indications that operative stabilization is the preferred method of management; but, again, this should only be undertaken under ideal conditions, as previously outlined.

Relative Shortening

Sarmiento (1981) has written that most longitudinally unstable tibial fractures of the short oblique or spiral variety do not excessively shorten when placed in a proper cast. He has based this assertion on both clinical and experimental observations, and we agree fully with him. However, there are instances, albeit rare, when unacceptable shortening is present at the initial examination (Fig. 17.11). The desirability of carrying out an open reduction, therefore, will depend entirely on the total personality of the injury, as discussed previously. The treatment will obviously differ for a young patient with 3 cm of shortening and high expectation of a cosmetically and functionally perfect result than for an elderly patient with a similar injury. In our opinion, when excessive shortening is present, the surgeon should discuss the treatment options with the patient, who in turn should share in the management decision, based on informed consent.

Segmental Fractures

In our view, proper open reduction will give more satisfactory results in select cases of segmental fracture than nonoperative means. Nonoperative

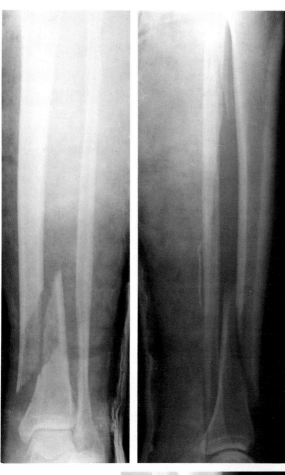

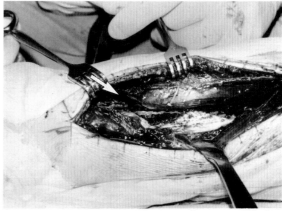

Fig. 17.11 a–f. Transition zone fracture of the tibia into the metaphysis with wide displacement and shortening. **a, b**. The anteroposterior and lateral radiographs of this 53-year-old man show a long spiral fracture extending from the lower third into the metaphysis. This fracture occurred during skiing. Two centimetres of shortening are noted. Because of the wide displacement of this fracture, associated with significant shortening, and in consultation with the patient, open reduction and internal fixation were felt to be the preferred treatment. The clinical photograph (**c**) shows the wide gap present at the time of surgery. **d** Reduction was easily obtained with the use of the AO distractor. Note the two interfragmental screws in position. **e, f** The final result, showing a medially placed neutralization plate and an anatomical reduction. Function returned quickly to the extremity, and the fracture was healed with in 10 weeks

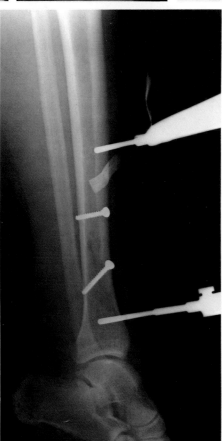

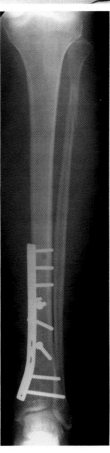

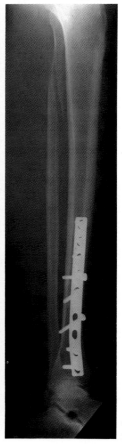

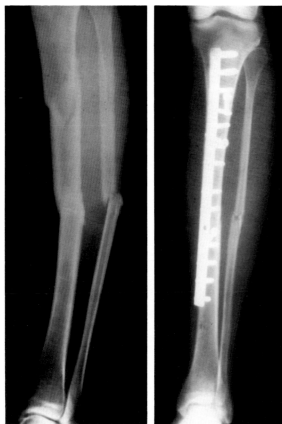

treatment of a segmental fracture is difficult, and, frequently, the final result is compromised by delayed union at one or other site, by malalignment, and by shortening (Fig. 17.12).

Fractures of the Tibia with Intact Fibula

The displaced fractured tibia associated with an intact fibula is difficult, though not impossible, to maintain in plaster. Drift of the tibia into varus is common and difficult to overcome; delayed union and nonunion are also common. Teitz et al. (1980) reviewed 23 patients of more than 20 years of age and found complications in 61%, including 6 with varus malunion and 6 with delayed union or nonunion. Therefore, early surgery should be considered for these cases. The key word is *displaced*; a relatively undisplaced fracture may be managed nonoperatively, but grossly displaced

Fig. 17.12a–f. Segmental fracture of the tibia. **a** Anteroposterior radiograph of a segmental fracture treated by open reduction and internal fixation (**b**). The patient in **c** and **d** was treated by a closed intramedullary nail distally locked, a preferred technique where technically possible (**e, f**)

a,
b

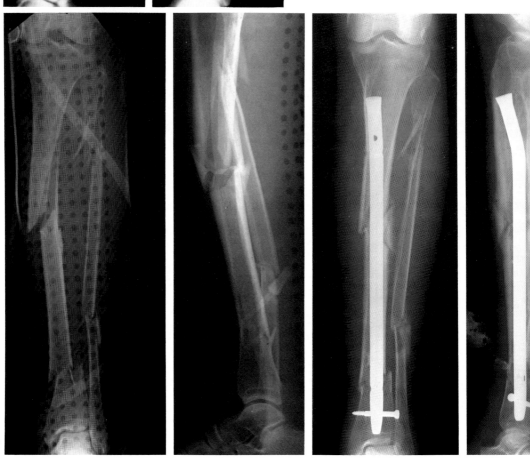

c,
d

e
f

fractures, often with disruption of the interosseous membrane up to and including the proximal tibiofibular joint, are best treated operatively. We favor this approach in most cases, allowing the patient to share in the decision. If closed treatment is used, remember that the plaster must extend above the knee in almost full extension until the fracture is healed, because this fracture may angulate *late* in the treatment cycle.

Transition Zone Fractures

Fractures through the transitional area between the metaphysis and diaphysis are mainly through cancellous bone, which contains large numbers of osteoblastic cells, and therefore, normally, few problems in healing should be encountered. However, we find that union in these particular fractures in any long bone, especially the tibia, may be delayed (Fig. 17.13).

In the young, the metaphysis and the transition zone between the diaphysis and metaphysis is strong; fractures of this area in young people therefore often mean an injury caused by high violence.

On initial inspection of the radiographs, some degree of comminution and gap may be present, which may persist even after reduction (Fig. 17.13 b). Since cancellous bone heals well if compressed, and often poorly if not, and since compression may be achieved quite simply by interfragmental compression, the entire outlook for the patient and his fracture may be changed dramatically by an early decision favoring surgery (see Fig. 17.11).

Fractures through this area may be of two distinct types, the shear type and the compression type, each with their own specific problems. The *shear* injury is characterized by gross instability indicated by a large gap between the fragments and marked comminution. If closed reduction fails to close the large gap often present in these fractures, we favor early stabilization by the appropriate means, usually internal fixation with interfragmental compression and a neutralization plate (Fig. 17.9) or a locked intramedullary nail, if technically possible (see Fig. 17.12c–f). In the elderly population, fractures through this region may almost be considered pathological, since the osteoporotic process has its greatest effect in the metaphysis. Although more commonly associated with delayed union and nonunion in humeral and femoral fractures, osteoporosis can play the same role in fractures of the tibia.

Compression injuries to the metaphysis caused by direct trauma may cause so great a crush that, when reduction has been performed, a large gap will be present at the site of bone compression. Such fractures are notoriously difficult to maintain in the reduced position and consideration should be given to early operative intervention with bone graft. Since this applies more to the so-called pilon fracture than to tibial fractures, it will be discussed more fully in Chap. 18.

Polytrauma

Current surgical practice strongly favors stabilization of lower extremity diaphyseal fractures in polytraumatized patients. This is especially true in patients in whom the erect position is necessary for treatment of the many chest complications often seen in these individuals. Several studies have shown that the morbidity rate in these patients is diminished if early stabilization of the fractures is performed and the patient is mobilized quickly (Border et al. 1975). Furthermore, these patients had better final functional results of the fracture itself. For the tibia, however, this is only a relative indication because patients with tibial fractures can be maintained in light plaster casts and mobilized early without resorting to surgery.

Conditions Requiring Prolonged Bed Rest

If the patient has a major pelvic ring disruption, or injury about the hip joint that will prevent early weight bearing on that extremity, consideration should be given to stabilization of the tibial fracture. However, this is only indicated if careful assessment of the fracture indicates an increased risk of delayed union.

High-Expectation Patient (Professional Athlete)

In some patients, the desire for a perfect result is so high that operative fixation of the fracture becomes preferable to nonoperative treatment. This would be especially true in the professional athlete requiring full knee and ankle motion, especially in sports such as skiing, basketball, or track and field sports. Socio-economic factors rarely play a part in the decision making for the tibia because most individuals can function very well with the functional weight bearing casts and splints now available.

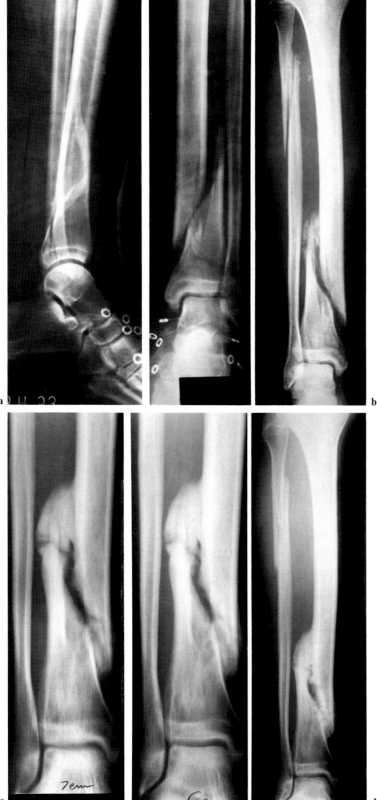

Fig. 17.13a–d. Transition zone fracture. **a** This 53-year-old man sustained a long spiral fracture of his tibia and fibula while skiing. He was treated in an above-knee plaster and began weight bearing immediately. In spite of early weight bearing union was delayed, as shown in **b**, taken at 5 months. The tomograms taken at 7 months (**c**) show union to be complete at the periphery but not at the center of the lesion. Bony union was complete at one year (**d**). The patient's ankle movement was good, but he continued to have tenderness and some pain on weight bearing at that stage; 1 cm of shortening was present. This type of long spiral fracture in the metaphysis, when associated with comminution, a large gap at the fracture site, and shortening, may be considerably delayed in union and therefore represents a relative indication for surgery. (From Tile 1980)

a

b

c

d

Delayed Primary Indications

Grossly unstable fractures of the tibia may be difficult to maintain in an acceptably reduced position. This is especially true if comminution is extreme. In those cases, shortening and/or angulation may occur in plaster. If this situation arises, we prefer early fracture stabilization when it becomes apparent that closed methods are failing.

Secondary Indications

a) Delayed Reduction

Patients referred late with an unacceptable reduction of their fracture will require open reduction if, as often occurs, closed reduction fails. Open reduction may be hazardous, since soft tissue contracture is the rule. The AO/ASIF distractor is an invaluable instrument in such cases, minimizing the need for excessive soft tissue stripping and achieving normal length at the fracture site (see Fig. 17.11).

b) Complications of Fractures

Open methods are required for the management of such complications as delayed union or non-union, malunion or sepsis.

We stress again, that *surgery should only be carried out according to the strict biological and biomechanical principles outlined in the next few pages, and by an experienced surgical team with a full surgical armamentarium.*

Having completed the decision-making process and having decided upon operative intervention, we must now decide when to intervene and how to fix the fracture.

17.4.2 Timing of Surgery

The exact timing of operative treatment is extremely important and will have a major bearing on the eventual outcome of the fracture. Ideally, we prefer early to late surgery in tibial fractures, but not if this means operating through excessively traumatized skin or soft tissue. Moreover, in this subcutaneous bone, closed intramedullary techniques are, where possible, preferred to open techniques. The surgeon must carefully weigh and balance the various factors influencing the decision, such as the following:
1. General Factors:
   – The severity of other injuries in the polytraumatized patient
   – The general medical state of the patient

2. Local Factors:
   – The time elapsed since injury
   – The state of the skin and soft tissues
   – The importance of the surgical indication
   – The type of surgical intervention planned

If the patient is seen shortly after injury and there is a strong indication for surgical treatment, then that surgery should proceed immediately. Swelling is usually minimal at this stage, so already traumatized skin will not be subjected to further damage by pressure, as would happen if treatment were delayed. For open methods, an atraumatic operative technique, evacuation of the fracture hematoma, stable fixation of the bone to prevent further soft tissue damage, and adequate postoperative suction drainage should lead to good wound healing with little trouble.

Closed intramedullary techniques are favored for closed fractures, since no incisions will be made at the fracture site. However, timing is important, since adding a reamed intramedullary nail to an already maximally swollen leg may give rise to a compartment syndrome.

One added advantage of early surgery is the ease of fracture reduction, since no fixed shortening of the soft tissues has occurred. Early restoration of the normal muscle length without contracture allows early painless motion of the extremity.

If, however, the patient arrives late, or for other reasons surgery is delayed beyond 8–24 h, after injury, the situation may change dramatically. The extremity may become very swollen and the skin ecchymotic, with areas of fracture blisters. Operative intervention through this type of skin is fraught with obvious danger and may lead to disaster. Therefore, unless a major absolute indication exists, such as an open fracture or a compartment syndrome, it is best to delay surgery until the skin has become revascularized or areas of skin loss have become apparent. The patient should remain in bed, with the limb elevated and inspected frequently. It is often necessary to delay the surgical intervention for 7–14 days, until it is safe to proceed. In this situation, the operative reduction of the fracture becomes difficult and may require the use of a distractor, as described below. If possible, where traumatized skin precludes a surgical incision, the surgeon should turn to closed nailing as the technique of choice, *if practicable*. Recent advances in nailing techniques, namely, the self-locking type of nail, have extended the indications for nailing in tibial fractures, making it a more viable option in this particular type of case (see Fig. 17.12c–f).

In summary, a careful analysis of the individual patient will lead the astute surgeon to the correct decision. Early operative intervention is ideal for patients with a major indication, but it should never be carried out through doubtful skin. In such cases, it is far safer to delay surgery and deal with the late technical difficulties by established techniques.

17.4.3 Surgical Methods

We have now decided which tibial fractures should be fixed and when to fix them. We now turn our attention to the surgical methods. Any operative intervention must be carried out according to strict biological and biomechanical principles with careful attention to detail. The skin incision must be

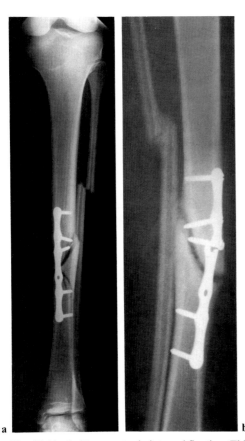

Fig. 17.14a, b. How not to do internal fixation. This fracture could have been treated nonoperatively, but the surgeon elected to perform operative intervention. Note that the posterolateral fragment has not been fixed with lag screws (**a**). The screws holding this inadequate plate also enter the fracture, thereby holding it apart. In spite of 16 weeks in plaster, the fracture failed to unite and the plate eventually broke (**b**). (From Tile 1980)

carefully planned and executed and all biological tissue handled with atraumatic techniques. The internal fixation should be stable enough to allow the surgeon to do without most external appliances such as casts or splints. In this decade, fixations such as those shown in Fig. 17.14 are inexcusable. The surgeon must always remember that the weak link in the system is the bone and, therefore, many of the techniques are not appropriate to patients with extremely osteoporotic bone. If the bone is porotic, but a strong indication for surgery exists, then special techniques must be used, such as cement augmentation followed by external protection of the fixation. Several conflicting factors often coexist, as, for instance, in the case of a displaced fracture in the knee in an elderly individual with osteoporotic bone; so that time and again, the surgeon is required to exercise sound judgment and choose the best treatment for his patient.

17.4.3.1 Incisions

The choice of incision is dependent upon many factors, including the degree of skin trauma, the presence of an open wound, the type and location of the fracture, and the type of surgical intervention.

As a general principle, *no incision should ever be made directly over a subcutaneous bone.* Even a relatively minor stitch abscess or small area of wound necrosis will assume much greater significance if the incision has been made directly over the subcutaneous surface rather than over soft tissue. Also, an incision over bone would limit the location of the implant, since the implant should not be placed directly under the incision, for obvious reasons. This is especially true in the tibia, since the skin over the subcutaneous border of the tibia is often poorly vascularized and skin breakdown not uncommon, but is also true for the ulna, the clavicle, and any other subcutaneous bone.

The periosteum and surrounding anterior muscle mass must be handled with extreme care. The fracture should always be exposed through its torn soft tissue envelope. Only as much intact periosteum should be stripped back as is necessary to expose the fracture. Any small fragments of bone with attached soft tissue should be carefully preserved, together with remaining periosteum and muscle.

a) Standard Anterolateral Approach

Our standard incision is made 1 cm lateral to the subcutaneous anterior border of the tibia, lying over the anterior compartment muscle mass (Fig. 17.15). This incision offers many advantages including:

1. Extensile exposure. The entire tibia from knee to ankle may be exposed through this incision. At the upper end, it may be carried laterally to expose the lateral tibial plateau, and at the ankle it may be carried either laterally or medially to expose the tibial articular surface. Therefore, it is truly an extensile approach and one can fix any tibial fracture through this incision. Since the incision is over soft tissue only and not over bone, minor problems in the incision assume less importance. The major potential problem is at the distal end, in the region of the anterior tibial tendon. In this area, the incision should curve just medial to the tendon. Great care is necessary to ensure that the tendon sheath remain closed if possible; if it is opened, it should be resutured so that the tendon itself is not directly under the incision.

2. Open wound treatment. In open fractures, the wound should be left open. If under excessive tension, the wound in a primary open reduction and internal fixation for a closed fracture must also be left open (see Fig. 17.8). With careful planning of the incision, the bone and implants will remain covered.

3. Medially based flap. Since the incision is lateral to the subcutaneous surface, the skin flap will be based medially, in an area of higher vascularity, and skin sloughs will not normally occur. It is important, however, that the subcutaneous tissues be handled with great delicacy. Since the skin is vascularized from its deep surface, it is essential that the entire subcutaneous layer be taken with the skin when the medially based flap is raised and the anterior surface of the tibia exposed; otherwise skin necrosis will ensue.

Note: *If the patient has had a recent incision along the posteromedial border of the tibia, do not make an anterolateral incision, as the area between the two incisions is poorly vascularized and major necrosis of the flap may ensue.* Under these circumstances, always use the previous incision.

b) Posteromedial

The posteromedial incision, made 1 cm posterior to the medial border of the tibia, is useful for decompression of the deep posterior compartment

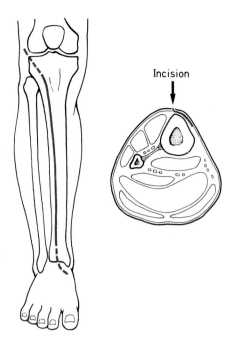

Fig. 17.15. Anterolateral approach to the tibia. The incision is made 1 cm lateral to the anterior crest of the tibia on the anterior tibial muscle mass. This incision allows the surgeon to raise a medially based flap which can then cover any internal fixation on either the lateral or medial surface of the tibia. If a wound breakdown occurs, this incision has the added advantage of not being directly over the fixation or the bone

of the leg. Open reduction may be performed using the subcutaneous surface or the posterior surface of the tibia if necessary (Fig. 17.16).

c) Posterolateral

The posterolateral approach with the patient in the prone or lateral position is excellent for secondary bone grafting procedures, especially if the anterior skin is badly traumatized (Fig. 17.17a, b). It may also be used in open fractures with skin loss and ensuing sepsis. Care should be taken not to violate the anterior compartment in those cases. An added advantage is the possibility of incorporating the fibula in the grafting procedures if there is a gap in the tibia due to bone loss (Fig. 17.17c–i).

d) Incision for Closed Nailing

In suitable cases, closed nailing techniques, with or without self-locking devices, will be ideal, with the added advantage of not further traumatizing the skin at the fracture site. We prefer a longitudinal incision just medial to the tibial tubercle, with

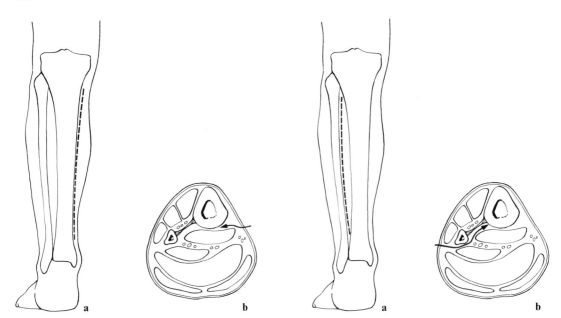

Fig. 17.16a, b. Posteromedial approach to the tibia. This approach should rarely be used in acute trauma. The incision is made 1 cm posterior to the medial border of the tibia over the muscle mass (a). The posterior surface of the tibia may be approached by raising a small skin flap, as shown in the cross-section (b)

Fig. 17.17a–i. The posterolateral approach to the tibia. The ▶ skin incision is shown in a, with the patient in the prone position. The dissection proceeds posterior to the peroneal muscles, along the interosseous membrane, to the posterior aspect of the tibia (b). Exposure of the posterior of the middle third of the tibia is excellent. This approach is excellent

the point of bone perforation dependent on a central siting on the preoperative radiograph. Thus, the entry may be central, by splitting the patellar tendon (Fig. 17.18) or medial, beside the tibial tubercle.

17.4.3.2 Fixation

We have stressed the importance of atraumatic techniques for the skin and soft tissues; careful handling of the skeletal tissue is equally vital. As the soft tissue cover on the tibia is sparse, indiscriminate handling of the bone may destroy all vestiges of soft tissue attachment, which in turn may lead to death of the skeletal tissue, delayed union, and, possibly, implant failure.

Rationale for Implant Selection

Careful planning is required to achieve stable fracture fixation. The preoperative radiographs must be of excellent quality, capable of showing all possible lines of comminution, as this will affect the type and position of the implants. Preoperative drawings should be made from these radiographs. With them the surgeon can carefully plan the internal fixation and instruct the operating room personnel about the necessary implants. The method

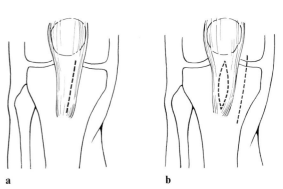

Fig. 17.18a, b. Incision for closed nailing. This incision should be longitudinal, just medial to the tibial tubercle and extending proximally to the patella, along the medial third of the patellar tendon (a). The deep portion of the incision is developed either along the medial subcutaneous border of the tibia, or through the split patellar tendon (b). The preoperative radiographic assessment will determine the entry point of the nail

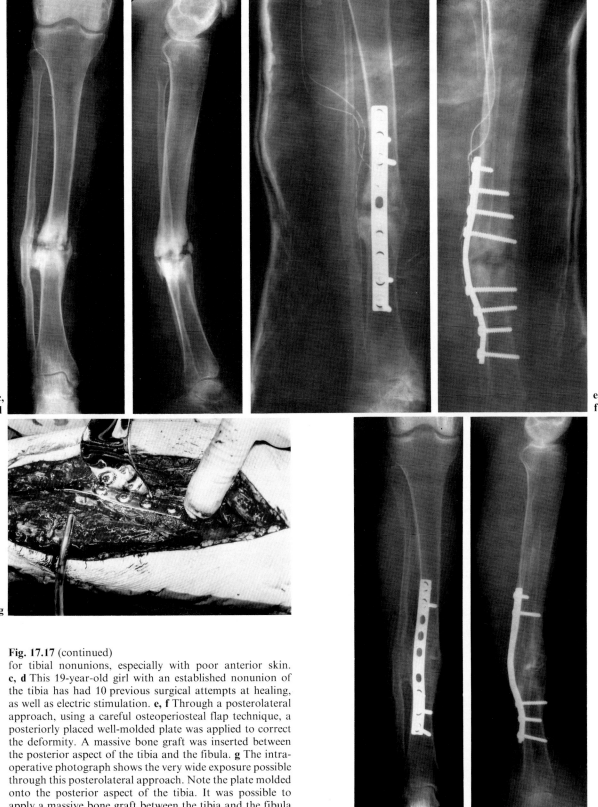

c, d

e, f

g

h   i

Fig. 17.17 (continued)
for tibial nonunions, especially with poor anterior skin.
c, d This 19-year-old girl with an established nonunion of
the tibia has had 10 previous surgical attempts at healing,
as well as electric stimulation. **e, f** Through a posterolateral
approach, using a careful osteoperiosteal flap technique, a
posteriorly placed well-molded plate was applied to correct
the deformity. A massive bone graft was inserted between
the posterior aspect of the tibia and the fibula. **g** The intraoperative photograph shows the very wide exposure possible
through this posterolateral approach. Note the plate molded
onto the posterior aspect of the tibia. It was possible to
apply a massive bone graft between the tibia and the fibula
through this approach. **h, i** The final result at 1 year shows
bony union with cross union to the fibula

of internal fixation chosen, will, in turn, direct the type of incision used. For the tibia, many methods are available for achieving stable fixation, including:

1. Splintage with intramedullary devices
   Rigid — Closed technique
        — Open technique
   Flexible
2. Internal Fixation
   Compression — Interfragmental lag screws
              — Axial compression with tension band plates
   Neutralization plates
   Buttress plates
3. External fixation — may compress, neutralize, or buttress
4. Combined methods of internal and external fixation

The selection of any particular method of stabilization depends upon a knowledge of the natural history of the fracture, namely, those factors which make up the personality of the injury. This includes a careful assessment of the fracture pattern and the soft tissue injury. Both must be considered in any management plan. Of equal importance in the decision-making process is the state of the bone, that is, whether it is normal or osteoporotic and therefore unable to hold screws.

The first step in this process is the determination of the location of the fracture, that is, whether it is articular, metaphyseal, or diaphyseal.

Associated Articular with Shaft Fracture

Displaced articular fractures of the ankle or knee require anatomical reduction of the joint surface whether associated with other fractures in the tibia or not.

In *closed* fractures, open reduction and internal fixation with interfragmental lag screws is the method of choice. Buttress plates are usually required for the metaphyseal component (see Fig. 17.8). If the diaphysis is involved, the plate fixation may be extended to that fracture from the metaphysis, or other combinations may be used, such as screws and plates at the joint and intramedullary devices in the shaft. Careful preoperative planning is essential if such combinations are to be used.

In *open* as in closed injuries, the principle of anatomical reduction of joint fractures must be adhered to. The above methods are valid, that is, interfragmental screw fixation and buttress plating. The major concern is timing. In general, for grade I or II open fractures, the joint should be fixed at the time of the initial surgery following cleansing and débridement. In severe grade III injuries, the surgeon must be guided by the circumstances of the case. Again, we favor immediate fixation of these injuries to allow early motion, but factors may militate against this and cause delay. These factors may be local, such as extreme contamination or vascular compromise, or they may be general factors precluding a complex, lengthy joint reconstruction.

Every effort should be made to close the joint with soft tissue and to stabilize the metaphyseal and diaphyseal components, allowing the joint to be managed with continuous passive motion.

Metaphyseal (Nonarticular)

Which method of internal fixation of metaphyseal fractures is the most favorable will depend on the exact location of the fracture (proximal or distal), the degree of comminution, the state of the bone, and the state of the soft tissues.

Closed. In *normal* bone, fractures close to the joint are best managed by one or two plates, depending on the degree of comminution. For unicortical comminution, one plate will suffice; for bicortical comminution, two plates (Fig. 17.19). Fractures within the metaphysis but more removed from the joint may be managed by plating or by a locked intramedullary nail, if careful preoperative planning indicates that this is technically possible (Fig. 17.20).

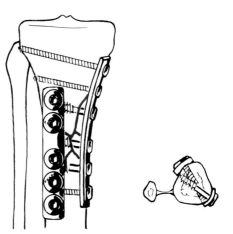

Fig. 17.19. Fixation of a metaphyseal fracture of the tibia. A fracture with severe bicortical comminution requires two plates for stability. Note the use of the large 6.5-mm fully threaded cancellous screws to fix the medial plate distal to the knee joint

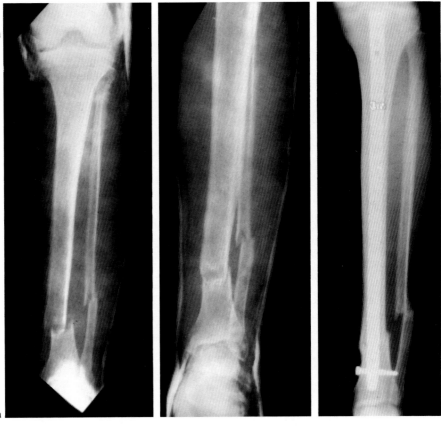

Fig. 17.20a–c. Closed nailing for metaphyseal fracture. **a** Anteroposterior radiograph of the tibia of a 22-year-old polytraumatized male; excessive valgus deformation is visible in **b**. **c** The closed nailing of this distal fracture was achieved with a single distal locking screw following careful preoperative planning

In *osteoporotic* bone, screws may not hold. Therefore, postoperative immobilization may be necessary if plates are used. Flexible intramedullary pins may be desirable in such cases.

Early open surgery should not be attempted through severely traumatized skin, which is often present in fractures of the distal tibia. In these cases, the limb should be elevated and immobilized in traction, and surgery performed after the blisters have disappeared and the skin has revascularized.

Open. In grade I and grade II open metaphyseal fractures, plating techniques may be used primarily. Careful planning should permit coverage of the implant. If a locked nail device is to be used, it should be delayed until soft tissue healing has taken place.

In grade III open fractures, external skeletal fixation is the method of choice.

Diaphyseal

Closed. The methods available include open reduction and internal fixation with interfragmental screws combined with neutralization plates, ten-sion band plates, or intramedullary devices, both rigid and flexible.

Since the circulation of the pretibial skin is so precarious, closed methods of internal fixation of closed fractures are preferable to open methods. A standard or locked intramedullary nail inserted by closed techniques offers good stability for all fracture types. Even fractures with extreme comminution may be statically locked at both ends to prevent shortening (see Fig. 17.25).

Reaming is required to achieve stability, especially with the standard nail. Therefore, the surgeon must be alert to the possibility of a postoperative compartment syndrome. The rigid intramedullary nail is technically demanding, but is relatively safe, can be inserted by closed techniques, and gives good stability, thereby allowing early motion and inspection of the soft tissues. It is the method of choice for closed shaft fractures requiring stabilization, especially if the skin or soft tissues are compromised.

Flexible rods have gained popularity but do not offer full stability except in relatively stable fracture types such as the transverse fracture. They

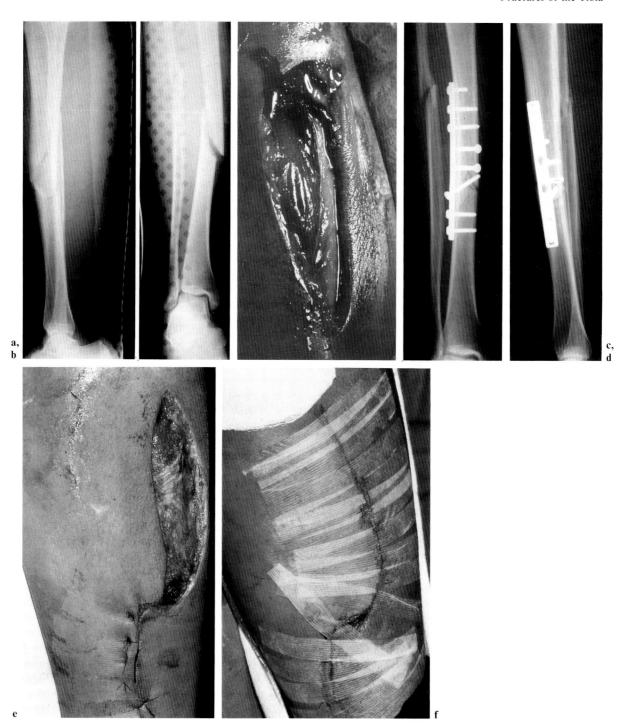

Fig. 17.21 a–i. Open fracture treated by internal fixation. **a** This 19-year-old sky diver was injured when her parachute opened only 200 feet from the ground. The radiographs show a high-energy, short, oblique tibial fracture with a butterfly fragment; the massive skin avulsion is shown in **b**. Very little muscle damage was found, and it was therefore elected to treat this fracture with cleansing, débridement, and primary internal fixation, using lag screws and a plate placed on the lateral surface of the tibia under the anterior tibial muscle mass (**c, d**). Note the interfragmental screws fixing the butterfly fragment and the lag screw across the fracture site through the plate, increasing the stability of the system. The laceration was left open postoperatively but the surgical incision was closed (**e**). **f** The avulsion flap 5 days after injury. The flap was viable and exhibited no swelling, with a good layer of granulation tissue covering the remainder of the wound. At that time skin tapes were used to close the wound. **g, h** The bone after metal removal. **i** The patient had an excellent functional result and returned to competitive sky diving. (From Tile 1980)

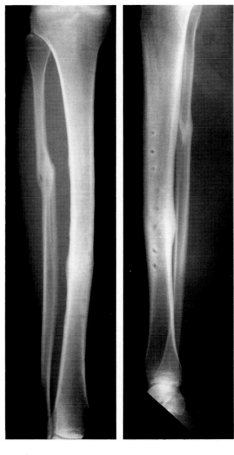
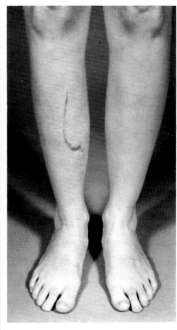

g   h

Fig. 17.21 g–i

i

are easy to insert and do not require reaming, but they require some postoperative external splintage.

Open. The management of the open diaphyseal fracture of the tibia requires careful surgical judgment; the consequences of the wrong initial decision may be very grave, in some instances leading to amputation. An open tibial fracture with a distal vascular injury leads to an amputation 60% of the time (Lange et al. 1985). Therefore, the initial decision must be the desirability or otherwise of *limb salvage*. This decision will depend on general factors in the polytraumatized patient and also on local factors, including the type of vascular trauma, the degree of bone and muscle loss, and the severity of nerve involvement. In polytraumatized patients with severe open tibial fractures associated with distal vascular injury and skin, muscle, and bone loss, amputation may be the most prudent choice.

Immediate Management. The methods available for the management of open tibial diaphyseal fractures include interfragmental screws and plates, intramedullary devices, rigid or flexible external fractures, or a combination of the above. Al-though theoretically all the methods of stabilization may be used, the following general principles should be followed:

1. Intramedullary devices requiring reaming should not be used primarily in the immediate management of open tibial fractures.

2. Open reduction and internal fixation using interfragmental screws and plates can be used for grade I or II open fractures (Fig. 17.21), but not for grade III fractures, where unacceptable infection rates have been reported (Chapman and Mahoney 1979; Tile et al. 1985). If this method is adopted, the implants should be buried under soft tissues, where possible.

3. Grade III open fractures are best provisionally stabilized by simple external skeletal frames (half frames).

Therefore, for grade I open diaphyseal fractures, *any of the above methods is suitable.* We favor immediate cleansing and débridement of the wound, intravenous antibiotics, and primary open wound care with secondary closure of the wound. Open reduction and internal fixation may be used primarily or, after good soft tissue healing, delayed closed intramedullary nailing may be carried out.

Alternatively, the patient may be managed non-operatively, as previously decribed (Sect. 17.4.1.1).

For grade II open fractures, we prefer either external skeletal fixation or immediate open reduction and internal fixation with screws and plates applied to the lateral surface of the tibia.

For severe open fractures (grade III), we recommend an external skeletal frame, usually a half-frame configuration with cross linkages. Primary internal fixation with plates or intramedullary nails has lead to an unacceptably high sepsis rate. Prior to application of the frame, a culture is taken from the wound, which is then cleansed and débrided. Intravenous antibiotics, usually cephalosporins, and adequate tetanus prophylaxis are given immediately. Following débridement, the wounds are left open and covered with a wetting agent such as acriflavine with glycerin.

Subsequent Management. The patient with a diaphyseal fracture of the tibia must be told that the initial treatment of the fracture is only the first step in the management and that many other procedures may be required. Subsequent treatment is dependent upon many factors, such as the degree of soft tissue injury and the degree of bone injury. All are influenced by the general state of the patient and the presence or absence of sepsis in the wound.

Specific considerations relating to soft tissue injury include whether the injury involved no skin loss, skin loss only, or skin, muscle, and other soft tissue damage. Similarly, assessment of the bony injury will take into account whether the injury has been anatomically reduced and stabilized, whether it is one with marked comminution precluding anatomical reduction, or whether it is one with both comminution and bone loss. In addition to the above, the presence or absence of sepsis must be taken into consideration.

Although we will describe the subsequent management of the soft tissue and bone elements separately, it is obvious that they require concurrent treatment.

1. Management of the Soft Tissues. Since the wounds will have been left open in virtually all cases, we recommend that the first dressing change be carried out in the operating room 2–5 days postoperatively. The treatment of the soft tissue depends upon the degree of soft tissue injury.

No skin loss. If the wound has been left open and there is no definite skin loss, the wound may be left to granulate and heal by secondary intent, or, if clean and not tense, it may be closed secondarily with suture or tapes by the 5th postoperative day (see Fig. 17.21). Good healing may be anticipated.

Skin loss. If the patient has sustained loss of skin, this loss may be either over muscle or over bone. If over muscle and small, it may be left to granulate by secondary intent; if larger, it should be managed with a split-thickness skin graft applied when the wound is granulating, usually 5–7 days after trauma. If it is over the subcutaneous border of the tibia and the bone is exposed, the same treatment may be implemented; that is, it should be allowed to granulate by secondary intent if the wound is small or a split-thickness skin graft should be applied directly onto the bone if granulation tissue has covered the bone. However, large split-thickness skin grafts applied directly to bone have a tendency to break down, and we have found the long-term outlook to be much better if a gastrocnemius muscle flap is rotated to cover the defect on the subcutaneous border of the tibia. Therefore, with bone exposed, the preferred treatment is to cover the exposed bone with muscle. We believe that this increases the vascularity to the bone and almost ensures bony union. This procedure should also be carried out in a granulating wound 5–14 days after trauma (Fig. 17.22).

Composite soft tissue loss. We have already indicated that in the polytraumatized patient with a vascular injury and a massive soft tissue wound involving skin and muscle, with or without neurovascular damage, there may be a case for primary amputation. In the isolated fracture, however, primary amputation is rare unless the soft tissue injury is unsalvageable.

In patients who have skin and muscle loss and whose limb has been revascularized, secondary treatment also depends upon whether or not the bone is exposed. If the bone is not exposed, split-thickness skin grafts should be applied to the granulating wound. For cases in which it is exposed, many sophisticated forms of management are now available. For smaller wounds in the diaphysis, a myofascial flap using the gastrocnemius muscle is the treatment of choice (Fig. 17.22). If the wound is too massive, precluding the above procedure, a free muscle flap using the latissimus dorsi muscle is indicated (Fig. 17.23). Finally, if the muscle and skin loss is associated with bone loss, a composite free flap from the iliac crest may be indicated.

None of these procedures can be carried out unless the wound is clean and granulating, for if

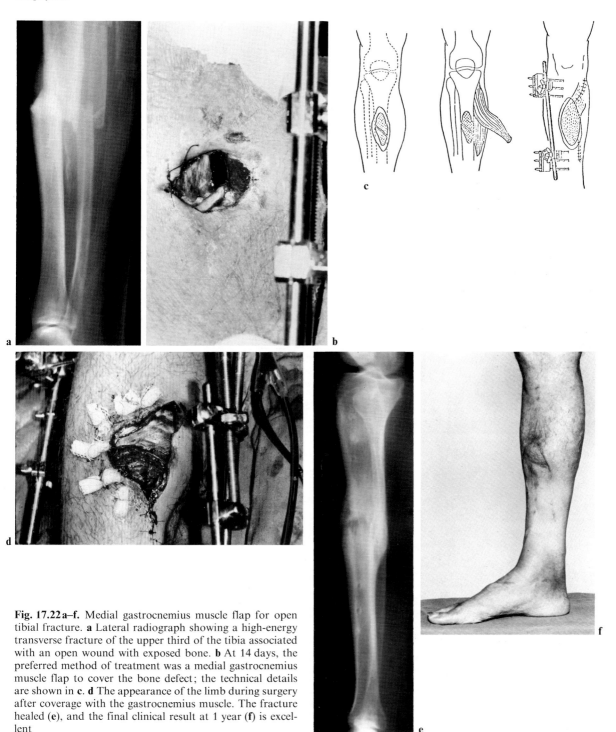

Fig. 17.22a–f. Medial gastrocnemius muscle flap for open tibial fracture. **a** Lateral radiograph showing a high-energy transverse fracture of the upper third of the tibia associated with an open wound with exposed bone. **b** At 14 days, the preferred method of treatment was a medial gastrocnemius muscle flap to cover the bone defect; the technical details are shown in **c**. **d** The appearance of the limb during surgery after coverage with the gastrocnemius muscle. The fracture healed (**e**), and the final clinical result at 1 year (**f**) is excellent

carried out in the face of sepsis they will undoubtedly fail.

2. Management of the Bony Injury. Subsequent management of the bony injury will also depend on many factors, not the least of which is the soft tissue component previously discussed.

For the bony injury, several possibilities also exist:

Anatomical reduction. If an anatomical reduction has been achieved and the fracture stabilized by either internal or external fixation, it is unlikely that further surgical intervention will be required.

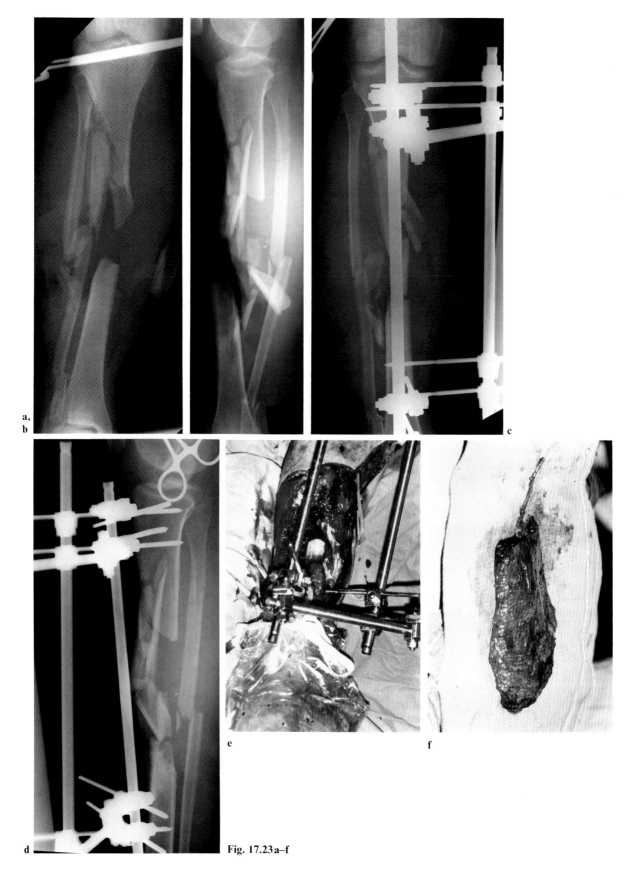

Fig. 17.23 a–f

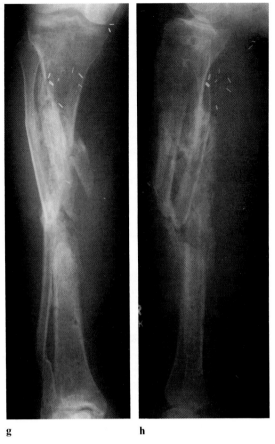

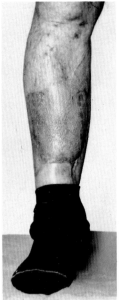

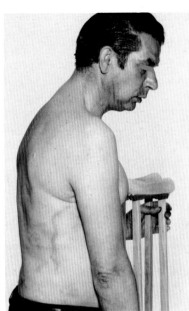

g   h

i   j

◀ **Fig. 17.23a–j.** Open fracture of the tibia with bone loss treated with a latissimus dorsi free muscle flap. **a, b** This 39-year-old male sustained an open fracture of the tibia and fibula with skin, muscle, and bone loss. Initial treatment consisted of wound cleansing, débridement, and removal of dead bone. The fracture was stabilized by external skeletal fixation using an anterior and medial half frame joined in a triangular fashion (**c, d**). Definitive management included a massive cancellous bone graft through a posterolateral approach as well as a free latissimus dorsi flap for anterior soft tissue coverage. **e** Intraoperative photograph showing the extent of soft tissue coverage by the free latissimus dorsi muscle flap (**f**). **g, h** Bone union was complete at 6 months. **i** The appearance of the limb. **j** The donor site of the latissimus dorsi free muscle graft. The patient's overall shoulder function was good

The vast majority of patients in this situation will heal their tibial fractures within an appropriate period, namely 16–20 weeks.

Comminuted fractures with no bone loss. If the patient has had a comminuted fracture with no bone loss, the need for subsequent bone grafting procedures will be dependent on the particular local circumstances. Factors influencing the decision include the degree of comminution, the original method of management, and the degree of soft tissue injury. Therefore, the decision regarding bone grafting must be individualized for each case.

If the wound is small (grade I) and the fracture has been fixed secondarily with a stable intramedullary nail, bone grafting will usually be unnecessary. For the comminuted fracture treated with open reduction and internal fixation but where the degree of comminution does not allow anatomical reduction, *bone grafting is highly desirable.* This is also true for cases treated with an external skeletal frame.

Bone loss. If fragments of bone have been lost due to the original trauma or subsequently due to débridement, bone grafting is essential, no matter whether treatment is open reduction and internal fixation or external skeletal fixation (see Fig. 17.10).

Method of Bone Grafting. Bone grafting may be performed anteriorly, posteriorly, or may be part of a composite free flap.

Anterior. If there has been no major skin or soft tissue loss anteriorly, a cancellous bone graft inserted through the original wound at the time of wound closure is acceptable. However, if the anterior soft tissues are poor, then the posterolateral approach is far more desirable.

Posterolateral. Because of the subcutaneous position of the tibia and the severe damage often inflicted upon the anterior subcutaneous soft tissues, the posterolateral route of bone grafting is usually far more desirable and physiologic than the anterior approach (see Fig. 17.17). The incision is made just posterior to the fibula. The cutaneous branch of the peroneal nerve must be protected. Access to the posterior compartment is between the peroneal and posterior compartment muscle masses; the interosseous membrane should not be violated. Osteoperiosteal flaps should be raised from the fibula to the posterior aspect of the tibia proximal and distal to the fracture. If major bone loss is present, the bone graft should be carried to the fibula. A massive amount of cancellous bone graft may be obtained from the posterosuperior iliac spine. If bone loss is minimal, the cancellous bone graft should placed only along the posterior aspect of the tibia.

This procedure should be preplanned and carried out approximately 3 weeks after injury, when much of the swelling has disappeared and the soft tissues have healed.

Massive Bone Loss. Cases with a major degree of bone loss in the tibia require careful individual decision making. If bone loss is partial, that is, unicortical, then the posterolateral cancellous bone graft is the procedure of choice (see Fig. 17.17). Most of these fractures will heal and good functional results should ensue. If the bone loss is massive and bicortical, the posterolateral cancellous graft still may be the procedure of choice. In such cases, we have often placed a massive posterolateral bone graft and secondarily, after anterior wound healing, placed a cancellous bone graft anteriorly as well (see Fig. 17.10). The more massive cases of bone loss are best healed by adequate soft tissue coverage followed by a vascularized fibular graft augmented with cancellous bone, or by a composite flap of bone muscle and skin from the anterior iliac crest (see Fig. 17.23).

It should be stressed that most cases can be adequately managed using the simpler posterolateral bone graft techniques.

Techniques

Having examined the rationale for implant selection, we will now examine fracture fixation techniques, including stable intramedullary nails inserted either open or closed, locked or unlocked, flexible intramedullary nails, open reduction and internal fixation using lag screws and plates, external skeletal frames and, finally, combinations of the above.

Intramedullary Nailing

Stable. The intramedullary nail is the ideal method of fixation for the transverse or short oblique fracture of the midtibial diaphysis.

With newer locking techniques, these indications have been extended to include more comminuted and more proximally or distally placed fractures. Locking the nail at one end prevents rotation, thus permitting its use in more proximal or distal fractures; locking it at both ends allows a severely comminuted fracture to be fixed with little chance of excessive shortening. Since this technique is relatively recent and requires expertise in closed nailing, considerable judgment must be exercised before it is applied to difficult cases.

We do not favour primary intramedullary nailing in open tibial fractures because of the possibility of introducing sepsis into the intramedullary canal. Delayed primary nailing after skin healing in grade I open fractures is acceptable.

If preoperative planning indicates that the intramedullary nail is the ideal treatment, then one must decide between closed and open methods.

Closed nailing has several advantages and is the preferred method where possible. It allows the surgeon to operate at a site proximal to the fracture and not interfere with the already traumatized and poorly vascularized skin on the anterior tibial border; therefore, skin necrosis leading to infection is rare. Theoretically, the infection rate should be lower than with open nailing, although this is controversial.

As we have mentioned, any remaining soft tissue is left attached to the bony fragments, so as to enhance healing. Intramedullary reaming will allow bone-forming cells in the reamed débris to be deposited at the fracture site, further enhancing healing. Since the tibia is a subcutaneous bone, the technique of closed nailing is relatively easy, although the addition of self-locking techniques is more difficult. Reduction may be aided by direct finger palpation. The major disadvantage with closed tibial nailing is that it requires an experienced surgeon, a fracture table, and an image intensifier. Since the indications for its use are limited, very few surgeons working outside major trauma centers gain enough experience with the technique to feel comfortable with it. This is one area where short courses or technique workshops would be beneficial to the practicing surgeon.

For closed nailing the patient is placed on the fracture table with the knee in the flexed position. A longitudinal incision is made, as previously de-

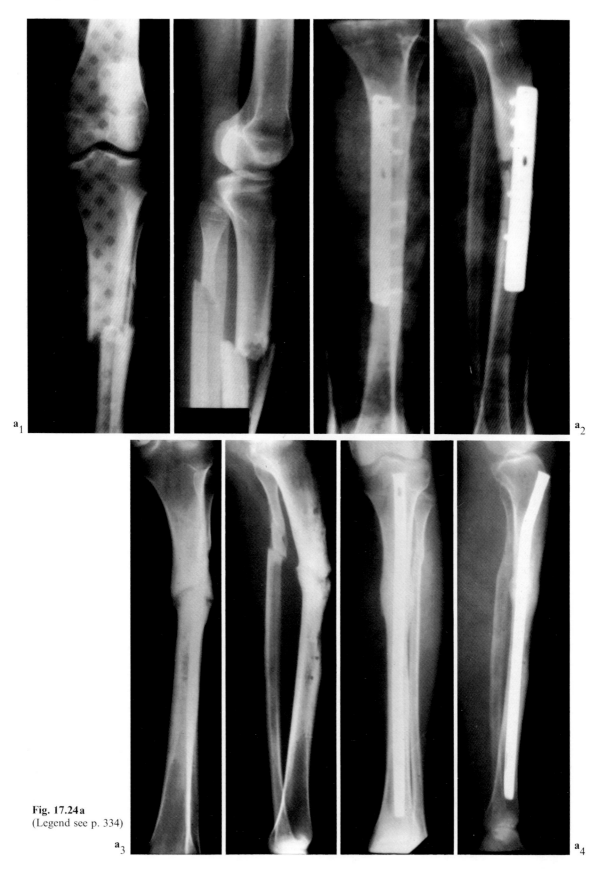

Fig. 17.24a
(Legend see p. 334)

a₃

a₄

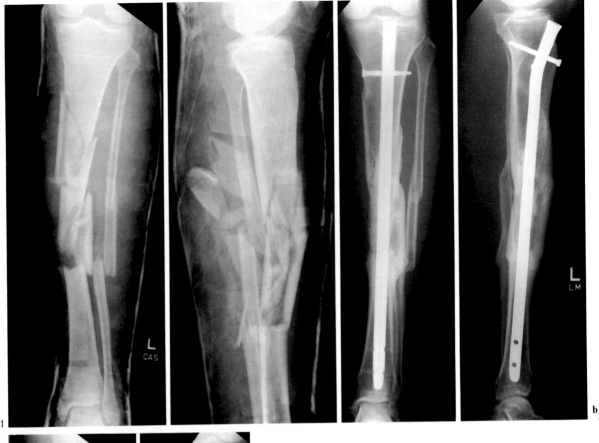

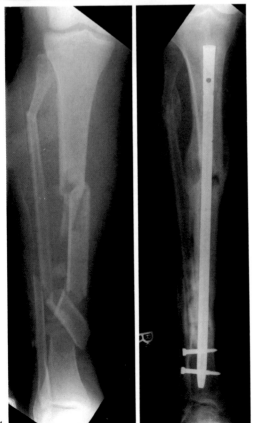

Fig. 17.24a–d. Examples of closed intramedullary nailing. **a** Intramedullary nail with no locking. *1:* Transverse fracture of the upper third of the tibia with significant displacement. *2:* Open reduction and internal fixation using a plate. *3:* Nonunion 9 months after fracture. No sepsis was present in this case. *4:* Treatment with a stable reamed intramedullary nail. No locking was necessary in this nail because of the extreme sclerosis at the fracture site allowing firm fixation of the nail. Solid union occurred and excellent function returned. **b** Fractured tibia with proximal lock. *1:* Anteroposterior and lateral radiographs showing a severely comminuted fracture of the middle third of the tibia. *2:* Treatment consisted of a closed intramedullary nail with a proximal lock. In this particular fracture configuration preoperative planning indicated sufficient fixation by the nail in the distal fragment for a distal lock not to be necessary. The proximal fragment required locking because of the proximal location of the fracture. Union was complete in 4 months. **c** Closed intramedullary nailing with distal lock. *1:* A severely comminuted segmental fracture of the middle to distal third of the tibia. *2:* Preoperative planning indicated reasonable stability in the proximal fragment, so only a distal lock was used. At 10 weeks, healing had progressed

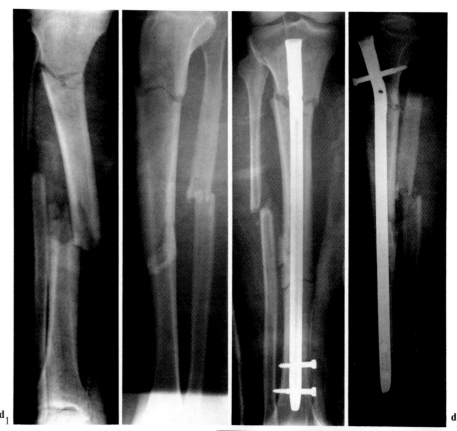

d_1 d_2

Fig. 17.24 (continued)
d Fracture of the tibia with proximal and distal lock. *1:* Anteroposterior and lateral radiographs of segmented tibial fracture. *2:* In this case it was felt that both a proximal and distal lock were necessary. The distal lock may not have been essential since the distal third of the bone is intact. *3:* The radiographs show sound healing at 6 months

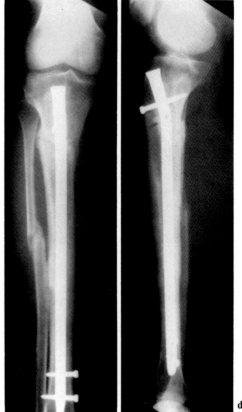

d_3

scribed. After bone perforation, a guide wire is placed into the medullary cavity and extended across the fracture site, which should be reduced. Visualization is afforded by the image intensifier. Reaming is essential to achieve stability, but the amount of reaming will be dependent on the fracture configuration, the amount of comminution, and the presence or absence of a segmental component. The size of the nail and therefore the amount of reaming can be determined by measurements with the ossimeter on the preoperative radiograph. In stable fracture configurations, the medullary canal should be reamed to a size necessary to achieve 2 cm of stable bone proximal and distal to the fracture. If this can be achieved, no locking techniques are necessary.

If reaming cannot achieve this stability because of unicondylar or bicondylar comminution, then the use of a proximal or distal locking screw is essential. If the fracture is proximal, the nail must be locked proximally to prevent rotation. Likewise, if distal, it must be locked distally to avoid rotation. However, if bicortical comminution is present, the nail must be locked both proximally and distally to prevent both rotation and shortening (Fig. 17.24).

Following reaming, the appropriate nail is assembled and driven across the fracture. The locking screws are inserted using the appropriate jigs and siting devices as necessary and the wound closed. Stability should be tested under the image intensifier so that proper postoperative planning can ensue.

The advantages of *open* intramedullary nailing of a tibial fracture are more theoretical than practical. Open reduction allows the surgeon to anatomically reduce the fracture, to add cerclage wires or antirotation plates as necessary, and to instantly check the stability he has achieved. Also bone grafts may be added if anatomical reduction has not been achieved. The major disadvantages are possible problems with the soft tissues, such as skin necrosis and sepsis, and possible devitalization of attached bone fragments; in our opinion, these outweigh the advantages. Also, the addition of the locked nail to our armamentarium has almost eliminated the need for open techniques.

Intramedullary nailing of the tibia is fraught with the same *complications* as it is in other long bones; there are, however, problems specific to the tibia, and these are outlined below.

1. Posterior Insertion. Because the point of insertion of the nail is anterior, the nail will naturally tend to be driven against the posterior cortex (Fig. 17.25). The surgeon may be lulled into a false sense of security by the ease with which the flexible reamers navigate the shaft. The more rigid nail, however, may be driven posteriorly, shattering the cortex, and forcing the surgeon to abandon the procedure and change the management to an external frame, internal fixation with a plate, or a cast. Changing the method of fixation to a plate, after the intramedullary blood supply has been destroyed by reaming, has obviously sinister implications and *must be avoided*. Usually, a cast will not confer enough stability to be used in this situation. This leaves an external frame as the treatment of choice.

The best choice of all, however, is prevention: no undue force should be used to drive in the tibial nail. The fracture must be continually visualized during nailing, either directly in open nailing or

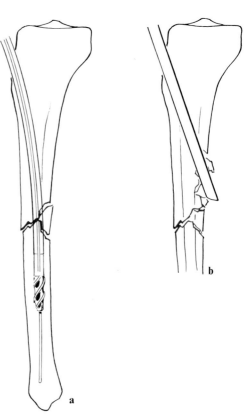

Fig. 17.25a, b. Posterior insertion of the intramedullary nail. The guide wire and the reamer, being flexible, may enter the distal fragment easily (**a**). However, when the relatively rigid nail is inserted, it may be driven posteriorly, shattering the cortex (**b**). This complication can be prevented by changing the entry point and by not using undue force in driving in the nail

radiographically in closed nailing. If resistance is met, the nail should be removed and a smaller nail used or further reaming performed. Moving the entry point proximally and fully flexing the knee may further aid the surgeon who meets this difficulty.

2. Rotational and Vertical Instability. These potential problems have been eliminated by careful planning and the use of the locked nail.

3. Compartment Syndrome. Reaming into a closed compartment may cause a compartment syndrome which must be dealt with by immediate decompression. This complication is relatively frequent, leading many centers to monitor the compartment pressures of all patients undergoing closed tibial nailing.

Flexible. The major advantage of flexible nails is ease of insertion, the major disadvantage, poor stability. No reaming is necessary, so the risk of precipitating a compartment syndrome is diminished. We have generally not used this technique because of its main problem, lack of sufficient stability to allow external splints and casts to be discarded.

Open Reduction and Internal Fixation

The use of open reduction and internal fixation techniques using screws and plates has sharply decreased in the past decade with the advent of the locking nail. However, there are still many situations where this technique must be used, and in many centers it remains the operative treatment of choice.

The incision is made as described above, 1 cm lateral to the anterior border of the tibia over the anterior tibial muscle mass (see Fig. 17.15). The most frequently used implants are the 4.5-mm DC plates and 4.5-mm cortical screws, used either as lag screws or to fix the plate to bone. In the metaphyseal area the 6.5-mm cancellous screws are also used, either the lag screw type, for interfragmental compression, or the fully threaded type, for fixation of the plate to the metaphyseal bone.

We favor placement of the plate on the lateral surface of the tibia, especially when used in open fractures. The plate will thus be buried under the anterior tibial muscle mass even when there is significant skin loss (Fig. 17.26). Seven cortices proximal and distal to the fracture are necessary to achieve stability.

The use of the implant depends on the fracture type. For purely transverse fractures, a properly molded DC plate is used to achieve axial compression and is placed on the lateral surface of the tibia. For short oblique fractures, a similar implant is used; where possible, a lag screw is placed through the plate across the fracture. For spiral or comminuted fractures, interfragmental compression with lag screws is essential before plate fixation. In these two types of fracture, the 4.5-mm DC plate is used as a neutralization plate with lag screws through the plate across the fracture wherever possible (see Fig. 17.26).

Because of the subcutaneous position of the tibia with its relatively poor blood supply, it is essential that atraumatic techniques be used during open reduction and internal fixation of this bone.

Preoperative planning should guide the surgeon's choice of incision and implants. Several types of comminution are recognized, such as the posterolateral, posteromedial, and anterior torsional butterfly. However, the principles of management remain the same for all.

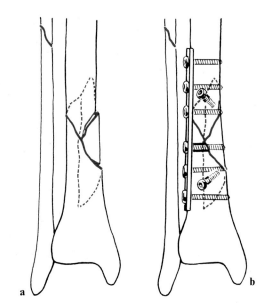

Fig. 17.26a, b. Fixation of tibial fracture with lateral plate. **a** Tibial fracture with posteromedial butterfly. **b** The butterfly fragment is fixed with two interfragmental screws. We favor placement of the plate (in this case a 4.5-mm DC plate) on the lateral surface of the tibia under the anterior tibial muscle mass. Any screws crossing the major fracture line should be lag screws, as shown

External Skeletal Fixation

The recommended method of frame configuration has changed considerably over the past decade. The double frame with pins crossing the anterior compartment of the tibia resulted in significant complications: anterior compartment syndromes, permanent impairment of dorsiflexion, and injury to neurovascular structures were not uncommon. In addition, the rigidity of the double frame significantly impaired bone healing. For that reason, a simple anterior half frame is now recommended, as shown in Fig. 17.27. In cases of bicortical comminution or major bone loss, a medial half frame may be added to the fixation and further stability achieved by triangulation, as shown in Fig. 17.28.

Combined Minimal Internal with External Skeletal Fixation

In some open fractures a combination of minimal internal fixation with interfragmental screws, followed by the use of external skeletal fixation as a neutralization frame, may be the most desirable. This combination should be employed when major fragments in the open fracture can be simply fixed with interfragmental screws without further soft tissue damage. In these instances, the use of the

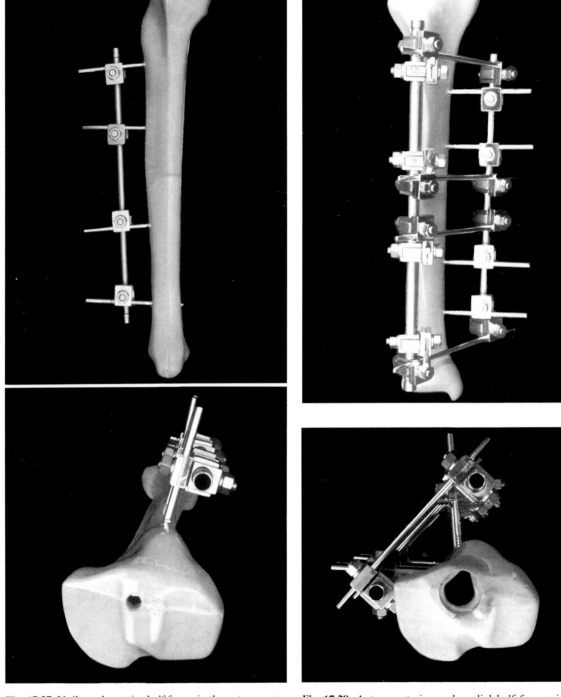

Fig. 17.27. Unilateral anterior half frame in the anteroposterior direction on the tibia. (From Hierholzer et al. 1985)

Fig. 17.28. Anteroposterior and medial half frames joined in a triangular fashion to increase stability. (From Hierholzer et al. 1985)

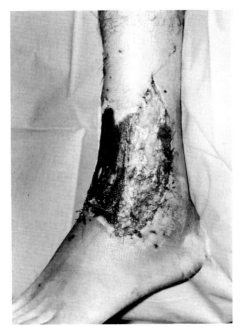

Fig. 17.29. A relaxing incision on the lateral aspect of the lower leg resulted in complete loss of the anterior flap. This necrotic flap was excised. Subsequently, the anterior tibial tendon also became necrotic and required excision

external skeletal frame as a neutralization frame may be preferable to the further soft tissue stripping necessary for application of a neutralization plate internally.

Bone Grafts

Cancellous bone grafts should be considered in all cases in which an anatomical reduction has not been achieved. They should always be performed where bone loss is present or where the area of comminution is so great that healing is likely to be retarded beyond the limits of the implant. In such circumstances, the stability of the system is provided only by the implant. Since anatomical reduction of all the fragments is technically impossible, they can provide no direct stability to the fracture. Devitalization of the fragments makes delayed union likely; therefore, the addition of a bone graft is necessary to prevent this delay and the implant failure which usually follows. As we have previously indicated, *in open fractures treated with an external fixator, delayed union is so common that we prefer early elective bone grafting in almost all cases,* usually to be performed 2–3 weeks after injury.

Since the posterior skin and soft tissues are usually the better preserved, we prefer the posterolat-

eral approach in most cases (see Fig. 17.17). This way, the grafts are under a muscle layer which will hasten their vascularization. If large gaps are present, the grafts may be used to bypass the tibia; this is done by applying them to the fibula proximal and distal to the fracture, creating a tibiofibular diastasis. The results of such posterior bone grafting are excellent, and the technique is therefore highly recommended.

17.4.3.3 Wound Closure

a) Primary

The next major decision to be made concerns skin closure. In closed fractures, if the skin can be closed with meticulous, tension-free, atraumatic techniques, then this is the preferable course. Suction drainage should always be used to prevent hematoma formation. Not infrequently, however, it is extremely difficult to close the skin without tension. In this situation, it is far safer to leave a portion of the wound open than to close it under tension and risk the possibility of skin necrosis and sepsis. Therefore, the dictum to be followed is, "Close if possible, but not at all cost."

If the incisions have been well planned and are away from the subcutaneous border, and if the implant has been carefully placed so that it is buried under soft tissue, then little harm will come from leaving the skin open. On the 5th day, when granulation tissue has appeared, it is usually a simple matter to either secondarily suture or tape the wound, if the swelling has subsided.

When two incisions have been used, one over the fibula and one over the tibia, the more important incision should be closed and the other one left open, to be closed secondarily when possible.

There are, however, exceptions to the above rule. Sensitive structures such as tendon, nerve, artery, and joint should not be left open (we do not consider bone to be a sensitive structure). Other techniques may be required to close the tissues over these sensitive structures. This is especially true at the distal end of the tibial incision, where the anterior tibial tendon may become exposed and, if it does, may die, with serious consequences.

Rotating a skin flap along the anterior border of the distal tibia in an acute injury is a dangerous procedure and cannot be recommended. Too often, we have seen loss of this flap and exposure and death of the underlying tendon, resulting in its death (Fig. 17.29).

b) Delayed Primary and Secondary

Wounds not associated with skin loss may be sutured on the 5th day after trauma if they are clean, granulating, and free of tension; if small, they may be left to heal by secondary intent.

Wounds associated with significant skin or muscle loss require careful consideration. In most cases, a simple split-thickness skin graft will be sufficient cover for the clean granulating wound and may be applied at the first or second dressing change.

If devitalized bone is exposed and granulation delayed, we favor an early muscle pedicle graft for coverage (see Fig. 17.22). Care must be taken to remove the area of devitalized bone. Cancellous bone grafting is almost always required to aid union.

Finally, the occasional open tibial fracture with major bone and soft tissue loss will be best treated by a free microvascular composite graft, but only in a well vascularized, noncontaminated bed (see Fig. 17.23).

17.4.3.4 Postoperative Course

a) Immediate

At the end of the operative procedure, the surgeon must realistically appraise the situation at hand. The skin must be carefully assessed, whether the wound is closed or open; if closed, the degree of tension, if any, must be gauged. The surgeon must be completely honest regarding the degree of stability achieved for that particular fracture.

If the surgeon feels that excellent stability of the fracture has been achieved and the bone is of normal strength, then motion of the extremity may be started early. The leg should be elevated with the ankle splinted at 95° dorsiflexion. Under ideal conditions, the splint may be removed on the 2nd postoperative day and the patient encouraged to move the ankle. The splint should be reapplied after exercise and at night until the patient has regained normal dorsiflexor function, otherwise a disastrous plantar flexion deformity will develop. Patients should sleep with their splints for at least 2–3 weeks following injury.

Early motion of the ankle should be delayed (a) if there is concern about the stability of the fracture or (b) if soft tissue healing would be jeopardized. In both of these situations, the leg should remain splinted until the surgeon is satisfied that the dangerous period is over. In some instances of severe porosis or comminution, a cast or cast

brace must be retained until union is complete. This is preferable to an otherwise inevitable implant failure with its related problems.

b) Follow-Up

Careful follow-up is required in order to monitor the race between implant failure and bone union. If the patient exhibits good soft tissue healing and sound stability of the internal fixation system, feather weightbearing can be started forthwith and gradually increased, depending on the radiographs, which should be taken at 3-weekly intervals. The average tibial fracture will be healed at 16–20 weeks, when more normal activities may be initiated.

Careful decision making according to these guidelines should make good functional results possible for the majority of patients with this difficult fracture (Allgöwer and Perren 1980; Karlstrom and Olerud 1974).

References

Allgöwer M (1967) Natl Acad Sci/Natl Res Council, pp 81–89
Allgöwer M, Perren SM (1980) Operating on tibial shaft fractures. Unfallheilk/Traumatology 83(5):214–8
American College of Surgeons (1981) Advanced trauma life support system. American College of Surgeons, Committee on Trauma
Böhler J (1936) Treatment of fractures. John Wright, Bristol, England, p 421
Border JR, LaDuca J, Seibel R (1975) Priorities in the management of the patient with polytrauma. Prog Surg 14:84–120
Brown PW (1974) Early weight bearing treatment of tibial shaft fractures. Clin Orthop 105:165–178
Chapman MW, Mahoney M (1979) The role of early internal fixation in the management of open fractures. Clin Orthop 138:120–131
Charnley J (1961) The closed treatment of common fractures, 3rd edn. Livingstone, Edinburgh
Dehne E, Metz CW, Deffer P, Hall R (1961) Nonoperative treatment of the fractured tibia by immediate weight bearing. J Trauma 1:514–535
Fraser RD, Hunter GA, Waddell JP (1978) Ipsilateral fractures of the femur and tibia. J Bone Joint Surg [Br] 60B:510–515
Gustilo, RB (1982) Management of open fractures and their complications. Saunders, Philadelphia (Monographs in Clinical Orthopaedics, vol 4)
Hierholzer G, Rüedi T, Allgöwer M, Schatzker J (1985) Manual of the AO/ASIF tubular external fixator. Springer, Berlin Heidelberg New York Tokyo
Karlstrom G, Olerud S (1974) Fractures of the tibial shaft: A critical evaluation of treatment alternatives. Clin Orthop 105:82–115
Lange RH, Bach AW, Hansen ST Jr, Hansen KH (1985)

Open tibial fractures with associated vascular injuries: Prognosis for limb salvage. J Trauma 25(3):203–8

McMurtry RY, Saibil E, Tile M (1984) General assessment and management of the polytraumatized patient. Williams and Wilkins, Baltimore, pp 41–56

Mubarek SJ, Owen GA, Hargens AR et al. (1978) Acute compartmental syndromes: Diagnosis and treatment with the aid of the Wick catheter. J Bone Joint Surg [Am] 60A:1091–1095

Müller ME et al. (1979) Manual of internal fixation, 2nd edn. Springer, Berlin Heidelberg New York

Nicoll EA (1964) Fractures of the tibial shaft. A survey of 705 cases. J Bone Joint Surg [Br] 46B:373–387

Rorabeck C (1977) Pathophysiology of the anterior compartment syndrome. Surg Forum 28:495–497

Rüedi TH, Webb JK, Allgöwer M (1976) Experience with a dynamic compression plate (DCP) in 418 recent fractures of the tibial shaft. Injury 7(4):252–257

Salter RB et al. (1980) The biological effect of continuous passive motion on the healing of full thickness defects in articular cartilage – An experimental investigation in the rabbit. J Bone Joint Surg [Am] 62A(8):1232–1251

Sarmiento A (1967) A functional below-knee cast for tibial fractures. J Bone Joint Surg [Am] 49A:855–875

Sarmiento A, Latta LL (1981) Closed functional treatment of fractures. Springer, Berlin Heidelberg New York

Teitz CC, Carter DR, Frankel VH (1980) Problems associated with tibial fractures with intact fibulae. J Bone Joint Surg [Am] 62A:770

Tile M (1980) Fractures of the tibia: Indications for open reduction of tibial fractures. In: Leach et al. (eds) Controversies in orthopaedic surgery. Saunders, Philadelphia

Tile M (1984) Fractures of the pelvis and acetabulum. Williams and Wilkins, Baltimore

Tile M, Beauchamp CB, Kellam JF (1985) Open fractures: Is primary stabilization desirable. In: Uhthoff HK (ed) Current concepts of infections in orthopaedic surgery. Springer, Berlin Heidelberg

Tscherne H, Gotzen L (1984) Fractures with soft tissue injuries. Springer, Berlin Heidelberg New York

Watson-Jones R, Coltart WD (1943) Slow union of fractures: with a study of 804 fractures of the shafts of the tibia and femur. Br J Surg 130:260–276

18 Fractures of the Distal Tibial Metaphysis Involving the Ankle Joint: The Pilon Fracture

M. TILE

18.1 Introduction

The pilon fracture, a metaphyseal injury extending into the ankle joint, is difficult to treat successfully by any method. If the fracture into the ankle joint is displaced, the basic principles of open anatomical reduction and stable internal fixation, followed by early motion *if technically possible*, are valid. It is in this particular area, to an extent equaled perhaps only by fractures of the acetabulum, that the words "if technically possible" loom large; for this fracture is often so comminuted that technical difficulties cannot be overcome.

The major problems affecting the natural history of this injury may be summarized as follows:
1. The nature of the injury
2. The state of the bone
3. The state of the soft tissues
4. Technical difficulties

18.2 Natural History

18.2.1 The Nature of the Injury

Fractures in cancellous bone are subject to either compressive or shearing forces, each inflicting its own particular type of lesion on the bone (see Figs. 18.1, 18.2). Compressive forces cause severe impaction, while shearing or tensile forces cause marked disruption of the bone and soft tissues without impaction, resulting in gross instability. A fracture caused by a combined shear and compressive load may present a lesion with both impaction of the articular surface and instability of the metaphysis.

In the distal tibia and ankle, an area predisposed to high energy trauma, either force may be operative. Severe compression injuries are seen in patients falling from a height; whereas shearing injuries are often seen in ski injuries, the so-called boot-top fracture, or major motor vehicle trauma.

It is with the complex force patterns of high energy motor vehicle trauma that both types of injuries may be seen.

18.2.1.1 Axial Compression

a) Tibia

Articular Cartilage

Severe compression (Fig. 18.1a) usually causes impaction of the articular surface, often with marked comminution (Fig. 18.1b, c). On some occasions, the comminution is so great that anatomical repair of the articular surface is virtually impossible. If surgical repair is attempted, small avascular pieces of articular cartilage and subchondral bone may have to be discarded, leaving gaps on the joint surface. Osteoarthritis will inevitably follow no matter what form of treatment is used.

Metaphysis

Fractures of the distal metaphysis caused by compression associated with a rotation force often severely impact the metaphyseal bone, causing unacceptable axial malalignment (Fig. 18.1d). The result of uncorrected axial malalignment in the lower extremity is abnormal stress on the distal joint, which in time will destroy it. Since the upper extremity is not subjected to the major weight-bearing stresses of the lower extremity, some leeway is permissible, especially about the shoulder. However, in the lower extremity, anatomical alignment is necessary to prevent these major forces of weight bearing from destroying the joint.

Therefore, when these impacted fractures are reduced by closed manipulation, an extremely large periarticular gap is formed (Fig. 18.1d–m). Nature abhors a vacuum – if treated nonoperatively, the distal fragment may tend to displace into that gap in the postreduction period, necessitating multiple reductions. Also, since the compression fracture has been disimpacted, and since cancellous bone heals poorly under such condi-

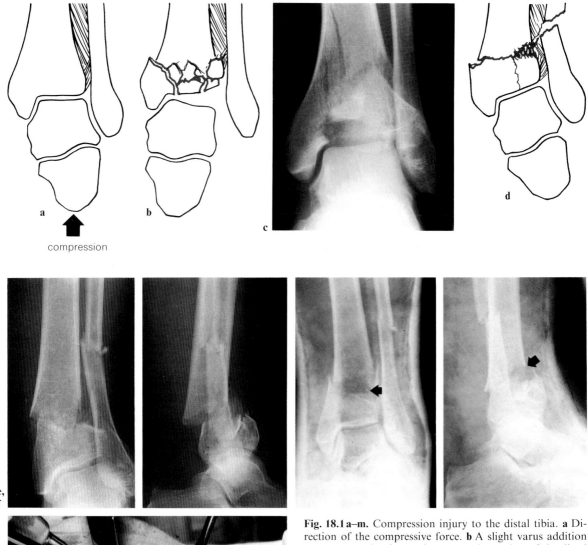

compression

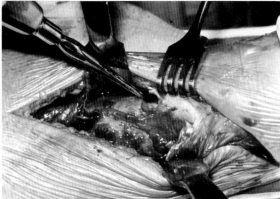

Fig. 18.1 a–m. Compression injury to the distal tibia. **a** Direction of the compressive force. **b** A slight varus addition to a compressive force often causes impaction of the distal tibial articular surface, leaving the fibula intact, as shown on the radiograph (**c**). **d** A valgus addition to the compressive force may cause impaction of the distal tibial metaphysis with a fracture of the fibula. **e, f** Radiographs of a 43-year-old woman who sustained the latter type of injury while skiing. Note the extreme valgus position of the distal tibia. A closed reduction under general anesthesia (**g, h**) restored axial alignment but resulted in an extremely large gap on the anterior and lateral surface of the distal tibia, as shown by the *arrows*. **i** Intraoperative clinical photograph showing the large gap, through which a curette has been passed. Operative treatment was undertaken to prevent loss of reduction and consisted of intramedullary fixation of the fibula, restoration of the articular surface, and bone grafting of the distal metaphysis of the tibia and stabilization with a cloverleaf plate (**j, k**). The final result after plate removal 3 years following injury is excellent (**l, m**)

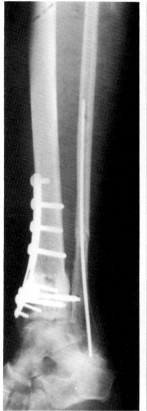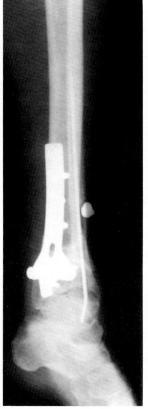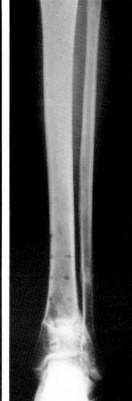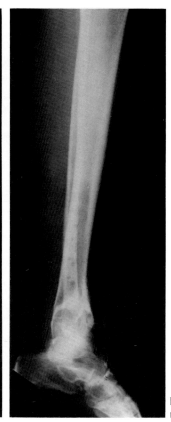

j,
k

l,
m

Fig. 18.1 j–m

tions, union may be delayed. This, in turn, will require prolonged immobilization of the limb with resultant poor ankle function.

b) Fibula

In many compression injuries the fibula may remain intact, which it never does in the shearing type injury. With an intact fibula, the ankle is often driven into varus with severe impaction of the medial part of the tibial plafond (Fig. 18.1 b, c).

18.2.1.2 Shear (Tension)

a) Tibia

Articular Cartilage

Pure shearing or tensile forces, free of axial loading and usually rotatory in nature, may spare the articular surface (Fig. 18.2 a, b). Minor cracks may appear at the joint surface, but severe impaction is rare. The long-term prognosis, therefore, is more favorable than for injuries with major articular compression.

Metaphysis

The shear injury to the distal tibia produces an unstable injury with a disrupted soft tissue envelope. Although the articular surface may be relatively intact, the unstable nature of the bony injury, if treated nonoperatively, often requires immobilization, with resultant stiffness of the ankle.

b) Fibula

The fibula is always fractured, usually as a result of a valgus external rotation force (Fig. 18.2 b). The fibular fracture is usually transverse or short oblique in nature, with a butterfly fragment. However, on occasion, the fibula is markedly comminuted, making any reconstruction difficult.

18.2.1.3 Combined

Severe high-energy trauma may produce a combined injury, with both shearing and axial compressive forces (Fig. 18.2 c, d). It is obvious that the lesion found in a particular patient – that is, the personality of the individual fracture – is the

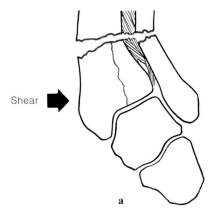

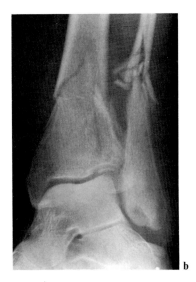

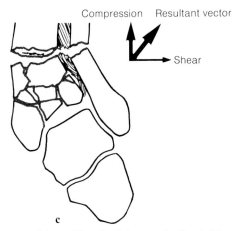

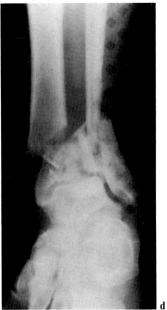

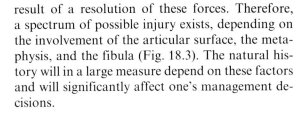

Fig. 18.2 a–d. Shearing injury to the distal tibia. **a** The shearing force in valgus which fractures the fibula as well as the distal tibial metaphysis. **b** Anteroposterior radiograph showing a fracture of this type with comminution of the fibula. **c** Shearing injury of the distal tibial metaphysis combined with a compression force, resulting in severe comminution of the articular cartilage. **d** Radiographic appearance of such a case

result of a resolution of these forces. Therefore, a spectrum of possible injury exists, depending on the involvement of the articular surface, the metaphysis, and the fibula (Fig. 18.3). The natural history will in a large measure depend on these factors and will significantly affect one's management decisions.

18.2.2 State of the Bone

In younger patients with good quality bone, the surgeon may expect that the holding power of the screws will be satisfactory. However, like fractures in many other areas of the body, metaphyseal frac-

tures of the distal tibia often occur in elderly patients with osteoporotic bone, which makes stable internal fixation difficult to obtain.

18.2.3 State of the Soft Tissues

The importance of the soft tissues in open fractures has been stressed in the medical literature for decades. Recently, Tscherne and Gotzen (1984) have written a book to stress the equal importance of the state of the soft tissues in closed fractures. Their grading system is particularly appropriate to the distal tibial fracture, where major soft tissue damage is so common and the consequences of

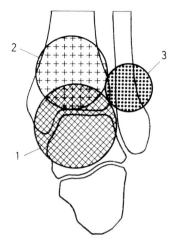

Fig. 18.3. The three important anatomical zones to be considered in the decision making and prognosis of the pilon fracture. *1*, articular surface; *2*, metaphysis; *3*, fibula

soft tissue loss so disastrous. Tscherne and Gotzen's grading of soft tissue injuries for closed fractures is as follows:

Grade 0 – Little or no soft tissue injury (Fig. 18.4a)

Grade I – Significant abrasion or contusion (Fig. 18.4b)

Grade II – Deep contaminated abrasion with local contusional damage to skin or muscle (Fig. 18.4c)

Grade III – Extensive contusion or crushing of skin or destruction of muscle; also subcutaneous avulsions, decompensated compartment syndrome, or rupture of a major blood vessel (Fig. 18.4d)

In this particular injury the state of the skin and subcutaneous tissue is of overriding importance. Notoriously poor soft tissue healing, often measured in months, is common about the distal tibia. Venous drainage is often inadequate, leading to chronic edema and stasis ulceration. A high-energy injury may severely traumatize this poorly vascularized tissue, either by direct or indirect forces. Since much of the tibia at the ankle is subcutaneous, the skin and subcutaneous tissues, lacking the protection of muscle, may be traumatized by the fracture fragments from within, without an open wound being present. The resultant massive swelling may lead to the early formation of post-traumatic bullae. Skin necrosis may ensue, especially if the surgeon has chosen to further traumatize the skin with an ill-advised surgical procedure. Therefore, the timing of the surgery and delicate, atraumatic handling of the soft tissues are of vital importance in the management of this fracture.

18.2.4 Technical Difficulties

We have already discussed some of the important technical difficulties, such as severe comminution of the articular surface, impaction of cancellous bone, weak osteoporotic bone, and the precarious state of the soft tissues. In addition to those factors, exposure of the distal tibia to fully visualize the articular surface of the ankle is difficult, which further compounds the problem.

18.2.5 The Dilemma

A classic "Catch 22"[1] situation is obvious: that is, nonoperative care may result in persistent joint

---

[1] Catch 22: the obvious solution to a difficult problem leads to further problems of its own, which may be greater than the original problem.

Fig. 18.4a–d. Grading system of soft tissue injury in closed fractures. **a** Grade 0 – little or no soft tissue injury. **b** Grade 1 – superficial abrasion (*shaded area*) with local contusional damage to skin or muscle. **c** Grade 2 – deep contaminated abrasion with local contusional damage (*shaded area*) to skin and muscle. **d** Grade 3 – extensive contusion or crushing of skin or destruction of muscle (*shaded area*). (From Tscherne and Gotzen 1984)

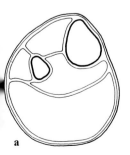
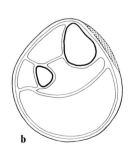
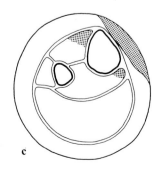
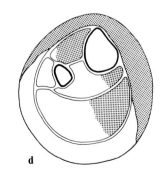

a   b   c   d

displacement and a poor outcome, but surgical treatment, in turn, is fraught with many difficulties. Good results may therefore be difficult to achieve by any method for some of these fractures.

The literature on this subject, sparse as it is, reflects this dilemma. Most reports indicate the need for anatomical restoration of the distal tibia but feel the difficulties and the risks involved are too great. Williams et al. (1967) and Ruoff and Snider (1971) therefore recommend traction methods as an alternative to open reduction, with the occasional use of percutaneous pinning in internal fixation of the fibula. However, their number of cases was too small to be significant.

Conrad (1970) described the lateral tibial plafond fracture associated with trimalleolar ankle fractures and made a plea for their anatomical open reduction. However, that injury is different from the so-called *explosion* or pilon fracture of the distal tibia, and the conclusions are therefore inapplicable.

The European literature is more extensive, but reaches similar conclusions. Bonnier (1961), De-Coulx et al. (1961), Fourquet (1959) all reported large series treated by both open and closed methods, with 43%, 45%, and 50% functional results. No definite trends were noted.

The reports of Rüedi and Allgöwer (1969) began to shed light on this dilemma. They adhered to the principles of the AO/ASIF group, i.e.:
1. Reconstruction of the fibula (if fractured)
2. Reconstruction of the articular surface of the tibia
3. Cancellous bone grafting of the gap in the distal tibial metaphysis, and
4. A medial or anterior tibial buttress plate to restore stability

and at a 4-year review were able to show good functional results in 74% of their 84 patients with pilon fractures.

The same group of patients were reviewed again 9 years after surgery: few had regressed and many had improved their previous rating (Rüedi 1973). For the first time in the literature, these reports indicated that this fracture was amenable to meticulous anatomical open reduction, stable internal fixation, and early motion.

Further reports by Heim and Naser (1977), Rüedi and Allgöwer (1979), and Szyszkowitz et al. (1979) confirmed these findings. The further publications by Rüedi and Allgöwer came from Basle, where 50% of the injuries were caused by high-energy motor vehicle trauma, unlike their original report in which most were caused by skiing inju-

Table 18.1. Treatment results of different types of fracture. (From Kellam and Waddell 1979)

Results	Compression type (in %)	Shearing type (in %)
Excellent	37 ⎫ 53	70 ⎫ 84
Adequate	16 ⎭	14 ⎭
Poor	47	16

ries. They were able to achieve excellent results in 69.4% of their cases, in spite of the shift of the injuries to a more high-energy type.

However, Kellam and Waddell (1979) indicated in a study of 26 distal tibial pilon fractures that results were more often linked to the type of fracture than to their management. With open reduction of the shearing type injury without major joint impaction, they achieved good results in 84% of the patients, a figure comparable to the Swiss group. However, in the severely impacted, comminuted compression type, they achieved only 53% good results (Table 18.1). However, the results obtained by operative treatment were superior to those by nonoperative treatment.

18.2.6 Summary

Have we, at this time, solved our dilemma? The answer, to a certain extent, is yes – but only to a certain extent. The final result of any lower extremity joint injury is dependent upon the ability of the surgeon to achieve an anatomical reduction of the joint surface. If this cannot be achieved by closed means, then open reduction is indicated. If we are to embark upon that course for the distal tibial fracture, it behooves us to pay particular attention to the timing of the operation, to the handling of the soft tissues, and to the precise details of the internal fixation. This, in turn, will avoid many of the complications, and should improve the functional results.

However, there will be some fractures in this area that by virtue of their articular cartilage destruction will defy even the most expert surgeon. In those cases, the prognosis resides more in the injury itself than in the treatment, and poor functional results, often ending in ankle arthrodesis, may be expected (see Fig. 18.11).

18.3 Classification

The Rüedi/Allgöwer (1969) classification of distal tibial fractures is based on the degree of displace-

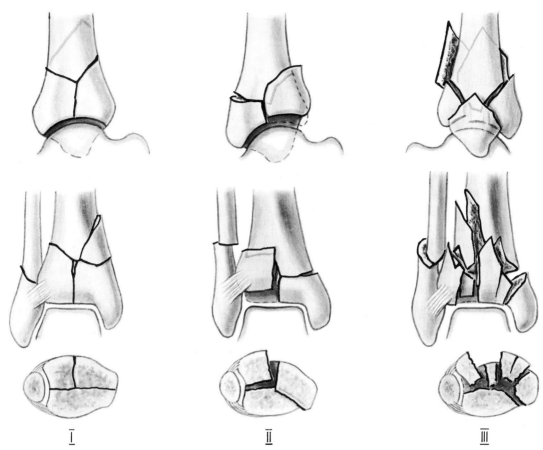

Fig. 18.5. Classification of distal tibial fractures (Rüedi and Allgöwer 1969). Grade I – articular fracture without significant displacement. Grade II – articular fracture with significant articular incongruity. Grade III – compression fracture with significant articular and metaphyseal incongruity. (From Müller et al. 1979)

ment of the articular fragments (Fig. 18.5). Fractures are graded as follows:

Grade I — Articular fracture without significant displacement

Grade II — Articular fracture with significant articular incongruity

Grade III — Severely comminuted and impacted articular fracture

This classification is satisfactory for discussion purposes and we recommend it. However, to help us with the management of the individual patient the classification must, as with other fractures, be expanded. Each case is different and must be individually assessed. We have learned that by answering a series of questions rather than by adhering to a precise unbending classification, logical decision making will follow. The important questions to ask are related to the state of the fibula, the articular surface of the tibia or talus, and the metaphyseal region of the tibia, as given in the following sections.

18.3.1 Fibula

Is the fibula fractured? In cases where it is intact, the injury has usually been caused by a severe varus compression force, often crushing the medial portion of the tibial articular surface (see Fig. 18.1 b, c). Also, the intact fibula acts as a post, stabilizing the important lateral aspect of the joint, the surgical implications of which are obvious. If the fibula is fractured, then the force involved is usually a valgus shear with resultant severe injury to the lateral aspect of the joint (see Fig. 18.1 d, e).

18.3.2 Articular Surface of the Tibia

Is the articular fracture displaced, and if so, is it a relatively uncomminuted fissue, or a grossly comminuted shattered lower end of tibia (Fig. 18.2)? Severe impaction and comminution of

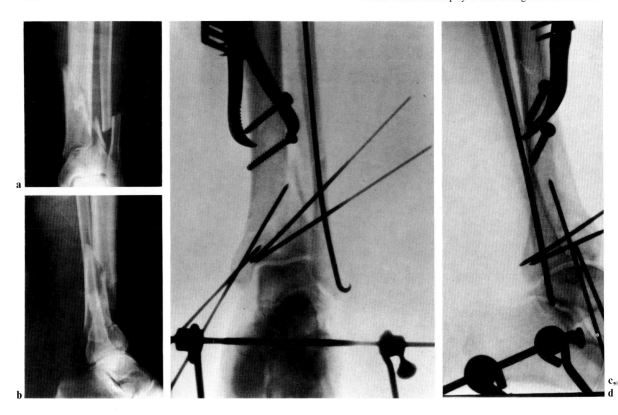

Fig. 18.6a–j. Pilon fracture with good prognosis. **a, b** Anteroposterior and lateral radiographs of a 32-year-old male injured while skiing. Note the comminution to the distal tibial metaphysis, the fracture of the fibula, and the valgus and anterior displacement. The distal tibial articular surface is relatively intact, with only one small undisplaced fracture through it. The intraoperative radiographs (**c, d**) show the fixation of the fibula with a Rush rod, the stabilization of the lower-third tibial fracture with two interfragmental screws, and the provisional stabilization of the articular surface with four Kirschner wires. No bone graft was required in this case. The postoperative radiographs at 6 weeks (**e, f**) show early union, and the patient's function at that time (**g, h**) shows almost normal ankle motion. The final result after plate removal (**i, j**) shows normal articular cartilage and normal axial alignment. The patient had an excellent end result

the articular surface may be irreparable; the final outcome of the case will therefore be more dependent on the answers to these questions than to any others.

18.3.3 Distal Tibial Metaphysis

Is the bone in the lower tibial metaphysis normal or osteoporotic? Is the fracture severely comminuted? Is there axial malalignment? Is there im-

paction of the cancellous bone which will cause a large gap following reduction?

18.3.4 Personality of the Fracture

The above are the important questions to ask before embarking upon the treatment of a pilon fracture. The answers will precisely define the personality of the fracture and will lead the surgeon to a logical management decision for each patient. Many permutations and combinations are possible. For example, an undisplaced fracture into the ankle joint with marked comminution and displacement of the metaphysis is suitable for careful reconstruction. Because the articular surface is not beyond repair, with ideal treatment one should expect an excellent result (Fig. 18.6).

By contrast, in the case of a severely comminuted impacted fracture of the articular surface of the ankle joint, with or without axial malalignment in the metaphysis, even the most careful open reduction may fail to restore joint congruity, which will inevitably lead to a poor result. In such a case, so much articular comminution is present that surgery cannot possibly restore it. Open reduction should therefore be avoided and traction methods employed (Fig. 18.7).

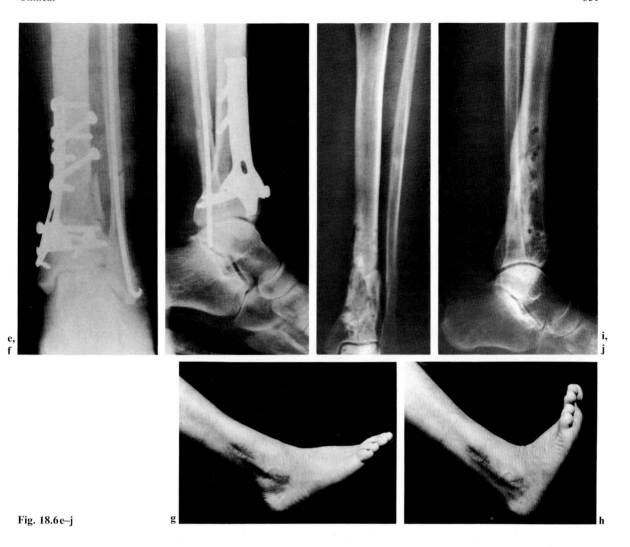

e,
f

i,
j

Fig. 18.6 e–j   g   h

All of these factors must be considered when comparing the results of different modalities, so as not to compare apples with oranges, as we have said before.

18.4 Assessment

Theoretically, the decision-making process should be relatively easy in this major weight-bearing joint fracture (Fig. 18.8). Since we believe that any *displaced* fracture of a major weight-bearing joint requires anatomical reduction, stable internal fixation, and early joint motion for optimal end results, then any such fracture in the distal tibia should be treated in that manner. However, because of the problems previously stated of severe bone comminution, osteoporosis, and poor soft tissues, exceptions have to be made.

As with all fractures, a careful assessment of the patient, the limb, and the injury, taking into account the expertise and experience of the surgeon, will aid in the decision-making process.

18.4.1 Clinical

General details of the medical history will reveal the chronological and physiological age of the patient and his or her general medical state and ambitions. The future expectations of the patient must be respected, especially in the case of the professional or amateur athlete.

The specific details of the mechanism of injury are important, as they will suggest to the surgeon the type of force involved. The violence exerted upon both the soft and skeletal tissues will vary considerably depending upon the mechanism of injury, whether a motor vehicle or motorbike acci-

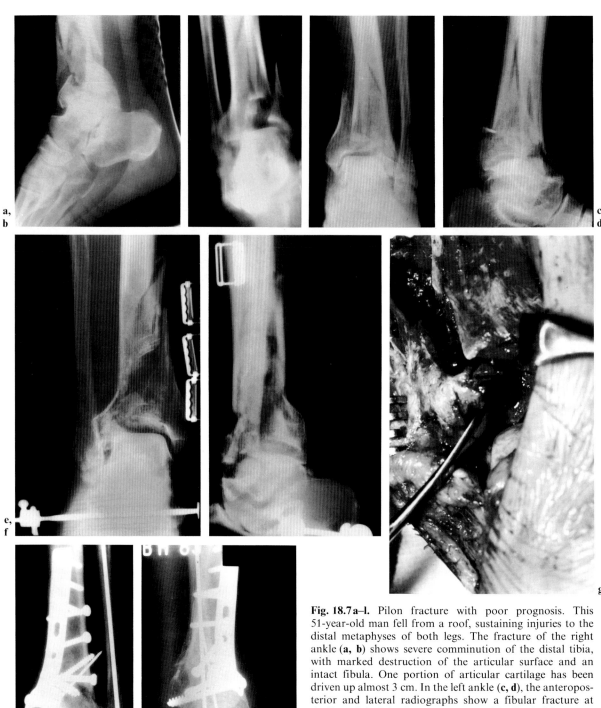

Fig. 18.7a–l. Pilon fracture with poor prognosis. This 51-year-old man fell from a roof, sustaining injuries to the distal metaphyses of both legs. The fracture of the right ankle (**a, b**) shows severe comminution of the distal tibia, with marked destruction of the articular surface and an intact fibula. One portion of articular cartilage has been driven up almost 3 cm. In the left ankle (**c, d**), the anteroposterior and lateral radiographs show a fibular fracture at the line of the joint but a reconstructable distal tibia.

The right ankle was treated with an os calcis pin and traction (**e, f**). At open reduction and internal fixation of the left ankle (**g**), note the severe comminution to the joint at the tip of the periosteal elevator. Osteosynthesis consisted of a Rush rod in the fibula, reconstruction of the articular surface, bone grafting, and stabilization with a T plate (**h, i**). The final result, 8 years later (**j–l**), shows good bony union bilaterally. Both ankles show osteophytes and joint narrowing and both are painful, the right being slightly worse than the left. The result in traction was almost equal to that afforded by internal fixation. The prognosis was determined more by the original injury to the articular cartilage than by the method of treatment

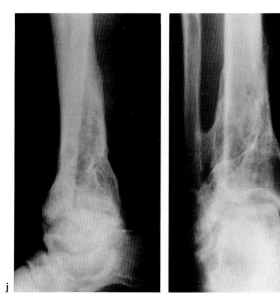
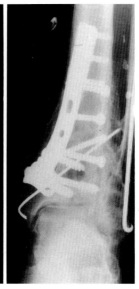
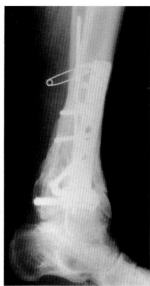

j
k,
l

Fig. 18.7j–l

dent, a fall from a height, or, in an older individual, a simple fall at home.

As always, a general physical examination is essential to assess the medical state of the patient.

Examination of the limb will reveal evidence of neurovascular damage and other skeletal injuries. A careful examination of the local area will reveal any lacerations at the fracture site. The degree of swelling and ecchymosis, as also the presence of fracture blisters, will have considerable bearing on the management decision, for an incision made through damaged skin may lead to a surgical disaster.

18.4.2 Radiological

In any articular fracture, it is imperative that a careful radiological assessment be carried out. All too often, major operative decisions are made on the basis of poor radiographs. The surgeon is then surprised during the operation by the number of fracture fragments present, and the injury may prove inoperable. The number of *surgical surprises* must be reduced, by surgeons demanding good anteroposterior, lateral, and oblique radiographs of the ankle as well as both anteroposterior and lateral tomograms. Computed tomograms (CTs) are invaluable in determining comminution of the articular surface.

A careful radiographic assessment will clearly reveal the number of articular fragments and will greatly aid in the treatment decision; then, if surgery is indicated, careful preoperative planning is possible.

After this careful assessment, the surgeon must fully discuss the injury with the patient, and allow him or her to share in the treatment decision. If the prognosis for that particular injury is poor, the patient should be so informed. If there is any chance that the surgeon may wish to do a primary ankle arthrodesis, the patient must be told of this prior to surgery, otherwise, misunderstandings (and possibly litigation) may follow.

18.5 Indications for Surgery

18.5.1 Minimal Displacement

If the preoperative assessment has indicated an *undisplaced* fracture, immobilization in a cast followed by a cast brace will lead to an acceptable result (Fig. 18.8). Patients with this kind of fracture usually have a partially intact soft tissue envelope, which favors rapid union and allows early motion.

18.5.2 Significant Displacement

If significant displacement is noted – that is, if large fragments of the articular surface of the joint

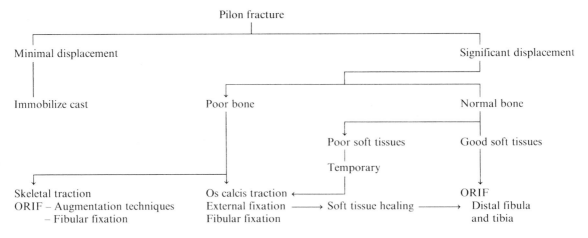

Fig. 18.8. Decision-making algorithm for pilon fractures

are displaced, or the metaphysis is grossly malaligned – surgery is indicated.

18.5.2.1 Operable

The determination of the operability of the fracture, employing logical surgical judgment, will be the next step in the decision-making process. If surgery is chosen, failure to achieve the stated goals of anatomical reduction and stable internal fixation will lead to the *worst of both worlds*, that is, the added trauma of the surgery inflicted upon an already severely injured extremity. It will also destroy all of the soft tissue hinges, so that nonoperative traction methods cannot be used successfully. Therefore, this initial decision is extremely important and must be based on a careful assessment of the radiographs, including the tomograms, as well of as the soft tissues.

If the *bone* is deemed to be normal, the degree of joint comminution not excessive, and the metaphysis reconstructible, then early operation is indicated, but only through satisfactory soft tissue (see Fig. 18.6).

a) Immediate Surgery

If the soft tissue is adequate for a major surgical procedure, then an open reduction and internal fixation should be carried out immediately. However, many patients are seen late and the skin and soft tissues are not suitable for surgery because of the presence of marked swelling or fracture blisters (see Fig. 18.7), and for these patients surgery must be delayed.

b) Delayed Surgery

Patients in whom surgery has to be delayed should be taken to the operating room, where under general anesthesia a *closed reduction* should be performed, correcting any angular displacement which may be impinging on the soft tissues. If the joint is subluxated, it must be reduced. If this reduction can be maintained in a plaster slab with a bulky dressing, the patient should be immobilized in this way. The limb should be elevated on several pillows and the patient encouraged to exercise limb and toes. If the instability is so marked that adequate alignment cannot be maintained, then an *os calcis traction pin* should be inserted and the patient kept on a Böhler–Braun frame to elevate the extremity (see Fig. 18.7e, f).

An excellent compromise in patients whose anterior skin is too poor for an early operative procedure but whose lateral skin is satisfactory is *immediate open anatomical reduction of the fibula with delayed tibial fixation*. This restores limb length, affords partial stability to allow the soft tissues to heal, and prevents the common drift to valgus of the tibia. The addition of a temporary os calcis traction pin is also desirable (Fig. 18.9).

In all of the above situations, the surgeon should wait until the skin and soft tissue have returned to a reasonable state before performing the surgical procedure on the tibia. This may require 7–10 days of elevation of the limb. During this period, revascularization of the traumatized soft tissues will occur. If the skin and soft tissues never return to an acceptable state, then traction must become the definitive treatment. In that particular

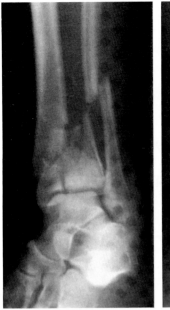 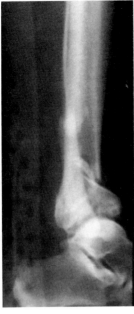 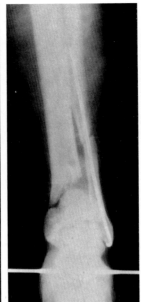 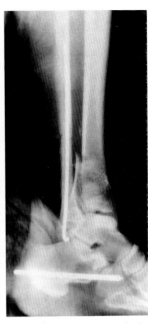

a,
b
c,
d

Fig. 18.9a–j. Immediate fibular fixation, delayed tibial fixation. This 42-year-old workman fell from a scaffold and sustained an open pilon fracture (**a, b**). On the night of admission, the wound was cleansed and débrided. The fibula was fixed with a Rush rod and an os calcis pin was inserted for skeletal traction on a Böhler–Braun frame (**c, d**). On the 7th day after injury, open reduction and internal fixation of the tibial fracture were performed. The postoperative radiograph (**e**) shows the excellent reconstruction of the joint surface with interfragmental screws, Kirschner wires, and a DC plate. A bone graft was used in this case. The original open portion of the wound was left open, the remainder sutured (**f**). Three years following injury, the bone has healed and the ankle joint has remained congruous and stable (**g, h**). The patient has 5° dorsiflexion to 20° plantar flexion (**i, j**)

situation, prior fibular fixation will prove markedly advantageous.

18.5.2.2 Inoperable

If the preoperative assessment indicates that the bone is so osteoporotic or the degree of comminution is so great that surgery, even by the most expert hands, cannot restore and stabilize the joint, then other methods of treatment must be sought.

a) Skeletal Traction

With the patient under general anesthetic a closed reduction should be carried out, the fracture being viewed under the image intensifier. If the fragments become reasonably aligned, a Kirschner wire should be inserted into the os calcis and the patient treated in traction for 6–8 weeks until the fracture has shown some consolidation. During this period, early motion of the ankle is encouraged.

Alignment must be maintained during this period, so frequent radiographs are necessary. If the alignment cannot be maintained because of a tendency to valgus deformation, fixation of the fibula, if fractured, should be considered as outlined above. This will prevent displacement and may greatly simplify the management in traction.

The surgeon must be certain that the ankle joint is not immobilized in the dislocated position. We have seen a number of patients treated nonoperatively with the ankle in the dislocated position – needless to say, with disastrous results.

Therefore, if a closed reduction is attempted but fails, the surgeon must discover the cause of this persistent dislocation. Usually, the medial soft tissues, such as the posterior tibial tendon, the neurovascular bundle, or the flexor digitorum longus, are caught in the fracture. In one such case, the surgeon even fixed the fibula but left the ankle joint dislocated in traction (Fig. 18.10). Further surgery at 4 weeks revealed the posterior tibial tendon to be interposed between the main tibial fragments.

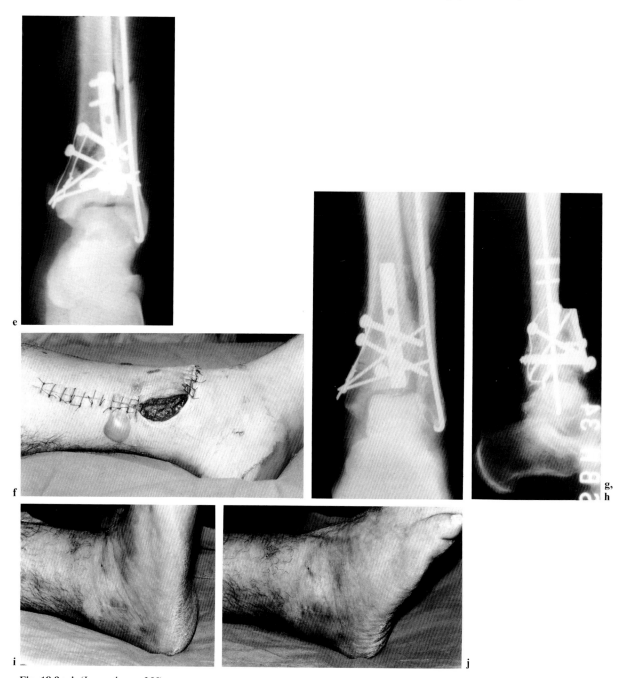

Fig. 18.9e–j. (Legend s. p. 355)

b) Primary Arthrodesis

If the patient has good bone but the degree of comminution is so excessive that an anatomical reduction cannot be carried out, then the surgeon could consider primary arthrodesis (Fig. 18.11). In our opinion, this is rarely indicated and, as stated previously, must be thoroughly discussed with the patient preoperatively to avoid misunderstanding and possible litigation. The advantage of primary arthrodesis is that it not only stabilizes the ankle, but allows early mobilization of the remainder of the foot, which is so important with ankle arthrodesis. However, with an os calcis traction pin and elevation, mobilization of the ankle and foot are also possible; therefore, unless the situation is

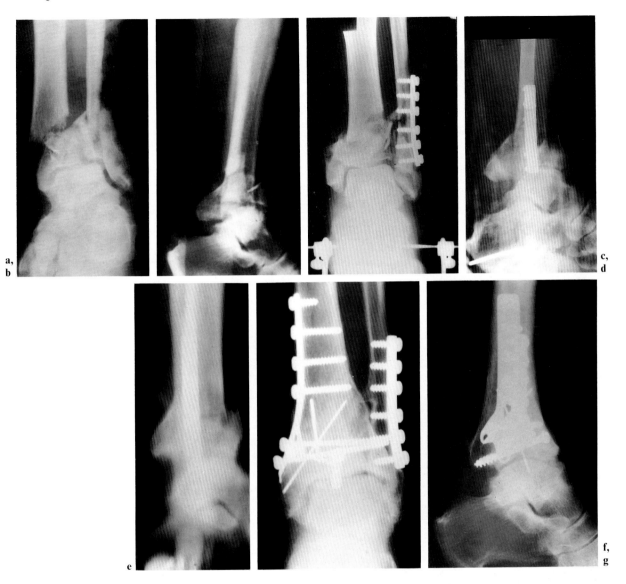

Fig. 18.10a–g. Posterior tibial tendon entrapment. This 29-year-old workman fell from a roof, sustaining a severely comminuted intraarticular open pilon fracture of the left ankle (**a, b**). Initial treatment consisted of débridement of the wound, stabilization of the lateral malleolus, insertion of an os calcis pin, and subsequent os calcis traction. The original medial wound was left open. The immediate postoperative radiographs (**c, d**) show the position of the fracture postoperatively. On the lateral radiograph (**d**), the ankle joint is clearly dislocated along with the anterior fragment of the distal tibia. This is better illustrated in the lateral tomogram (**e**). The posterior tibial tendon was interposed between the two bone fragments of the distal tibia and was not seen at the initial débridement. The dislocation was subsequently recognized at 3 weeks and open reduction, replacement of the posterior tibial tendon to its anatomical position, and internal fixation of the distal tibia were performed. Two years following injury, some joint narrowing and sclerosis is noted, indicative of an early osteoarthritis. The patient's function at that time was fair (**f, g**)

completely hopeless we prefer this approach to primary arthrodesis.

18.6 Surgical Technique

18.6.1 Timing

If possible, the surgery should be performed soon after the injury, before the development of severe soft tissue swelling and fracture blisters. Open fractures should also be dealt with immediately. The wounds should be cleansed and débrided. Precise preoperative planning is required to safely incorporate the wounds into the surgical incisions and to optimally place the implants.

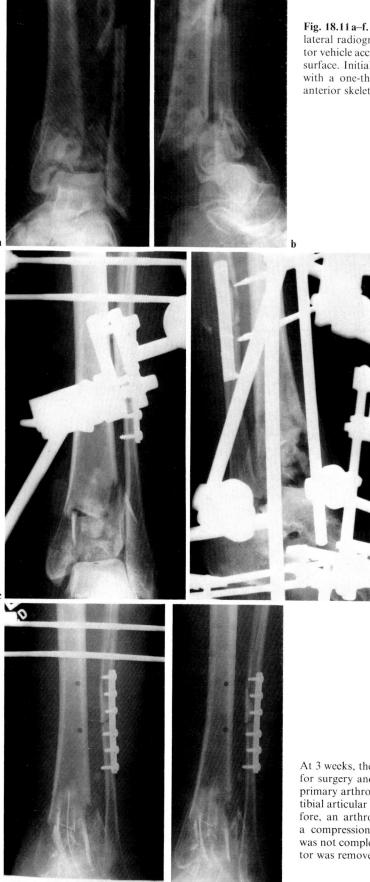

Fig. 18.11 a–f. Primary arthrodesis. **a, b** Anteroposterior and lateral radiographs of a 26-year-old man involved in a motor vehicle accident. Note the severe crushing of the articular surface. Initial treatment consisted of fixation of the fibula with a one-third semitubular plate and application of an anterior skeletal frame (**c, d**).

At 3 weeks, the patient's soft tissues were deemed adequate for surgery and the patient was forewarned that a delayed primary arthrodesis would probably be required. The distal tibial articular surface was impossible to reconstruct. Therefore, an arthrodesis was performed using bone graft and a compression technique (**e**). At 4 months, consolidation was not complete but was progressing and the external fixator was removed (**f**). The arthrodesis subsequently healed

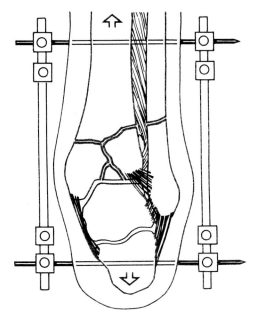

Fig. 18.12. External fixator to maintain temporary traction in a pilon fracture

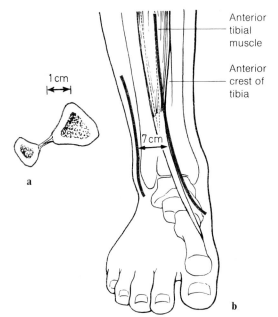

Fig. 18.13a, b. Surgical approach to fractures of the distal tibia (*pilon fractures*). The incision for the distal tibia should be medial to the tibialis anterior tendon, crossing the ankle joint and then curving slightly medially. This incision should be well lateral to the anterior subcutaneous surface of the tibia (**a**). The lateral incision should be posterior to the most prominent portion of the lateral malleolus and fibula, the surgeon being certain to keep as wide a bridge of skin as possible between it and the medial incision (**b**). (Adapted from Müller et al. 1979)

In situations where massive swelling and traumatic bullae are already present, *surgery is hazardous and must be avoided*. As previously mentioned, any dislocation must be reduced, and the limb should be elevated in a bulky dressing if stable, or, if unstable, with a traction pin in the os calcis.

An *external fixator* will serve the same purpose, that is, immobilization to allow soft tissue healing and traction to maintain length (Fig. 18.12). One or two pins in the tibia joined to one pin in the os calcis will be sufficient to maintain traction on a temporary basis. Usually 7–10 days are required for the soft tissues to recover sufficiently to allow safe reconstruction of the fracture.

18.6.2 Approach

18.6.2.1 Soft Tissue

Careful planning of the skin incision is essential. Given the choice, the favored incision runs just lateral to the anterior surface of the tibia and just medial to the tibialis anterior tendon, extending distally over the anterior portion of the medial malleolus (Fig. 18.13). However, the incisions might have to be modified depending upon the presence of lacerations or traumatized skin. The lateral incision for the fibular fracture should be posteriorly placed to increase the bridge between the two incisions (Fig. 18.13b).

Delicate handling of the skin in this area is imperative. It is relatively avascular, and improperly raised flaps and traumatic handling of the skin will result in necrosis with its ensuing problems. The surgeon must take great pains to be certain that the flap raised over the lower tibia is full thickness, that is, contains both skin and subcutaneous tissue right to the periosteum. If the subcutaneous layer is entered, the blood supply will be compromised and necrosis of the skin may ensue. This in turn often leads to sepsis and a disastrous result.

18.6.2.2 Skeletal Tissue

As in all metaphyseal fractures, especially those involving a joint surface, exposure of the joint should be through major tears in the soft tissue envelope (see Fig. 18.14a, b). This will preserve the remaining soft tissue attachments to the fracture fragments and facilitate stabilization of the comminuted metaphyseal fragments. Also, these soft tissue attachments must be preserved in order to maintain bone viability.

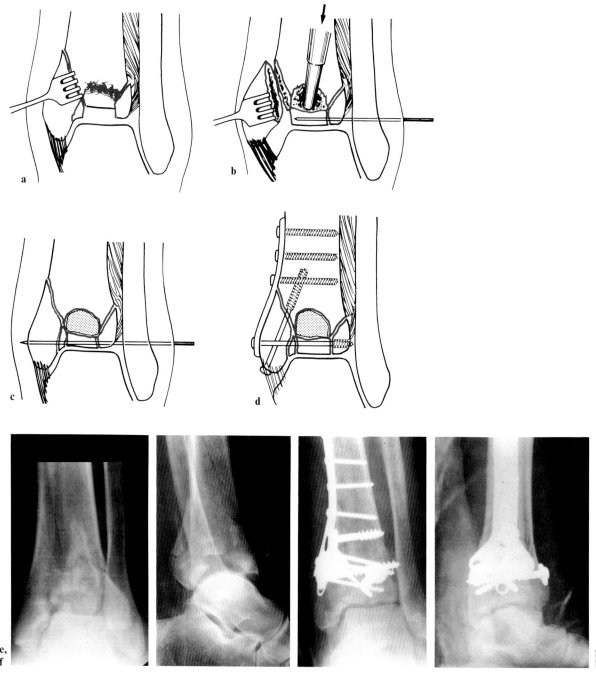

Fig. 18.14a–h. Technique of open reduction and internal fixation in a pilon fracture with an intact fibula. Since the fibula is intact, lateral stability of the ankle mortise is maintained. A large tibial fragment usually remains with the fibula and is used as a guide to articular reconstruction. The large medial vertical fragment is retracted with a rake retractor (**a**). Working through the fracture in order not to destroy soft tissue, the articular fragments are restored to their anatomical position and provisionally fixed with 2-mm Kirschner wires (**b**). Any gap is filled with cancellous bone to hold the articular fragments in place (**c**). The tibia is then buttressed with a medial buttress plate and lag screws as indicated (**d**). **e, f** Anteroposterior and lateral radiograph of a 23-year-old male involved in a motor vehicle accident. Note the intact fibula and the articular crush. **g, h** Reconstruction by the above method using a cloverleaf plate, with excellent articular reconstruction

18.6.3 Technique of Internal Fixation

18.6.3.1 *Without Fibular Fracture*

If the fibula is intact, lateral stability of the ankle mortise is maintained. Usually, however, the tibial fracture exhibits comminution and impaction of the joint surface (see Fig. 18.2c).

A large intact fragment usually remains with the fibula and is used as a guide to the articular reconstruction. The large medial vertical fragment may be carefully retracted with a rake retractor, thus exposing the articular surface (Fig. 18.14a, b). All soft tissue attachments to this fragment must be retained. If a central depressed articular fragment is found, it must be restored to its anatomical position and provisionally fixed with Kirschner wires (1.6–2.0 mm) (Fig. 18.14b). A cancellous bone graft will hold the articular fragments in place, then the medial vertical fracture is reduced, thus "closing the book" (Fig. 18.14c). This type of fracture is akin to the usual type of depressed proximal lateral plateau fracture. The large medial fragment is stabilized with interfragmental lag screws and a medial buttress plate, usually the T or cloverleaf type (Fig. 18.14d–h).

18.6.3.2 *With Fibular Fracture*

If the fibula is fractured (Fig. 18.15a), the four steps in the reconstruction are as follows:
1. Reconstruction of the fibula (Fig. 18.15b)
2. Open reduction of the tibial articular surface and metaphysis (Fig. 18.15c)
3. Cancellous bone grafting of the metaphyseal defect (Fig. 18.15c)

4. Application of a buttress plate to the anterior or medial cortex of the tibia (Fig. 18.15d)

a) Fibular Reconstruction

The fibular reconstruction should be performed using standard AO/ASIF techniques (Fig. 18.15b).

If the fracture is transverse, an intramedullary Steinmann pin or Rush rod may be used. This has the added advantage of a short incision and minimal dissection on the lateral side, which makes the medial approach and closure much simpler. Restoration of fibular length is essential, but less than perfect rotational stability of the fibula is acceptable in the pilon fracture since stability of the tibia is restored. In the usual bi- or trimalleolar ankle fracture, it is imperative to achieve rotational stability of the fibula, and therefore intramedullary devices in the fibula are contraindicated. However, in the particular type of fracture with which we are dealing here, that is, the pilon fracture, intramedullary devices in the fibula are ideal if the fibular fracture is transverse and not comminuted.

If the fibula is comminuted, the fracture should be fixed with interfragmental compression screws

Fig. 18.15a–d. Pilon fracture reconstruction with fibular fracture. **a** Pilon fracture with intra-articular comminution and fibular fracture. **b** Step 1: reconstruction of the fibula by either an intramedullary rod or a one-third semitubular plate. **c** Steps 2 and 3: reconstruction of the articular surface of the distal tibia and provisional fixation with Kirschner wires. The resultant gap is filled with cancellous bone graft. **d** Step 4: application of a medial buttress plate (T plate). (Adapted from Müller et al. 1979)

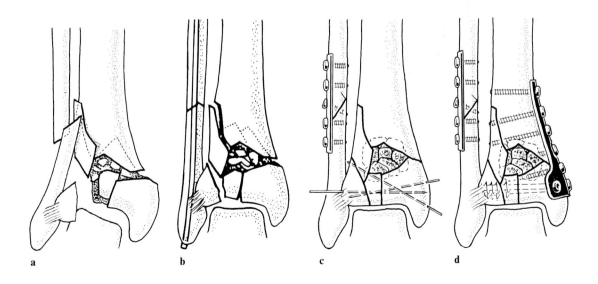

a   b   c   d

and a one-third semitubular plate as a neutralization plate. If the fibula is grossly comminuted, it
is extremely important to be certain that full length
is restored to the fibula. The fibula is connected
to the lateral articular fragment of the tibia; therefore, its proper length is the key to the reduction
of this tibial articular surface. *Shortening of the
fibula will cause malreduction of the major tibial
fracture.*

In rare instances, there may be so much comminution of the fibula that primary fixation of this
bone is impossible. In those circumstances, articular reconstruction of the tibia should proceed first,
and fixation of the fibula be undertaken after-
wards if technically possible. However, failure to
reconstruct the fibula at all is a major error in
judgement and may jeopardize the tibial reconstruction, as the tendency of the ankle to drift into
valgus will be difficult to overcome. Stabilization
of the fibula is therefore an essential part of the
treatment (Fig. 18.19).

b) Articular Reconstruction of the Tibia

After fixation of the fibula, articular reconstruction should proceed in a logical fashion.

Visualization of the fragments may be extremely difficult, and under these circumstances we recommend the intraoperative insertion of an os calcis pin with an attached stirrup, so that the assistant may maintain constant traction while the surgeon works. To obviate the need for a second assistant, the surgeon may choose to insert a tibial
pin and use the external frame as a distractor,
thereby achieving the same end (see Fig. 18.12).

The key to the articular reconstruction is the
lateral fragment, which should be in the anatomically correct position if connected by the inferior
tibiofibular ligament to the already anatomically
fixed fibula. Each of the major fragments should
be reduced and carefully fixed with Kirschner
wires. If only major fragments are involved, the
reduction is relatively easy and should be anatomical (Fig. 18.15c).

If gross comminution of the metaphysis is present, the surgeon should first focus his attention
on an accurate reconstruction of the articular surface. The articular fragments should be provisionally fixed with 1.6 mm Kirschner wires, then held
with large cancellous screws if possible. Following
articular reconstruction, the distal and proximal
fragments are realigned and provisionally held
with Kirschner wires, awaiting definitive fixation.

c) Cancellous Grafting

A cancellous bone graft, which may be taken prior
to surgery or simultaneously by a second operative
team, is now impacted into the large metaphyseal
gap (Fig. 18.15c). Small fragments of articular cartilage which have not been fixed with Kirschner
wires and are not small enough to discard may
be held in place between the cancellous bone graft
and the dome of the talus. Their stability, however,
must be ensured, so that they do not fall out into
the joint and act as a loose body. The cancellous
bone graft should be fully impacted to restore stability to the distal fragment.

d) Medial Tibial Cortex Buttress Plate

To ensure the anatomical reduction of this provisionally fixed tibia, a buttress plate must be applied either anteriorly or medially, depending upon
the area of comminution (Fig. 18.6). The medial
buttress plate may be either of the T plate or cloverleaf variety (see Fig. 18.6). The cloverleaf plate
is weak and should only be used in those situations
where the comminution is so great that multiple
screw holes are required for the fixation of the
articular surface. In most cases, the T plate is a
better implant. If the comminution is anterior, the
anterior or spoon plate will give far better fixation
and is recommended (Fig. 18.16). These general
principles are well illustrated in Fig. 18.17.

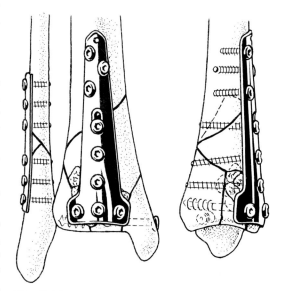

Fig. 18.16. Spoon plate as an anterior buttress plate. As
the situation dictates, an anterior buttress may be more
desirable than a medial buttress, and for this situation the
spoon plate is an excellent implant. (From Müller et al.
1979)

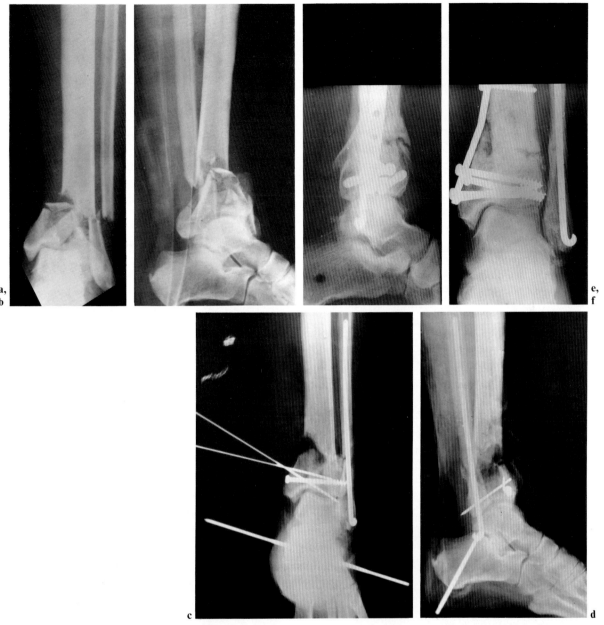

Fig. 18.17 a–f. This 48-year-old male fell from a hayloft to the barn floor. He sustained a severe pilon fracture (**a, b**). The intraoperative films (**c, d**) illustrate the initial steps in the reduction. The fibula was fixed with a Rush rod. An os calcis traction pin allowed visualization of the articular surface, which was provisionally fixed with Kirschner wires and an interfragmental screw. Note the extremely large medial and anterior gap. This gap was subsequently filled with cancellous bone graft and a medial buttress plate applied restoring the anatomy (**e, f**)

If it becomes obvious to the surgeon after the start of the surgical procedure that the bone is too weak to hold a screw, the situation may be improved by using low viscosity polymethyl methacrylate bone cement in the screw hole or at the fracture site. However, we would recommend this procedure only in older individuals. In those cases, the Kirschner wires should be retained as definitive forms of internal stabilization and should not be removed until union is complete. Early motion will not be possible, so the final result may be compromised.

18.6.4 Wound Closure

If both incisions can be closed without tension, this should be done, primarily over suction drains.

Very commonly, however, suturing both incisions will cause undue tension on one or other wound. When this is the case, it is far better to leave a portion of one wound open than to close it under tension, since this will undoubtedly result in skin necrosis. It is best to close the tibial wound because of its proximity to the anterior tibial tendon, the subcutaneous border of the tibia, and the major metal implant. The lateral wound may be left open along all or a part of its length. If the lateral skin incision has been correctly made, posterior to the fibula, then the fibular plate will be covered by the skin flap and few problems will ensue. This lateral wound may then be closed on the 5th–10th postoperative day with fine sutures or skin tapes.

Note: *in this area, do not attempt to rotate skin flaps to ensure skin closure.* The skin in this area may be so traumatized that the entire flap may be rendered avascular and become necrotic, causing a major surgical disaster (Fig. 18.18). It is far better to leave one wound open and close it sec-

ondarily than to undertake ill-advised primary plastic procedures.

18.6.5 Postoperative Care

18.6.5.1 Early

In the immediate postoperative period a bulky dressing and posterior slab are applied to the ankle in the neutral position and the extremity elevated to reduce swelling.

The course of the patient's postoperative care will depend upon the surgeon's honest appraisal of the stability achieved by surgery. If the bone quality is good and the surgeon has been able to achieve stable internal fixation, then the dressing and splint are removed on the 2nd postoperative day and motion is encouraged. The stabilized fracture is relatively painless, many patients being able to move their ankle comfortably as early as the 2nd postoperative day. To prevent a troublesome equinus deformity from developing, the ankle must be maintained in a right-angled splint when the patient is not exercising; once an equinus deformity has developed, attempts at correction by rehabilitation may be tedious and prolonged, and are often unsuccessful.

If the surgeon is in doubt about the stability of the fracture at the conclusion of the operation,

Fig. 18.18. a Radiograph of 29-year-old male with an open fracture of the right ankle due to a gunshot. After débridement, the surgeon attempted a relaxing incision, resulting in complete necrosis of the skin and anterior tibial tendon (**b**). The fracture was secondarily fixed with two interfragmental screws and the wound débrided and skin grafted (**c**)

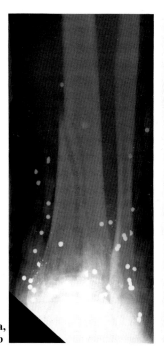
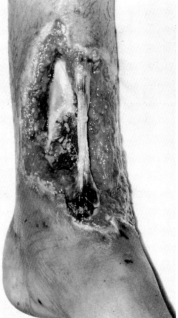
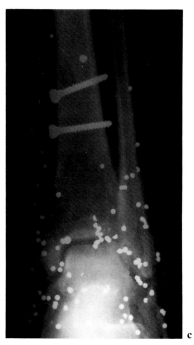

a,
b

c

he should insert an os calcis pin for skeletal traction to protect the osteosynthesis. Preservation of the anatomical reduction is essential to the long-term result and should not be compromised by early motion.

The use of the traction pin will allow early motion of the ankle while affording protection to the internal fixation. The pin is generally required for 4–6 weeks, when healing of the cancellous bone has usually progressed sufficiently to remove it. A cast brace with a moving ankle piece may then be applied until bone union is complete.

18.6.5.2 Late

The patient must be carefully monitored clinically and radiologically. A patellar-bearing weight-relieving caliper may be used after 6 weeks if healing is progressing well. This allows the patient to bear partial weight with the aid of crutches. The splint should be regularly removed for ankle exercises. If the patient has no pain and the radiograph indicates no problems with the implant, bone union is usually complete at 10–16 weeks and full weight bearing may be resumed. This will, of course, de-

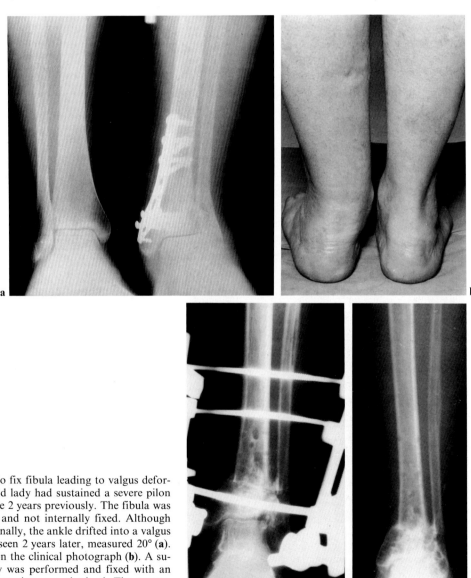

Fig. 18.19a–d. Failure to fix fibula leading to valgus deformation. This 41-year-old lady had sustained a severe pilon fracture to her left ankle 2 years previously. The fibula was extremely comminuted and not internally fixed. Although anatomically fixed originally, the ankle drifted into a valgus deformity which when seen 2 years later, measured 20° (**a**). The deformity is seen on the clinical photograph (**b**). A supramalleolar osteotomy was performed and fixed with an external fixator (**c**). Correction was obtained. The anteroposterior radiograph (**d**) shows the osteotomy healed and the good position of the ankle joint

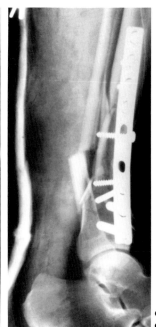
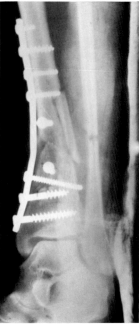

a,
b

c,
d

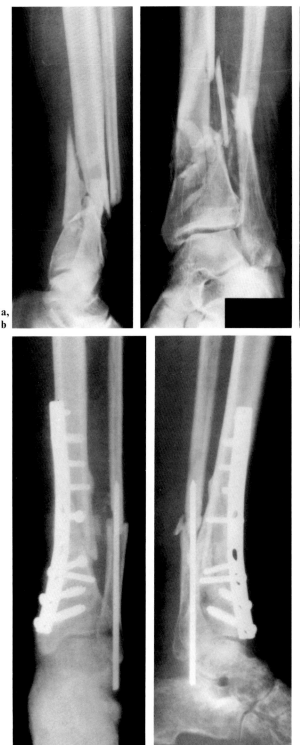

e   f

Fig. 18.20 a–f. Failure to fix fibula with varus deformation. **a, b** Lateral and anteroposterior radiographs of a 27-year-old female with a pilon fracture involving both the tibia and the fibula. **c, d** Immediate postoperative radiographs showing the varus position of the distal tibia. The fibula was not fixed. Note the recurvatum deformity in **d**. An attempt to secondarily fix the fibula failed to anatomically reduce the tibial fracture (**e, f**). The final result was fair

pend upon other factors, such as the degree of comminution, the size and incorporation of the bone graft, and the state of the soft tissues.

18.7 Common Pitfalls of Treatment

Since the pilon or distal tibial metaphyseal fracture is fraught with major problems in management, it seems relevant to mention here many of the common pitfalls we have encountered in our practice, when the principles stated above have been compromised.

18.7.1 Poor Decision Making

This is probably the commonest cause of grief with this fracture. In some cases, operable fractures are treated nonoperatively, with poor results; while in others, shattered fractures, obviously nonoperable, are treated operatively, with a similar outcome.

18.7.2 Operating Through Poor Skin

Operating through severely traumatized skin with fracture blisters constitutes a great error of judgement, and often leads to a major disaster, occasionally even an amputation.

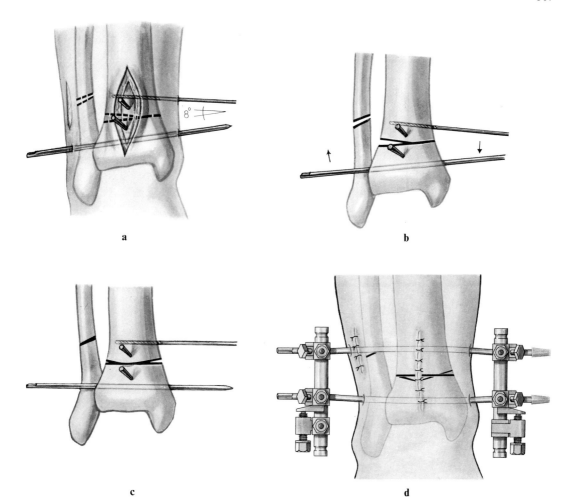

Fig. 18.21 a–d. Stable fixation with two Steinmann pins and external fixators. **a** Resect a small segment of the fibula and insert a Steinmann pin parallel to the distal articular surface of the tibia. From the medial side and proximal to the planned osteotomy insert a 3.2-mm drill bit into the tibia. This drill bit should subtend the desired angle of correction with the Steinmann pin. Into the anterior crest insert two Kirschner wires, one on each side of the osteotomy. They will serve to control the rotational alignment as well as the angulation of the osteotomy. **b** Carry out the osteotomy between the Kirschner wires. **c** Correct the deformity. **d** Remove the drill bit and replace it with a Steinmann pin. Reduce the osteotomy and compress it with two external fixators. (From Müller et al. 1979)

18.7.3 Technical Difficulties with the Fibula

If the fibula length is not restored, the ankle will tend to drift into valgus (Fig. 18.19), while if the normal valgus curve of the fibula is not restored, the ankle will assume to varus position (Fig. 18.20). The resulting axial malalignment will cause difficulty with the gait and eventual degenerative arthritis in the ankle.

18.7.4 Technical Difficulties with the Tibial Fracture

There is a tendency among surgeons to fix the articular position of the joint and ignore the metaphyseal crush; that is, to do only one half of the job. This is a common error, usually leading to axial malalignment and a poor final result.

Furthermore, failure to fill the large metaphyseal gap with bone graft may allow the articular fracture to displace, with adverse late consequences.

18.7.5 Poor Postoperative Care

Over-optimistic assessment of the operative stabilization and the state of the bone often leads the surgeon to institute early motion of the ankle. If the assessment was wrong, the inevitable result will be collapse of the fixation and loss of the anatomical reduction.

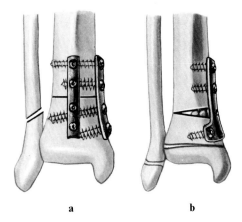

◀ **Fig. 18.22. a** Two semi-tubular plates used for the fixation of a supramalleolar osteotomy in an adult. **b** In children where the deformity results from a premature partial closure of the epiphyseal plate, we prefer an open wedge osteotomy which restores some length and corrects the deformity. The defect is bone grafted and the osteotomy fixed with a small T plate. (From Müller et al. 1979)

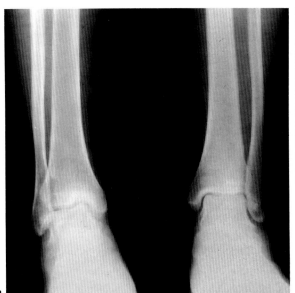

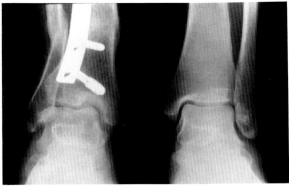

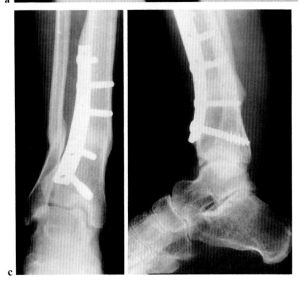

Fig. 18.23a–c. Varus deformation requiring supramalleolar osteotomy. **a** Comparative standing anteroposterior radiographs of both ankles showing the severe varus deformation of the right ankle, due to an impacted fracture of the distal tibial articular surface. The patient had severe pain and difficulty walking with the right foot. A supramalleolar osteotomy was performed with fibular osteotomy, and the tibial osteotomy was internally fixed. The comparative radiograph (**b**) now shows correction of the varus deformity. **c** Anteroposterior and lateral radiographs taken at 1 year showing the healed osteotomy and the excellent anatomical position. Eight years following osteotomy, the patient's ankle is still functioning well with only minimal discomfort

A major cause of grief is failure to splint the ankle at 90° postoperatively. The resulting equinus deformity may be difficult to deal with. There is no excuse for this preventable complication.

18.8 Late Reconstruction: Supramalleolar Osteotomy

If the patient has continuing pain following union of a pilon fracture, careful clinical and radiographic assessment will determine whether the articular cartilage of the ankle joint has been so damaged that arthrodesis of the ankle is the only alternative, or whether the articular surface is satisfactory and axial malalignment is the major cause of the problem. In instances of the latter, a supramalleolar osteotomy will restore axial alignment, usually restore normal foot mechanics, and be very helpful to the patient. Careful preoperative planning is essential to the correct performance of this operative procedure. The osteotomy may be fixed with an external fixation device under compression, or with internal fixation (Figs. 18.21, 18.22). Even in instances where there is damage to articular cartilage, supramalleolar osteotomy may prove to be of major help to the patient without resorting to arthrodesis. The patient in Fig. 18.23, a 29-year-old school teacher, had a marked varus deformation with a medial indentation of the distal tibial articular surface. She had great difficulty in walking. A supramalleolar osteotomy was performed, correcting the varus deformity, and in spite of the articular defect, her ankle continues to function well 8 years after surgery.

References

Bonnier P (1961) Les fractures du pilon tibial. Thesis, Lyons

Conrad RW (1970) Fracture dislocations of the ankle joint in the impaction injury of the lateral weight bearing surface of the tibia. J Bone Joint Surg 52A:1337

DeCoulx P, Razemon JP, Rouselle Y (1961) Fractures du tibial pilon. Rev Chir Orthop 47:563

Fourquet D (1959) Contribution à l'étude des fractures récentes du pilon tibial. Thesis, Paris

Heim U, Naser K (1977) Fractures du pilon tibial: resultats de 128 osteosynthèses. Rev Chir Orthop 63(1):5–12

Kellam JF, Waddell JP (1979) Fractures of the distal tibia. J Trauma 8:593–601

Müller ME, Allgöwer M, Schneider R, Willenegger H (eds) (1979) Manual of internal fixation, 2nd edn. Springer, Berlin Heidelberg New York

Rüedi T (1973) Fractures of the lower end of the tibia into the ankle joint: results 9 years after open reduction and internal fixation. Injury 5:130

Rüedi TP, Allgöwer M (1969) Fractures of the lower end of the tibia into the ankle joint. Injury 1:92

Rüedi TP, Allgöwer M (1979) The operative treatment of intraarticular fractures of the lower end of the tibia. Clin Orthop 138:105–110

Ruoff AC, Snider RK (1971) Explosion fractures of the distal tibia with major articular involvement. J Trauma 11:866

Szyszkowitz R, Marti R, Wilde CD, Reschauer R, Schloffmann W (1979) Die offene Reposition und Verschraubung der Talusfrakturen. Hefte Unfallheilkd 133:41–48

Tscherne H, Gotzen L (1984) Fractures with soft tissue injuries. Springer, Berlin Heidelberg New York Tokyo

Williams CW, Langston J, Sander A (1967) Comminuted fractures of the distal tibia into the ankle joint. J Bone Joint Surg 49A:192

19 Fractures of the Ankle

M. Tile

19.1 Introduction

19.1.1 Basic Principles

As in all fractures through the articular surface of a major weight-bearing joint, optimal treatment for fractures of the ankle follows the basic tenet: restoration of the normal anatomy is required to prevent development of secondary arthritis. The anatomical reduction may be obtained by closed means, but often, in unstable fractures, it cannot be maintained. The most precise method of restoring and maintaining the anatomy of the unstable ankle injury is open reduction and internal fixation. As an added advantage, modern stable internal fixation will allow early motion and usually ensure a satisfactory outcome.

19.1.2 Anatomical Considerations

19.1.2.1 Stability

Stability is imparted to the ankle by its bony configuration and its complex ligamentous system. The dome of the talus is held snugly in the ankle mortise by a cup-like structure consisting of the adjacent articular surfaces of the tibia and fibula. At the ankle, these two bones are held together by the interosseous membrane and the strong syndesmotic ligaments, the anterior tibiofibular ligaments, and the strong posterior tibiofibular ligaments (Fig. 19.1 a). Only minor degrees of motion are possible at the intact distal tibiofibular joint. Further stability is imparted by the medial and lateral collateral ligaments and the intervening joint capsule.

The medial or deltoid ligament is a fan-shaped structure consisting of two portions, a superficial and a deep (Pankovich and Shivaran 1979; Fig. 19.1 b). The deep portion, in turn, consists of two parts: the deep anterior talotibial ligament, originating from the anterior aspect of the medial malleolus and distally inserting on the medial side of the talus, and the deep posterior talotibial ligament, running from the posterior aspect of the medial malleolus posteriorly to the medial aspect of the talus. The superficial portion, the tibiocalcaneal band, consists of a continuous fan-like structure connecting the anterior colliculus of the medial malleolus to the navicular bone, calcaneus, and talus. The tendon sheaths of the posterior tibial and flexor digitorum communis muscles are contiguous with the deltoid ligament.

On the lateral aspect, stability is maintained by the complex lateral collateral ligament, consisting of three portions (Fig. 19.1 c). Functioning as the anterior cruciate ligament of the ankle, the anterior talofibular ligament connects the anterior portion of the fibula to the talar tubercle, thereby preventing anterior displacement of the talus in the ankle mortise. The importance of this ligament in ankle pathology has been greatly underestimated. The calcaneofibular ligament limits inversion by its attachments from fibula to calcaneus. The posterior talofibular ligament runs horizontally and medially, completing the lateral stabilizing mechanism and limiting posterior and rotatory subluxation of the talus.

19.1.2.2 Congruity

The ankle joint is fully congruous in all positions of the talus, from full plantar flexion to full dorsiflexion (Inman 1976). Previous teaching held that the talus, narrower posteriorly than anteriorly, would be unstable in the ankle mortise when plantar-flexed. However, Inman postulated that both the talar and tibial articular surfaces are segments of a cone or frustum, with the apex located medially (Fig. 19.2a); therefore, during the normal ankle motion of dorsiflexion to plantar flexion, the dome of the talus rotates around its laterally placed base (Fig. 19.2b). The smooth and congruous motion of the normal ankle depends upon an anatomical and stable lateral malleolar complex,

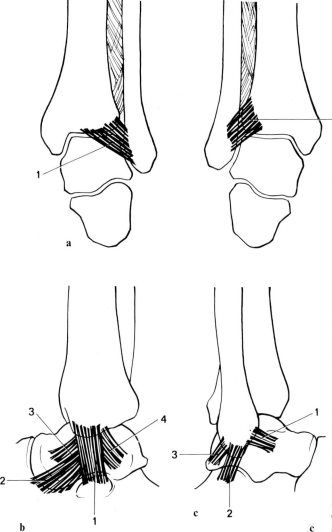

Fig. 19.1. a *Left:* The anterior (*1*) and posterior (*2*) tibiofibular ligaments (syndesmotic ligaments). *Right:* cross section of the ankle showing the syndesmotic ligaments. *1* anterior tibial tendon, *2* neurovascular bundle: anterior tibial nerves and vessels, *3* extensor hallucis longus, *4* extensor digitorum longus, *5* saphenous vein, *6* tibia, *7* posterior tibial tendon, *8* flexor digitorum longus tendon, *9* neurovascular bundle: posterior tibial nerves and vessels, *10* flexor hallucis longus tendon, *11* Achilles tendon, *12* sural nerves, *13* posterior syndesmotic ligament, *14* peroneous longus tendon, *15* peroneous brevis tendon, *16* fibula, *17* anterior syndesmotic ligament.

b The medial (deltoid) ligament. Note the fan-shaped insertion of this ligament, which contains two portions, a superficial (*1*) (the tibiocalcaneal band) and a deep one, a part of which becomes the spring ligament (*2*). The deep portion has two parts, a deep anterior talotibial ligament (*3*) and a deep posterior, talotibial ligament (*4*).

c The lateral ligament. This ligament has three parts, the anterior talofibular ligament (*1*), the posterior talofibular ligament *3*, and the calcaneofibular ligament *2*

to accommodate the longer excursion of the larger lateral border of the talus. As each segment of the cone rotates, full congruity is maintained in all positions. Further work in our laboratory using latex injection into the joint confirmed the congruous nature of the joint.

Using standard radiographic techniques in normal subjects, Gollish et al. (1977) also ascertained that the normal ankle has no talar tilt either in valgus or varus in the stance phase of gait and is fully congruous in that position (see Fig. 19.8 a, b).

19.1.2.3 Physiology

Although the ankle joint remains congruous, some motion does occur at the distal tibiofibular joint during normal gait. In the stance phase, a lateral

thrust occurs from the talus to the lateral malleolus. This force is then transferred back to the tibia through the interosseous membrane (Fig. 19.3). The lateral malleolus, therefore, is a weight-bearing structure, maintaining approximately one-sixth of the body weight (Elmendorff and Petes 1971).

19.1.2.4 Pathoanatomy

Several important clinical considerations arise from the preceding comments. First, since the ankle ligaments are vital for the stability of the joint, they must be considered as important as the bone in the assessment of the injury. On clinical examination, the presence of local tenderness, ecchymoses, and swelling at the site of a ligamentous attachment, in the absence of a radiologically

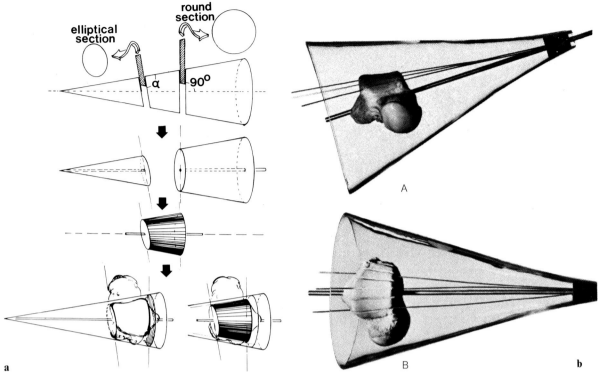

Fig. 19.2. a Pictorial representation of present concept of construction of trochlea of talus. A frustum is cut from a cone. The section cut at 90° to the axis of the cone is circular when projected onto a transverse plane of the cone; this corresponds to the fibular (lateral) facet. The section cut obliquely is elliptical; this corresponds to the tibial (medial) facet. Note that the fibular facet, being farther from the apex of the cone, possesses greater dimensions. With minor modifications, a section of the frustum is converted into the trochlea of the talus. The anteroposterior curve of the fibular facet is an ellipse because of the oblique orientation of the conical surface of the trochlea when viewed from above. **b** *A* Talus mounted inside transparent glass cone and oriented so it is viewed from front. Note that while the superior surface of the trochlea is horizontal, the axis is oblique, causing both the glass cone and the conical surface of the trochlea, as outlined by the Kirschner wires, to be slanted. *B* View from above the glass cone with enclosed talus, which has not been moved. Note that because of the obliquity of the axis and the slant of the glass cone (*A*), the open base of the glass cone is now viewed as an ellipse. Attention is called to the resultant parallelism between the edge of the glass cone and the curvature of the lateral edge of the trochlea. (From Inman 1976)

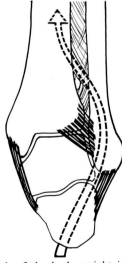

Fig. 19.3. Approximately one-sixth of the body weight is transferred through the fibular malleolus to the tibia

proven fracture, should alert the surgeon to a major ligamentous disruption. Demonstration of a subluxation of the talus in the ankle mortise, occasionally under a general anesthetic, will confirm the resultant instability. Secondly, since the joint is fully congruous in all positions of ankle motion, it follows that even minor abnormalities in the ankle mortise will alter the biomechanics of the joint and may result in major long-term problems. Therefore, restoration of ankle congruity is imperative if secondary osteoarthritis is to be avoided.

Finally, contrary to previous belief, the lateral side of the joint is of vital clinical importance for both stability and congruity, and must therefore be anatomically restored. Shortening or rotatory displacement of the fibula will markedly affect the articular contact area between the talus and the tibia.

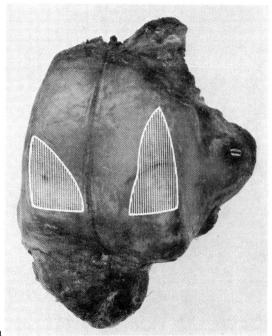
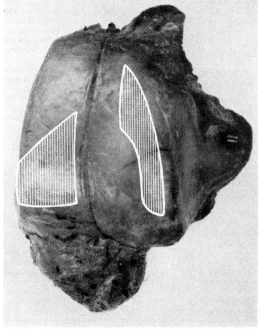

a   b

Fig. 19.4a, b. Reduction in the contact area of the talar dome with the tibial plafond by **a** a tilt in the vertical axis of the lateral malleolus and **b** a posterior displacement of the vertical axis of the talus. (From Müller et al. 1965)

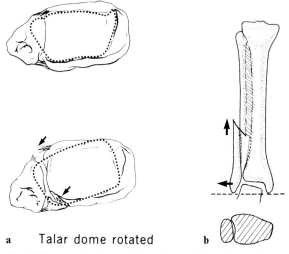

a   Talar dome rotated   b

Fig. 19.5a, b. A shortened malrotated lateral malleolus places the joint in a subluxated position, as shown in cross-sectional drawings (**a**) and diagram (**b**). (**b** From Müller et al. 1965)

bination with dye techniques, Gollish et al. (1977) found similar results.

Ramsay and Hamilton (1976), using a black carbon transference technique, determined the contact area in 23 dissected tibiotalar articulations, with varying displacements of the talus laterally. The greatest reduction in contact area occurred during the initial 1 mm of lateral shift, the average reduction being 42%.

Therefore, the incongruity resulting from a malunited lateral malleolus places the joint in a subluxated position (Fig. 19.5). This will in turn decrease the joint surface contact area, with a concomitant rise in the surface pressure, and lead inevitably to degenerative changes.

Displacements on the medial side, with an intact lateral malleolus, do not have the same biomechanical significance.

19.1.3 Natural History

Are these theoretical facts borne out clinically? The answer is a definite *yes*. The final result clearly relates more to restoration of joint congruity than to any other single factor. Minor degrees of incongruity usually lead to early symptoms and eventual osteoarthritis, gross incongruity to early dissolution of the joint (Figs. 19.6, 19.7). Many surgeons have argued that the case for careful restoration

Willenegger and Breitenfelder (1965) showed that a 2°–4° tilt in the vertical axis of the lateral malleolus displaced the talus 2 mm laterally, while a 2–3 mm posterior displacement of the lateral malleolus moved the vertical axis of the talus by 10°, both reducing the contact area on the talar dome significantly (Fig. 19.4). Using latex in com-

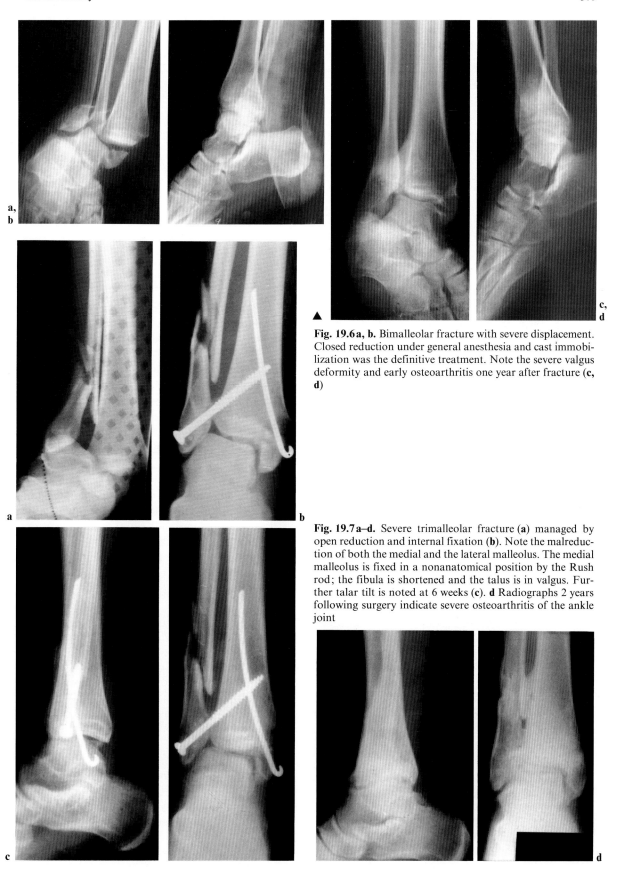

Fig. 19.6a, b. Bimalleolar fracture with severe displacement. Closed reduction under general anesthesia and cast immobilization was the definitive treatment. Note the severe valgus deformity and early osteoarthritis one year after fracture (**c, d**)

Fig. 19.7a–d. Severe trimalleolar fracture (**a**) managed by open reduction and internal fixation (**b**). Note the malreduction of both the medial and the lateral malleolus. The medial malleolus is fixed in a nonanatomical position by the Rush rod; the fibula is shortened and the talus is in valgus. Further talar tilt is noted at 6 weeks (**c**). **d** Radiographs 2 years following surgery indicate severe osteoarthritis of the ankle joint

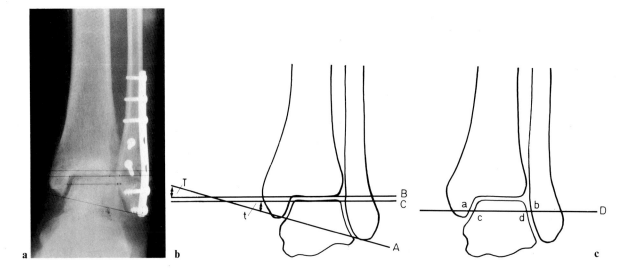

Fig. 19.8a–c. Measurement of valgus talar tilt and mortise width. **a** Radiograph showing lines of measurement. **b** For the measurement of talar tilt three lines are used: one line is drawn to join the tips of the medial and lateral malleoli (*A*), another parallel to the surface of the tibial plafond (*B*), and a third parallel to the talar surface (*C*). Two angles (*T, t*) are measured, with the difference between them constituting the talar tilt. **c** Calculation of the mortise width. A line (*D*) is drawn 5.0 mm distal and parallel to the talar dome. This intersects four cortices, *a, b, c, d*. The mortise width is calculated as the length *ab* minus *cd*, measured in millimeters

of the anatomy has been overstated, since few cases of ankle fracture eventually require an arthrodesis or arthroplasty. Although it is true that patients tend to tolerate symptoms in the ankle better than in the knee or hip joint, a plausible explanation may be that the ankle acts in tandem with the complex hindfoot mechanism and may in part be protected by an intact and functioning subtalar joint. However, patient complaints following ankle fracture are frequent, especially when the anatomy has not been restored (Gollish et al. 1977).

Willenegger and Breitenfelder (1965) reported that all cases of inadequate reduction showed signs of secondary osteoarthritis within 18 months of injury.

Hughes (1980) reported a comparative series of ankle fractures from three major centers. Poor restoration of the anatomy led to poor results, no matter what treatment method was employed. As one might expect, fractures treated by closed means had significantly poorer results than those treated by open means, because of the difficulty

in maintaining the reduction. However, some fractures treated by open reduction also had a poor outcome, due to inadequate anatomical restoration.

Gollish et al. (1977) found similar results. Objective criteria were used to assess the adequacy of reduction achieved and to correlate that with the clinical outcome. The parameters chosen were talar tilt and mortise width. Twenty-five patients with normal ankles had these two parameters measured on a standard 15° internal oblique view as illustrated in Fig. 19.8a.

For the measurement of talar tilt, three lines are used (Fig. 19.8b). One line was drawn to join the tips of the medial and lateral malleoli, another parallel to the surface of the tibial plafond, and a third parallel to the talar surface. Two angles (*T, t*) were then measured, with the difference between them constituting the talar tilt. The mean (valgus or varus) talar tilt in the control group was not significantly different from 0.00, the normal range being from −1.5° to +1.5°.

The mortise width was calculated as follows: a line drawn 5.0 mm distal and parallel to the talar dome intersects four cortices at points *a, b, c, d* (Fig. 19.8c). The mortise width was then taken as the length *ab − cd*, measured in millimeters. The normal mortise width was 4.0 mm, with a range of 2.0–6.0 mm.

The results of 77 prospectively documented ankle fractures were as follows. Out of 36 cases in which both talar tilt and mortise width were normal, 35 (97.2%) had a good clinical result. In 41 cases the measurement of either or both parameters was outside the normal range; of these, 21 (51.2%) had a result rated fair or poor. The difference between these two groups is statistically highly significant. This demonstrates that the final result of the treatment of an ankle fracture is chiefly dependent upon anatomical joint restoration.

Surgical reconstruction has improved the final results in fractures of the ankle, but precise attention to all details, especially anatomical reduction, is of course mandatory. The result of a lateral malleolus fixed with shortening or malrotation will be poor. Careful study of the parameters, talar tilt, and mortise width on the *intraoperative films* will avoid these errors.

19.1.4 Mechanism of Injury

In a series of experiments using fresh amputation specimens, Lauge-Hansen clearly described the mechanisms of ankle injury and the resultant pathological anatomy (Lauge-Hansen 1942). From his studies, he proposed a classification of ankle injury based on the position of the foot at the moment of trauma and the direction of the injurious force. Essentially, he described two major directional forces acting upon the ankle, supination and pronation. These are complex forces:
– *Supination* of the foot is a combination of inward rotation at the ankle, adduction of the hindfoot, and inversion of the forefoot. This combined force may be called adduction, internal rotation, or inversion (Fig. 19.9a).

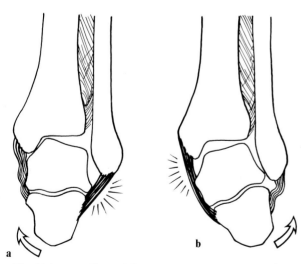

Fig. 19.9a, b. Effect of foot position. **a** Supination of the foot causes laxity of the medial ligament and tension in the lateral ligament of the ankle. **b** Pronation of the foot causes tension in the medial ligament and laxity in the lateral ligament of the ankle

– *Pronation* of the foot is a combination of outward rotation at the ankle, abduction of the hindfoot, and eversion of the forefoot. This combined force is usually called abduction, external rotation, or eversion (Fig. 19.9b).

These forces, which act in opposite directions, produce markedly different injury patterns in the ankle.

Pankovich (1979) has interpreted the above terminology as follows: pronation and supination indicate the position of the foot as it rotates around the subtalar joint axis; internal (inversion) and external (eversion) rotation of the talus are rotational movements around the vertical axis of the tibia. Abduction and adduction are rotational movements of the talus around its long axis. Adduction forces acting upon the ankle produce avulsions of the lateral malleolus below the ankle mortise, or its equivalent lateral ligament. The most common injury to the ankle, the "ankle sprain", is due to this force.

The particular injuries produced by abduction or eversion forces acting upon the ankle joint will depend upon the position of the foot at the moment of trauma.

Lauge-Hansen described these patterns as follows:
– In the *supinated* foot, the medial ligament is relaxed during the initial phase of the injury; therefore, the lateral complex is injured first and the medial last.
– In the *pronated* foot, with the medial ligament under tension during injury, the sequence of injury is reversed, that is, the medial complex is injured first and the lateral last. Biomechanical studies have emphasized the injury sequence, which is helpful in predicting the degree of instability.

The following account of the pattern of ankle injury, based on Lauge-Hansen, helps us to understand the bony and soft tissue pathological anatomy and should therefore be studied by all surgeons treating ankle injuries. Of special importance is Lauge-Hansen's emphasis on ligamentous injury and, therefore, hidden instability. In this description the position of the foot is indicated first, and the force involved second.

19.1.4.1 Supination–Adduction

In the first stage of supination–adduction injury (Fig. 19.10), a transverse avulsion fracture of the fibula may occur distal to the syndesmosis or the lateral ligament may rupture. Since the lateral injury is distal to the mortise, the syndesmotic ligaments remain intact.

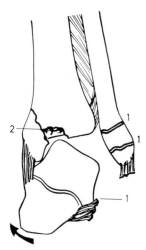

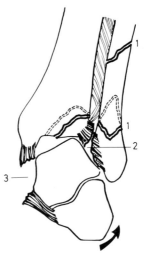

Fig. 19.10. Mechanism of injury: supination–adduction force. In the first stage, a transverse avulsion fracture of the fibula may occur distal to the syndesmosis or the lateral ligament may rupture (*1*). With a continuing adduction force, a vertical fracture of the medial malleolus occurs, often with impaction of the joint surface (*2*)

Fig. 19.11. Mechanism of injury: eversion–abduction force. A shearing, rotational injury to the lateral joint complex is produced, including *1* a spiral rotational fracture of the fibula, *2* a disruption of the syndesmotic ligament, and *3* a disruption of the medial ligament or medial malleolus

If the adduction force continues, a vertical fracture of the medial malleolus occurs, often with impaction of the joint surface by the subluxating medial talar dome. The posterior structures are usually intact. Occasionally, a fracture may occur in the posteromedial aspect of the tibia, posterior to the medial malleolus. Two types of dome fracture of the talus may occur as the ankle subluxates into varus: on the lateral side, a shear osteochondral fracture, on the medial side, an articular crush (Berndt and Harty 1959).

19.1.4.2 Eversion–Abduction

The combination of eversion and abduction forces produces a shearing rotational injury to the lateral joint complex and avulsion of the medial complex (Fig. 19.11). Three mechanisms are recognized:

a) Supination–Eversion

This common injury pattern is caused by external rotation of the supinated foot. The following injury sequence occurs:

1. Rupture of the anterior syndesmotic ligament or avulsion of the anterior portion of the fibula (Wagstaffe's fracture) or the anterior tubercle of the tibia.
2. A spiral fracture of the fibula at or above the joint. The fracture begins distally from an anteromedial position and spirals in a posterolateral superior direction.

3. Rupture of the posterior tibiofibular ligament or avulsion of its posterior tibial insertion.
4. Lastly, as tension is applied to the medial aspect of the joint, avulsion of the medial malleolus or rupture of the deltoid ligament.

b) Pronation–Abduction

With the foot in pronation, the deltoid ligament is under tension and the sequence of injury is therefore reversed. A lateral injury in this pattern always signifies medial instability. In the pronation–abduction pattern, the sequence of injury is as follows:

1. Rupture of the deltoid ligament or avulsion fracture of the medial malleolus.
2. Rupture of the syndesmotic ligaments or bony avulsion of one of their attachments.
3. Oblique fracture of the fibula at or above the syndesmosis. This fracture is more oblique or transverse and is grossly unstable. The interosseous membrane is ruptured up to the level of the fibular fracture. Dome fractures of the talus are common in this shearing fracture.

c) Pronation–Eversion

A pronation–eversion injury is very similar to the previous type, but with subtle differences. The stages are as follows:

1. Fracture of the medial malleolus or rupture of the deltoid ligament.

2. Rupture of the anterior tibiofibular ligament or avulsion of one of its bony insertions.
3. Fracture of the fibula, at or above the syndesmosis. The fracture is more spiral anterosuperiorly to posteroinferiorly. The interosseous ligament is ruptured up to the level of the fracture.
4. Rupture of the posterior tibiofibular ligament or fracture of the posterior tubercle of the tibia (Volkmann's triangle), leading to instability of the mortise.

A carefull perusal of the above descriptions of the injury types will indicate the orderly sequence of the bony and ligamentous injury and will help in the subsequent decision-making process.

19.2 Classification

19.2.1 Introduction

A classification is only useful if it aids in our management of the fracture and if it allows us to compare the results of treatment of similar injuries. For the individual patient and his attending surgeon, the former is the more valuable. Unfortunately, none of the existing classifications is wholly satisfactory, and it is far better to precisely define the personality of each individual fracture and use suitable treatment than to memorize an arbitrary classification and attempt to make all injuries fit the common molds.

Although the work of Lauge-Hansen (1942) has allowed us to understand the injury patterns, his classification is cumbersome and difficult to apply clinically. It suggests that the forces acting upon the ankle will always produce a "classic" pattern, and will be identifiable from the radiographs: a suggestion difficult to reconcile with the variants seen in clinical practice.

Brunner and Weber (1982), representing the views of the AO/ASIF group, have classified ankle fractures according to the position of the fibular fracture, stating that "the higher the fibular fracture, the more extensive the damage to the tibiofibular ligaments; and the greater the damage, the greater the danger of ankle mortise insufficiency" (Fig. 19.12). A type A fracture is located at or below the syndesmosis, type B at the syndesmosis, and type C above it. However, this classification seems to imply that C-type fractures, above the syndesmosis, are more dangerous and, therefore, may have a poorer prognosis than B-type; also, by inference, that surgery is always required for

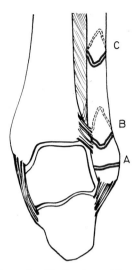

Fig. 19.12. AO/ASIF classification of ankle fractures. The AO/ASIF classification depends upon the position of the fibular fracture, below (type A), at (type B), or above (type C) the ankle mortise

such injuries. However, in a recent review we found no statistical difference between the final results of B- and of C-type fractures (Gollish et al. 1977). Also, the work of Lauge-Hansen (1942), Pankovich (1979), De Souza Dias and Forester (1974), and Monk (1969) have shown that the supination, external rotation injury may involve the fibula above the syndesmosis without significant medial damage. This common fracture may be stable, may not require surgery, and usually has a good prognosis, in spite of the location of the fibular fracture proximal to the syndesmosis. The key to its stability is the integrity of the posterior tibiofibular ligament or its bony attachments.

Both classifications are useful, the Lauge-Hansen for outlining the sequence of injury and the importance of ligamentous damage to the stability of the ankle, and the AO/ASIF classification of Brunner and Weber for stressing the importance of the lateral joint complex. However, neither can be used in deciding the treatment for any individual fracture. All Lauge-Hansen's types of fracture may be either stable or unstable and therefore, may require either closed or open treatment; the same may be said for all the AO/ASIF types.

Clearly, there are two distinct types of injury (see Table 19.1), type I due to an adduction–inversion force causing a lateral injury below the syndesmosis (see Fig. 19.9a), and type II caused by an external rotation–abduction force, producing an injury to the lateral complex at or above the syndesmosis (Fig. 19.9b).

Table 19.1. Proposed classification of fractures of the ankle

Type I:	Stable
	Unstable
Type II:	Stable
	Unstable
Isolated medial malleolus fracture	

The type I injury corresponds to the Lauge-Hansen supination–adduction injury and the AO/ASIF type A injury, and is characterized by an avulsion fracture of the lateral malleolus and a shear on the medial side. The type II injury, corresponding to the Lauge-Hansen types supination–eversion, pronation–eversion, and pronation–abduction, and to the B and C types of the AO/ASIF classification, is characterized by a torsion or shear fracture of the lateral joint complex and an avul-

Fig. 19.13a–d. Ankle stability. **a** The stability scale. The stability of the ankle is dependent upon the four bony and ligamentous structures depicted in **b, c, d**. These structures include the lateral malleolus or lateral ligament (*1*), the medial malleolus or medial ligament (*2*), the anterior syndesmotic ligament or its bony attachments (*3*), and the posterior syndesmotic ligament or posterior malleolus (*4*). If only one of these groups is lost, stability of the ankle will be maintained. As each successive group is lost, no matter what the mechanism of injury, the ankle is pushed along the stability scale. When all four groups are lost, the ankle is completely unstable, held together only by skin

sion of the medial malleolus. With this mechanism, an *isolated* fracture of the medial malleolus or equivalent rupture of the deltoid ligament may also, rarely, occur.

As important as the position of the fibular fracture is the *stability* of the ankle mortise. Both type I and type II fractures may be stable or unstable; therefore, it is obvious that a clear understanding of the factors causing instability is mandatory.

Stable injuries may be defined as those that cannot be displaced by physiological forces. Simple symptomatic treatment is all that is required for a good result. If physiological forces are applied to an *unstable* fracture, however, it will displace. Anatomical reduction of unstable injuries by closed means may therefore be easy to obtain, but difficult to maintain.

Stability is not a matter of black or white but rather shades of gray, depending on the degree of soft tissue and skeletal damage. Thus, the same fibular fracture above the syndesmosis may be stable or unstable or any grade in between, depending on the amount of ligamentous and capsular damage associated with it. This is the reality of daily medical practice. Our proposed classification must reflect this and be helpful in management decisions.

Therefore, our proposed classification (Table 19.1) is based on two main factors: first, the

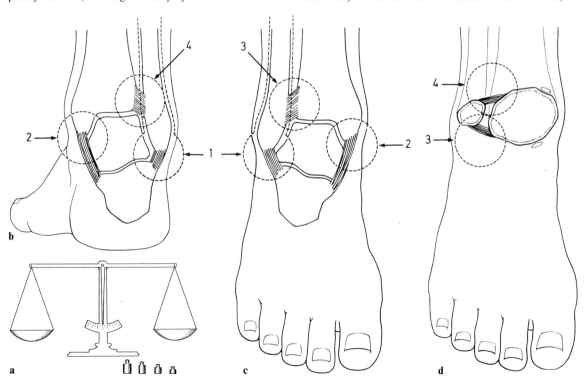

position and character of the injury on the lateral aspect of the joint, and, secondly, a clinical and radiological assessment of joint stability.

If stability is defined as the ability of the injured ankle to withstand physiological stress without displacement, what are the factors leading to instability? The stability of the normal ankle (Fig. 19.13) is dependent upon:

1. The lateral malleolus or lateral ligament
2. The medial malleolus or medial ligament
3. The anterior syndesmotic ligaments or their bony equivalents (anterior tibia or fibula)
4. The posterior syndesmotic ligaments or the posterior malleolus

If only one of the above groups is lost, stability of the ankle will be maintained. As each successive group is lost, no matter what the mechanism of the injury, the ankle is pushed further along the stability scale (Fig. 19.13a). When all four groups are lost, the ankle is completely unstable, held together only by skin. There is thus a spectrum of instability, and all ankle injuries may be placed anywhere along the stability scale.

19.2.2 Classification

19.2.2.1 Type I

a) Stable

Type I injuries are caused by adduction or inversion forces. The lateral injury is an avulsion fracture of the fibula below the syndesmotic ligament, or an equivalent rupture of the whole or part of the lateral ligament (Fig. 19.14). The syndesmotic ligament is always intact; therefore, no instability occurs at the syndesmosis.

b) Unstable

With continuing inversion, disruption of the anterior capsule occurs, allowing displacement of the fibular avulsion fracture and varus subluxation of the talus in the mortise. At this stage, the varus instability may be recognized on a stress radiograph. With further inversion, the entire talus may be subluxated out of the mortise, rotating only on the intact medial ligament. The entire anterior capsule is torn and the ankle, although congruous, is grossly unstable.

If the ankle is simultaneously subjected to axial loading, a vertical fracture of the medial malleolus may occur together with crushing of the medial talar and tibial articular cartilage. Eventually, the

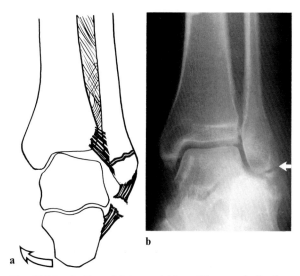

Fig. 19.14a, b. Type I injury, stable. **a** Diagram indicating a fracture of the lateral malleolus below the mortise or its equivalent, a rupture of the lateral ligament. **b** Radiographic example of such a fracture (*arrow*)

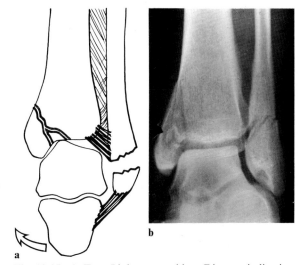

Fig. 19.15a, b. Type I injury, unstable. **a** Diagram indicating a displaced lateral malleolar fracture associated with a vertical fracture of the medial malleolus and impaction of the medial aspect of the tibial plafond. **b** Radiographic example of such a case

continuing force causes a posteromedial tibial fracture (Fig. 19.15).

Displacement of the talus is indicative of both *incongruity* and *instability* of the ankle. Since both the lateral and medial joint structures are disrupted, the ankle is unstable. Compression of the talus or medial tibial plafond may cause impaction of the articular cartilage, thereby altering the prognosis.

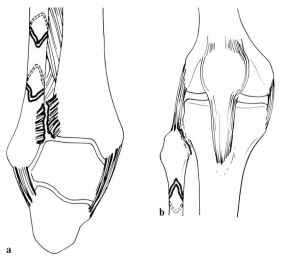
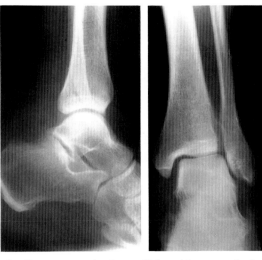

Fig. 19.16a–d. Type II injury, stable. **a, b** Diagrams showing the fibula fractured at or above the syndesmosis. In this injury the anterior tibiofibular ligament is torn but the pos-terior ligament remains intact. This stable pattern is shown in the radiographs (**c, d**)

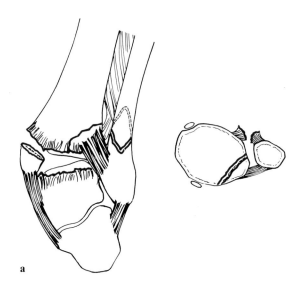
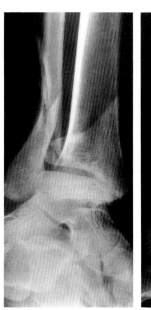

Fig. 19.17a–c. Type II injury, unstable. The key to the sta-bility of the ankle mortise is the posterior syndesmotic liga-ment complex, that is, the posterior syndesmotic ligament or its equivalent bony attachment, the posterior malleo-lus (**a**). **b, c** Anteroposterior and lateral radiographs of inju-ry to this complex resulting in instability of the ankle

19.2.2.2 Type II

a) Stable

Type II injuries are characterized by a fractured fibula at or above the syndesmosis (Fig. 19.16). The forces producing this fracture are vectors of abduction or external rotation around a foot fixed in either supination or pronation.

If the fibula is fractured at or above the syndes-mosis, the *anterior* tibiofibular ligament or its equivalent bony attachment must be disrupted. At this stage, the ankle mortise is relatively stable if the *posterior* syndesmotic ligament and the medial structures are intact.

b) Unstable

The key to the stability of the ankle mortise is the posterior syndesmotic ligament complex, that is, the ligament or its equivalent bony attachment, the posterior tibial tubercle or malleolus (Fig. 19.17).

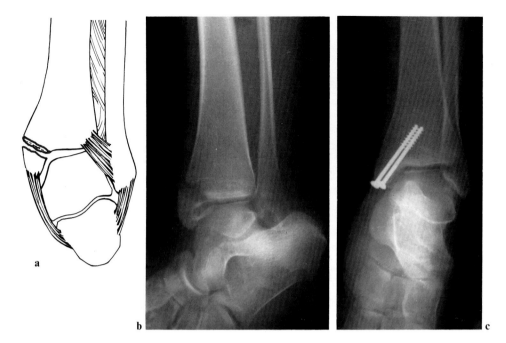

The presence of a posterior lesion always indicates a degree of instability, whether or not the medial structures are disrupted. *Complete disruption of the medial structures, associated with a displaced lateral complex, is definite evidence of gross instability.*

Remember also that the position of the foot at the moment of injury will determine the sequence of injury, the pronated foot receiving a medial injury first, the supinated foot a medial injury last. However, no matter what the mechanism, instability must be assumed when an injury to both sides of the joint is accompanied by a posterior syndesmotic ligament injury.

19.2.2.3 Isolated Medial Malleolus Fracture

This rare injury (Fig. 19.18) is the first stage of the pronation–eversion injury described by Lauge-Hansen. With that particular mechanism, the medial malleolus or the deltoid ligament is avulsed, but no further injury occurs. Although the ankle is stable, the medial malleolus may be displaced, with resultant incongruity. Since congruity is essential for a satisfactory result, open reduction and internal fixation for the *displaced* medial malleolus fracture is essential.

19.3 Assessment of Stability

Prior to treatment, a careful clinical and radiological assessment of the ankle is necessary in order

Fig. 19.18a–c. Isolated fracture of the medial malleolus: **a** diagram; **b** clinical example. Because of the unacceptable degree of displacement, this fracture was fixed with two 4.0-mm cancellous screws (**c**)

to determine the degree of congruity and stability of the joint. These two factors are interrelated but not synonymous: joint congruity is an absolute concept and is essential for a long-term satisfactory result, whereas stability is a relative concept.

These factors may be determined by a precise examination in logical sequence.

19.3.1 Clinical

19.3.1.1 History

The mechanisms of injury will suggest the degree of violence. Of special importance is the ability of the patient to walk after the injury. A normal patient able to walk reasonably well on the injured ankle is unlikely to have a degree of instability that requires surgery; nevertheless, surgery is occasionally, and perhaps unnecessarily, carried out on such patients. On the other hand, a severe, shearing, high-energy injury due to motor vehicular trauma, for instance, is almost certain to be unstable.

19.3.1.2 Physical Examination

1. Signs of Injury. Local tenderness, ecchymosis, and swelling, if confined to one side of the ankle,

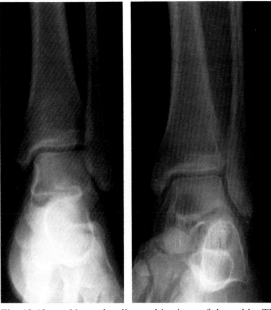

a,
b

c

Fig. 19.19 a–c. Normal radiographic views of the ankle. The anteroposterior view (**a**), the mortise view, taken at 15° of internal rotation (**b**), and the lateral view (**c**) are essential for proper visualization of the ankle joint

whether lateral or medial, are usually indicative of a stable injury, whereas if these local signs of injury extend to both sides of the joint, instability can be presumed.

2. Displacement. Obvious clinical displacement always indicates instability.

3. Instability. Abnormal motion of the talus in the ankle mortise may be felt on clinical examination, either in the conscious patient or during an examination under anesthesia.

19.3.2 Radiological

Standard radiological assessment must include anteroposterior, lateral, and mortise views (Fig. 19.19). The mortise view, taken at 15° of internal rotation, is *essential* for proper visualization of the inferior tibiofibular syndesmosis.

Tomograms may be of value in assessing the degree of comminution and in outlining talar dome fractures, if present.

For the purpose of this description of the radiographic picture it is necessary for a moment to divide the ankle into its component parts (see Fig. 19.13).

19.3.2.1 Lateral Complex: Fibula and Tibiofibular Syndesmosis

Two factors are of importance in the injury to the lateral joint complex: (a) the amount of *short-*

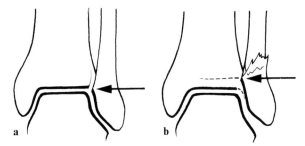

a   b

Fig. 19.20 a, b. The tibiofibular line. The subchondral bone plates of the distal tibia and fibula form a continuous line, the tibiofibular line (**a**). Any disruption of that line caused by shortening or rotation of the fibula is cuidence of displacement of the lateral malleolus (**b**)

ening or *displacement* and (b) the *location* and *shape* of the fibular fracture.

The amount of shortening or displacement of the fibular fracture as seen on both the mortise or lateral view is significant. On the mortise view, any break or gross displacement of the tibiofibular line should be viewed with suspicion (Fig. 19.20). Shortening or lateral displacement of the lateral malleolus is presumptive evidence of a tear in a portion of the syndesmotic ligaments; the presence of an avulsion fracture at one of its attachments is definite evidence of the same (Fig. 19.21). The lateral radiograph will indicate any posterior displacement and shortening of the fibula. Also, posterior subluxation of the talus in the mortise may be associated with a posterior tibial lip fracture or a posterior tibiofibular ligament tear (see Fig. 19.17b).

The location of the fibular fracture, i.e. below, at, or above the syndesmosis, is also significant, although less so than the degree of shortening or displacement. A transverse fracture below the syndesmosis indicates an avulsion of the lateral complex by inversion forces. External rotational forces disrupt the fibula at or above the syndesmosis. The exact site of the fibular fracture does not indicate the degree of instability present, but the shape

of the fracture may: spiral fractures at or above the joint indicate low-energy rotation injuries, whereas short oblique or comminuted fractures at or above the syndesmosis are usually caused by high-energy abduction injuries and are more likely to be unstable (Fig. 19.22).

19.3.2.2 Talus

The talus should be carefully examined for several abnormalities, as follows:

1. Talar Tilt. The normal ankle has *no* valgus talar tilt, any degree of tilt constitutes the most important sign of tibiotalar incongruity due to instability of the lateral complex (Fig. 19.23). The incongruity may be due to lateral shift of the talus or, more commonly, to external rotation of the talus in the mortise (see Fig. 19.5a). It should be measured on the mortise view as shown in Fig. 19.19b.

2. Subluxation of the Talus. The talus may be subluxated either posteriorly or posterolaterally, accompanying the distal fibular fracture, or, rarely, extending into the syndesmosis to lie between the tibia and the displaced fibula (see Fig. 19.2b).

3. Dome Fractures. Fractures of the dome of the talus are common, and can best be seen on the mortise view.

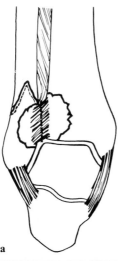

a

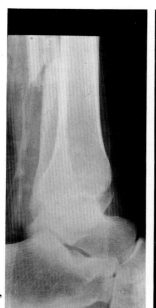
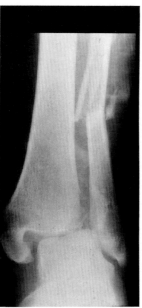
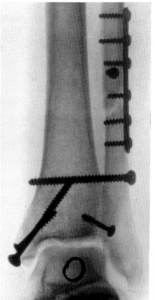
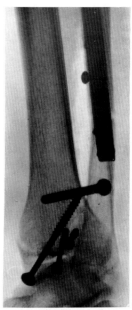

b,
c

d,
e

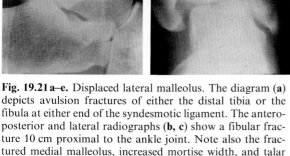

Fig. 19.21 a–e. Displaced lateral malleolus. The diagram (**a**) depicts avulsion fractures of either the distal tibia or the fibula at either end of the syndesmotic ligament. The anteroposterior and lateral radiographs (**b, c**) show a fibular fracture 10 cm proximal to the ankle joint. Note also the fractured medial malleolus, increased mortise width, and talar tilt, as well as the avulsion fracture of the tibial end of the anterior syndesmotic ligament. Postoperative radiographs (**d, e**) show an anatomical reduction of the fibula and medial malleolus as well as a single screw in the avulsion fracture

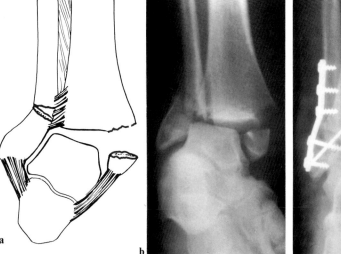
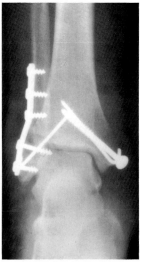

Fig. 19.22a–c. Abduction injury. **a** Diagram showing an almost transverse fracture just above the mortise, of the kind usually caused by a high-energy abduction force. **b** Anteroposterior radiograph of such a fracture. Note the transverse nature of the fibular fracture just above the syndesmosis. **c** Postoperative radiograph showing an anatomical reduction

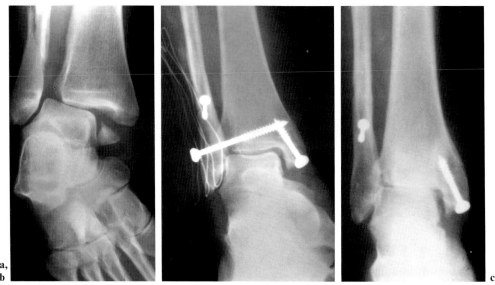

Fig. 19.23a–c. Talar tilt. Note the severe lateral displacement of the talus in the anteroposterior radiograph (**a**). The fibula is fractured above the mortise and is rotated. The immediate postoperative radiograph (**b**) clearly shows a lack of anatomical reduction. There is increased mortise width and a lateral talar tilt due to shortening and malreduction of the fibula. The end result at 3 years (**c**) indicated severe osteoarthritis requiring an ankle arthrodesis

19.3.2.3 Posterior Tibial Process

The surgeon must carefully assess this area for the size and location of the posterior fracture. If associated with a type II fibular fracture, the posterior tibial fragment is always attached to the distal fragment of that fracture by the posterior syndesmotic ligament (see Fig. 19.17b). The posterior fracture may vary in size from a small posterior tibial avulsion to a large triangular fragment of the posterolateral margin of the tibia (Volkmann's triangle). The latter is probably related to high axial loading as well as rotation at the moment of impact.

If the posterior syndesmotic complex is disrupted, the ankle joint must be unstable.

19.3.2.4 *Medial Complex*

The following points are of importance:

1. The direction of the fracture
2. The size of the fragment
3. The presence of articular comminution
4. The amount of displacement of the fracture
5. The presence of a posterior fracture

Vertical fractures are indicative of inversion injuries and are often associated with comminution of the medial tibial articular surface. If displaced and associated with a lateral injury, rotatory instability and incongruity must be present (see Fig. 19.15 b).

Transverse fractures at or below the joint level are avulsion types, and, if displaced and associated with a lateral injury, are always definite evidence of an unstable mortise (see Fig. 19.22).

Undisplaced fractures of the medial malleolus without evidence of a lateral injury are stable, although they may be minimally displaced (see Fig. 19.18).

In summary, careful radiological assessment may show definite evidence of instability of the ankle mortise. Of special significance is the degree of talar tilt, either varus or valgus; and the displacement of either the medial or the lateral complex associated with a posterior injury, or both. By combining the radiographic with the clinical assessment, supplemented by examination under anesthesia when necessary, an adequate appraisal of the degree of instability may be made.

19.4 Management

19.4.1 Decision Making

Many ankle fractures can and should be treated nonoperatively; however, a physician is distinguished not by his ability to treat relatively minor injuries, but by his ability to recognize and adequately treat those which, if untreated, will lead to poor results.

The prognosis of the stable types of injury is excellent no matter what treatment is given, but, with improper treatment, that of the unstable types is poor. Very often, in a busy emergency department, the physician is so distracted by mundane problems that the important injuries are not recognized; i.e., he or she cannot recognize the trees for the forest.

Once the important clinical and radiographic features of the ankle injury have been assembled, they must be ordered and considered in logical fashion. It should be remembered that the management decision also depends upon other factors, including the general medical state and expectations of the patient, as well as the condition of the limb, and the expertise of the surgical team – that is, on a careful assessment of the whole personality of the injury and the context of its treatment.

The first step in the decision-making process is to look at the lateral aspect of the joint and determine whether the patient has sustained a type I or type II injury.

19.4.1.1 *Type I*

If the fracture in the fibula is at or below the syndesmosis and is transverse, it is a type I fibular fracture of the avulsion kind (see Fig. 19.12a). Since the syndesmotic ligaments are intact, the ankle mortise must be stable. However, rotatory instability may occasionally occur in injuries of this type if the medial structures are involved. *Warning:* occasionally a shearing, rotational type II injury may appear at the syndesmotic level and lull the surgeon into believing it is a simple transverse avulsion fracture (type I), when in reality it is a dangerous type of type II fracture (see Fig. 19.22).

If the avulsion fracture of the fibula is undisplaced or minimally displaced, and *no* lesion is recognized clinically or radiologically on the medial side, then application of a walking cast until the fibula has healed (usually 6–8 weeks) will achieve an excellent result.

If the clinical and radiological examination has revealed an injury to the medial aspect of the joint as well, surgery may be indicated. Surgical indications for the type I injury (see Fig. 19.15) include:

1. A displaced, unstable, lateral malleolar avulsion fracture with major soft tissue disruption, which remains displaced after closed reduction. Failure to close the gap in the lateral malleolar fracture may lead to delayed union or even nonunion, and a compromised clinical result.

2. A displaced fracture of the medial joint complex, including the vertical-type medial malleolus fracture, with or without a fracture of the posteromedial aspect of the tibia.

3. An osteochondral fracture of the medial articular surface of the tibia or the talus.

Although a crush injury to the medial articular surface of the tibia or the talus is listed as an indication for surgery, it must be recognized that precise reconstruction of the joint may be impossible. If the fragments are large enough, they may be supported by cancellous bone graft in the subchondral area; if small, they should be removed. If the articular crush has occurred in isolation, with no medial complex fracture, little can be accomplished by surgery, and early motion, if possible, should be started.

19.4.1.2 Type II

A type II fibular fracture at or above the syndesmosis may be stable or unstable; careful clinical and radiological assessment will reveal which it is in any given case. If the surgeon is still uncertain about the stability of the ankle after clinical and radiological assessment, an examination under anesthesia may be found helpful. Under anesthesia, the ankle may be stressed in the presumed direction of injury and checked radiographically with an image intensifier or plain radiographs (Fig. 19.24). If the ankle is stable, very little displacement will occur at the lateral complex with

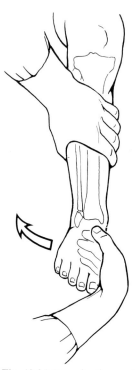

Fig. 19.24. Examination under anesthesia. If uncertainty exists about the stability of the ankle, examination under anesthesia is helpful. In this type II fracture, manipulation of the ankle into valgus may cause a marked opening in the ankle mortise, indicating instability

stress abduction and eversion, and nonoperative treatment will be satisfactory.

a) Stable

If little or no displacement is present in the fibula (see Fig. 19.16), and there is no clinical or radiographic evidence of a posterior or a medial injury, nonoperative treatment is indicated, as no further displacement will occur. A good result may be anticipated with merely symptomatic treatment, namely, a below-knee walking cast retained until fibular union is complete. Note that this stable type of ankle injury may occur with a fibular fracture at any level, be it *at or above* the syndesmosis. The most common type II injury, the supination–eversion variety without medial disruption, may be associated with a fibular fracture at or above the ankle mortise, including an injury to the proximal tibiofibular joint, and still be classified as stable. Therefore, the proximal position of the fibular fracture is not presumptive evidence of mortise instability.

b) Unstable

If the original clinical assessment reveals massive swelling, ecchymoses, and tenderness on both the medial and lateral sides of the joint, the surgeon should assume instability of the ankle mortise. This will be confirmed by the radiological examination, which may reveal any of the unstable fracture patterns. If instability remains uncertain, it may be confirmed at examination under anesthesia. The radiographic signs of instability include abnormal valgus talar tilt, increased mortise width associated with shortening and displacement of the fibula, subluxation of the talus, and a fracture of the posterior or medial malleolus or their ligamentous equivalents (see Fig. 19.17). These unstable fractures require *stabilization*, otherwise incongruity will occur, with malunion and poor outcome to be expected. This does not imply that surgery is the only method of stabilization, but in our opinion, it is the best method for most cases.

Having determined that the type II injury is unstable, the surgeon should now assess the medial injury, as this injury may influence the management decision as outlined below.

With Medial Malleolar Fracture

Surgical stabilization is the method of choice for the unstable type II fracture with an associated medial malleolar fracture. Closed reduction requires a reversal of the mechanism of injury, so

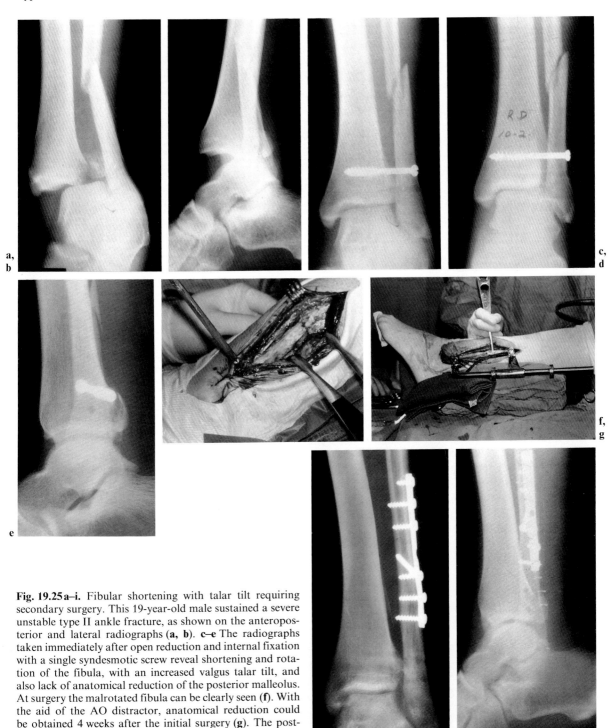

Fig. 19.25a–i. Fibular shortening with talar tilt requiring secondary surgery. This 19-year-old male sustained a severe unstable type II ankle fracture, as shown on the anteroposterior and lateral radiographs (**a**, **b**). **c–e** The radiographs taken immediately after open reduction and internal fixation with a single syndesmotic screw reveal shortening and rotation of the fibula, with an increased valgus talar tilt, and also lack of anatomical reduction of the posterior malleolus. At surgery the malrotated fibula can be clearly seen (**f**). With the aid of the AO distractor, anatomical reduction could be obtained 4 weeks after the initial surgery (**g**). The postoperative radiograph shows the anatomical reduction of the ankle mortise following fixation of the fibula with an interfragmental screw and a one-third tubular plate (**h**, **i**)

the ankle must be immobilized in internal rotation. Not only is this a poor position for the ankle, but the lack of a stable medial post makes redisplacement a common occurrence.

Nonoperative management of this fracture is so fraught with the danger of redisplacement that proper operative treatment is actually the more conservative approach. We believe that an immediate decision favoring open reduction and internal fixation should be made for almost all such fractures; there should be few exceptions.

With Deltoid Ligament Rupture

The presence of a deltoid ligament tear with a type II lateral injury also indicates mortise instability, the only difference being a ligament disruption instead of an avulsion fracture of the medial malleolus. Since the implications are the same, the treatment should also be the same. The surgeon should not be lulled into a false sense of security by this injury. Examination under anesthesia will quickly reveal the degree of mortise instability present.

We favor operative stabilization for the fibular fracture, to restore its length and ensure joint congruity. Anatomical reduction of the fibula restores stability to the mortise and greatly simplifies the management of the injury.

We have no quarrel with surgeons who feel that this fracture may be managed by closed means. In this injury, internal rotation of the ankle may anatomically reduce the fibular fracture. The presence of a medial post, namely the intact medial malleolus, *may* ensure that redisplacement will not occur. A word of caution is in order, however: if the postreduction radiograph shows any degree of valgus talar tilt or increased mortise width, a posterior injury with talar subluxation or interposition of the medial ligament or posterior tibial tendon should be suspected, and operative treatment reverted to immediately (Fig. 19.25).

If treated nonoperatively, patients with this injury must be observed closely, at weekly intervals, so that the surgeon may be certain that the reduction is maintained once the soft tissue swelling has subsided. The original cast must be above the knee so as to maintain the internal rotation of the ankle,

and must be changed frequently in order to maintain this position. A successful outcome may be expected if careful attention to detail is followed. However, in our opinion the surgical management is simpler, allows early rehabilitation of the ankle, and will in most instances, if done correctly, ensure far better results.

19.4.1.3 Isolated Medial Malleolar Fracture

If displaced, isolated avulsion fractures of the medial malleolus should be treated by surgical stabilization. This will ensure rapid union of the compressed cancellous bone, and allow early motion to the joint, with the expectation of an excellent result.

19.4.2 Surgical Technique

19.4.2.1 Tourniquet

We feel that a bloodless field is important for precision surgery, and a tourniquet is therefore recommended.

19.4.2.2 Timing

Ideally, surgery should be carried out as soon as possible following injury. However, skin problems abound in the vicinity of the ankle, especially over the medial malleolus. If the patient is seen late or if skin viability is questionable, surgery must be delayed to avoid skin necrosis. We have found it prudent on occasion to fix just one injury, if the skin on that aspect of the joint is satisfactory, and delay fixation of the other injury until the condition of the skin improves. *If surgery is delayed, any ankle subluxation must be reduced immediately to eliminate pressure on the skin medially* (Fig. 19.26).

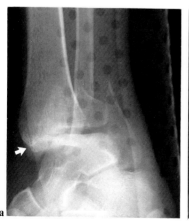
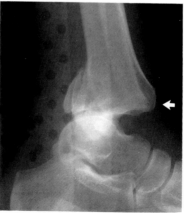

a   b

Fig. 19.26a, b. Subluxation of the ankle. Note the severe ankle subluxation on the anteroposterior (**a**) and lateral (**b**) radiographs. In this situation, the skin may be severely traumatized by pressure from the protruding medial malleolus (*arrows*). Closed reduction should be performed immediately to eliminate pressure on the skin

19.4.2.3 Incisions

a) Lateral

We prefer an anterolateral to a posterolateral incision (*a* and *a¹* respectively in Fig. 19.27a). The skin posterior to the fibula is thin and may necrose easier than the thicker anterior skin. Remember also that incisions should never be made over the subcutaneous border of any bone but adjacent to it. This is as true in the distal fibula as it is elsewhere. If skin necrosis does occur, the implant will usually remain covered. In the upper portion of the wound, the superficial peroneal nerve is in jeopardy as it tracks anteriorly across the fibula. It must be protected to prevent injury which would result in a painful neuroma.

b) Medial

If a longer exposure is required for a vertical fracture, a long anteromedial incision is preferred (Fig. 19.27b, *b*). The skin flap, formed with its base posteromedially, usually heals well because of its blood supply from the posterior tibial artery. The saphenous nerve lying adjacent and immediately lateral to the saphenous vein must be avoided. If a longer anteromedial incision is required, the lateral incision should be made posteriorly to increase the bridge area of skin between them. Usually, in these instances, a small lateral approach will suffice for the avulsion fracture.

For the more typical medial malleolar avulsion fracture, a short anteromedial incision is sufficient to allow fixation of the fracture and inspection of the medial talar dome. If the medial malleolus fracture is associated with a large posteromedial fragment, the posteromedial approach is preferred (Fig. 19.27b, *c*).

The skin on both sides of the ankle is very thin and its condition precarious; therefore it must be treated very gently to avoid disastrous complications.

c) Posterolateral

For patients with a large posterolateral fragment associated with a fibular fracture, the posterolateral approach is preferred, with the patient in the prone position (Fig. 19.27c, *d*).

19.4.2.4 Open Reduction and Internal Fixation

Although we have chosen to describe the technique according to the anatomical parts of the ankle, remember that careful preoperative planning of the entire injury is required in order to plan the incisions and the type of internal fixation required.

Type I

Lateral Complex

Since the lateral complex (that is, the lateral malleolus, the syndesmosis, and the posterior tibial tubercle) is the key to the stability of the ankle, it should be inspected first, and if the lateral mal-

Fig. 19.27a–c. Surgical approaches for malleolar fractures. **a** For exposure of the lateral malleolus we prefer an anterolateral (*a*) to a posterolateral (*a'*) incision. The skin incision follows the anterior border of the fibula and runs parallel to the superficial branch of the peroneal nerve. **b** Incisions for exposure of the medial malleolus: anteromedial (*b*) or posteromedial (*c*). The anteromedial incision affords excellent exposure of the ankle joint and is preferred. The posteromedial incision should be used for simultaneous exposure of the medial malleolus and a large posteromedial fragment which may be fixed by retrograde interfragmental screws. **c** Posterolateral incision (*d*) for posterior exposure and internal fixation of a fibular fracture associated with a large posterolateral malleolar fracture. The patient is usually in the prone position for maximum exposure. (Adapted from Müller et al. 1979)

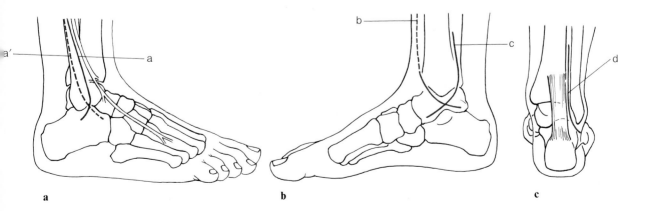

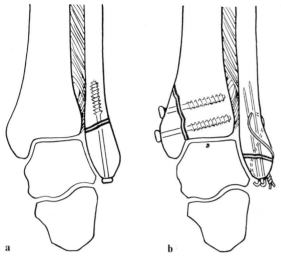

leolar fracture is transverse and below the syndesmosis, the following method is recommended. As this injury is truly an avulsion fracture with a ligamentous attachment, dynamic compression cannot be obtained; it may therefore be fixed by a screw or with a tension band wire, which will achieve static compression (Fig. 19.28). We prefer the latter for small fragments and for osteoporotic bone, in which screw fixation is usually unsatisfactory.

Fig. 19.28a, b. Fixation of a transverse avulsion fracture of the lateral malleolus. **a** Fixation with a lag screw. **b** Fixation of the lateral malleolar fragment with a tension band wire and the vertical medial malleolar fracture with two interfragmental lag screws

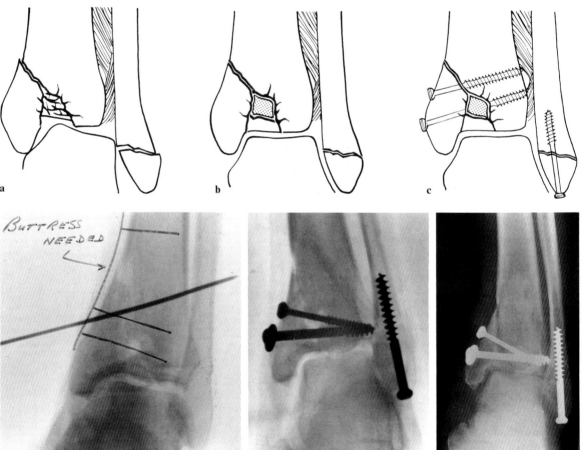

Fig. 19.29 a–f. Fixation of a type I vertical medial malleolar fracture with impaction. **a** Drawing of such a fracture. Note the marked varus talar tilt with the medial dome of the talus impacting on the articular surface of the distal tibia. **b** The displaced articular fracture must be reduced and held with a bone graft. Provisional fixation with Kirschner wires follows. **c** Definitive fixation with interfragmental screws. **d** Intraoperative anteroposterior polaroid radiograph of such a fracture in a 18-year-old female. Preoperative planning would have shown the surgeon that a buttress plate was required. **e** Fixation proceeded with an interfragmental lag screw for the fibular fracture and two lag screws for the medial malleolar fracture. No buttress plate was used. The end result was poor because of a varus deformation of the medial fracture and consequently the dome of the talus (**f**)

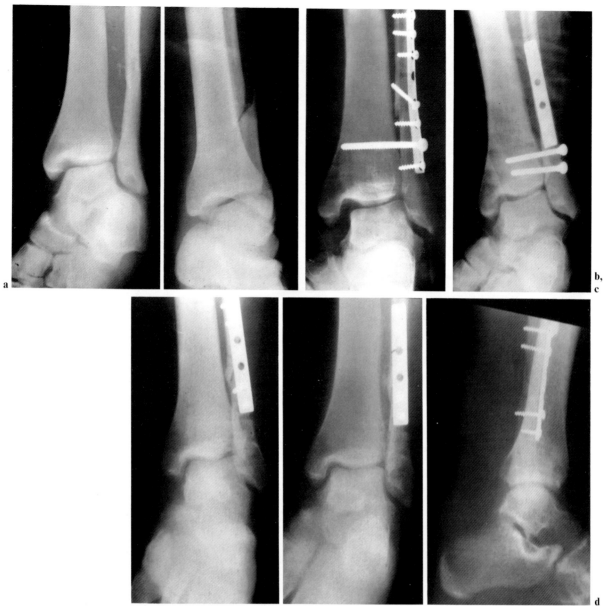

Fig. 19.30a–d. Failure to restore fibular length. The antero-lateral and oblique radiographs (**a**) of this 19-year-old male show a fibular fracture with shortening and rotation result-ing in a valgus talar tilt. Open reduction of the fibular frac-ture was performed immediately. The postoperative radio-graph (**b**) shows the internal fixation of the fibula with a syndesmotic screw. Note the marked mortise widening be-tween the medial malleolus and the medial border of the talus. The obvious reason was a malreduced and poorly fixed fibular fracture. This potentially disastrous complica-tion was recognised and the patient reoperated upon at 7 days, with accurate fixation of the fibula (**c**) and restora-tion of the ankle mortise. The final result at 1 year after removal of the syndesmotic screws was excellent (**d**). *If such a malreduction is noted on the postoperative radiographs, the surgeon must notify the patient and reoperate to rectify the situation as soon as safety permits*

The lateral talar dome should always be in-spected for osteochondral fragments which, if present and small, should be discarded, and if large, should be replaced and fixed with articular pins or a small screw. As much of the torn anterior capsule and synovium as possible should be resu-tured.

Medial Complex

If the type I injury is a medial fracture, it is usually of the vertical shear variety. This should be care-fully inspected for the following important lesions:

1. Articular crush of the medial surface of the tibia or talar dome

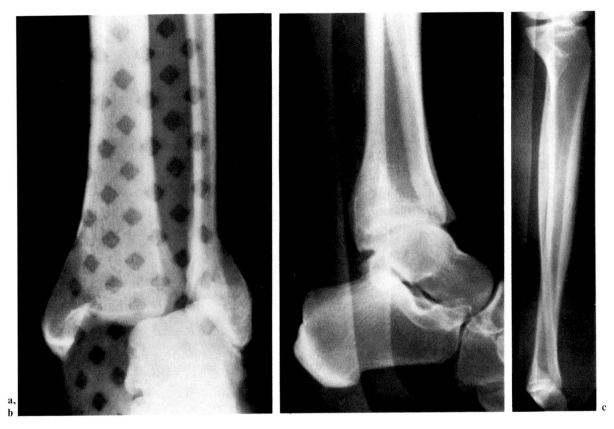

Fig. 19.31 a–c. Fracture dislocation of the ankle with anterior dislocation of the fibula. **a** Anteroposterior radiograph of a 57-year-old man showing a short oblique fracture of the lateral malleolus with diastasis of the distal tibiofibular joint and lateral dislocation of the talus. **b** Lateral radiograph showing the oblique fracture and anterior displacement of the proximal fibular fragment. **c** Full-length lateral radiograph of the tibia showing the distal portion of the fibula displaced anteriorly, the key radiographic finding in this injury. (From Schatzker and Johnson 1983)

2. Comminution of the cortex
3. Posteromedial fracture of the tibia

Careful preoperative planning and intraoperative inspection is required to arrive at the most appropriate method of fixation. If the fracture is a single cleavage through good bone, with no comminution, then screw fixation with at least two malleolar or large cancellous lag screws will suffice (Fig. 19.28 b).

If inspection reveals an articular crush to the tibia, considerable surgical judgement is required. If the crushed area is large enough to affect joint congruity, then the articular surface should be restored and a bone graft inserted above it to maintain this position (Fig. 19.29 a, b). Any small, loose fragments should be discarded. If the crushed area

is small and does not affect joint congruity or joint biomechanics, it should be left alone in the hope that early motion will allow adequate healing of the area.

If the medial talar dome is crushed, the same principles apply. However, elevation of the crushed talar dome is difficult and the result may be unsatisfactory. A crush to either the tibia or the medial talar dome will adversely affect the prognosis, and the patient should be so informed.

If the proximal portion of the vertical fracture is comminuted, a buttress plate is required. Failure to apply this will result in redisplacement and loss of joint congruity, as shown in Fig. 19.29 d–f. The plate may be a small DC plate, a one-third, a T, or a clover-leaf plate.

If the bone is too small for screw fixation, multiple Kirschner wires should be retained as definitive fixation, with, of course, postoperative cast immobilization.

b) Type II

With the type II pattern (that is, a fibular fracture at or above the syndesmosis), ankle stability will depend upon anatomical reconstruction and stable fixation of the lateral complex, and, therefore, this area should be fixed first.

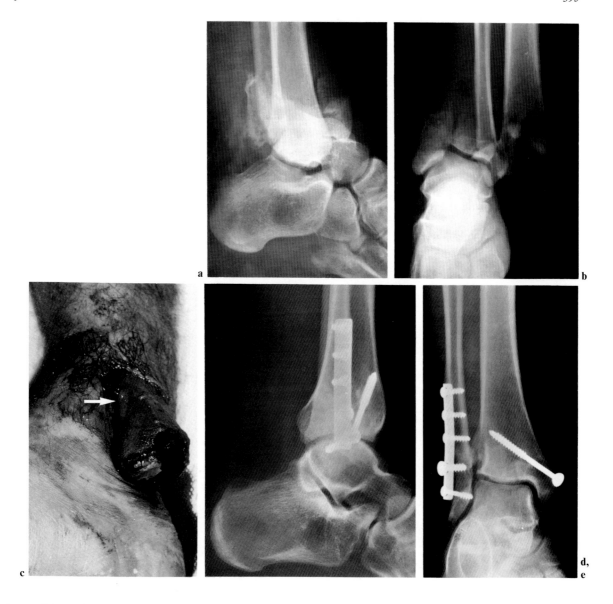

Lateral Complex

Anatomical reduction of the lateral joint complex is essential to ensure normal ankle biomechanics. It should therefore be approached first and provisionally fixed. Fibular length must be restored – the most satisfactory method for this is by open reduction and internal fixation of the fibula. When open reduction and internal fixation are accomplished, the lateral malleolus will return to its normal position in the ankle mortise. Failure to restore the normal length and rotation of the fibula is the commonest error made in surgery for ankle trauma, unfortunately leading to many poor results (Fig. 19.30).

Although the first step is reduction of the fibular fracture, the surgeon may find this impossible.

Fig. 19.32a–e. Soft tissue interposition blocking reduction. **a, b** Lateral and anteroposterior radiographs of an 18-year-old male injured in a motorbike accident. The tibia protruding through the skin is shown in **c**. An attempt at closed reduction failed because of the interposition of the posterior tibial tendon and the neurovascular bundle (*arrow*). **d, e** Radiographs taken 1 year after anatomical reduction, bone graft, and internal fixation

If the fibula *cannot* be reduced, the cause may be one of the following:
1. The lateral malleolus may be stuck behind the tibia and only be removable manually at surgery, often with considerable difficulty (Schatzker and Johnson 1983; Fig. 19.31).
2. Soft tissue may be interposed on the medial side, blocking reduction. The entrapped soft tissue

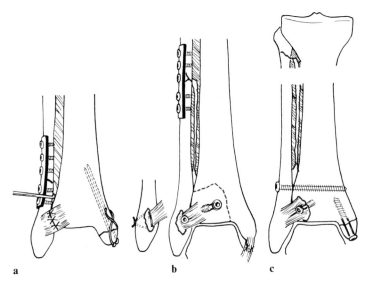

Fig. 19.33a–c. Fixation of the fibular diaphysis. **a** If the fracture is distal, the one-
third tubular plate is the preferred implant.
The stability of the syndesmosis should be
tested and its anatomical reduction assessed.
If anatomical reduction cannot be maintained, a position screw is indicated. The
syndesmotic ligament may be resutured.
b Fractures in the fibular diaphysis may be
fixed with a 3.5 mm DC plate or a one-third
tubular plate, depending on the size of the
bone. Avulsions of bone from either end of
the syndesmotic ligaments should be fixed
with lag screws. **c** For fractures of the proximal fibula too high for internal fixation or
dislocations of the proximal joint, a syndesmotic position screw may be indicated.
(From Müller et al. 1979)

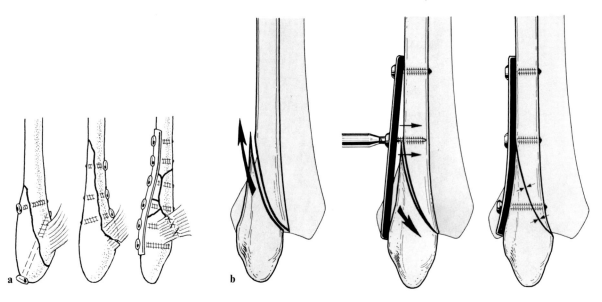

Fig. 19.34a, b. Fixation of the fibular malleolus. **a** Various
methods for fixation of the fibular malleolus using interfragmental lag screws and a one-third tubular plate. A plate
is essential in all cases of comminution or osteoporosis.
b Antiglide plate with supplementary interfragmental compression. A one-third tubular plate applied to the posterior
surface of the fibula is attached first proximally, then distally. The plate prevents proximal gliding of the distal fragment. If possible, a lag screw should be inserted through
the plate to provide supplementary interfragmental compression. (**a** From Müller et al. 1979; **b** from Brunner and
Weber 1982)

is usually an avulsed deltoid ligament which re-
tracts into the joint, or, less commonly, the posteri-
or tibial tendon caught in the medial malleolar
fracture. Occasionally, all of the medial structures
may be driven through the disrupted syndesmosis
(Fig. 19.32).

In these situations, it is necessary to correct the
medial interposition problem before completing
the lateral stabilization, otherwise an anatomical
reduction will be impossible to obtain.

Fibula

The fibular fracture must be carefully assessed. If
it is in the *diaphysis,* the basic rules for diaphyseal
fractures apply. A transverse fracture is fixed with
a tension band plate, a comminuted or spiral fracture by interfragmental screws, and a neutralization plate. The most satisfactory implant is the
3.5-mm DC plate and the new 3.5-mm cortical
screws (Fig. 19.33), or the one-third tubular plate
for smaller patients.

If the fibular fracture is in the *metaphysis* (that
is, the lateral malleolus), it is usually spiral and

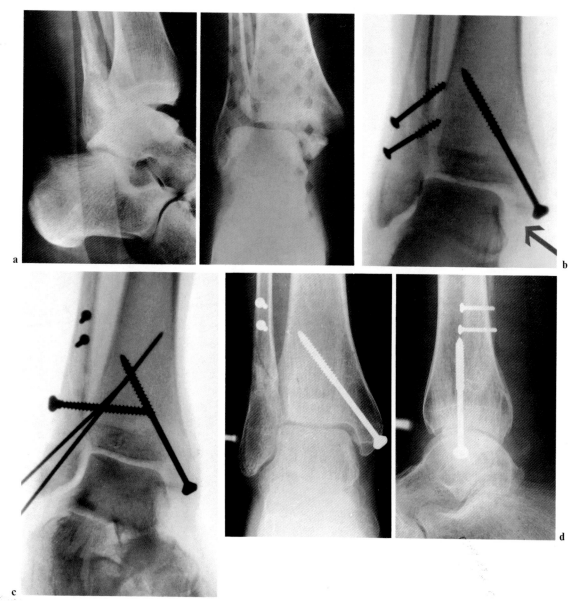

Fig. 19.35a–d. Fixation of the lateral malleolus in osteoporotic bone. **a** Lateral and anteroposterior radiographs of a 44-year-old male with a type II unstable fracture of his ankle. The immediately postoperative polaroid radiograph (**b**) shows a malreduced fibula with a marked talar tilt and increased mortise width. The patient has referred for further treatment 5 weeks following the first operation. Reoperation was planned through the fibula which was now osteoporotic. The intraoperative polaroid film (**c**) shows the use of Kirschner wires to fix the distal fibula as well as a position screw and interfragmental screws on the main fractures. The final result at 5 years is good. The ankle is anatomical (**d**), but the patient has some stiffness and discomfort in the joint

comminuted. Open reduction is performed directly, and provisionally held by Kirschner wires. If the bone is *good* and will hold a screw, stabilization can be obtained by interfragmental compression with lag screws and a neutralization plate placed posteriorly if possible, to prevent the fracture from slipping. The most commonly used implants are the one-third tubular plate, the 3.5-mm and 4.0-mm cancellous screws, and the 3.5-mm cortical screws (Fig. 19.34a). Where possible, the plate should be applied posterolaterally to achieve the antiglide function (Brunner and Weber 1982) (Fig. 19.34b).

Poor or *osteoporotic* bone is, however, common in the lateral malleolus, and the screws may not hold securely. In this case, the Kirschner wires used for provisional fixation should be retained and supplemented with further Kirschner wires across the fracture into the tibia (Fig. 19.35). Fixation will not be entirely stable, but anatomical reduction will be maintained if a supplemental external cast is applied. Since maintenance of anatomical reduction is vital to a satisfactory final result, it *must not* be sacrificed to early motion, which, in our opinion, is of secondary importance in the ankle. Attempted early motion with imperfect lateral fixation, whether by a plate or by Kirschner wires, has ruined many otherwise satisfactory operations and created many difficult problems for both patient and surgeon.

Once the fibula is reduced and fixed, we must turn our attention to the other part of the lateral joint complex. An intraoperative radiograph at this point will confirm the anatomical reduction and is recommended. No talar tilt should remain, the mortise should be anatomical, and the tibiofibular articular line should be restored. If the fibula is not anatomically reduced, the fixation *must* be removed and the cause found and rectified at this stage. The surgeon who fails to do so is deceiving himself and dooming his patient's ankle, for fixation of the fibula in a shortened or rotated position will often cause rapid dissolution of the ankle joint (see Fig. 19.23). The usual reason for persistent valgus talar tilt is a comminuted fibular fracture in which proper length has not been restored.

Posterior Lesion

If the fibular length has been restored and anatomically fixed, any posterior malleolar avulsions which are attached to the distal fibular fracture should be anatomical. If the fragments are small, no treatment is indicated, but if large, they should be dealt with surgically. This will eliminate any gap in the articular surface, reduce postoperative pain, allow early motion, and, most importantly, make certain that posterior displacement of the talus cannot occur. Fragments larger than 20% of the joint surface should be viewed with suspicion and those larger than 33% of the articular surface should be definitely fixed.

The approach to the posterior fracture will depend upon its size and location. If the fragment is thick and on the medial side, fixation is best done by a retrograde cancellous screw inserted from the anterior tibial surface to the posterior malleolar fragment (Fig. 19.36a). It should be remembered, however, that the posterior fragment may be thin, and the cancellous screw threads inserted in a retrograde manner may cross the fracture, thereby displacing it. Therefore, if the posterior fragment is thin or is lateral, a direct posterolateral approach is preferable (Fig. 19.36b). The patient is placed in the prone position. Both the fibular and posterior malleolar fractures may be exposed posterolaterally. Exposure is not difficult, and fixation of the fibular fracture is relatively straightforward. Fixation of the posterior malleolar fracture is much easier in this way than by a retrograde anterior screw, since compression can be obtained directly with cancellous lag screws.

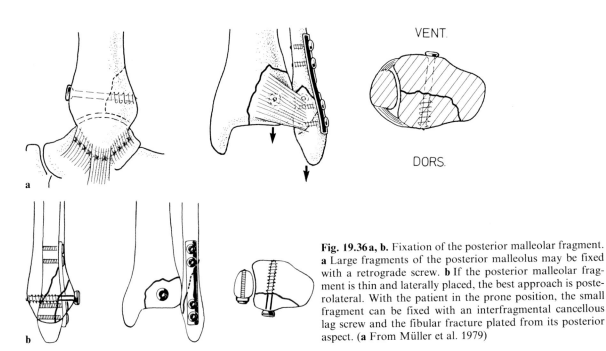

Fig. 19.36a, b. Fixation of the posterior malleolar fragment. **a** Large fragments of the posterior malleolus may be fixed with a retrograde screw. **b** If the posterior malleolar fragment is thin and laterally placed, the best approach is posterolateral. With the patient in the prone position, the small fragment can be fixed with an interfragmental cancellous lag screw and the fibular fracture plated from its posterior aspect. (**a** From Müller et al. 1979)

Syndesmosis

After reduction and stabilization of the fibula and the posterior fragments, the syndesmosis should now be inspected openly (see Fig. 19.33a). If all the fractures have been anatomically fixed, the distal tibiofibular joint should be anatomical; if it is not, as previously stated, the fibular reduction must be inspected. The distal tibiofibular joint, if anatomically reduced, should be stable and rarely requires a screw to hold it. Large avulsion fragments from the fibula or tibia should be internally fixed (see Fig. 19.33b, c). On rare occasions, the entire interosseous membrane and both anterior and posterior ligaments are disrupted. In those cases, if one is concerned about the stability of the joint, a screw may be inserted from the fibula into the tibia. The screw must not be a lag screw but a position screw, tapped on both sides in order not to compress the distal joint, which might limit ankle motion (see Fig. 19.33c). This screw should be removed prior to unprotected weight bearing, usually at 6–8 weeks.

High Fibular Fracture

It has been suggested that the high fibular fracture should not be fixed but the mortise restored by a low screw from the fibula to the tibia. Considerable danger exists in this approach. If the fibula was shortened, it is difficult to be certain that length has been restored, and the screw may therefore fix it in a shortened position. We believe that all displaced fibular fractures except those in the upper third should be openly fixed directly, rather than the surgeon relying on a mortise screw to restore fibular length (see Fig. 19.25a–d). In the upper third of the fibula, direct fixation is impractical and dangerous to the peroneal nerve, so a syndesmotic screw is the only alternative there, but care must be taken to ensure normal fibular length.

Medial Complex

Having fixed the important lateral joint complex, we can now turn our attention to the medial malleolus. Two possibilities are present.

Deltoid Medial Collateral Ligament Tear. With an anatomically restored lateral complex, little is gained by resuture of the medial ligament, so we recommend repair only if the ligament is interposed between the medial malleolus and the talus, blocking reduction of the talus.

Medial Malleolar Avulsion. An avulsed and displaced medial malleolus is ideally treated by open

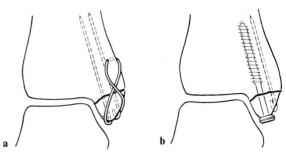

Fig. 19.37a, b. Fixation of the medial malleolar avulsion. If the fragment is small, a tension band wire technique is preferable (**a**). If the fragment is larger, a 4.0-mm cancellous screw or a malleolar screw supplemented with an antirotation Kirschner wire (**b**) will afford good fixation

reduction and internal fixation. If the bony fragment is small or osteoporotic, the best technique is tension band wiring using two 2-mm Kirschner wires and no. 18 gauge wire (Fig. 19.37a). If the bony fragment is large and through good bone, a malleolar screw beginning anteriorly and directed posterolaterally will stabilize the fragment. Rotational stability may be maintained by a second screw, usually a 4.0-mm cancellous screw, or by a Kirschner wire (Fig. 19.37b). Great care should be exercised in handling the medial malleolus, as it is small and may shatter. The surgeon usually has only one opportunity to fix this fracture and he should plan for it carefully. The medial malleolus will not respond well to multiple attempts at fixation.

19.4.3 Wound Closure

Atraumatic wound closure is required for the thin skin of this area. A small suction drain is helpful in the lateral incision to prevent hematoma formation.

19.4.4 Postoperative Program

19.4.4.1 Immediate

A well-padded dressing supported by a splint holding the ankle at a right angle is *imperative*. Failure to provide this will result in an equinus deformity because of the disruption of the anterior capsule. In our experience, this is one of the major errors made in the treatment of ankle injuries, and may ruin even the most expert internal fixation. During the early postoperative period, the limb should be elevated in order to prevent edema. When the patient has regained active control of the dorsiflexor muscles, usually on the 2nd–4th postoperative day, the splint may be removed for exercises. However, it must be retained at night or when not exercising to prevent equinus deformity.

19.4.4.2 Early Motion

In the ankle, anatomical reduction should never be compromised for early motion. The final results of treatment depend more on joint congruity than on early motion. If the surgeon is concerned about the stability of the internal fixation or the quality of the bone, especially in the lateral malleolus, the system should be protected until union is well advanced. Failure to do so will court disaster. We have seen expertly fixed lateral malleoli fall apart due to injudicious early motion, while a recent study in our center showed little difference between the final results of fractures moved early and those moved late (Gollish et al. 1977).

If the internal fixation is stable and the bone is good, then motion may be started as outlined above, and continued until rehabilitation is complete.

The patient is carefully monitored for clinical and radiological signs of implant failure. If none are present, partial weight bearing may be started by the 4th–6th week, and full weight-bearing by the 12th week, after which the patient may complete his rehabilitation program.

At the first sign of impending implant failure, corrective measures must be applied. As mentioned previously, congruity of the joint is all-important. If therefore, the implant seems to be in danger of failing, but congruity is present, the patient should be put in a nonweight-bearing plaster until union has occurred. If congruity has been lost by implant failure, then further surgery must be performed (see Fig. 19.35). However, this surgery may be extremely difficult because of the high porosity of the bone, and only stabilization with Kirschner wires may be possible. Postoperative immobilization is imperative until bony union has occurred.

19.5 Special Problems in Ankle Fractures

19.5.1 Open Ankle Fractures

The principles of management of open fractures of the ankle have been previously stated and do not differ from the principles of closed ankle trauma. Anatomical reduction is essential. After careful wound débridement and cleansing the ankle fracture should be fixed stably and anatomically with the smallest amount of implant possible. The trauma wounds should be left open, while the incisions may be closed. This treatment protocol will result in good results as reported by Franklin et al. (1984).

19.5.2 Ankle Fractures in the Elderly

While the same principles apply to the management of joint injuries in the elderly, the achievement of stable internal fixation by standard technique in them is extremely difficult. This is especially true in articular or periarticular fracture, since the cancellous bone of the metaphysis is often osteoporotic and cannot hold a screw. Also, vascularity in the lower extremity may be compromised, resulting in wound necrosis.

Open reduction and internal fixation in this age group must therefore be approached with care. If vascularity to the limb is diminished, standard techniques of open reduction and internal fixation should be avoided. Instead, percutaneous techniques through small stab wounds may suffice to restore some stability to the ankle while not compromising the skin on the limb. Since screws do not hold in the osteoporotic bone, techniques of Kirschner wire fixation supplemented by tension band wires are preferable. We have also used Rush rods inserted percutaneously into the lateral malleolus to restore some stability and length to the lateral joint complex. While perfect rotatory stability cannot be obtained by this method, the addition of a cast will usually be sufficient to prevent displacement of the mortise (Fig. 19.38).

In the ankle, as elsewhere in fracture of the elderly, caution is advised before embarking on standard techniques of open reduction and internal fixation. Beauchamp et al. (1983) have recently reported on the results of ankle fracture management in the elderly. Complications in this group were higher with open than with closed treatment, which resulted in poorer results in those treated by open means. We believe that by careful planning, including assessment of the vascular status of the limb, by using techniques of Kirschner wires or Rush rods inserted percutaneously or through small incisions, and by the addition of plaster casts, complications can be avoided and satisfactory results obtained.

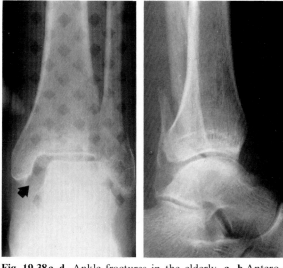
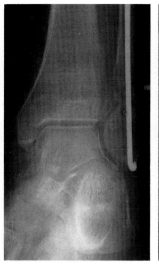
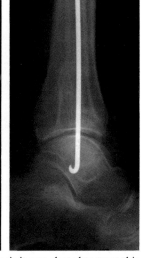

Fig. 19.38a–d. Ankle fractures in the elderly. **a, b** Antero-posterior and lateral radiographs of a type II unstable fracture of the ankle in a 78-year-old male. The *arrow* in **a** points to the noticeable increase in the mortise width. Because of the marked osteoporosis it was elected to treat this fracture with closed manipulation, anatomical reduction, and fixation of the fibula with a percutaneously inserted Rush rod. The final result at 1 year (**c, d**) was excellent

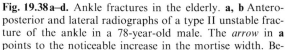
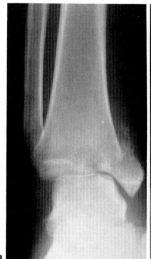
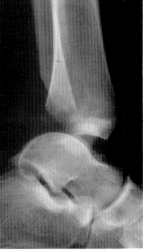
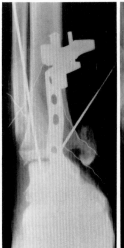
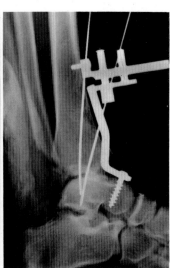
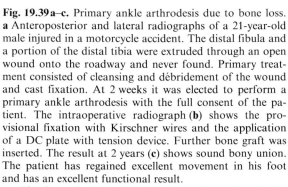
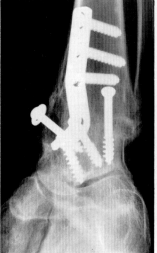
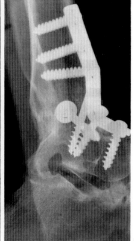

Fig. 19.39a–c. Primary ankle arthrodesis due to bone loss. **a** Anteroposterior and lateral radiographs of a 21-year-old male injured in a motorcycle accident. The distal fibula and a portion of the distal tibia were extruded through an open wound onto the roadway and never found. Primary treatment consisted of cleansing and débridement of the wound and cast fixation. At 2 weeks it was elected to perform a primary ankle arthrodesis with the full consent of the patient. The intraoperative radiograph (**b**) shows the provisional fixation with Kirschner wires and the application of a DC plate with tension device. Further bone graft was inserted. The result at 2 years (**c**) shows sound bony union. The patient has regained excellent movement in his foot and has an excellent functional result.

This form of ankle arthrodesis gives a high rate of fusion and allows the surgeon to obtain and maintain excellent position for the arthrodesis

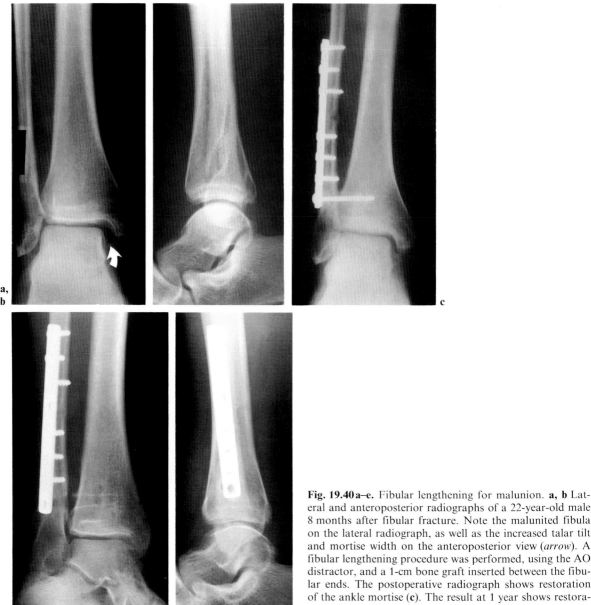

Fig. 19.40a–e. Fibular lengthening for malunion. a, b Lateral and anteroposterior radiographs of a 22-year-old male 8 months after fibular fracture. Note the malunited fibula on the lateral radiograph, as well as the increased talar tilt and mortise width on the anteroposterior view (*arrow*). A fibular lengthening procedure was performed, using the AO distractor, and a 1-cm bone graft inserted between the fibular ends. The postoperative radiograph shows restoration of the ankle mortise (c). The result at 1 year shows restoration of the ankle mortise and union of the osteotomy (d, e). The final clinical result is good

19.5.3 Primary Ankle Arthrodesis

Primary ankle arthrodesis is rarely indicated in the management of ankle trauma. Even in cases of severe comminution in osteoporotic bone, one does better to revert to os calcis traction and early motion than primary fusion. It is only in the rare instance where reconstruction of the joint is impossible, especially in open fractures with bone loss, that early ankle arthrodesis may be desirable (Fig. 19.39). However, this must never be done without prior discussion and consent of the pa-

tient, otherwise serious medicolegal problems may arise.

Techniques of primary arthrodesis will depend upon the situation at hand, and include external fixation and various types of internal fixation with bone grafts.

19.5.4 Fibular Lengthening for Malunion

While it is beyond the scope of this book to discuss late reconstruction procedures, one such procedure in the ankle is worthy of note, namely, fibular

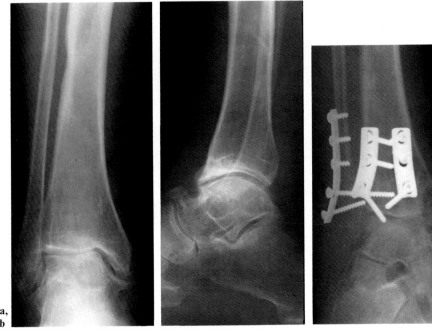

a,
b

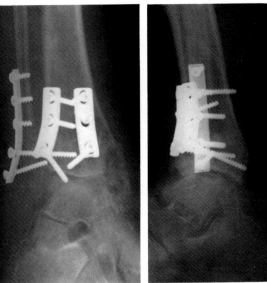

c,
d

lengthening for malunion. The major cause of a malunited ankle fracture is a shortened, externally rotated fibula, resulting from either operative or nonoperative treatment (Fig. 19.40a, b). Radiographs will show an increased valgus talar tilt, giving the appearance of a smaller joint space, which implies early cartilage loss. This loss of joint space radiographically does not, however, reflect cartilage loss in the first several months following injury. If lengthening is performed in carefully selected cases of fibular malunion, joint congruity can be restored and a good long term result anticipated. Of course, this depends on the state of the articular cartilage at the time of surgery. If doubt exists about the suitability of a malunited ankle for this procedure, preoperative ankle arthroscopy is indicated.

The technical aspect of the procedure must be carefully planned preoperatively. The exact technique will depend upon the type of malunion. If the fibular fracture is high, the best approach is to osteotomize the lower third of the fibula, distract the osteotomy site to the desired length, insert an iliac crest cortical-cancellous bone graft, and apply a 3.5-mm DC plate (Fig. 19.40c–e). The restoration of the normal ankle mortise must be verified on intraoperative radiographs. If the fibular fracture is low, osteotomy through the fracture site may be required. In both instances, the use of distractors is essential to achieve the lengthening.

Fig. 19.41 a–d. Supramalleolar osteotomy for malunion. This 56-year-old woman had sustained a fracture of her tibia and medial malleolus while skiing 12 years prior to presentation. Note the varus deformation of the tibial fracture and the severe varus tilt to the talus (a). The lateral radiograph (b) shows advanced osteoarthritis with a large anterior osteophyte and joint narrowing. The patient had severe pain. A supramalleolar osteotomy associated with joint débridement and removal of the anterior osteophyte restored her alignment, increased her motion, and relieved much of her pain (c, d)

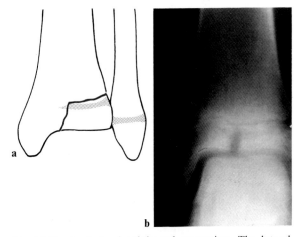

a

b

Fig. 19.42a, b. Lateral epiphyseal separation. The lateral epiphyseal fragment attached to the anterior tibiofibular ligament (Juvenile Tillaux fracture) is shown in the diagram (a). The radiograph (b) depicts such a fracture

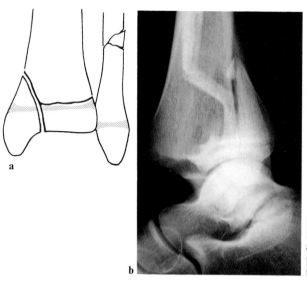

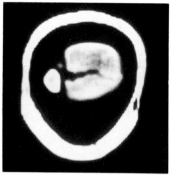

Fig. 19.43a–c. Triplane fracture of the distal tibia. a A three-fragment triplane fracture of the distal tibial epiphysis with an associated fibular fracture. b Lateral radiograph of triplane fracture and c CT scan showing the coronal split proximal to the physis. (Courtesy of Dr. Philip Spiegel)

19.5.5 Supramalleolar Osteotomy

Malunion of an ankle fracture may result in a major varus or valgus deformation. If the articular surface is still satisfactory, a supramalleolar osteotomy may restore alignment and preserve ankle function (Fig. 19.41). Careful preoperative planning is essential. The osteotomy is performed through the metaphysis of the tibia and fixation is usually by internal fixation, occasionally by external fixation.

19.5.6 Ankle Fractures in Adolescents

Specific fracture patterns may occur in children at the end of their growth period, usually between the ages of 13 and 15 years. At that particular stage of development, the distal tibial epiphyseal plate may exhibit partial closure, usually on the lateral side. Two types of fracture patterns have been identified, the lateral epiphyseal avulsion (the Juvenile Tillaux fracture; Bonnin 1970), and the triplane fracture (Spiegel et al. 1984).

The lateral epiphyseal avulsion is characterized by a fracture line extending from the articular surface of the tibia proximally across the epiphyseal plate, then laterally along the physis (Fig. 19.42). This fracture is caused by the anterior tibiofibular ligament in full external rotation.

The triplane fracture (Fig. 19.43) is characterized by two, three, or four fragments in the distal tibial metaphysis. The first fragment is the anterolateral portion of the distal tibial physis (similar to the Tillaux fracture), the second the remainder

of the physis extending into the distal tibial metaphysis, and the third the remainder of the distal tibial metaphysis (Fig. 19.43a). Frequently, the fibula is fractured above the ankle mortise, implicating an external rotation mechanism.

The principle of management for these fractures remains the same as before; that is, anatomical reduction is essential for good long-term results. Therefore, if the fracture is displaced and closed reduction is not successful, anatomical open reduction and internal fixation, using lag screws and Kirschner wires, are essential.

References

Beauchamp CG, Clay NR, Thexton PW (1983) Displaced ankle fractures over 50 years of age. J Bone Joint Surg 65(3)B:329–332
Berndt AL, Harty M (1959) Transchondral fractures (osteochondritis dissecans) of the talus. J Bone Joint Surg 41A:988
Bonnin JG (1970) Injuries to the ankle. Darien, Connecticut
Brunner CF, Weber BG (1982) Special techniques of internal fixation. Springer, Berlin Heidelberg New York
De Souza Dias L, Forester TP (1974) Traumatic lesions of the ankle joint. Clin Orthop 100:219–224
Elmendorff H, Petes D (1971) Late results of fractures of the ankle. Acta Orthop Unfall Chir 69:220
Franklin JL, Johnson KD, Hansen ST Jr (1984) Immediate internal fixation of open ankle fractures. A report of 38 cases treated with standard protocol. J Bone Joint Surg 66A:1349–1356
Gollish JD, Tile M, Begg R (1977) Fractures of the ankle. J Bone Joint Surg 59B:510
Hughes J (1980) The medial malleolus in ankle fractures. Orthop Clin North Am 2(3):649–660
Inman VT (1976) The joints of the ankle. Williams and Wilkins, Baltimore

Lauge-Hansen N (1942) Ankelbrud I. Genetisk diagnose og reposition. Dissertation, Munksgaard, Copenhagen

Monk CJ (1969) Injuries of the tibiofibular ligaments. J Bone Joint Surg 51B:330

Müller ME, Allgöwer M, Willenegger H (1965) Technique of internal fixation of fractures. Springer, Berlin Heidelberg New York, p 115, Fig. 117b, c

Müller ME, Allgöwer M, Schneider R, Willenegger H (1979) Manual of internal fixation, 2nd edn. Springer, Berlin Heidelberg New York

Pankovich AM (1979) Adult ankle fractures. J Con Ed Orthop 7:17

Pankovich AM, Shivaran MS (1979) Anatomical basis of variability in injuries of the medial malleolus and the deltoid ligament. I: Anatomical studies; II: Clinical studies. Acta Orthop Scand 50:217–223

Ramsay PL, Hamilton W (1976) Changes in tibiotalar area of contact caused by lateral tibia shift. J Bone Joint Surg 59A:356

Schatzker J, Johnson R (1983) Fracture-dislocation of the ankle with anterior dislocation of the fibula. J Trauma 23(5):420–423

Spiegel PG, Mast JW, Cooperman DR, Laros GS (1984) Triplane fractures of the distal tibial epiphysis. In: Spiegel P (ed) Topics in orthopaedic trauma (Techniques in orthopaedic surgery). University Park, Baltimore, pp 153–171

Willenegger H (1979) Evaluation of ankle fractures non-operative and operative treatment. Clin Orthop 138:111

Willenegger H, Breitenfelder (1965) Principles of internal fixation. Springer, Berlin Heidelberg New York

20 Fractures of the Talus

M. TILE

20.1 Introduction

Injuries to the talus occur infrequently, but, when they do, the consequences can be grave. Misconceptions about this injury abound, due mainly to poor comprehension of the blood supply to the talus, and to the common practice of comparing dissimilar cases.

Disability arising from talar fractures is due to the major complications of avascular necrosis and of malunion from nonanatomical reduction, which in turn leads to osteoarthritis of the subtalar joint and altered biomechanics of the foot. Also, skin problems are common, often worsened by injudicious surgery. Sepsis may ensue, with severe disability or amputation the likely outcome.

In 1832, Sir Astley Cooper gave in dramatic detail one of the first accounts of the natural history of dislocation of the talus. He describes vividly how "Mr. Downes, on the 24th of July, 1820, had the misfortune to dislocate the astragalus by falling from his horse." In consultation he observed "that I would not operate and that perhaps the skin might give way and the bone become exposed – when we would be justified in removing it." Previous treatment was therefore further pursued: "On the 29th the leeches were repeated and the lotion continued." – "On the 20th of August – ... there was a great discharge of pus and the astragalus became loose ... . On Oct. 5, 1820, finding the astragalus very loose, I removed it" (i.e., 10 weeks after the accident). In October, 1821, the patient "had slight motion at the ankle which was gradually increasing."

Syme (1848) recorded 13 patients, of whom only two survived. He recommended primary amputation for open injuries of the talus. Anderson (1919) collected 18 cases of talar injuries occurring in air crashes and named this injury "aviator's astragalus."

Coltart, in 1952, wrote the then definitive work on this subject. He recorded 228 cases, of which 106 were fractures or fracture dislocations of the talar neck. Most of the subsequent reviews reflect the principles in Coltart's series. He described the natural history of fractures of the talar neck with no displacement, with subtalar dislocation, and with complete dislocation of the body of the talus, and indicated the prognosis of each.

As in all fractures, sound management depends upon a return to basic principles. Fractures of the talar neck with displacement demand anatomical reduction and stable internal fixation if closed reduction fails, otherwise the subtalar joint will be adversely affected. However, surgery must not jeopardize the already precarious blood supply to the body of the talus.

Therefore, a precise knowledge of the blood supply to the talus is essential for logical management.

20.2 Anatomical Considerations

The talus is an unique bone, in that 60% of it is covered by articular cartilage and it has no muscular or tendinous attachments (Fig. 20.1).

20.2.1 Vascular Anatomy

The surgical significance of the vascular anatomy cannot be overemphasized. Because of the association of certain fractures and dislocations with avascular necrosis of the body of the talus, the extraosseous and intraosseous vascular anatomy has been the subject of considerable investigation. Lexor et al. (1904), Sneed (1925), Phemister (1940), McKeever (1943), Watson-Jones (1946), Kleiger (1948), and Wildenauer (1950) were pioneers in this field.

Wildenauer (1950) fully described the blood supply of the talus and is credited with being the first to describe the important artery arising from the posterior tibial artery and coursing through the tarsal canal, which is now known to be the most important vessel to the body of the talus.

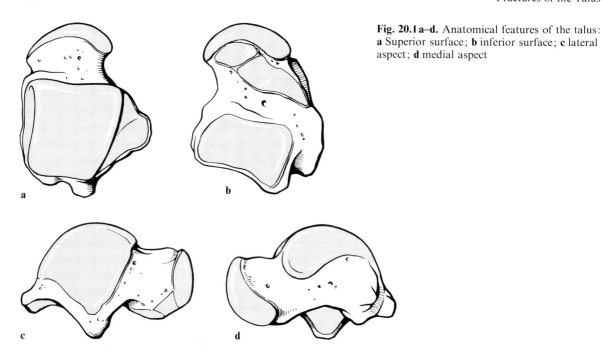

Fig. 20.1a–d. Anatomical features of the talus: a Superior surface; b inferior surface; c lateral aspect; d medial aspect

He also pointed out the anatomical distinction between the tarsal sinus and the tarsal canal. The tarsal canal is formed by the sulcus of the talus and the sulcus of the os calcis. It lies obliquely from a posterior medial to an anterior lateral position and opens into the tarsal sinus. In the canal one finds the interosseous talocalcaneal ligament and the artery of the tarsal canal. Wildenauer believed the most important vascular contributions

came from the arteries of the tarsal sinus, tarsal canal, and the medial periosteal network.

Further studies by Coltart (1952), Lauro and Purpura (1956), Haliburton et al. (1958), and Montis and Ridola (1959) added to our knowledge by confirming the studies of Wildenauer, especially the importance of the medial blood supply.

Mulfinger and Trueta (1970) have written the classic work on this subject, again reaffirming the

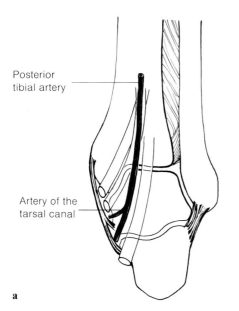

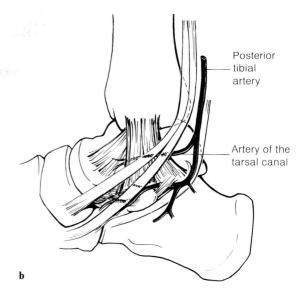

Fig. 20.2a, b. Extraosseous blood supply to the talus. a The artery of the tarsal canal arising from the posterior tibial artery. Note its position along the interior surface of the

deltoid ligament. From there, it can be seen entering the tarsal canal (b)

Fig. 20.3a, b. The deltoid branch. **a** Blood supply to the talus in sagittal sections. The artery of the tarsal canal is shown with the deltoid artery branch arising from it, lying close to the inner surface of the deltoid ligament and entering the body of the talus.

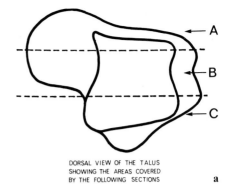

DORSAL VIEW OF THE TALUS
SHOWING THE AREAS COVERED
BY THE FOLLOWING SECTIONS

a

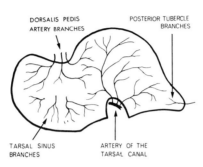

DORSALIS PEDIS
ARTERY BRANCHES
DELTOID
BRANCHES
POSTERIOR
TUBERCLE BRANCHES

TARSAL SINUS
BRANCHES
ARTERY OF THE
TARSAL CANAL
POSTERIOR
TIBIAL ARTERY

BLOOD SUPPLY TO THE
MEDIAL ONE - THIRD
OF THE TALUS

DORSALIS PEDIS
ARTERY BRANCHES
POSTERIOR TUBERCLE
BRANCHES

TARSAL SINUS
BRANCHES
ARTERY OF THE
TARSAL CANAL

BLOOD SUPPLY TO THE
MIDDLE ONE - THIRD
OF THE TALUS

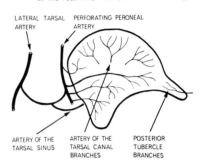

LATERAL TARSAL
ARTERY
PERFORATING PERONEAL
ARTERY

ARTERY OF THE
TARSAL SINUS
ARTERY OF THE
TARSAL CANAL
BRANCHES
POSTERIOR
TUBERCLE
BRANCHES

BLOOD SUPPLY TO THE
LATERAL ONE - THIRD
OF THE TALUS

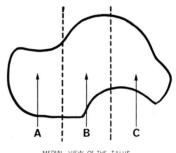

MEDIAL VIEW OF THE TALUS
SHOWING THE AREAS COVERED
BY THE FOLLOWING SECTIONS

b

b Blood supply to the talus in coronal sections. The deltoid branch arising from the artery of the tarsal canal is clearly seen with its relationship to the deltoid ligament and medial malleolus. The other arterial supply, including the perforating peroneal artery, the lateral tarsal artery, the artery of the tarsal sinus, and the dorsalis pedis artery, is also clearly indicated. (From Mulfinger and Trueta 1970)

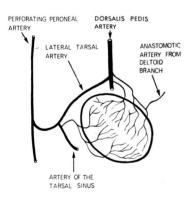

PERFORATING PERONEAL
ARTERY
DORSALIS PEDIS
ARTERY

LATERAL TARSAL
ARTERY
ANASTOMOTIC
ARTERY FROM
DELTOID
BRANCH

ARTERY OF THE
TARSAL SINUS

BLOOD SUPPLY TO THE
HEAD OF THE TALUS

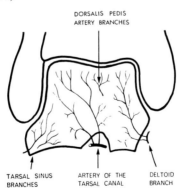

DORSALIS PEDIS
ARTERY BRANCHES

TARSAL SINUS
BRANCHES
ARTERY OF THE
TARSAL CANAL
DELTOID
BRANCH

BLOOD SUPPLY TO THE
MIDDLE ONE - THIRD
OF THE TALUS

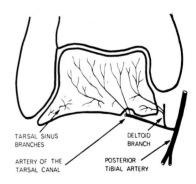

TARSAL SINUS
BRANCHES
DELTOID
BRANCH

ARTERY OF THE
TARSAL CANAL
POSTERIOR
TIBIAL ARTERY

BLOOD SUPPLY TO THE
POSTERIOR ONE - THIRD
OF THE TALUS

earlier findings of Wildenauer. Their experimental technique ensured that only the arterial blood supply was injected with contrast medium, offsetting criticism of previous studies.

The important arterial supply to the talus is described in the following sections.

20.2.1.1 Extraosseous Arterial Supply

a) From the Posterior Tibial Artery

Artery of the Tarsal Canal. This important artery usually arises from the posterior tibial artery, 1 cm proximal to the origin of the medial and lateral plantar arteries (Fig. 20.2). From that point, it passes anteriorly between the sheath of the flexor digitorum longus and the flexor hallucis longus muscles to enter the tarsal canal, in which it lies anteriorly close to the talus. Many branches enter the body of the talus from the arterial network in the tarsal canal. Continuing through the tarsal canal into the tarsal sinus, this artery anastomoses with the artery of the tarsal sinus, forming a rich vascular sling beneath the talar neck.

Deltoid Branch

A substantial artery supplying a portion of the medial half of the body of the talus hugs the inner surface of the deltoid ligament of the ankle (Fig. 20.3). This vessel arises most commonly from the artery of the tarsal canal, or directly from the posterior tibial artery; less frequently from the medial plantar branch of the posterior tibial artery. The surgical significance of this vessel is obvious. First, since most injuries of the talus occur with dorsiflexion and inversion, the medial soft tissues, including this artery, may remain intact and ensure the viability of the body of the talus. Secondly, medial surgical approaches to the talus may interfere with this vessel, thereby possibly injuring the only remaining blood supply to the talus.

b) From the Anterior Tibial Artery

Superior Neck Branches. The dorsalis pedis artery, a continuation of the anterior tibial artery, sends branches to the superior surface of the neck of the talus.

Artery of the Tarsal Sinus. This artery is always present, large, and always anastomoses with the artery of the tarsal canal. It is formed by an anastomosis of a branch of the dorsalis pedis artery with a branch of the perforating peroneal artery. This lateral blood supply is profuse, with many direct branches into the bone.

c) From the Peroneal Artery

Small branches from the peroneal artery join with branches of the posterior tibial artery to form the posterior plexus around the talus. The perforating peroneal artery contributes to the artery of the tarsal sinus, but in general the peroneal supply to the talus is not considered to be important.

20.2.1.2 Intraosseous

a) Head of Talus

The head of the talus is supplied by two sources, medially by branches of the dorsalis pedis artery, and laterally by branches of the arterial anastomosis in the artery of the tarsal sinus (Fig. 20.4).

b) Body of Talus

The *anastomotic artery* in the tarsal canal supplies most of the talar body, through four or five branches on the medial side. This vessel usually supplies almost all of the middle third of the body, except for the extreme superior aspect, and all of the lateral third, except for the posterior aspect.

The *deltoid artery* supplies the medial third of the body (see Fig. 20.4).

Rich anastomoses within the bone were found in almost all cases, especially between the superior neck vessels and the vessels arising from the tarsal canal. In some people, the artery of the tarsal sinus and the tarsal canal may anastomose within the bone.

20.2.1.3 Summary

From these studies, it may be deduced that:

1. The body of the talus has a rich blood supply through several anastomoses.
2. The major blood supply enters posterior to the talar neck, so that an isolated neck fracture, unless it extended posteriorly into the body, would be unlikely to interfere with the blood supply.
3. An important vessel lies adjacent to the inner surface of the deltoid ligament. Except in cases of total dislocation of the talus and posterior extrusion of the body, this vessel maintains the viability of the talar body, if it is not interfered with surgically.

20.2.2 Mechanism of Injury
20.2.2.1 Common Pattern

Most fractures of the talar neck are caused by a severe dorsiflexion force (see Fig. 20.5). In the Royal Air Force studies (Coltart 1952), forced

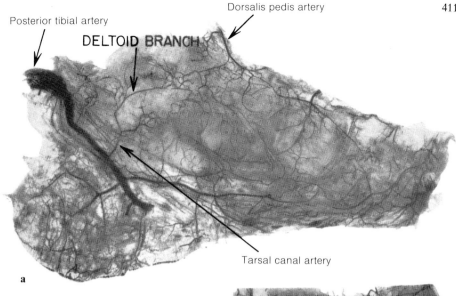

Posterior tibial artery

DELTOID BRANCH

Dorsalis pedis artery

Tarsal canal artery

a

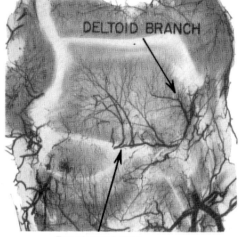

DELTOID BRANCH

Tarsal canal artery

b

Fig. 20.4a, b. Interosseous blood supply to the talus. **a** Sagittal section of the middle third of the tarsal bone. Anastomoses between the deltoid branches and dorsalis pedis artery can be seen. **b** Coronal section through the middle third of the talus, again showing the anastomotic links. (From Mulfinger and Trueta 1970)

Fig. 20.5a, b. Talar neck fractures. Most talar neck fractures are caused by a severe dorsiflexion force. The talar neck abuts the anterior portion of the tibia and the continuing force fractures the talar neck (**a**). A continuing inversion force (**b**) ruptures the lateral subtalar ligaments and often the lateral ligament of the ankle, or causes an avulsion of the lateral malleolus

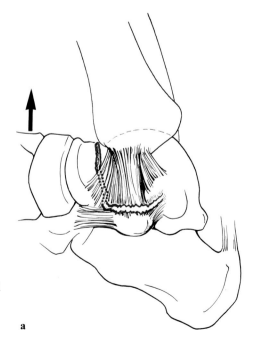

a

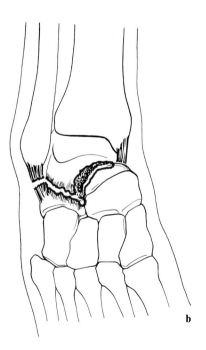

b

dorsiflexion of the foot against the rudder bar caused the fracture of the talar neck: hence the term "aviator's astragalus." In our society, most injuries are caused by the complex high-energy forces associated with motor vehicle accidents.

Rotation forces may be added to those of dorsiflexion to complete the injury. Following the talar neck fracture, the body of the talus locks in the ankle mortise. The remainder of the foot, including the head of the talus and the os calcis, displaces medially through the subtalar joint (Fig. 20.5).

Continuation of the dorsiflexion force ruptures the intraosseous ligaments between the talus and os calcis as well as the posterior talofibular and talocalcaneal ligaments. The body of the talus is forced posteromedially out of the mortise with the neck fracture, pointing laterally and superiorly. In more than 50% of such cases the medial malleolus fractures obliquely or vertically (see Fig. 20.12).

Thus, the body of the talus rotates around the intact or partially intact deltoid ligament, and eventually rests posterior to the medial malleolus, anterior to the tendo Achilles. The neurovascular structures are rarely injured primarily, but may be secondarily if pressure on them is not rapidly removed.

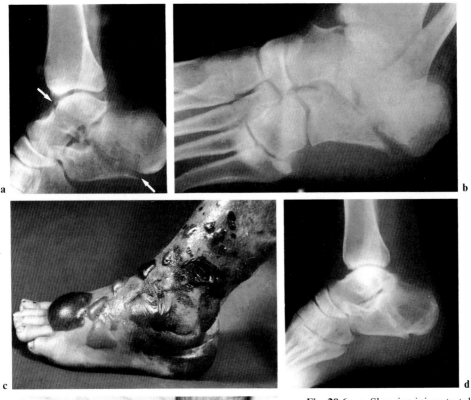

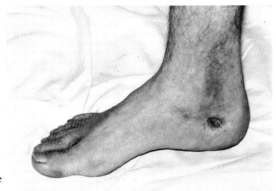

Fig. 20.6a–e. Shearing injury to talus. This 32-year-old male had his foot caught in the jaws of a logging machine. His body was then rotated around the stabilized os calcis and talus, creating an open shear fracture through both bones (a). The oblique radiograph of the foot (b) shows the shearing oblique fracture through the talar neck and calcis. Within 48 h, massive fracture blisters and contusion were evident on the foot and ankle (c). Nonoperative treatment was the only option, because of the soft tissue crush. The lateral radiograph (d) and the clinical photograph (e) show the final result 5 years following injury. The fractures have healed, but there was evidence of patchy avascular necrosis of the body of the talus with no collapse. The function of the foot is good. An area on the medial aspect of the os calcis required a split thickness skin graft

20.2.2.2 Atypical Patterns

Instead of the usual injury of dorsiflexion, shearing forces may occasionally produce an unusual injury. Shearing forces, acting perpendicular to the cancellous trabeculae, are usually associated with marked instability and displacement, as in the case shown in Fig. 20.6. In that example, the patient's foot was caught in the jaws of a logging machine and his body rotated around the stabilized os calcis and talus, creating an open shear fracture through both bones.

20.2.2.3 Total Dislocation of the Talus

This severe injury is usually caused by forced, violent, internal rotation and plantar flexion. As the foot displaces, the anterolateral capsule and the collateral ligaments rupture. Further inversion causes a rupture of the talocalcaneal ligaments allowing the talus to extrude from the ankle mortise, often with rupture of the overlying skin (Fig. 20.7; see also Fig. 20.14).

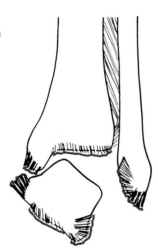

Fig. 20.7. Total dislocation of the talus with disruption of all soft tissue attachments

20.3 Classification and Natural History

Armed with a knowledge both of the rich blood supply of the talus and also of the mechanisms of injury, it is possible to develop a classification of fractures of the talus of considerable prognostic value. The most widely accepted classification of these fractures is a variation on that originated by Coltart (1952), as shown in Table 20.1. Excluded from this classification are the common avulsion fractures of portions of the talus and frac-

tures of the talar dome – so-called osteochondritis dissecans of the talus – since both of these injuries differ in their behavior from the more uncommon fractures of the body and neck.

Clearly, the outcome of these injuries is dependent upon the *type of fracture* and the *degree of violence* causing it. These aspects will also affect the *talar blood supply* and the degree of *subluxation or dislocation of the talar body*, the major factors influencing the prognosis of this injury.

20.3.1 Fractures of the Body of the Talus

Simple linear cracks in the body should pose few management problems; the results should be uniformly good with simple treatment.

Major violence may cause severe comminution to the body of the talus, usually defying primary reconstruction. Areas of avascular necrosis and marked incongruity of the subtalar and even the ankle joint combine to make this injury potentially disastrous (Fig. 20.8). Late pain, deformity, and collapse of the talus are common, often requiring secondary reconstruction procedures.

20.3.2 Fractures of the Talar Neck

20.3.2.1 Type I: Undisplaced Fractures of the Talar Neck

Linear fractures of the talar neck with *no* subluxation of the subtalar joint usually have an excellent prognosis with simple management (Fig. 20.9). Ample blood supply is retained in most cases to maintain the viability of the body, and if the hindfoot is truly anatomical, no biomechanical abnormalities will ensue. All major literature reports confirm this, including the reviews of Coltart (1952), Pennal (1963), Hawkins (1970), and Kenwright and Taylor (1970).

Table 20.1. Classification of fractures of the talus

Fractures of the talar body
Fractures of the talar neck
Type I: Undisplaced fracture of the talar neck
Type II: Displaced fracture of the talar neck with subtalar joint subluxation
Type III: Displaced fracture of the talar neck with dislocation of the body
Subtalar dislocation
Total dislocation of the talus

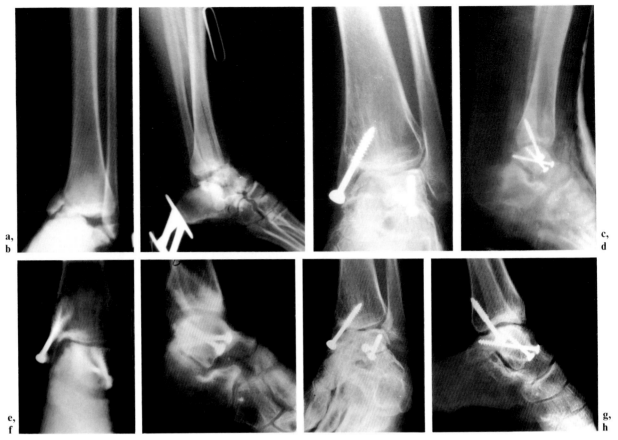

Fig. 20.8a–h. Fracture through the body of the talus. **a** Anteroposterior and **b** lateral radiographs of this 19-year-old female show a comminuted fracture of the talar neck extending through the body, together with a fracture of the medial malleolus. Treatment consisted of open reduction and internal fixation. At 3 months, the anteroposterior and lateral radiographs (**c, d**) show union of the medial malleolus. The medial aspect of the talus appears vascularized, whereas the lateral aspect of the talus is sclerotic and avascular. Anteroposterior and lateral tomography (**e, f**) show a defect in the distal tibia, allowing varus deformation. **g, h** At 5 years, the talus has not collapsed but shows a patchy avascular necrosis. The patient has restricted ankle motion, minimal discomfort, and functions well in spite of the avascular necrosis

20.3.2.2 Type II: Displaced Fractures of the Talar Neck with Subluxation of Subtalar Joint

Any degree of displacement of the fracture through the neck of the talus must be accompanied by a corresponding subluxation of the subtalar joint (Fig. 20.10). Most often, the os calcis and the remainder of the foot subluxate medially, thereby preserving the medial soft tissues even if the medial malleolus is fractured. In this particular type of injury, avascular necrosis leading to collapse of the body is uncommon, but anatomical reduction is required to prevent malunion with resultant foot problems.

a) Avascular Necrosis

Although portions of the talar body may become avascular, collapse is rare. The intact medial soft tissue envelope usually retains sufficient vascularity to the body to maintain partial viability. The process of *creeping substitution* is able to strengthen the dead bone at a speed which more than compensates for the tendency of that bone to collapse (see Figs. 20.8, 20.10).

It is wrong to believe that this injury usually results in late problems associated with avascular necrosis. Therefore, aggressive treatment modalities for this injury, such as primary subtalar fusion, should be avoided because the outlook with proper management is favorable. Peterson and Goldie (1975) pointed out in an experimental study that division of the talar neck *with displacement* disrupted the talar blood supply. However, the clinical reviews are clear on this point: that is, the majority of cases will not develop clinically

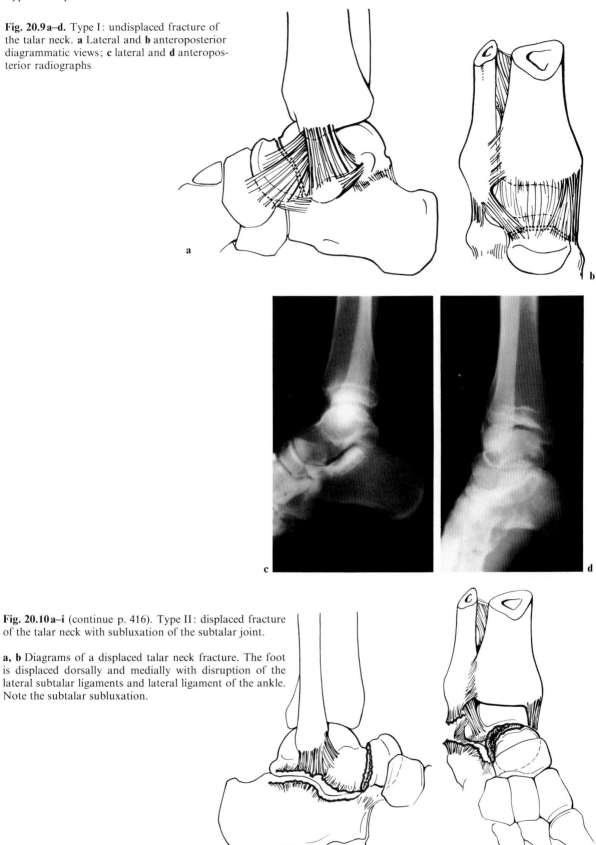

Fig. 20.9 a–d. Type I: undisplaced fracture of the talar neck. **a** Lateral and **b** anteroposterior diagrammatic views; **c** lateral and **d** anteroposterior radiographs

Fig. 20.10 a–i (continue p. 416). Type II: displaced fracture of the talar neck with subluxation of the subtalar joint.

a, b Diagrams of a displaced talar neck fracture. The foot is displaced dorsally and medially with disruption of the lateral subtalar ligaments and lateral ligament of the ankle. Note the subtalar subluxation.

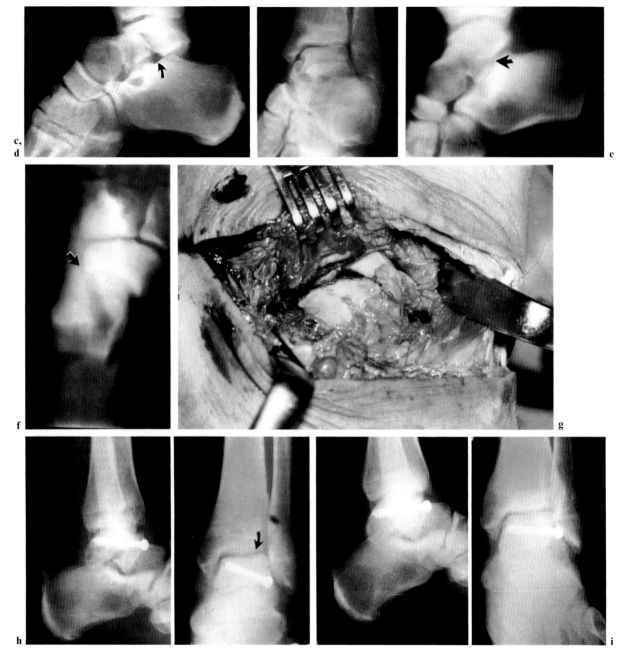

Fig. 20.10 (continued). **c** Lateral and **d** anteroposterior radiographs of a 43-year-old male showing a comminuted oblique fracture of the talar neck extending posteriorly into the body. The *arrow* in **c** shows the subtalar subluxation, clearly seen in the lateral tomograms (**e**, *arrows*). **f** Anteroposterior tomogram showing the oblique nature of the fracture (*arrow*), confirmed at the time of surgery (**g**). Through a lateral approach, the fracture was reduced and internally fixed with a single cancellous bone screw. The anatomical appearance is shown in the lateral and anteroposterior radiographs (**h**). At 10 weeks, no evidence of radiolucency is noted in the talus, indicating avascular necrosis (*arrow*). **i** At 62 weeks, increased density is still noted in the talus but there is no evidence of collapse. The patient's talar body never collapsed and he has gone on to an excellent long-term result

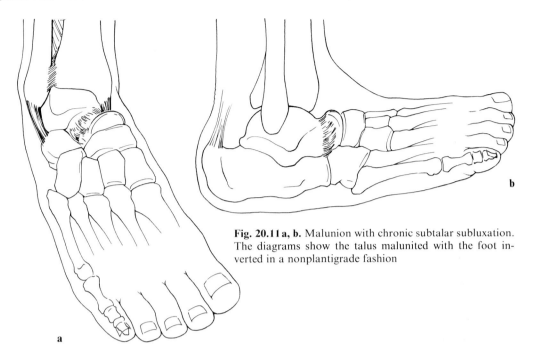

Fig. 20.11 a, b. Malunion with chronic subtalar subluxation. The diagrams show the talus malunited with the foot inverted in a nonplantigrade fashion

significant avascular necrosis. Although the reported incidence of avascular necrosis of the talar body in type II injuries is 20%–50%, all authors agree that most cases proceed to bony union with no collapse of the avascular bone. Pennal (1963) reported three cases (33%) of patchy avascular necrosis with no collapse, Kenwright and Taylor (1970) four cases (36%) with no collapse, and Hawkins (1970) 42% with no significant collapse.

b) Malunion with Chronic Subtalar Subluxation

In a talar neck fracture, malunion is of greater clinical significance than avascular necrosis. If an anatomical reduction is not obtained and maintained, the neck of the talus will heal in an abnormal position (Fig. 20.11). Of necessity, the subtalar joint will remain chronically subluxated. This in turn causes two major problems leading to a poor result: secondary degenerative arthritis and altered foot mechanics.

Secondary Degenerative Arthritis of the Subtalar Joint

This condition may occur early because of the altered joint biomechanics, and is the most frequent cause of unsatisfactory results in type II injuries. Of Pennal's ten cases, the six treated nonoperatively developed these changes, whereas the four treated operatively did not.

Altered Foot Mechanics

If the talar neck heals in the malunited position, the subluxated os calcis at the subtalar joint is usually displaced inwards. Since the remainder of the foot rotates around the subtalar axis through the talar neck and the os calcis, the net effect is a varus heel and foot (Fig. 20.11 b). The normal plantigrade position of the foot is lost, markedly altering the patient's gait pattern.

Therefore, *if the talar neck fracture is not anatomically reduced by closed means, open reduction and internal fixation are absolutely imperative.*

20.3.2.3 Type III: Displaced Fractures of the Talar Neck with Posterior Dislocation of the Body

Avascular necrosis of the body is inevitable in these injuries (Fig. 20.12), and plays the major role in determining the outcome. The incidence of avascular necrosis approaches 100%, the occasional exception being those cases which retain the deltoid ligament attachment to the talus. I have seen this ligament retained even in an open fracture, as illustrated in Fig. 20.12c–h. Pennal (1963) reported avascular necrosis in 14 out of 14 cases (100%); however, in one it was patchy in nature. Kenwright and Taylor (1970) reported 3 out of 4 (75%) with surprisingly good results. Hawkins reported 18 out of 20 (90%), with 3 nonunions. Treatment of this injury by all methods re-

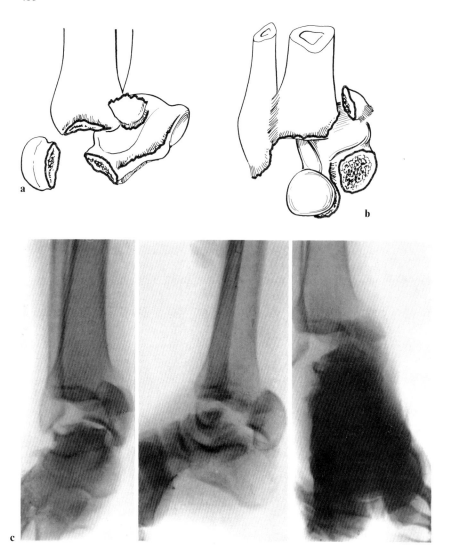

Fig. 20.12a–h. Type III: displaced fracture of the talar neck with posterior dislocation of the body of the talus. **a** Lateral and **b** anteroposterior diagrams showing a talar neck fracture with displacement of the body posteriorly and medially. Note the fracture of the medial malleolus, a common associated injury. **c** Oblique, lateral, and anteroposterior radiographs of an 18-year-old male with this injury. Note the posteromedial position of the talar body and the fracture of the medial malleolus as shown in the drawing. The clinical photograph (**d**) clearly shows the talar body posteromedially just under the posterior tibial tendon. The neurovascular bundle is posterior to the articular cartilage which is indicated by the probe. This was an open fracture laterally. A posteromedial incision was made and a Steinmann pin inserted in the os calcis for traction. The intraoperative radiographs (**e**) show the reduction prior to insertion of a lag screw fixation. In this case, there was soft tissue attachment to the displaced body and we felt vascularity would be maintained to the body of the talus (**f**). Note also the position of the medial malleolar fracture. The talar fracture was fixed with a single screw, as shown in the clinical photograph (**g**) and the postoperative radiograph (**h**). At 8 weeks, there is a clear radiolucent line along the dome of the talus, indicating vascularity. The patient developed a patchy avascular necrosis with no collapse ▶

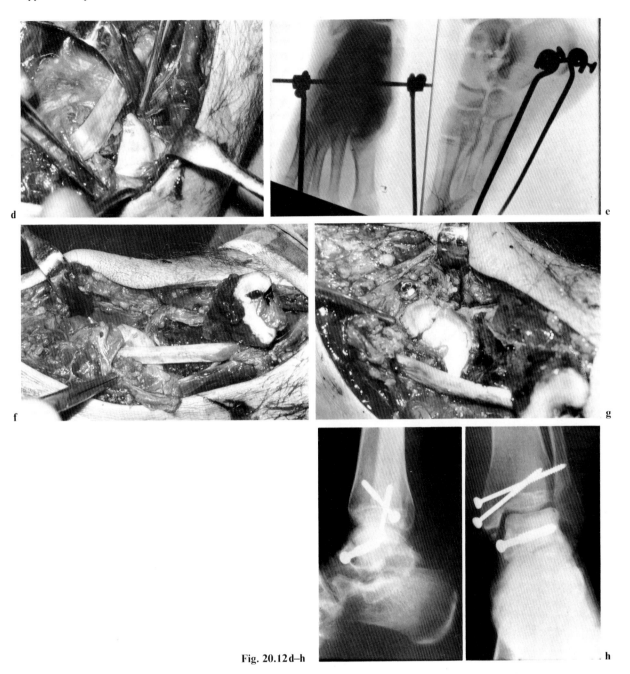

Fig. 20.12 d–h

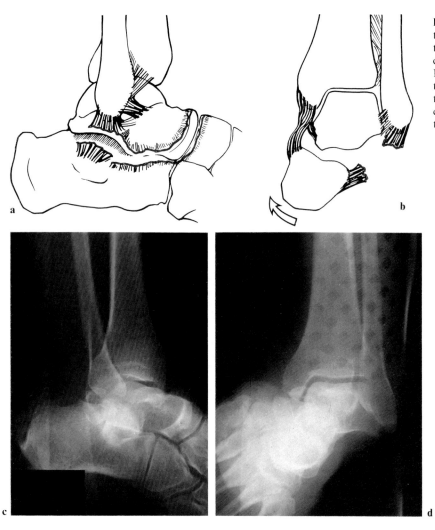

Fig. 20.13a–d. Subtalar dislocation. **a** Lateral and **b** anteroposterior diagrammatic views of a complete subtalar dislocation. Note the disruption of the subtalar and lateral ligaments. **c** Lateral and **d** anteroposterior radiographs of subtalar dislocation

sulted in only 3 satisfactory results. None of the attempts to revascularize the talus early showed any significant effect; therefore, the ultimate prognosis for this injury must be guarded.

Even more sinister is the *open* type III fracture, in Hawkins' series 50% of the total.

20.3.3 Subtalar Dislocation

This injury (Fig. 20.13), if reduced quickly and anatomically, usually results in good function of the foot and no avascular necrosis of the talus. Late osteoarthritis of the subtalar joint may occur in some cases.

20.3.4 Total Dislocation of the Talus

This injury (Fig. 20.14) is usually caused by violent inversion forces, completely extruding the talus

laterally. Most often, the dislocation is *open*. Usually, all soft tissues are stripped from the bone, and therefore avascular necrosis is certain. Sepsis and skin necrosis are common in the open injury. Of Pennal's ten cases, two required tibiocalcaneal fusion and one an amputation. Detenbeck and Kelly (1969), reporting on nine such cases of which seven were open, failed to reduce the dislocation closed in all cases. Their dismal results emphasize the seriousness of this injury:

– Eight out of nine patients developed sepsis.
– Seven out of nine patients required talectomy, five with tibiocalcaneal fusion.
– Nine out of nine patients required an amputation for sepsis.

Therefore, this injury has the greatest potential for disaster; often that potential is realized.

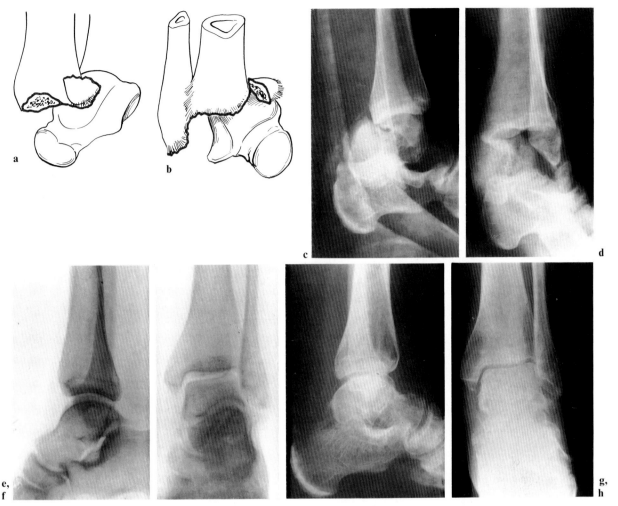

Fig. 20.14a–h. Total dislocation of the talus. **a** Lateral and **b** anteroposterior diagrams showing a complete dislocation of the talus with a fracture of the medial malleolus. This injury is clearly seen on the lateral (**c**) and anteroposterior (**d**) radiographs of a 29-year-old man involved in a mo- tor vehicle accident. Closed reduction failed to reduce the total dislocation of the talus, and therefore open reduction was necessary. The intraoperative Polaroid radiographs (**e, f**) indicate the reduction. At 6 months, patchy avascular necrosis is evident (**g, h**) but no collapse occurred

20.4 Management

20.4.1 Assessment

Prior to instituting management of the fracture, a careful assessment is mandatory.

20.4.1.1 Clinical

As always, a complete medical history and physical examination are essential in order to reveal the mechanism of injury, the general medical profile of the patient, and the state of the limb. Of great importance is the state of the soft tissues, either the presence of an open wound or, if the wound is closed, the presence of severe skin damage heralding the early onset of fracture blisters and necrosis. Injudicious surgery through such skin may prove disastrous.

20.4.1.2 Radiological Assessment

Standard views of the hindfoot should be supplemented with tomograms and special views, in order to clearly outline the subtalar joint.

Standard views include an anteroposterior, a lateral, and two oblique views of the foot (see Fig. 20.12).

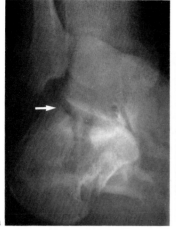
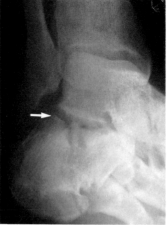

a

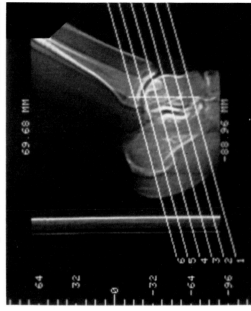

b

Fig. 20.15a–f. Broden's view of the subtalar joint. The subtalar joint is best seen on Broden's view (**a, b**; *arrows*). In this case, one of an os calcis fracture, one notes the precise relationship between the talus and os calcis. **c–f** CT scans of the same case. Again, note the relationship between the os calcis and the talus

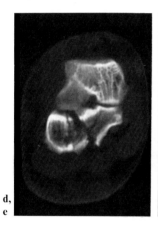
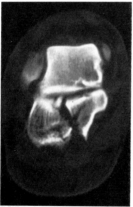
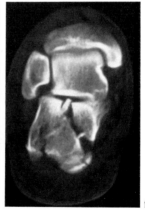

d,
e

f

Tomograms are in our opinion invaluable (as they are in other fractures) for revealing comminution of the neck and body and incongruity of the subtalar joint (see Fig. 20.10e, f).

Broden's view (Broden 1949) is excellent for viewing the subtalar joint, especially after a closed reduction (Fig. 20.15a, b).

Computed tomograms (CT) of the foot will afford excellent visualization of the fracture pattern, as well as the degree of comminution (Fig. 20.15c–e).

20.4.2 Decision Making

Careful assessment will reveal the personality of the injury. Following this, the management should become logical.

20.4.2.1 Fractures of the Body

a) Undisplaced

For this kind of fracture only symptomatic treatment is required, usually a below-knee cast for 6–8 weeks. A good result may be expected.

b) Displaced

If the fracture is comminuted and displaced, as is too often the case, the surgeon must assess whether it can be operatively stabilized. If the body is split, it may be possible to perform an open reduction and stable internal fixation using cancellous screws (Fig. 20.16). If the body is completely shattered, the surgeon may immobilize the foot until pain subsides and then begin a rehabilitation program. Most often, the patient will require a

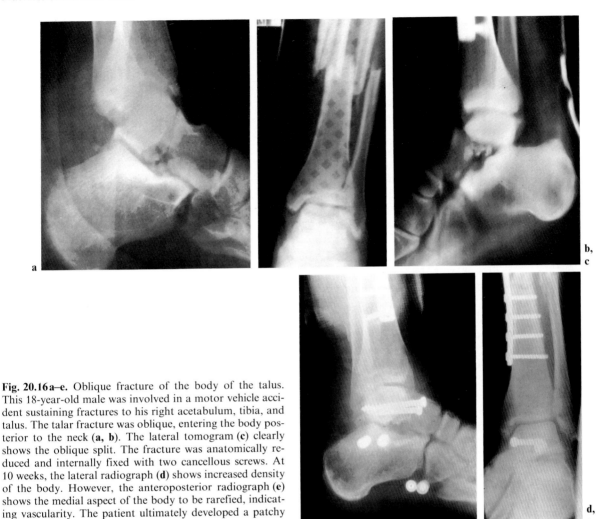

Fig. 20.16a–e. Oblique fracture of the body of the talus. This 18-year-old male was involved in a motor vehicle accident sustaining fractures to his right acetabulum, tibia, and talus. The talar fracture was oblique, entering the body posterior to the neck (**a, b**). The lateral tomogram (**c**) clearly shows the oblique split. The fracture was anatomically reduced and internally fixed with two cancellous screws. At 10 weeks, the lateral radiograph (**d**) shows increased density of the body. However, the anteroposterior radiograph (**e**) shows the medial aspect of the body to be rarefied, indicating vascularity. The patient ultimately developed a patchy avascular necrosis but no collapse

secondary reconstructive procedure, such as a tibiocalcaneal fusion.

As an alternative for the worst cases, we favor primary excision of the body of the talus and either a Blair-type fusion (Crenshaw 1971, p. 502) or tibiocalcaneal fusion. This procedure should only be performed through skin which has healed sufficiently to avoid necrosis.

20.4.2.2 Fractures of the Talar Neck

a) Type I

If an assessment of the injury indicates an undisplaced linear type fracture through the talar neck, i.e., a type I injury, simple treatment consisting of immobilization in a plaster cast until the fracture is healed (usually 6–8 weeks) is adequate. The expected result of such treatment is a healed fracture in perfect position, with no abnormality of the subtalar joint. Avascular necrosis is a rarity and late secondary arthritis of the subtalar joint is also uncommon.

A word of warning however: the assessment of the subtalar joint must be *extensive and accurate* and include all of the radiographic views previously mentioned. If there is any question about displacement of the subtalar joint, the injury should be considered a type II injury, which requires anatomical reduction.

b) Type II

If the fracture of the talar neck is associated with a subluxation of the subtalar joint (type II fracture), anatomical restoration of the neck is essential to restore congruity to the subtalar joint, which, in turn, will restore the normal plantigrade position of the foot. A closed reduction with general anesthesia may accomplish this task. However, it is again essential that the closed reduction of the talar neck is absolutely anatomical. In our opinion, this is rarely accomplished, so that a common final result with such fractures treated non-operatively is malunion and chronic subluxation of the subtalar joint (see Fig. 20.10).

In order to avoid this, we recommend *early anatomical open reduction and internal fixation* of this injury, if the patient's general state allows. This injury should be considered like any other fracture-dislocation of a weight-bearing joint, of which anatomical open reduction and stable internal fixation are the hallmarks of treatment.

If the surgical approach does not interfere with the remaining medial blood supply, significant avascular necrosis will be rare. Furthermore, since the anatomical reduction of the subtalar joint restores congruity between the dome of the os calcis and the talus, secondary problems in that joint and in the foot will be avoided, resulting in a satisfactory outcome.

In a type II injury there is no indication for primary subtalar fusion in an attempt to restore blood flow to the body of the talus, since the flow is usually ample.

c) Type III

A fracture of the talar neck with dislocation of the talar body (i.e. type III: see Fig. 20.12), whether open or closed, constitutes a surgical emergency. The extruded body lies posterior to the medial malleolus. Although the neurovascular bundle is rarely injured primarily, pressure on these structures may cause secondary nerve injury or vascular impairment, either arterial or venous. It is therefore urgent that the body of the talus be reduced.

Even under general anesthesia and with a pin inserted in the os calcis, less than 10% of these injuries can be reduced closed, so little time should be wasted with this maneuver. One or two attempts under image intensification should convince the surgeon that open reduction will be necessary.

Since more than 50% of patients with this injury have an associated fracture of the medial malleolus, open reduction should be performed medially by turning down the bony fragment (see Fig. 20.12). Care should be taken to preserve any medial soft tissue attachment to the body of the talus, as this may be its only remaining blood sup-

ply. Reduction of the body of the talus is then performed manually. This may be a difficult task, requiring full reenactment of the injury in forced dorsiflexion with a Steinmann pin in the os calcis for traction.

Once the body of the talus has been restored to its normal position, the talar neck fracture should then be stably fixed with cancellous lag screws. We favor stable internal fixation, even in cases where the body is free of all soft tissue, unless the body is comminuted or contamination of the wound would make sepsis likely in an open fracture. In those cases, the body of the talus should be discarded and a Blair-type fusion (Crenshaw 1971, p. 502) or a tibiocalcaneal fusion should be performed at the earliest safe opportunity.

Revascularization of the Talus. Is there any method now available to increase the blood supply to an avascular talar body? Phemister (1940) experimentally denuded the articular cartilage from the talus and found that the bone could then be revascularized much more quickly than if the articular cartilage remained. This led some surgeons to perform primary subtalar fusion in an effort to enhance the blood supply to the talar body and prevent collapse of that structure. Sporadic reports in all of the published papers do not support the clinical application of this basic principle. The results are very unpredictable, and therefore the method cannot be recommended at this time (Fig. 20.17).

Perhaps in the future direct microvascular techniques to restore the arterial supply of the talus will become possible, and will eliminate avascular necrosis. Until then, tibiocalcaneal fusion, giving a good stable hindfoot, or fusion from the tibia to the talar head (Blair fusion), are better than talectomy, except in cases of total dislocation of the talus. The condition of the talus in that injury – usually open and completely devoid of all blood supply – is such that it cannot safely be salvaged. Attempts to do so have led to an extremely high rate of sepsis and amputation. "Suitable" treatment would consist of total excision of the talus, either as definitive treatment or combined with a primary or a delayed primary tibiocalcaneal fusion. If sepsis can be avoided by proper soft tissue management, the final result should be satisfactory.

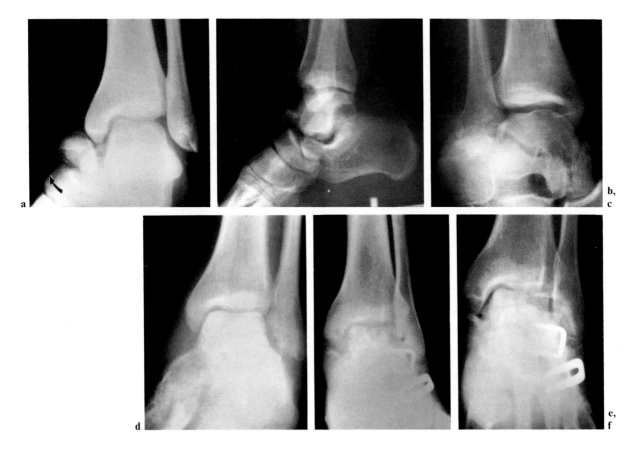

Fig. 20.17 a–f. Avascular necrosis of the talus. The **a** antero-posterior, **b** lateral, and **c** oblique radiographs show a fracture through the talar neck with displacement (*arrow* in **a**). At 24 weeks, the anteroposterior radiograph (**d**) shows a dense sclerotic talar body. At this time, a triple arthrodesis was performed in an attempt to bring vascularity to the body of the talus. At 2 years (**e**), and 3 years (**f**) some degree of collapse of the body is noted. The patient has subsequently required further reconstructive surgery and has a poor result

20.4.3 Surgical Technique

20.4.3.1 Timing

The timing of the operative procedure, if operating is indicated, is of vital importance. Obviously, if the fracture is open, immediate surgery is indicated. However, if the fracture is closed, careful assessment and planning are required. Dislocation of the body of the talus or the entire talus constitutes a surgical emergency, and if closed reduction does not succeed, immediate open reduction is called for. The soft tissues must be handled with extreme care. In this situation the wound, if under tension, must be left open.

In a type II fracture-dislocation, the surgeon has more leeway. If the skin is obviously traumatized, surgery should be delayed until the swelling has subsided and the skin improves. Incisions should never be made through areas of fracture blister, since the inevitable outcome will be skin necrosis and sepsis (see Fig. 20.6c). In such cases, the fracture subluxation should be reduced closed, the extremity elevated, and surgery delayed until local conditions are safe.

20.4.3.2 Antibiotics

In this area, we favor the use of prophylactic antibiotics, administration of which should be started prior to the operative procedure. A single intravenous dose of 1 g cefazolin at the time of induction of narcosis, prior to inflation of the tourniquet, will be adequate and should be used for 48 h postoperatively.

20.4.3.3 Tourniquet

In order to achieve an accurate anatomical reduction of the femoral neck, use of a tourniquet, though not mandatory, is desirable.

20.4.3.4 *Skin Approaches*

The skin on both the medial and lateral aspects
of the foot is extremely delicate and to avoid skin
breakdown must be handled with great care. The
approach to each individual fracture will be dic-
tated by the conditions of the case. Important factors are the type of fracture, the presence or absence of an open wound, and the presence of a
medial malleolar fracture.

a) Lateral

If there is no fracture of the medial malleolus, we
favor the lateral approach to the talar neck. Two
incisions are possible; anterolateral longitudinal
(Fig. 20.18a), and lateral oblique.

The anterior incision is safe and physiological.
Unlike the lateral oblique incision, it rarely causes
skin breakdown, and for this reason we strongly
favor it. In the anterolateral approach, the exten-

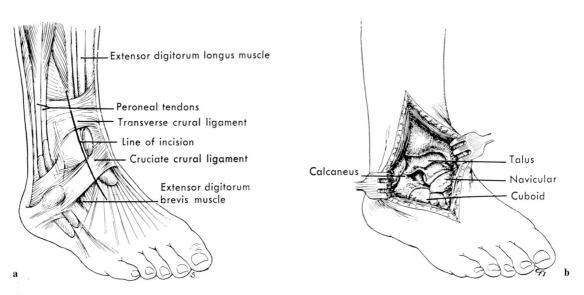

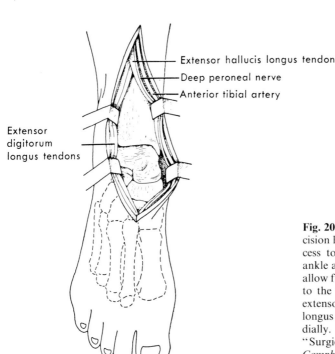

Fig. 20.18a–c. Anterolateral approach to the talus. **a** Incision lateral to the extensor digitorum longus muscle. **b** Access to the talus by dividing the anterior capsule to the
ankle and talonavicular joint. Extension of the incision will
allow full view of the talar neck and body. **c** Alternate access
to the talus may be gained through a portal between the
extensor digitorum longus tendon and the extensor hallucis
longus tendon with the neurovascular bundle retracted medially. (Reproduced by permission from: A.H. Crenshaw
"Surgical Approaches," in Edmonson and Crenshaw (eds.),
Campbell's Operative Orthopaedics, 6th edn., St. Louis 1980,
The C.V. Mosby Co.)

sor tendons and neurovascular structures are retracted medially and the ankle joint capsule is divided, allowing exposure of the entire talus (Fig. 20.18b). Access may also be gained through the interval between the extensor hallucis longus tendon together with the neurovascular bundle medially and the extensor digitorum longus tendons laterally (Fig. 20.18c), but the advantage of the increased medial exposure through this route is offset by the risk of damage to the neurovascular structures, and the lateral portal is therefore preferred.

The oblique lateral incision (Fig. 20.19) affords excellent exposure but is more apt to lead to skin breakdown and should be avoided unless access to the posterior aspect of the talus is required. This approach follows the skin lines obliquely across the talar neck, ending posterior to the fibular malleolus.

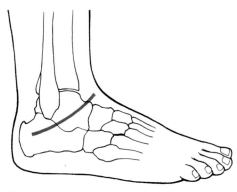

Fig. 20.19. Oblique lateral approach to the talus. (Adapted from Crenshaw 1971)

The major advantages of these lateral approaches are twofold. First, the lateral is the easiest approach to the fracture of the talar neck, since simple division of the skin and subcutaneous tissues usually leads one directly into the fracture site, as most of the deep capsular structures are torn. Secondly, a lateral incision avoids damage to the deltoid artery, which may be present with an intact deltoid ligament. In some cases, this may be the only blood supply to the body of the talus and medial approaches could damage it.

If increased exposure is required on the lateral side, a transverse osteotomy of the fibula may be carried out at the level of the mortise. Full access can then be obtained to the body of the talus. At the end of the procedure, the malleolus can be fixed with a malleolar screw through predrilled holes.

b) Medial

If the medial malleolus is fractured, or if the body of the talus is posteriorly dislocated, a medial approach is indicated. A longitudinal incision is made just anterior to the medial malleolus, extending distally across the talar neck, curving slightly posteriorly, long enough to give access to both the talar neck and the ankle joint. The medial malleolus should be retracted posteriorly. Great care must be taken to preserve the attachment, if any, of the deltoid ligament to the malleolus and the talus. If reduction of the dislocated body is difficult, a Steinmann pin should be inserted into the calcaneus so that traction may be applied. At the end of the procedure the medial malleolus should be fixed back with malleolar screws or tension band wires.

20.4.3.5 Stable Internal Fixation

Whether the lateral or medial approach is chosen, stabilization of the fracture is the same. As always, it is extremely important to operate through the fracture site, great care being taken to preserve all soft tissue attachments. This is especially important in comminuted fractures. The talar neck should be reduced anatomically and provisionally fixed with 2.0-mm Kirschner wires. In cases of extreme comminution, the Kirschner wires will serve as definitive fixation, but in all cases it is preferable to fix the fracture with a 6.5-mm cancellous lag screw under compression; this is usually possible from either the medial or the lateral side. A second screw, usually a malleolar screw or a 4.0-mm cancellous lag screw with a washer, or else one or two Kirschner wires should be used to prevent rotation (Fig. 20.20; see also Figs. 20.10, 20.12, 20.16). Cannulated cancellous screws which may be inserted over the Kirschner wires are helpful in this situation. In some cases of extreme comminution, a bone graft will be required to fill the gap. In all cases, the subtalar joint should be exposed to ensure perfect congruity.

The cancellous fracture fixed with interfragmental compression should heal rapidly in an anatomical position.

After an osteotomy of the lateral or medial malleolus, or if the medial malleolus is fractured, the bones affected should be stabilized using standard techniques.

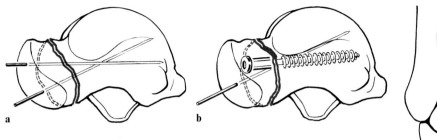

Fig. 20.20 a–c. Stable internal fixation of talar neck fracture. **a** Provisional fixation is achieved with Kirschner wires. **b, c** A cancellous lag screw is used to compress the talar neck fracture. A Kirschner wire may be retained or a second screw inserted to increase the stability. The direction of the screw, from medial to lateral or from lateral to medial, will depend on the obliquity of the talar neck fracture as it extends into the body. If the fracture extends anterolaterally to posteromedially, as is usual, the screw should be inserted from the medial aspect of the talar head. If the obliquity is the opposite, from anteromedial to posterolateral, the screw should be inserted laterally from the talar head. If the fracture is transverse, the screws can be inserted in either direction

20.4.3.6 Postoperative Care

Wound Closure

In dealing with open fractures, it is best to leave the lacerated portion of the wound open.

Many wounds, even in closed fractures, will be under extreme tension. In these cases, no attempt should be made to close the wound. Areas of sensitive tissue, such as tendon, should ideally be covered, but in some instances it is better even to leave the joint open than to attempt closure under tension. If possible, the patient may return to the operating room on the 5th day for wound closure or skin graft.

A bulky dressing with a plaster splint immobilizing the foot in neutral rotation and the ankle at 90° should be applied.

Follow-up Care

Recognition and Management of Avascular Necrosis. The specific follow-up care of the patient will depend upon the type of injury and its management. In type I or type II talar neck fractures, the risk of avascular necrosis is minimal, whereas in type III injuries necrosis is virtually certain.

Avascular necrosis of the body of the talus may be suspected as early as 6–8 weeks following injury. Evidence of bone resorption, shown by the presence of subchondral atrophy in the dome of the talus, is de facto evidence of an *intact* blood supply (Fig. 20.21 a, b). In cases in which the blood supply to the talar body is interrupted, bone resorption is impossible; therefore, no subchondral atrophy is seen on the early radiograph and the talar body appears relatively dense (Fig. 20.21 c–e).

Technetium polyphosphate bone scanning, if performed early, may be of some prognostic importance. Also, magnetic resonance imaging (MRI) is a very sensitive indicator of avascular necrosis and will become important clinically as its availability increases.

Type I talar neck fractures treated nonoperatively should remain in plaster until bony union has occurred, i.e., usually for 6–12 weeks. Weight bearing may be started early (after 2–4 weeks) if the fracture is stable.

The postoperative management of *type II* fractures with cancellous screw fixation will depend upon the degree of stability of the subtalar joint at the conclusion of surgery. If the joint is stable, motion may be started early, but in cases with an unstable subtalar joint, the foot must be kept in plaster for 8–12 weeks until the capsule has healed. In this group of patients, the final outcome is usually good, even if patchy avascular necrosis of the body of the talus develops. Late collapse of the body is rare, although radiographs and bone scans should nevertheless be carefully monitored. If avascular necrosis is suspected, restricted weight

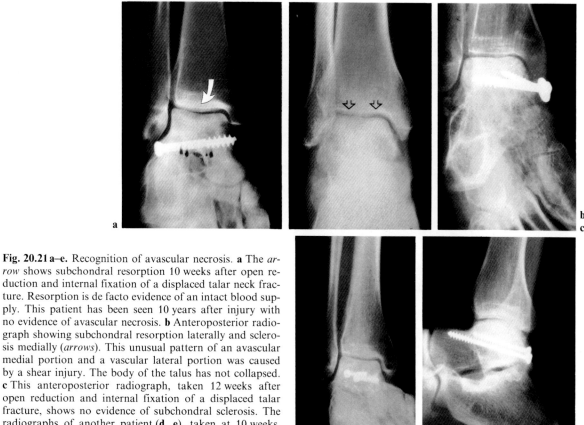

Fig. 20.21 a–e. Recognition of avascular necrosis. **a** The *arrow* shows subchondral resorption 10 weeks after open reduction and internal fixation of a displaced talar neck fracture. Resorption is de facto evidence of an intact blood supply. This patient has been seen 10 years after injury with no evidence of avascular necrosis. **b** Anteroposterior radiograph showing subchondral resorption laterally and sclerosis medially (*arrows*). This unusual pattern of an avascular medial portion and a vascular lateral portion was caused by a shear injury. The body of the talus has not collapsed. **c** This anteroposterior radiograph, taken 12 weeks after open reduction and internal fixation of a displaced talar fracture, shows no evidence of subchondral sclerosis. The radiographs of another patient (**d, e**), taken at 10 weeks, also show no evidence of subchondral sclerosis. Both of these patients developed complete avascular necrosis of the talar body

bearing in a patellar-bearing caliper is advised, although these devices are not completely effective.

In *type III* injury, with the inevitable avascular necrosis (see Fig. 20.17), the follow-up care is controversial. At this time, there is no evidence that attempts at revascularization of the body of the talus will be successful. Bone forage operations and subtalar fusion have been attempted with equivocal results. In our opinion, management should be nonoperative, the patient being fitted with a weight-relieving caliper. If collapse of the body does occur, the treatment options include:

1. Excision of the body with fusion of the tibia to the head of the talus (Blair fusion; see Crenshaw 1971, p. 502)
2. Excision of the talus and tibiocalcaneal fusion
3. Tibio-talar-calcaneal fusion through a lateral approach

It is beyond the scope of this book to describe the surgical techniques of these reconstructive procedures in detail.

20.4.4 Special Problems

20.4.4.1 Open Fractures and Fracture-Dislocations

Open type I and type II talar neck fractures should be managed as previously indicated. Following careful wound cleansing and débridement, the talar neck fracture should be primarily stabilized with cancellous bone screws and Kirschner wires. All soft tissue attachments to the bone must be retained. The wound should be left open and closed secondarily when possible. On occasion, it is safer to let the wound heal by secondary intent than to attempt plastic procedures or wound closure. If the fracture has been stabilized, a careful assessment should be made of the stability of the subtalar and ankle joint. If it is stable, early motion may be initiated, the fracture usually being protected with a below-the-knee splint and hinged ankle device while at rest.

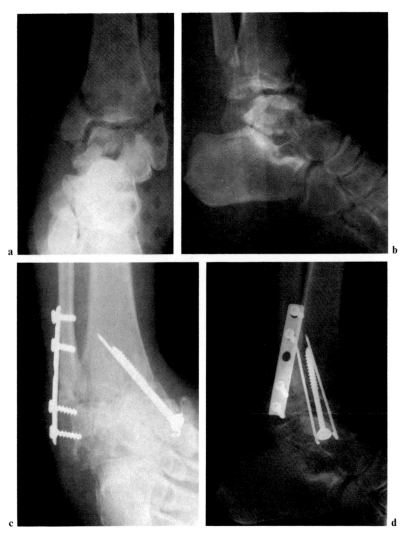

Fig. 20.22 a–d. Comminuted fracture of the body of the talus. **a** Antero-posterior and **b** lateral radiographs showing severe comminution of the body of the talus as well as a fracture of the medial and lateral malleoli of the ankle. This patient also had a se-vere head injury. The talar fracture was open. Many small fragments of bone had to be discarded, including areas of the articular surface (**b**). At 9 months, areas of collapse of the ta-lus are seen on the anteroposterior and lateral radiographs (**c, d**). The patient's head injury precluded fur-ther reconstructive surgery

In type III open fractures with total dislocation of the talus, or in open fractures with a shattered talar body, the situation changes drastically (Fig. 20.22). In these cases, with complete strip-ping of all soft tissues from the displaced frag-ments, it is safer to discard the body of the talus and proceed to a tibiocalcaneal fusion. The risk entailed by leaving a large dead talar body in situ in a potentially contaminated wound is too great, and sepsis is a frequent outcome.

Obviously, each case is different and requires careful assessment, but, in general, the above are the principles favored by us.

20.4.4.2 Comminuted Fractures of the Talar Body

In closed, extremely comminuted fractures of the body of the talus, open reduction and stable inter-nal fixation may be impossible (Fig. 20.23). The late results of this fracture are poor and in some instances, when the skin in the region allows, it is preferable to carry out a delayed primary tibio-calcaneal fusion (Fig. 20.23 a, b). We favor the lat-eral approach, dividing the fibula 6–8 cm proximal to the ankle joint and rotating it posteriorly. This allows excellent exposure of the entire lateral as-pect of the ankle and subtalar joint and the avascu-lar, comminuted talar body can be removed. The fibula can then be used to stabilize the tibia to the os calcis. An iliac crest cancellous graft should supplement the fusion (Fig. 20.23 c, d).

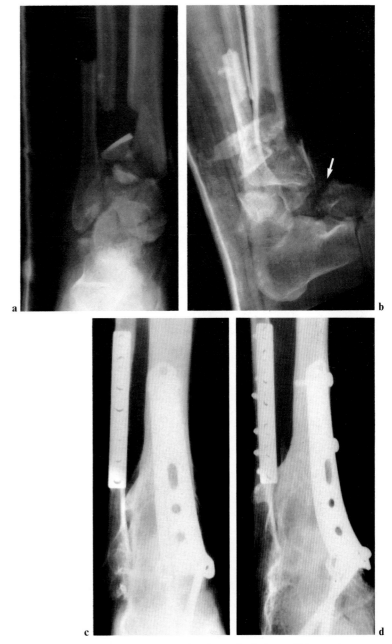

Fig. 20.23a–d. Tibiocalcaneal fusion. This patient, a 40-year-old male, had a severe fracture of the distal tibia and talar neck (**a, b**). Note the severe displacement of the talar neck fracture (*arrow*). He eventually developed avascular necrosis and required a tibiocalcaneal fusion (**c, d**)

References

Anderson HG (1919) The medical and surgical aspects of aviation. London, Oxford Medical Publications

Broden B (1949) Roentgen examination of the subtaloid joint and fractures of the calcaneus. Acta Radiol 31:85–91

Coltart WD (1952) "Aviator's astragalus". J Bone Joint Surg [Br] 34B:545–566

Cooper A (1832) Treatise on dislocations and fractures of the joints. London, pp 341–342

Crenshaw AG (ed) (1971) Campbell's operative orthopaedics, vol 1, 5th edn. Mosby, St. Louis

Detenbeck LC, Kelly PJ (1969) Total dislocation of the talus. J Bone Joint Surg [Am] 51A(2):283

Haliburton RA, Sullivan CR, Kelly PJ, Peterson LFA (1958) The extra-osseous and intra-osseous blood supply of the talus. J Bone Joint Surg [Am] 40A:1115–1120

Hawkins LG (1970) Fractures of the neck of the talus. J Bone Joint Surg [Am] 52A(5):991

James S (1848) Contributions to the pathology and practice of surgery, 1st edn. Sutherland and Knox, Edinburgh, p 126

Kenwright J, Taylor RG (1970) Major injuries of the talus. J Bone Joint Surg [Br] 52B:36–48

Kleiger B (1948) Fractures of the talus. J Bone Joint Surg [Am] 30A:735

Lauro A, Purpura F (1956) La trabecolatura ossea e l' irrorazione sanguina nell'astragalo e nel calcagno. Minerva Chir 11:663–667

Lexor E, Kuliga, Turk W (1904) Untersuchungen über Knochenarterien. Hirschwald, Berlin, Sect 4

McKeever FM (1943) Fracture of the neck of the astragalus. Arch Surg 46:720

Montis S, Ridola C (1959) Vascolarizzazione dell'astragalo. Quad Anatomia Practica 15:574

Mulfinger GL, Trueta J (1970) The blood supply of the talus. J Bone Joint Surg [Br] 52B:160–167

Pennal GF (1963) Fractures of the talus. Clin Orthop 30:53–63

Peterson L, Goldie I (1975) The arterial supply of the talus. Acta Orthop Scand 46:1026–1034

Phemister DB (1940) Changes in bone and joints resulting from interruption of circulation. Arch Surg 41:436

Sneed WL (1925) The astragalus: a case of dislocation excision and replacement; an attempt to demonstrate the circulation in this bone. J Bone Joint Surg 7:384–399

Syme (1848) Contribution to the pathology and practice of surgery. 1st edn, 126 pp. Sutherland and Knox, Edinburgh

Watson-Jones R (1946) Fractures and joint injuries, vol 2, 3rd edn. Livingstone, Edinburgh, pp 821–843

Wildenauer E (1950) Die Blutversorgung des Talus. Z Anat Entwicklungsgesch 115:32

Subject Index

M. E. Müller, M. Allgöwer, R. Schneider, H. Willenegger

Manual of Internal Fixation

Techniques Recommended by the AO Group

In collaboration with W. Bandi, A. Boitzy, R. Ganz, U. Heim,
S. M. Perren, W. W. Rittmann, T. Rüedi, B. G. Weber, S. Weller

Translated from the German by J. Schatzker

2nd, expanded and revised edition. 1979. 345 figures, 2 templates for
preoperative planning. X, 409 pages.
ISBN 3-540-09227-7

Contents: Introduction. – General Considerations: Aims and Funda-
mental Principles of the AO Method. Means by Which Stable Internal
Fixation Is Achieved. Preoperative, Operative and Postoperative
Guidelines. – Special Part: Internal Fixation of Fresh Fractures:
Closed Fractures in the Adult. Open Fractures in the Adult. Fractures
in Children. – Appendix: Reconstructive Bone Surgery. Delayed
Union. Pseudarthroses. Osteotomies. Arthrodeses.

The second edition of this popular manual has been expanded and
revised, facilitating full comprehension and flawless execution of internal fixation procedures. Particular attention is devoted in this edition
to correlating the various fractures, their prognosis and the appropriate
therapeutic technique.

The first section explains the basic biomechanic principles of the
AO/ASIF method of stable internal fixation. It deals with the function
and use of AO implants, AO instruments, and with the essentials of
the operative technique and postoperative care. It also discusses the
handling of the most important postoperative complications.

The second edition deals at length with the AO recommendations for
operative treatment of the most common closed fractures in the adult.
This is organized in anatomical sequence. A discussion of closed fractures is followed by a discussion of open fractures in the adult, then by
one of fractures in children and finally, of pathological fractures.

The third part is a condensed presentation of the application of stable
fixation to reconstructive bone surgery. An appendix is devoted to
pseudarthroses, osteotomies, and arthrodeses.

Based on clinical experience with over 50,000 operatively treated cases,
this manual offers orthopedic surgeons, traumatologists, and general
surgeons current and comprehensive information on this significantly
successful technique.

Springer-Verlag
Berlin Heidelberg New York
London Paris Tokyo

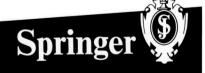

J. Schatzker, Toronto

The Intertrochanteric Osteotomy

1984. 204 figures. VII, 205 pages. ISBN 3-540-10719-3

This book outlines the principle features of the AO tubular system of external fixation developed by the Working Group for Osteosynthesis of the AO/ASIF. The main advantage of tubular external fixation is that only four basic elements are necessary for assembling various models. It is thus easy to use and extremely versatile.

The book opens with a discussion of the basic mechanical prerequisites for tubular external fixation. The indications for its use are then discussed. The steps for actual technical application are presented, accompanied by numerous drawings. Various models of tubular external fixation are systematically shown; each has its own special advantages and justification. The AO tubular system is especially recommended for the treatment fractures that present particular problems. The indications for the use of tubular external fixation make it not a rival of, but rather a necessary supplement to the standard methods of screw and plate fixation.

G. Hierholzer, Duisburg; T. Rüedi, Chur; M. Allgöwer, Basel; J. Schatzker, Toronto

Manual on the AO/ASIF Tubular External Fixator

1985. 104 figures, some in color. V, 100 pages.
ISBN 3-540-13518-9

Contents: Introduction and Basic Indications for the Use of External Skeletal Fixation. – Mechanical Principles of External Skeletal Fixation. – Remarks Concerning the Pathophysiology of Compound Fractures. – Indications for External Skeletal Fixation Versus Internal Fixation. – Four Building Components of the AO Tubular System and the Accompanying Surgical Instruments. – Basic Assemblies and Their Use. – Technical Details for Construction. – Clinical Application of External Skeletal Fixator. – Appendix: Special Indications for the Tubular External Fixator. – References. – Subject Index.

C. F. Brunner, B. G. Weber

Special Techniques in Internal Fixation

1981. 91 figures. X, 198 pages. ISBN 3-540-11056-9

F. Séquin, R. Texhammar

AO/ASIF Instrumentation

Manual of Use and Care

Introduction and Scientific Aspects by H. Willenegger

Translated from the German by T. C. Telger

1981. Approx. 1300 figures, 17 separate checklists. XVI, 306 pages.
ISBN 3-540-10337-6

B. G. Weber, F. Magerl

The External Fixator

AO/ASIF-Threaded Rod System Spine-Fixator

With a chapter by C. Brunner

Foreword by A. Sarmiento

Translated from the German by T. C. Telger

1985. 362 partly colored figures. XV, 373 pages.
ISBN 3-540-13756-4

Springer-Verlag
Berlin Heidelberg New York
London Paris Tokyo

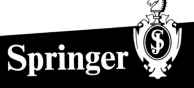